EBERSOLE AND HESS'

Gerontological Nursing & Healthy Aging

SECOND CANADIAN EDITION

Theris A. Touhy, DNP, GCNS-BC
Professor
Christine E. Lynn College of Nursing
Florida Atlantic University
Boca Raton, Florida

Kathleen F. Jett, PhD, GNP-BC
Gerontological Nurse Practitioner
College of Nursing
University of Florida
Gainesville, Florida

Veronique Boscart, PhD, RN
CIHR/Schlegel Industrial Research Chair for Colleges in Seniors Care
Director, Schlegel Centre for Advancing Seniors Care
Conestoga College
Kitchener, Ontario

Lynn McCleary, PhD, RN
Associate Professor
Department of Nursing
Brock University
St. Catharines, Ontario

ELSEVIER

ELSEVIER

Library and Archives Canada Cataloguing in Publication

Touhy, Theris A., author
   Ebersole and Hess' gerontological nursing & healthy aging / Theris A. Touhy, DNP, GCNS-BC (Professor, Christine E. Lynn College of Nursing, Florida Atlantic University, Boca Raton, Florida), Kathleen F. Jett, PhD, GNP-BC (Gerontological Nurse Practitioner, College of Nursing, University of Florida, Gainesville, Florida), Veronique Boscart, PhD, RN (CIHR/Schlegel Industrial Research Chair for Colleges in Seniors Care, Director, Schlegel Centre for Advancing Seniors Care, Conestoga College, Kitchener, Ontario), Lynn McCleary, PhD, RN (Associate Professor, Department of Nursing, Brock University, St. Catharines, Ontario). – 2nd Canadian edition.

Includes bibliographical references and index.
ISBN 978-1-77172-093-9 (softcover)

   1. Geriatric nursing–Textbooks.   2. Aging–Textbooks.   3. Older people–Health and hygiene–Textbooks.
4. Textbooks.   I. Jett, Kathleen Freudenberger, author   II. Boscart, Veronique, author   III. McCleary, Lynn, author   IV. Title.   V. Title: Ebersole and Hess' gerontological nursing and healthy aging.   VI. Title: Gerontological nursing & healthy aging.

RC954.T68 2018   618.97′0231   C2017-905542-9

VP Medical and Canadian Education: Madelene J. Hyde
Content Strategist (Acquisitions): Roberta A. Spinosa-Millman
Content Development Manager: Laurie Gower
Content Development Specialist: Martina van de Velde
Publishing Services Manager: Julie Eddy
Senior Project Manager: David Stein
Cover Designer: Brett J. Miller, BJM Graphic Design and Communications
Book Designer: Margaret Reid
Cover Photo Credits: women stretching: Monkey Business Images/Shutterstock.com; man on bicycle: lightpoet/Shutterstock.com; couple doing tai chi: Tom Wang/Shutterstock.com; background image: mythja/Shutterstock.com
Typesetting and Assembly: Toppan Best-Set Premedia Limited

Elsevier Canada
420 Main Street East, Suite 636, Milton, ON, Canada L9T 5G3
Phone: 416-644-7053

1   2   3   4   5   23   22   21   20   19

Ebook ISBN: 978-1-77172-089-2

Working together to grow libraries in developing countries

www.elsevier.com • www.bookaid.org

To my beautiful grandchildren, Colin and Molly Touhy.
Thanks for merry-go-round rides, tea parties, Barney, cannonballs in the pool,
scuba divers, and Twinkle Twinkle Little Star. Being your Gramma TT makes
growing older the best time of my life and I love you.
To the older people I have been privileged to nurse, and their caregivers,
like Peggy Bennett and Joan Belton, thanks for making the words
in this book a reality for the elders you care for and for teaching me
how to be a gerontological nurse.
To Pat and Priscilla, thanks for entrusting us with the care
of this very special book.

Theris Touhy

To my husband Steve, who is a source of never-ending support.
Without his willingness to keep me supplied with food,
the long hours sitting in front of the computer and writing
would not have been possible.
To the older adults who have opened their lives to me so that I may learn.
To our four children and four wonderful grandchildren, Haley, Amelia, Emory, and
Logan, who always remind me that the best part of life is the time we spend
together and that the older we get, the more we have loved
and the more adventures we have shared.

Kathleen Jett

To my exquisite grandmothers, for instilling a healthy respect for older adults and
teaching me that a person's wisdom, interest, and enthusiasm can keep a passion alive.
To Dr. Dorothy Pringle and Dr. Katherine McGilton, for their knowledge, guidance, and untold
support in guiding me in my gerontological career. I share this accomplishment with them.

Veronique Boscart

To Elsa Marziali, Lynn McDonald, and Dot Pringle.
Thank you for introducing and welcoming me to gerontological nursing and social work.

Lynn McCleary

Contents

Reviewers

Beryl Cable-Williams, RN, BNSc, MN, PhD
Professor, Sir Sandford Fleming College
Faculty Member, Trent/Fleming School of Nursing
Trent University
Kingston, Ontario

Erica Cambly, RN, MN
Assistant Professor, Teaching Stream
Lawrence S. Bloomberg Faculty of Nursing
University of Toronto
Toronto, Ontario

Sharon Clarke, RN, DipEd, MHScN
Program Coordinator
Practical Nursing Program
Conestoga College ITAL
Kitchener, Ontario

Heidi Holmes, RN, BA, BScN, MScN, GNC, SANE
Professor of Nursing
Conestoga College
Kitchener, Ontario

Sue Ann Mandville-Anstey, RN, PhD
Faculty Instructor
Centre for Nursing Studies
Memorial University
St. John's, Newfoundland

Katherine Poser, RN, BScN, MNEd
Professor
School of Baccalaureate Nursing
St. Lawrence College
Kingston, Ontario

Elizabeth Ubaldi, RN, BA, MN
Professor of Nursing
Sault College
Sault Ste. Marie, Ontario

Preface

Gerontological nurses have always led the way in promoting health and improving health care for older adults. The specialty continues to grow in influence and importance, with gerontological nursing competencies increasingly recognized as basic educational requirements for all nurses. All nurses need specialized knowledge of aging and health. The vast majority of our clients are older, whether we work in the community, in acute-care hospitals, or in residential or long-term care settings. This text provides knowledge nurses need to be prepared to promote healthy aging and meet the complex health care needs of the growing number of older Canadians.

We are delighted to bring you the Second Canadian Edition of *Ebersole and Hess' Gerontological Nursing & Healthy Aging*. This well-respected, established, and valued textbook has been thoroughly revised for Canadian students, nurses, and educators, providing the most current Canadian and international evidence for gerontological nursing practice. The content is consistent with the Canadian Gerontological Nursing Association's *Standards of Practice*, the *Prescriptions for Excellence in Gerontological Nursing Education* issued jointly by the Canadian Gerontological Nursing Association and the American National Gerontological Nursing Association, and the *Core Interprofessional Competencies for Gerontology* established by the National Initiative for the Care of the Elderly (NICE).

ORGANIZATION

The organization of the First Canadian Edition and the recently revised Fourth US Edition is retained in this Second Canadian Edition. The content is organized in four major divisions. In **Section I**, the foundations of healthy aging and the foundations of gerontological nursing are examined. Healthy aging, culture and aging, and communication in health and illness are described. Historical and current trends in gerontological nursing are explained. In **Section II**, changes associated with normal aging are presented, including issues older adults may experience as they adapt to these changes. The nurse's role in health promotion and implications for working in partnership with older adults to maintain or restore wellness are described. **Section III** focuses on common health problems experienced by older adults. Implications for practice are described, including how nurses can help older adults living with persistent health problems that are more common in older age. This section does not provide the in-depth coverage of the health problems that one would find in a medical-surgical nursing textbook. The emphasis is on the unique experiences of older adults and implications for nursing with older adults experiencing the health problems. In **Section IV**, social, psychological, economic, and legal issues that affect healthy aging are presented. Health and social policies that affect how health care is delivered and the continuum of care are described. Issues related to mental health and wellness are examined. Transitions in relationships, roles, loss, grief, and death are discussed.

The text is organized for optimal student learning. Each chapter begins with the phenomenological consideration of the lived experience of the older adult. Key concepts, glossaries, learning activities, and discussion questions summarize the chapter and relate directly to the objectives of the chapter. Sources of additional information and reputable websites are provided at the end of each chapter.

NEW TO THIS EDITION

- Updated statistics on global and Canadian population aging
- Updated information about health disparities associated with ethnicity, including information

from the Truth and Reconciliation Commission of Canada

- New resources for incorporating spirituality in nursing with older persons
- Description of the teach-back method for health education and improving health literacy
- New Canadian research about delirium in long-term care homes
- Explanation of the genetics of Alzheimer's disease
- New resources for understanding the experience of dementia and nonpharmacological approaches for dementia care
- New resources for preventing, identifying, and intervening in cases of abuse and neglect of older persons, including new content regarding institutional abuse
- New and more detailed information about experiences of LGBTQ older persons
- Updated information about pensions and the social security system in Canada
- Information about Medical Assistance in Dying laws and the nursing role

ANCILLARIES

(Available at http://evolve.elsevier.com/Canada/Ebersole/gerontological/)

FOR INSTRUCTORS

- **TEACH for Nurses:** Lesson plans tie together every chapter resource you need for the most effective class presentations, with sections dedicated to objectives, teaching focus, instructor chapter resources, answers to chapter questions, and an in-class case study discussion. Teaching strategies include content highlights, student activities, online activities, and large group activities.
- **PowerPoint Presentations:** PowerPoint slide presentations to accompany each chapter.
- **Test Bank:** Approximately 300 NCLEX examination questions.
- **Image Collection:** Illustrations and photos that can be used in a presentation or as visual aids.

FOR STUDENTS

- **Additional Resources:** Print, electronic, and visual resources are included to help in further research, study, and understanding of the material presented in each chapter.
- **Examination Review Questions:** Approximately 300 questions in NCLEX format, for practice and self-assessment, designed to reinforce content from each textbook chapter.
- **Glossary**

Acknowledgements

We would like to thank Priscilla Ebersole and Patricia Hess for the opportunity to author this book and to share their beautiful words and passion for gerontological nursing. We hope that our work honours them and the specialty we all love. It has been a real privilege for us to be a part of the work of two gerontological nurses from whom we have learned how to care for older persons.

Theris Touhy
Kathleen Jett

We are, likewise, honoured and privileged to have had the opportunity to author this Second Canadian Edition. We are grateful for the opportunity to contribute to the continued growth of gerontological nursing in Canada.

Veronique Boscart
Lynn McCleary

Introduction to Healthy Aging

LEARNING OBJECTIVES

Upon completion of this chapter, the reader will be able to:

- Identify factors that influence the aging experience.
- Define *health* and *wellness* within the context of aging and chronic illness.
- Describe the trends seen in global aging today.
- Apply the principles of primary health care to gerontological nursing.

GLOSSARY

Centenarian A person who is at least 100 years old.

Cohort A group whose members share some common experience.

Determinants of health Factors and conditions that influence the health status of individuals, communities, and populations.

Fertility rate The average number of children born to a woman in her lifetime; reported for countries and global regions.

Holistic health care Care in which the whole person is considered, as well as the interaction with and between the various components of a person's life.

Interprofessional collaboration Collaboration among individuals in different professions, including health professions and other professions.

Life expectancy The average number of years a person is expected to live. Life expectancy is based on mortality rates and can be calculated for newborns (life expectancy at birth) or for people who have survived to a particular age (e.g., life expectancy at age 65 years).

Old Age Security pension A Canadian federal government pension provided to persons who are aged 65 years and older who have lived in Canada for at least 10 years.

Sector A part of the economy (for example, the health care sector, the education sector, and the social services sector).

Wellness A state of health (including physical, psychological, spiritual, and economic well-being) that is optimal for an individual at any point in time.

THE LIVED EXPERIENCE

I believe a human life is like a river, meandering through its course, rushing through rapids, flowing placidly over the plains, twisting and turning through countless bends until it spends itself. It is the same river; yet it looks very different from one place to another. So it is with our lives; circumstances vary from one time to another in the course of a life, but I think each stage has its own value.

Georgia, 35 years old

Providing nursing care to older persons is a reward-ing, life-affirming vocation. Through this textbook, we hope to provide students with the basics of beginning a career as a gerontological nurse. Most nurses care for older people. "Older adults are not one subgroup of patients, but rather the core business of health care systems" (Terry Fulmer, cited in The John A. Hartford Foundation, n.d., ¶2). This chapter presents an over-view of aging, the health care needs of older persons, and the vital and exciting role of the nurse in facilitat-ing healthy aging.

AGING IN CANADA

Although all of us begin aging at birth, both the meaning of aging and those who are identified as older persons are determined by society and culture and are influenced by history and gender. For example, in ancient times, Eastern cultures influenced by Confucianism and Taoism revered older persons, but in ancient Western civilizations this was not the case. Older people were sometimes valued for their wisdom, but the physical decline of old age was viewed as a disease (Achenbaum, 2005). Achenbaum notes that while people as young as 40 years may have been viewed as "old" in some ancient societies, "old age" was typically seen to start much later. Since at least 1700 in Europe and North America, "old age" has started "at around 65, give or take 15 years either way" (Achenbaum, 2005, p. 24).

The terms *senior* and *elderly* refer to older persons. In this book, the preferred term is *older person*. As discussed in Chapters 6 and 7, there is no absolute threshold age at which a person becomes "old." In Canada, one standard for the designation of *old* is the age of eligibility for the **Old Age Security pension**, which was 70 years when Old Age Security was established in 1952, and was reduced to 65 years in the 1960s. Currently, people as young as 60 years of age can apply for Old Age Security. Retirement age, another marker of "old age," varies considerably; some people are able to retire in their fifties and others con-tinue to work into their eighties. Most Canadian sta-tistical summaries define *older persons* as those aged 65 years and older. World aging statistics from the United Nations (UN) use 60 years of age as a cutoff (United Nations, 2015).

Psychologists have divided the "old" into three groups: the "young-old," roughly 65 to 74 years old; the "middle-old," 75 to 84 years old; and the "old-old," over 85 years old. A fourth group, persons aged 100 years and older (**centenarians**), is growing rapidly. Currently, about 1.5% of the Canadian population is at least 100 years old. The total number is expected to increase from 8,100 persons in 2015 to 16,200 persons in 2031. The majority of centenarians will continue to be women (Hudon & Milan, 2016).

The proportion of the population aged 65 years or older has been steadily increasing since the early 1970s. In 1966, older persons accounted for 7.7% of the population; in 2015, 16.1% of the population was aged 65 years and older. This increase is due to a relatively low **fertility rate** of about 1.6 children per woman and an increased **life expectancy** in the 1900s (Statistics Canada, 2016a). Female Canadians born today have a life expectancy of 83 years, and males have a life expectancy of 78.3 years. Among those who are 65 years old now, men can expect to live another 18.5 years and women another 21.6 years (Statistics Canada, 2012).

Life expectancy varies across the country. Life expectancy in the territories and in Newfound-land and Labrador is lower than in other regions of Canada, and the highest life expectancy is in British Columbia (Statistics Canada, 2012). Lower life expec-tancy among Inuit and First Nations Canadians accounts for at least some of these geographic differ-ences (Wilson, Rosenberg, & Ning, 2015). The pro-portion of older people in the population is expected to increase dramatically over the coming years as "baby boomers" born between 1946 and the early 1960s retire (Statistics Canada, 2014). Fig. 1.1 shows the projected increase in the population aged 65 years and older by region in Canada.

Those born within the same decade and country may share a common historical context and are usually referred to as a **cohort**. For example, men born between 1920 and 1930 were very likely to have been active participants in World War II or the Korean War. In comparison, men born between 1940 and 1950 are not likely to have been in the military. That these two groups of men have different perspec-tives and different health problems is not surprising. Likewise, privileged women born between 1920 and

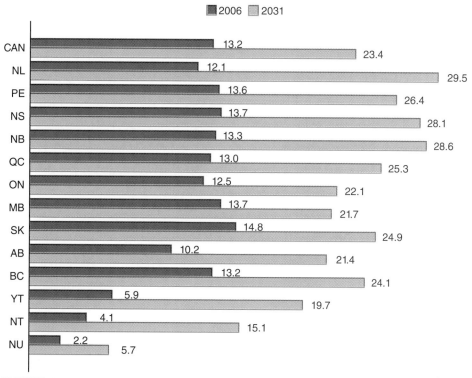

■ 2006 □ 2031

Region	2006	2031
CAN	13.2	23.4
NL	12.1	29.5
PE	13.6	26.4
NS	13.7	28.1
NB	13.3	28.6
QC	13.0	25.3
ON	12.5	22.1
MB	13.7	21.7
SK	14.8	24.9
AB	10.2	21.4
BC	13.2	24.1
YT	5.9	19.7
NT	4.1	15.1
NU	2.2	5.7

FIGURE 1.1 Percentage of population aged 65 years and older in Canada and regions, 2006, and projected, 2031. Statistics Canada. (2010). *Canadians in context—Aging population.* Retrieved from http://www4.hrsdc.gc.ca/.3ndic.1t.4r@-eng.jsp?iid=33.

1930 were raised with what are known as traditional values and roles; they may never have worked outside the home, or they were limited to what was considered "women's work," such as housekeeping, teaching, and nursing. In contrast, similar women born between 1940 and 1950 experienced social pressure to work outside of the home and had considerably more career opportunities as adults, partially as a result of the feminist revolution of the 1960s and 1970s.

Gender can have a significant effect on various aspects of aging. Women usually live longer than men and live alone in widowhood. Men who survive their wives often remarry. Women's social networks outside the work environment are usually larger than those of men, which could potentially reduce women's social isolation after the death of a spouse or partner.

Finally, North America is experiencing a "gerontological explosion" of ethnically diverse older persons. By 2031, at least 1 in 4 Canadians will be an immigrant and about 1 in 3 will belong to a visible minority (Statistics Canada, 2010). Only a relatively small proportion (8%) of Indigenous Canadians are seniors (Statistics Canada, 2016b). However, Indigenous seniors have a high prevalence of chronic health conditions and poor access to services (Fruch, Monture, Prince, & Kelley, 2016). Increasing the number of health care providers from different cultures, as well as ensuring the cultural competence of all providers, is essential to meeting the needs of a rapidly growing and ethnoculturally diverse aging population (see Chapter 4).

GLOBAL AGING

Historically, living to old age was rare; as little as 2% of the world's population were older people (Achenbaum, 2005). Life expectancy increased dramatically in the 1900s, increasing the number of older people

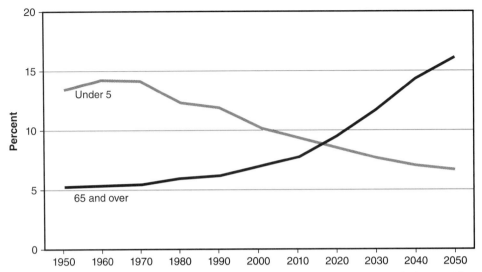

FIGURE 1.2 Average annual percent growth of older population in developed and developing countries, 1950 to 2050. From Kinsella, K., & Wan, H. (2009). U.S. Census Bureau, International Population Reports, P95/09-1, *An aging world: 2008*. Washington DC: U.S. Government Printing Office.

in society. At the same time, the global fertility rate decreased substantially (Fig. 1.2) and is projected to continue to decrease, from 2.5 children per woman in 2010–2015 to 2 children per woman in 2045 (United Nations, 2013). As a result of these two trends, the ratio of older people to younger people is increasing. More-developed countries have the highest percentage of population over 60 years of age because of their higher life expectancy and lower birth rate. For example, more than 25% of people in Germany, Italy, and Japan are over the age of 60 years (United Nations, 2015).

Worldwide, by 2045 the number of persons aged 60 years and older is likely to exceed that of persons younger than the age of 15 years. This phenomenon occurred in Europe in 1995 and in Canada in 2015 (Statistics Canada, 2015). By 2050, older persons will outnumber children worldwide (United Nations, 2014). The UN predicts that by 2050, 1 in 3 people in developed regions and 1 in 5 people in less-developed countries will be 60 years of age or older (United Nations, 2013). Although developed countries have a higher proportion of older people within their populations, the majority (62%) of older people in the world live in less-developed regions, and the population is aging at a much faster rate in these regions (United

Nations, 2014). These changes pose major challenges in meeting the needs of the global aging community.

Africa stands out as the only major region in which the population is still relatively young and where the number of older persons, although increasing, will remain relatively low compared to the number of younger persons. By 2050, 6% of the population in Africa will be 60 years of age or older (United Nations, 2015).

HEALTH, WELLNESS, AND AGING

The definitions of *health* vary greatly and are influenced by culture and by where one is in regard to lifespan. The strong emergence of the **holistic health care** movement has resulted in even broader definitions of health and **wellness**. Wellness involves one's whole being—its physical, emotional, mental, and spiritual components, all of which are vital (Fig. 1.3). In his classic work, Dunn defined the holistic approach to health as "an integrated method of functioning which is oriented toward maximizing the potential of which the individual is capable within the environment where he is functioning" (Dunn, 1961, p. 4). A holistic view of health incorporates the components shown in Fig. 1.3. Wellness involves achieving a balance

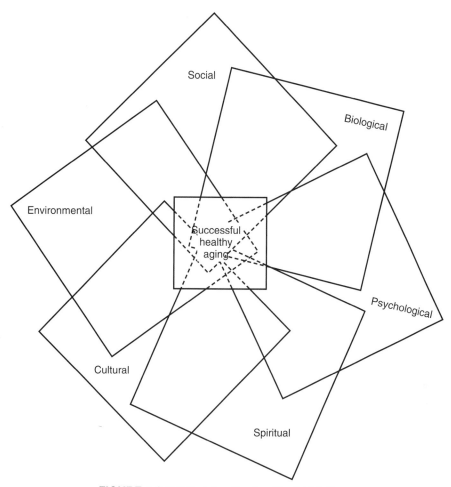

FIGURE 1.3 Healthy aging. Developed by Patricia Hess.

between one's internal and external environments and one's emotional, spiritual, social, cultural, and physical processes.

Wellness is a state of being and feeling that one strives to achieve through effective health practices. It involves the realization of the individual's full potential physically, psychologically, spiritually, and economically and is "the fulfillment of one's role expectations in the family, community, place of worship, workplace and other settings" (World Health Organization, n.d., p. 5). An individual must work hard to achieve wellness. In working toward wellness, an individual may reach plateaus in his or her ascension to higher-level wellness. The person may also regress because of an illness, acute event, or crisis, but these events can be a potential stimulus for growth and a return to moving along the wellness continuum (Fig. 1.4).

According to Dunn, health in later life is often thought of in terms of functional ability rather than the absence of disease—that is, the ability to do what is important to a given person (Dunn, 1961). This may mean one's ability to live independently or the ability to enjoy one's great-grandchildren when they visit at a long-term care home. However, what is important to a person is always individually determined.

In approaching aging from a viewpoint of health, a person's strengths, resilience, resources, and capabilities are emphasized rather than the person's existing pathological conditions. A wellness perspective is based on the belief that every person has an optimal

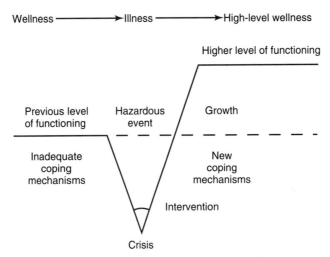

Wellness ──────→ Illness ──────→ High-level wellness

Higher level of functioning

Previous level of functioning   Hazardous event   Growth

Inadequate coping mechanisms   New coping mechanisms

Intervention

Crisis

FIGURE 1.4 Growth potential: Crisis as a challenge.

level of health independent of his or her situation or functional ability. Even in the presence of persistent illness, potentially disabling conditions, or impending death, it is possible to move toward higher wellness. This can be attained as long as the emphasis of care is placed on the promotion of well-being in the least restrictive environment, with support and encouragement for the person to find meaning in the situation.

PROMOTING HEALTHY AGING

Well-being for those older than 60 years is strongly related to functional status but is also affected by determinants of health. **Determinants of health** are the underlying causes of illness or wellness. They have long been recognized as important in Canada. In 1974, the Minister of Health, Marc Lalonde, argued that socioeconomic, environmental, and biological factors are equally or more important than health care in their influence on the health of the Canadian population. The Public Health Agency of Canada has identified 12 key determinants of health: (1) income and social status, (2) social support networks, (3) education and literacy, (4) employment and working conditions, (5) social environments, (6) physical environments, (7) personal health practices and coping skills, (8) healthy child development, (9) biology and genetic endowment, (10) health services, (11) gender, and (12) culture (Public Health Agency of Canada, 2011). All of these determinants of health have an

effect on older persons and are discussed in more detail throughout this book. Income and poverty are powerful determinants of health. (Economic issues related to aging are discussed in Chapters 4 and 22.) To promote healthy aging and individualize nursing care for older persons, gerontological nurses must assess and address the impact of determinants of health.

PRIMARY HEALTH CARE PRINCIPLES

The primary health care approach is a way to build health and attend to determinants of health. This approach was adopted by the World Health Organization in 1978 (World Health Organization & United Nations Children's Fund, 1978). Primary health care is sometimes confused with *primary care*, "the first contact people have with the health care system to seek out primary care services for the diagnosis, treatment and follow-up for a specific health problem, or to access routine screening such as an annual check-up. Primary care is a core component of primary health care, yet primary health care extends beyond the traditional health care system to include services that influence determinants of health such as income, housing, education and environment" (College & Association of Registered Nurses of Alberta [CARNA], 2016, ¶4–5). The principles of primary health care are accessibility, public participation, health promotion, appropriate technology, and intersectoral collaboration. Box 1.1 provides questions

BOX 1.1 Questions to Consider for Principles of Primary Health Care

Accessibility: What issues (e.g., hours, transportation, disability, cultural, economic factors) affect the ability of the older person to access your services? How can your services be made more accessible?

Health promotion: What are the effects of social, economic, and environmental factors on the health of the older person? Do you take these factors into account when you develop your interventions?

Interprofessional, interdisciplinary, and intersectoral collaboration: Do you work as a team with other health care providers or professionals from non-health disciplines? Could services or support from outside the health sector make a difference for the older person? Do you work as a team with people who work outside the health sector? What could be done to make these relationships more effective?

Use of appropriate skills and technology: Are the skills of different health care and social service providers used in the most effective way to support older persons? Are models of service provision based on the best evidence?

Public participation: Does the community you work with have input into the kinds of programs you offer or the way in which these programs are delivered? Do older persons and their families have a say in how services are organized and delivered in their community?

Source: Adapted from Canadian Nurses Association. (2005). *Primary health care: A summary of the issues.* Ottawa, ON: Author (p. 4). Retrieved from https://www.cna-aiic.ca/~/media/cna/page-content/pdf-en/bg7_primary_health_care_e.pdf?la=en.

related to each principle. Nurses can use these questions to strengthen their practice in any setting where they work with older persons and their families.

Accessibility refers to the availability of health services to all Canadians regardless of their age or geographic location (Canadian Nurses Association [CNA], 2005). Accessibility to services for older persons is limited in rural and remote regions. There is a need to improve accessibility to services for older ethnocultural minorities and for those who do not speak English or French.

Health promotion is "the process of enabling people to increase control over and to improve their health" (Canadian Nurses Association [CNA], 2005,

p. 1). Health promotion addresses the determinants of health; it includes health education, public education, nutrition, sanitation, and the prevention and control of diseases. Most of the chapters in this book include examples of ways to promote the health of older persons.

In gerontological nursing practice, *public participation* refers to individual older persons and their communities being "active partners in making decisions about their health care and the health of their communities" (Canadian Nurses Association [CNA], 2005, p. 1). Partnership with individuals is important in all nursing care. Public participation goes beyond nurse–community partnership. It means that citizens are involved in the identification of the health needs of the community. It results in flexible, responsive health care.

Appropriate technology "includes methods of care, service delivery, procedures and equipment that are socially acceptable and affordable" (Canadian Nurses Association [CNA], 2005, p. 1). An example of an innovative model of care for older persons, based on research evidence, is the Hospital Elder Life Program described in Chapter 21 (Hospital Elder Life Program, 2016).

Intersectoral collaboration "recognizes that health and well-being are linked to both economic and social policy. Intersectoral collaboration means experts in the health **sector** working with experts in other sectors such as education, housing, employment, immigration, etc. It also means that health care professionals from various disciplines collaborate and function interdependently to meet the needs of Canadians" (Canadian Nurses Association [CNA], 2002, p. 3). Gerontological nurses work in collaboration with health care providers from many disciplines. The Age-Friendly Communities initiative described in Chapter 26 is an example of a model that depends on collaboration across multiple sectors and incorporates all of the principles of primary health care.

IMPLICATIONS FOR GERONTOLOGICAL NURSING AND HEALTHY AGING

It is the responsibility of the nurse to assist older persons in achieving the highest level of wellness in relation to whatever situation exists. Through knowledge and affirmation, the nurse can empower, enhance, and support the older person's movement toward the highest level of wellness possible. The nurse assesses and can help explore the underlying situation that may be interfering with the achievement of wellness and works with the person and significant others to develop affirming and appropriate plans of care. The nurse and the older person collaborate on interventions to achieve individual goals and evaluate effectiveness. Gerontological nurses often work with other health care providers to support the health of older persons. **Interprofessional collaboration**, inter-disciplinary collaboration, and intersectoral collabo-ration are important parts of gerontological nursing. By incorporating the principles of primary health care into their practice, nurses can improve older persons' access to health promotion and health care services. Intersectoral collaboration and public participation are required to promote health and prevent illness and disability.

KEY CONCEPTS

- Gerontological nursing is an opportunity to make a significant difference in the lives of older persons.
- The meaning of aging is influenced by many factors.
- Nurses have a responsibility to contribute to accessible health care and the reduction of health disparities.
- Health, history, and gender are among the major factors influencing the aging experience.
- Each age cohort is distinctly different from others.
- Individual persons become more unique the longer they live. Nurses must be cautious in attributing any specific characteristics of older persons to "old age."
- All persons, regardless of age, illness, or life situa-tion, can be supported to achieve a higher level of wellness that is uniquely and personally defined.
- Primary health care principles can be used as an organizing framework for health promotion, regardless of a person's age or situation.
- Gerontological nurses have key roles in providing the highest quality of care to older persons in a wide range of settings and situations.

ACTIVITIES AND DISCUSSION QUESTIONS

1. Discuss the ways in which older persons contrib-ute to society today.
2. Interview an older person and ask how he or she has changed since being 25 years old.
3. Discuss health and wellness with your peers. Develop a definition of aging.
4. Discuss the dimensions of wellness and which ones you think may be most important.
5. Explain wellness in the context of chronic illness.
6. Discuss how you seek wellness in your own life.
7. Discuss what you can do to enhance the quality of life for the older persons to whom you provide care.
8. Discuss how older persons are portrayed in popular TV shows, commercials, and movies.

RESOURCES

Age pyramid of the population of Canada, 1956 to 2006
http://www12.statcan.gc.ca/census-recensement/2011/ dp-pd/pyramid-pyramide/his/index-eng.cfm

Canadian Association of Retired Persons (CARP)
http://www.carp.ca

Health Canada. Healthy living: Seniors
https://www.canada.ca/en/health-canada/services/ healthy-living/seniors.html

For additional resources, please visit *http://evolve .elsevier.com/Canada/Ebersole/gerontological/*

REFERENCES

Achenbaum, W. A. (2005). Ageing and changing: international perspective on ageing. In M. L. Johnson, V. L. Bengtson, P. G. Coleman, et al. (Eds.), *The Cambridge handbook of age and ageing* (pp. 21–29). New York, NY: Cambridge University Press.
Canadian Nurses Association (CNA). (2002). *Primary health care: A new approach to health care reform.* Ottawa, ON: Author. Retrieved from https://www.cna-aiic.ca/~/media/cna/page-content/pdf -fr/phc_presentation_kirby_6602_e.pdf?la=en.
Canadian Nurses Association (CNA). (2005). *Primary health care: A summary of the issues.* Ottawa, ON: Author. Retrieved from https://www.cna-aiic.ca/~/media/cna/page-content/pdf-en/ bg7_primary_health_care_e.pdf?la=en.
College & Association of Registered Nurses of Alberta (CARNA). (2016). *Primary health care.* Retrieved from http://www.nurses

.ab.ca/content/carna/home/current-issues-and-events/advocacy-initiatives/primary-health-care.html.

Dunn, H. L. (1961). *High-level wellness*. Arlington, VA: Beatty.

Fruch, V., Monture, L., Prince, H., et al. (2016). Home to die: Six Nations of the Grand River Territory develops community-based palliative care. *International Journal of Indigenous Health*, 11(1), 50–74. doi:10.18357/ijih111201615303.

Hospital Elder Life Program. (2016). *Hospital Elder Life Program*. Retrieved from http://www.hospitalelderlifeprogram.org/.

Hudon, T., & Milan, A. (2016). *Women in Canada: A gender-based statistical report* (Catalogue no. 89-503-X). Ottawa, ON: Statistics Canada. Retrieved from http://www.statcan.gc.ca/pub/89-503-x/2015001/article/14316-eng.pdf.

Lalonde, M. (1974). *A new perspective on the health of Canadians: A working document*. Ottawa, ON: Ministry of Supply and Services Canada. Retrieved from http://www.hc-sc.gc.ca/hcs-sss/alt_formats/hpb-dgps/pdf/pubs/1974-lalonde/lalonde-eng.pdf.

Public Health Agency of Canada. (2011). *What determines health?* Retrieved from http://www.phac-aspc.gc.ca/ph-sp/determinants/index-eng.php.

Statistics Canada. (2010). *Projections of the diversity of the Canadian population 2006 to 2031*. (Catalogue No. 91-551-X). Ottawa, ON: Author. Retrieved from: http://www.statcan.gc.ca/pub/91-551-x/91-551-x2010001-eng.pdf.

Statistics Canada. (2012). *Life expectancy, at birth and age 65 by sex and by province and territory*. Retrieved from http://www.statcan.gc.ca/tables-tableaux/sum-som/l01/cst01/health72a-eng.htm.

Statistics Canada. (2014). *Population projections: Canada, the provinces and territories, 2013 to 2063. The Daily*, September 17. Retrieved from http://www.statcan.gc.ca/daily-quotidien/140917/dq140917a-eng.pdf.

Statistics Canada. (2015). *Canada's population estimates: Age and sex, July 1, 2015*. Retrieved from http://www.statcan.gc.ca/daily-quotidien/150929/dq150929b-eng.htm.

Statistics Canada. (2016a). *Fertility: Fewer children, older moms*. Retrieved from http://www.statcan.gc.ca/pub/11-630-x/11-630-x2014002-eng.htm.

Statistics Canada. (2016b). *Aboriginal peoples in Canada: First Nations People, Métis and Inuit*. Retrieved from https://www12.statcan.gc.ca/nhs-enm/2011/as-sa/99-011-x/99-011-x2011001-eng.cfm.

The John A. Hartford Foundation. (n.d.). *The John A. Hartford Foundation Institute for Geriatric Nursing: Older adults are the core business of health care*. Retrieved from http://www.jhartfound.org/ar2006html/introduction_p3.html.

United Nations. (2013). *World population aging, 2013*. New York, NY: United Nations Department of Economic and Social Affairs. Retrieved from http://www.un.org/en/development/desa/population/publications/pdf/ageing/WorldPopulationAgeing2013.pdf.

United Nations. (2014). *Population aging and sustainable development. Population Facts*. No. 2014/4. Retrieved from http://www.un.org/en/development/desa/population/publications/pdf/popfacts/PopFacts_2014-4.pdf.

United Nations. (2015). *World Population Aging, 2015*. New York, NY: United Nations Department of Economic and Social Affairs. Retrieved from http://www.un.org/en/development/desa/population/publications/pdf/ageing/WPA2015_Report.pdf.

Wilson, K., Rosenberg, M. W., & Ning, A. (2015). Aboriginal health and development: two steps forward and one step back? In R. B. Kerr & I. Luginaah (Eds.), *Geographies of health and development* (pp. 61–71). New York, NY: Taylor & Francis Group.

World Health Organization. (n.d.). *Health promotion glossary update*. Retrieved from http://www.who.int/healthpromotion/about/HPR%20Glossary_New%20Terms.pdf.

World Health Organization & United Nations Children's Fund. (1978). *Report of the International Conference on Primary Health Care*. Alma-Ata, USSR: Author. Retrieved from http://whqlibdoc.who.int/publications/9241800011.pdf.

Gerontological Nursing History, Education, and Roles

LEARNING OBJECTIVES

Upon completion of this chapter, the reader will be able to:

- Discuss the history of gerontological nursing and the factors influencing the development of this specialty practice.
- Identify elements of the Canadian Gerontological Nursing Association Nursing Competencies and Standards of Practice.
- Examine the recommended competencies for gerontological nursing practice.
- Recognize and discuss the importance of certification.
- Discuss the professional nursing leadership role in the care of older people across the continuum of care settings.
- Describe several gerontological nursing roles and the educational preparation for practising them.
- Discuss formal gerontological organizations and their significance to the gerontological nurse.

GLOSSARY

Ageism This term incorporates two concepts: "way[s] of thinking about older persons based on negative attitudes and stereotypes about aging; and a tendency to structure society based on an assumption that everyone is young, thereby failing to respond appropriately to the real needs of older persons" (Ontario Human Rights Commission, 2011, ¶1).

Almshouse A historic charitable home providing accommodation for frail older people. Also known as a poorhouse.

Alternate level of care (ALC) Care to hospital patients who no longer require acute care services but who remain in hospital awaiting a suitable discharge destination such as residential care or a home with home care.

Health care aide (HCA) An unregulated health care provider. The term is used in this book to refer to nursing assistants, personal support workers, health care assistants, and continuing care assistants.

Knowledge translation The process of moving knowledge from research to practice, defined as "an active exchange of information between the researchers who create new knowledge and those who use it" (Canadian Institutes for Health Research, 2008, ¶7). Examples include the creation and dissemination of research syntheses and practice guidelines.

Minimum data set An instrument designed to collect the minimum amount of data required for care planning and monitoring; used as a quality indicator and in quality improvement. There are minimum data set versions for home care, long-term care, mental health, and rehabilitation settings.

THE LIVED EXPERIENCE

As I look back over my student clinical placements, it seems as though most of them, in a seemingly divine manner, have been working with older adults. I am drawn to this population. I feel as though I can actually help them, that I can really make a difference. ... This population needs us desperately; they are drastically underserved and present issues and complications that nurses, especially, can help. Many of the issues facing seniors can be alleviated, treated or effectively managed with nursing care ... this is nursing. To make life better and empower people to better their lives.

> **Third-year nursing student. From Noon, T. (2009). My journey into gerontological nursing: We are each on unique journeys as gerontological nurses. *Perspectives*, 33(2), 20–22 (p. 20).**

To know that I have made them feel they are human, that they're loved ... that someone still cares about them. I believe that lots of times they feel ignored and as if they have no value. It's very important to me that they feel valued and they know that they still contribute not only to society but to the personal growth of everyone that comes into interaction with them.

> **Gerontological nurse working in a long-term care home.**

CARE OF OLDER PERSONS: A NURSING IMPERATIVE

Older people make up a significant and growing proportion of the population worldwide. Older people today are healthier, better educated, and expect a much higher quality and greater quantity of life as they age than did the previous generation of older persons. Healthy aging is an achievable goal for many, and it is essential that we have the knowledge and skills to help people of all ages, races, orientations, and cultures achieve this goal.

Most nurses care for older people during the course of their careers. In addition, the public looks to nurses to be care providers who have the knowledge and skills to help people age well. Every older person should expect to receive care provided by nurses with competence in gerontological nursing. Gerontological nursing is not only for a specialty group of nurses. Knowledge of aging and gerontological nursing is core knowledge for the entire profession of nursing (Canadian Gerontological Nursing Association & National Gerontological Nursing Association, 2008).

Care of older persons is the fastest growing employment segment in the health care industry. Older persons are the core consumers of health care, having higher rates of outpatient visits, hospitalizations, home care, and long-term care service use than any other age groups. Despite this high demand, the number of health care workers who are interested in and prepared to care for older people remains low. Less than 1% of registered nurses (RNs) are certified in gerontology (Canadian Nurses Association [CNA], 2010a, 2010b).

It is essential to enhance interest and to increase the recruitment of students and practising nurses to care for older persons across the continuum of health care settings. Factors that motivate nurses to specialize in gerontological nursing often include positive interactions with older people over the course of a nurse's life, faculty and practice role models, a deep commitment to caring, and an appreciation of how a nursing model of care contributes to the well-being of older people. Box 2.1 presents the views of some gerontological nursing pioneers, as well as of current leaders, on the practice of gerontological nursing and what drew them to care of older persons.

HISTORY OF GERONTOLOGICAL NURSING

Historically, nurses have always been on the frontlines of caring for older people. They have provided hands-on care, supervision, administration, program development, teaching, and research, and are to a great extent responsible for the rapid advance of gerontology and gerontological nursing. Nurses have been and continue to be the mainstay of care of older persons (Baumbusch, Dahlke, & Phinney, 2012). Gerontological nurses have made substantial contributions to the

| BOX 2.1 | Reflections on Gerontological Nursing From Gerontological Nursing Pioneers and Current Leaders in the Field |

Vera McIver, Canadian Gerontological Nursing Pioneer
"A transformation took place in my psyche as I began working at the St. Mary's Priory. I saw needless degradation and knew changes had to be made to enrich the lives of these unfortunate patients. I kept striving for excellence, not only in efficiency and economy but also in improvements to the patient's environment and daily living experience. This feeling was so profound I simply had to express it.… Latent forces and talents must have come to the fore as my consciousness expanded and I came alive with this new endeavour.…I was single-minded. I was consumed by a passion to bring humanity to all those who became my responsibility." (Mantle & Funke-Furber, 2003, pp. xi–xii)

Elaine Gallagher, Canadian Gerontological Nursing Pioneer
"I chose to go to Duke University in 1975 because of a woman named Stone, Virginia Stone, and she was going around the world and was quite influential in Canada in terms of talking about personalizing care; giving people autonomy; treating them like people, like human beings as opposed to cases or patients or whatever. And was really optimistic about the fact that, you know, if you developed a really individualized care plan for someone, and encouraged them to get active and to get involved that you could actually reverse some of what people thought were some of the negative changes of aging." (Roberts, 2008, p. 27)

Terry Fulmer, Dean of the College of Nursing and Co-Director of the John A. Hartford Institute for Geriatric Nursing, New York University
"I soon realized that in the arena of caring for the aged, I could have an autonomous nursing practice that would make a real difference in medical outcomes. I could practice the full scope of nursing. It gave me a sense of freedom and accomplishment. With older patients, the most important component of care, by far, is nursing care. It's very motivating." (Ebersole & Touhy, 2006, p. 129)

Mathy Mezey, Independence Foundation Professor of Nursing Education, Division of Nursing, Steinhardt School of Education, and Director of the John A. Hartford Institute for Geriatric Nursing, New York University
"Because geriatric nursing especially offers nurses the unique opportunity to dramatically impact people's lives for the better and for the worst, it demands the best that you have to offer. I am very optimistic about the future of geriatric nursing. Increasing numbers of older adults are interested in marching into old age as healthy and involved. Geriatric nursing offers a unique opportunity to help older adults meet these aspirations while at the same time maintaining a commitment to the oldest and frailest in our society." (Ebersole & Touhy, 2006, p. 142)

Dorothy Pringle, RN, PhD, Professor and Dean Emeritus, Faculty of Nursing, University of Toronto
"When I started out in gerontological nursing, it was in its early days. We all came to it from other specialties. I was the mental health nursing coordinator in an acute care teaching hospital and essentially none of the professions was interested in older people. When we had an older person with dementia or psychotic depression, none of the psychiatrists or the social workers was very interested so it was left to the nurses and, frankly, we didn't know what to do. I thought, 'I need to go back to school. Somebody has to know how to work with these people.' I learned gerontology in my PhD education, where I worked with good practitioners and researchers who were an inspiration in terms of what was possible. Now gerontological nursing has matured enormously into a very clearly defined area of expertise, with nurses who take pride in what they are doing, and a community of interprofessional practitioners working together. Demographics dictate that all graduating nurses need to know about aging and age-related changes. They need to know what the research says and what best practices are, and be able to adapt that knowledge to the unique context of each older person. All nurses take into account the uniqueness of the people they work with, but with older people there's so much more life history influencing their values, their goals, and the kind of care they want. That's the special contribution of gerontology, and gerontological nurses bring that orientation to all the care they provide." (Dorothy Pringle, personal communication, December, 2010)

Sandra Hirst, RN, PhD, Director of the Brenda Strafford Centre for Excellence in Gerontological Nursing, and Associate Professor at the Faculty of Nursing, University of Calgary
"I started working in gerontological nursing by chance. I was inspired by the stories I heard from my older patients. The people I cared for had serious health challenges and a sense of humour that inspired me. It also gave me opportunities to reflect upon my own attitudes and behaviours towards older adults. I gained tremendous respect and value for seniors. Being a gerontological nurse has given me wonderful opportunities to grow—in community practice, educating

BOX 2.1 Reflections on Gerontological Nursing From Gerontological Nursing Pioneers and Current Leaders in the Field—cont'd

students, creating programs, working with older adults to prevent falls, leadership initiatives, and so many other ways. The range of possibilities for making a real difference is huge. To me, gerontological nursing is what nursing is really about; taking knowledge to the bedside, drawing on everything you've learned, connecting with people in a real way, caring, and commitment. It's like a puzzle. The sense of satisfaction you get from completing a puzzle is the same as when you work with older adults. That frustration you have when there is a missing puzzle piece is solved with nursing knowledge. Gerontological nursing knowledge is unique and special and makes it possible to feel like you're not just doing a good job; you're influencing quality of life. One of the important changes I've seen recently is that we're beginning to overcome ageism in nursing and nursing education. We're the largest specialty group within CNA [Canadian Nurses Association]. Individual faculty members are taking initiative to improve curriculum. Students are interested in gerontological nursing. We still have a way to go, but it's a big improvement." (Sandra Hirst, personal communication, January, 2011)

BOX 2.2 Gerontological Nursing in Canada: a Timeline

1950	International Association of Gerontological Societies (currently International Association on Gerontology and Geriatrics [IAGG]) founded
1950s	Home care programs established by the Victorian Order of Nurses (VON)
1967–68	The Priory Method Restorative Care Model created by Vera McIver
1971	Canadian Association on Gerontology (CAG) founded
1974	Gerontological Nursing Association (GNA), the first provincial gerontological nursing association, founded in Ontario
1976	*Perspectives, The Journal of the Gerontological Nursing Association* established
1983	First Canadian gerontological nursing conference, held in Victoria, British Columbia
1985	Canadian Gerontological Nursing Association (CGNA) founded
1987	Standards of Gerontological Nursing established by Ontario GNA and subsequently adopted by CGNA
1993	*Promoting Healthy Aging: A Nursing and Community Perspective* (Beckingham & DuGas) published
1995	Standards of Practice for gerontological nursing established by CGNA
1999	Canadian Nurses Association (CNA) included Gerontological Nursing Specialty Certification
2004	Sandra Hirst, first nurse elected president of CAG
2008	Brenda Strafford Centre for Excellence in Gerontological Nursing established, University of Calgary
2010	*Nursing Competencies and Standards of Practice* for gerontological nursing established by CGNA

body of knowledge guiding best practice in the care of older people. In examining the history of gerontological nursing, one must marvel at the advocacy and perseverance of nurses who have remained deeply committed to the care of older persons despite struggling against insurmountable odds over the years. Box 2.2 presents a timeline of significant accomplishments in the history of gerontological nursing and gerontology in Canada.

The history and development of gerontological nursing in Canada is tied to the history and development of the field of gerontology in Canada, as well as to the development of gerontological nursing and gerontology in the United States and internationally. Canadian nurses have benefited from leadership in gerontological nursing in the United States and from collaboration between American and Canadian nursing scholars and nursing bodies. For example, gerontological nursing textbooks, journals, and graduate education programs were available in the United States before they were available in Canada. Since 1996, The John A. Hartford Foundation has substantially funded gerontological nursing research, **knowledge translation**, and educational initiatives, resulting in significant development in the field of gerontological nursing.

Gerontological nursing originated when Florence Nightingale, the founder of modern nursing, accepted a position as superintendent in an institution similar to what we would think of as an early version of a long-term care home, the Institution for the Care of Sick Gentlewomen in Distressed Circumstances (Wykle & McDonald, 1997). Historically in Canada, care of older persons and care of the ill were provided by female family members at home. In the early years of the transition to hospital treatment for illness, inhumane hospital conditions could be avoided by the wealthy, who hired nurses to care for older persons at home (Dahlke, 2011).

Awareness of the need for education in gerontological nursing, as well as the need for improvement in the care of older persons in **almshouses**, first appeared in the American nursing literature in the early 1900s. In a 1903 article published in the *American Journal of Nursing*, Bassell wrote about care of older persons in Labrador (Hirst, King, & Church, 1996). An *American Journal of Nursing* editorial in 1908 focused on the need for better training in the care of older persons (Dock, 1908). The first book on gerontological nursing was written by Newton and Anderson in 1950 in the United States. In the 1950s, several articles about the need to improve nursing care of older persons appeared in the *Canadian Nurse,* and another two appeared in the *Alberta Association of Registered Nurses* newsletter, contributing to the emergence of gerontological nursing in Canada (Dahlke, 2011; Hirst et al., 1996).

In 1967, Vera McIver, who was to emerge as a leader in innovative gerontological nursing care and who is discussed in Box 2.3, took a position at St. Mary's Priory Hospital in Victoria, British Columbia. In Canada, the first provincial gerontological nursing association was formed in Ontario in 1974, followed by the establishment of the Canadian Gerontological Nursing Association (CGNA) in 1985. A few years later, in 1987, gerontological nursing standards were established by the CGNA. In 1993, the first Canadian gerontological nursing textbook was published (Beckingham & DuGas, 1993). Whereas most specialties in nursing practice developed from those identified in medicine, this was not the case with

---

BOX 2.3   Vera McIver and the Priory Model

St. Mary's Priory Hospital in Victoria, British Columbia, was a long-term care (LTC) facility providing 24-hour nursing care to women. It followed a custodial care model typical of LTC facilities at that time. The model was based on acute care models in which "the care of the physical body received preference over the care of the person" (Mantle & Funke-Furber, 2003, p. 7). Patients were expected to be dependent; medications and restraints were used if patients were too active. In 1967, Vera McIver was appointed Director of Nursing. She came to this position from acute care and, like most nurses of the time, had no extra educational preparation for caring for older persons. She quickly came to believe that "the end result of custodial care [was] a cascade of effects set in motion," and that immobility and lack of attention to social, emotional, and spiritual needs caused further physical deterioration, "mental deterioration and death of the human spirit" (Mantle & Funke-Furber, 2003, p. 8). McIver transformed care and management approaches at the Priory, creating a restorative care model that became known as the Priory Method. This approach was far ahead of its time and influenced care models in North America and further afield (Roberts, 2008). As described by Mantle and Funke-Furber (2003), the five overall strategies of the Priory Method restorative care model were as follows:

- Attention to the whole person, not just the disability
- Environment and staff behaviours designed to "convey positive expectations of wellness and the maximum use of remaining abilities" (Mantle and Funke-Furber, 2003, p. 23)
- Humanized, de-institutionalized environment
- Normalization of activities of daily living through environmental changes and physical strengthening
- Strengthening of residents' egos, owing to staff support of residents carrying out their own activities of daily living

---

gerontological nursing, since health care of older persons was traditionally considered to fall within the domain of nursing (Davis, 1984).

Gerontological nurse educators, scholars, and clinicians continue their commitment to and advocacy for older people. As will be seen throughout this book, gerontological nursing research provides a strong evidence base for practice across settings. Gerontological nursing research has gained wide acceptance in the scientific community and has made significant contributions to improved care and to policy decisions that influence care outcomes.

Research has shown that better care for older persons is possible and should be expected. The task ahead is to communicate this knowledge to all nurses who care for older persons and to create environments that support nurses' ability to use that knowledge in practice (Dahlke, 2011; Fox et al., 2012). Dahlke reported that workload pressures and a focus on efficiency often inhibit nurses' ability to provide holistic care, noting that "as in the past, current day nurses are providing older persons with routine physical care, rather than care that incorporates the older adults' holistic and diverse needs" (Dahlke, 2011, p. 5). May Wykle and Ruth Tappen—gerontological nursing scholars, educators, and researchers—have provided suggestions for future research (Box 2.4).

STANDARDS OF GERONTOLOGICAL NURSING PRACTICE

In order to develop accurate and informed attitudes, gerontological nursing organizations have established standards, legitimized the specialty, upgraded the knowledge base, enhanced the image of gerontological nurses, and identified the many benefits of working with older persons. In Canada, nursing practice competencies and standards are regulated by provincial organizations. Provincial regulatory bodies collaboratively developed a national set of entry-to-practice competencies in 2006 (Black et al., 2008). The entry-to-practice competencies specify that nurses should be able to provide care for persons of all ages and across practice settings (College of Registered Nurses of British Columbia, 2015). The regulatory bodies do not set out specific competencies for gerontological nursing. In 1989, the CGNA adopted the Standards of Gerontological Nursing developed by the Gerontological Nursing Association of Ontario (Gerontological Nursing Association [Ontario], 1987) and then embarked on a consultative process of developing national standards for gerontological nursing; the standards of practice were published in 1996. In 2010, a new set of standards, *Gerontological Nursing Competencies and Standards of Practice*, was published (Canadian Gerontological Nursing Association, 2010). There are six broad standards, each supported by a set of competencies. The standards are outlined

| BOX 2.4 | Future Directions for Gerontological Nursing Research as Suggested by Wykle and Tappen |

- Staffing patterns and the most appropriate mix to improve care outcomes in long-term care (LTC) settings
- The influence of culture, diversity, and ethnicity on aging
- Health disparities and health literacy
- Factors contributing to successful aging, health promotion, and wellness in the "baby boomer" generation
- Retirement decisions of the "baby boomers": how they are made and how they are changing
- Dementia as a chronic illness, and staying well in the presence of the disease
- Caregiving, particularly intergenerational
- Values and attitudes of the current generation toward aging, and the expectations of that generation
- Interventions to assist with the increasing prevalence of drug and alcohol abuse and other mental health problems of the current and future generations of older persons
- Integration of current best-practice protocols and guidelines into settings along the continuum in cost-effective and care-efficient models
- Models of acute care designed to prevent negative outcomes in older persons
- Strategies to increase preparation in gerontological nursing and increase recruitment of the brightest and best into gerontological nursing
- Models of interprofessional practice
- Health promotion and illness-management interventions in the assisted-living setting; role of professional nurses and advanced-practice nurses in this setting; aging in place
- Development of models for end-of-life care in home and in LTC homes

Source: Ebersole, P., & Touhy, T. (2006). *Geriatric nursing: Growth of a specialty.* New York: Springer (pp. 246–247).

in Box 2.5. Established in Canada by the National Initiative for Care of the Elderly and the Geriatric Education and Recruitment Initiative, *Core Interprofessional Competencies for Gerontology* contains 49 interprofessional competencies in nine categories: clinician; communicator; collaborator; supervisor/ leader; advocate; scholar; professional; educator; and health system (staff) member (National Initiative for

BOX 2.5   Canadian Gerontological Nursing Association Competencies and Standards of Practice

Standard I: Physiological Health
Gerontological nurses assist clients to maintain homeostatic regulation through assessment and management of physiological care to minimize adverse events associated with medications, diagnostic or therapeutic procedures, nosocomial infections, or environmental stressors.

Standard II: Optimizing Functional Health
Gerontological nurses promote older adults to optimize functional health that includes an integration of abilities that involve physical, cognitive, psychological, social, and spiritual status (AACN & Hartford, 2000).

Standard III: Responsive Care
Gerontological nurses provide responsive care that facilitates and empowers client independence through life-course changes. A responsive care approach recognizes that certain behaviours are not necessarily related solely to pathology, but instead may be related to circumstances within the physical or social environment surrounding well older persons and those with dementia and may be an expression of unmet need (Wiersman & Dupuis, 2007).

Standard IV: Relationship Care
Gerontological nurses develop and preserve therapeutic relationship care. Relationship-centred care is an approach that recognizes the importance and uniqueness of each health care participant's relationship with every other and considers these relationships to be central in supporting high-quality care, a high-quality work environment, and superior organizational performance (Safran, Miller, & Beckman, 2006).

Standard V: Health System
Gerontological nurses are aware of economic and political influences by providing or facilitating care that supports access to and benefit from the health care delivery system. Systems to support and sustain practice changes should be in place, including ongoing education, policies and procedures, and job descriptions (Crandall et al., 2007).

Standard VI: Safety and Security
Gerontological nurses are responsible for assessing the client and the environment for hazards that threaten safety, as well as planning and intervening appropriately to maintain a safe environment (Potter et al., 2009).

Source: Canadian Gerontological Nursing Association. (2010). *Gerontological Nursing Competencies and Standards of Practice* (pp. 9–12). Vancouver, BC: Author.

Care of the Elderly [NICE] and the Geriatric Education and Recruitment Initiative [GERI], 2010; also see http://www.nicenet.ca/resources).

Certification

Certification is a means of assuring the public that an individual has pursued some specialized study in a given area, has successfully demonstrated the requisite knowledge and competencies, and has been awarded recognition of this achievement. Canadian Nurses Association certification in gerontological nursing verifies professional competency and assures nursing colleagues, the public, and employers that the nurse possesses specialized knowledge that meets predetermined standards. In 2015, 2,557 registered nurses (RNs) were certified as gerontological nurses. (For additional information on certification, see http://www.cna-aiic.ca).

GERONTOLOGICAL NURSING EDUCATION

Ensuring gerontological nursing competency in all students graduating from a nursing program is imperative for the improvement of health care to older persons. Adequacy of preparation of students and the need for improved gerontological nursing education in Canada have been discussed in the gerontological nursing literature for many years (Baumbusch et al., 2012; Boscart et al., 2016; Burns et al., 1986; McCleary et al., 2009). The necessity of stand-alone courses, as provided for specialty practice areas such as maternal–child or mental health nursing, is under debate. Some educators advocate stand-alone courses and the integration of gerontological content in other courses (McCleary et al., 2017). There is evidence that gerontological content in nursing education is insufficient (Boscart et al., 2016; Hirst, Lane, & Stares, 2012; McCleary et al., 2017; Wagner et al., 2013). Reasons for this deficiency may include unsupportive faculty; insufficient gerontological nursing expertise among faculty; gerontological content being regarded as an extra requirement that overloads the already extensive informational requirements for accreditation of nursing education programs; assumptions that such content is integrated throughout the program; and a lack of interest from students and faculty. Deficient gerontological content and coursework in the

BOX 2.6 Prescriptions for Excellence in Gerontological Nursing Education

1. All students require core knowledge specific to the health and well-being of older adults. This knowledge should include current evidence about the social, psychological, spiritual, developmental, and biological changes associated with aging.
2. A gerontology-specific practicum should be required of every student.
3. Infuse gerontological content into current nursing courses.
4. Gerontological content should be taught by a nurse educator with experience, interest, and knowledge of older adults' health. We recommend certification. Interest and involvement in research is an asset in maintaining currency of content.
5. Develop and implement a mentor program between nursing students and nursing professionals with a commitment to gerontological nursing practice.

Source: Canadian Gerontological Nursing Association & National Gerontological Nursing Association. (2008). *Prescriptions for excellence in gerontological nursing education: A joint position statement* (pp. 3–4). Retrieved from http://www.cgna.net/uploads/CGNANGNAJointPosition-Statement.pdf.

education of health care providers can be viewed as a form of **ageism** and discrimination.

The CGNA and the US National Gerontological Nursing Association issued *Prescriptions for Excellence in Gerontological Nursing Education*, a joint position statement, in 2008. The recommendations are summarized in Box 2.6.

Some colleges and universities have incorporated dynamic courses in aging into their curricula (Boscart et al., 2016), and several resources to improve curricula and teaching are available. The John A. Hartford Foundation in the United States has been responsible for some of the most significant advances in gerontological nursing, education, and research. Between 1996 and 2007, the foundation granted $67 million in various educational and clinical demonstrations of effective programmatic changes in the provision of care to older people (https://hign.org/). John A. Hartford Foundation nursing initiatives include the Institute for Geriatric Nursing at New York University and Centers for Geriatric Nursing Excellence at nine American universities. The clinical

nursing website of the Hartford Institute for Geriatric Nursing (https://consultgeri.org) contains abundant evidence-informed resources for gerontological nurses and nurse educators.

The Hartford Institute for Geriatric Nursing and the American Association of Colleges of Nursing (AACN) collaborated in developing gerontological nursing competencies, curriculum materials for baccalaureate programs, and training for faculty members to enhance teaching and curricula (http://www.aacn.nche.edu). The National Initiative for Care of the Elderly and the Canadian Institutes for Health Research funded knowledge-exchange institutes for Canadian nursing faculty members (McCleary, 2010; McCleary et al., 2009). The Institutes provided faculty with Canadian and US evidence-informed resources to improve gerontological nursing education. A publicly accessible wiki was also created to share resources (http://kumu.brocku.ca/geriatricnursingeducation/Main_Page). With such resources now available, nursing educators must seriously consider specific minimum requirements for the care of older persons at each level of education in order to fulfill the responsibility of nurses to the public and the profession and to meet accreditation criteria.

Beyond course curriculum development, a large amount of research and practice innovation is available to gerontological nurses. Considering the rate of expansion of this knowledge and the fact that many nurses do not have sufficient knowledge about caring for older persons with complex needs, continuing education resources are important. Resources listed on the previously cited wiki can be used for continuing education in health care facilities. Many colleges offer continuing education courses and postgraduate certificates in gerontological nursing.

ROLES IN GERONTOLOGICAL NURSING

Gerontological nursing roles encompass every imaginable venue and circumstance. The opportunities are limitless because this is a rapidly aging society. The impact of gerontological nursing on the health and well-being of older persons and their families can be seen across various practice settings—in communities; in people's homes; and in acute care, rehabilitation, and long-term care environments. Gerontological nurses work directly with older persons and their families, linking them to needed services. Through leadership and research, gerontological nurses influence improvements in services and policies.

A gerontological nurse may be a generalist or a specialist. The generalist functions in a variety of settings (primary care, acute care, home care, rehabilitation and LTC homes, and the community), providing nursing care to individuals and their families. The gerontological nursing specialist is an advanced practice nurse, typically with education at the master's level.

SPECIALIST ROLES

Advanced practice nurses (APNs), sometimes referred to as clinical nurse specialists, perform all of the functions of generalists but possess advanced clinical expertise, understand health and social policy, and are proficient in planning, implementing, and evaluating health programs. Nurse practitioners (NPs) have additional education, usually at the graduate level, and function in an extended nursing role. APNs and NPs have demonstrated their skill in improving health outcomes and cost-effectiveness in primary, acute, and continuing care settings; community settings; retirement homes; hospices; LTC homes; and units that provide specialized care of older persons.

Research has demonstrated the positive outcomes associated with APNs and NPs, including increased patient satisfaction, decreased costs, fewer hospitalizations and emergency room visits, and improved quality of care (Newhouse et al., 2011; Kaasalainen et al., 2016). NPs in LTC homes provide primary care and advanced nursing care, resulting in improved quality of care (Martin-Misener et al., 2015). Some Canadian universities offer graduate courses in gerontological nursing but have no specialty programs. Mezey and Fulmer suggested that all graduate programs be "gerontologized" so that all APNs and NP graduates would have gerontological nursing competencies to meet the health care needs of an aging population (Mezey & Fulmer, 2002).

GENERALIST ROLES

Hospital-Based Care

Even though most nurses work in acute care with older persons and their families, many have not had specialized gerontological nursing in their nursing education programs. Older persons account for 60% of hospital days (Senior Friendly Hospitals, 2014). Older persons who experience episodic or acute illnesses frequently have multiple chronic conditions and comorbidities and have complex care needs. Exacerbations of persistent, chronic illnesses and injuries are often the cause of hospitalization for older persons. The most common reasons for older persons being admitted to Canadian hospitals are chronic obstructive pulmonary disease, heart failure, knee replacement, pneumonia, and myocardial infarction (Canadian Institute of Health Information, 2012). Common iatrogenic complications of hospitalization for older people include functional decline, new-onset incontinence, malnutrition, pressure ulcers, medication interactions and adverse effects, delirium, and falls (Senior Friendly Hospitals, 2014). Many of these conditions are directly related to and influenced by nursing care, reinforcing the need for nurses to be competent in the care of older persons.

Because of problems accessing home care, rehabilitation, or long-term care after hospitalization, some older patients can be ready for discharge but unable to leave the hospital. This group of older people are classified as receiving an **alternate level of care (ALC)**. About 14% of hospital beds are ALC beds (McCloskey et al., 2014). The vast majority of ALC patients are older persons, and a significant proportion have dementia. Acute care hospital settings are not suited to their needs, and rapid functional decline while they are waiting for discharge is common (McCloskey et al., 2014; Sutherland & Crump, 2013).

Nurses caring for older persons in hospitals may function as direct care providers, care coordinators, educators, and discharge planners, as well as fill leadership, research, quality improvement, and management positions. The complex needs of older persons who require hospital-based care means that in order to provide competent care, all nurses in hospital settings need to have a depth of knowledge about the various conditions associated with aging, the ability to distinguish normal aging from pathology, and well-developed critical thinking, care planning, intervention, and evaluation skills.

Some health care organizations have made organization-wide commitments to excellent care for older persons. The Nurses Improving Care for Health System Elders (NICHE) program was developed by the Hartford Institute for Geriatric Nursing in 1992. It emphasizes institutional commitment, collaboration, and nursing leadership to achieve improved safety and outcomes for hospitalized older persons (Capezuti et al., 2012). More than 500 hospitals in the United States and 13 in Canada are involved in NICHE programs (http://www.nicheprogram.org).

A key component of the NICHE program is the geriatric resource nurse model, whereby nurses are trained by advanced-practice gerontological nurses and then function as clinical resource experts on geriatric issues for other nurses on their unit. This is an innovative role for a hospital staff nurse interested in the care of older persons. The NICHE Acute Care of the Elderly Medical-Surgical Unit is based on patient- and family-centred approaches. The physical environment is adapted to meet the needs of older persons and to enhance functional independence. Staffing consists of an interprofessional team with expert knowledge in the care of older persons. Older persons are discharged to the least restrictive environment. Outcomes in hospitals using NICHE models include enhanced nursing knowledge and skills related to the treatment of common geriatric syndromes, improved patient satisfaction, decreased length of stay, reductions in admission rates, and reductions in hospital costs (Capezuti et al., 2012).

Community- and Home-Based Care

Nurses provide care and services for older persons in hospitals, rehabilitation settings, and LTC homes, but the majority of older persons live in the community. Community-based care settings include home care, independent older-adult housing, retirement communities, adult day health programs, primary care clinics, and public health departments. The growth in home- and community-based health care is expected to continue, since older people prefer to age in place, a perspective that is increasingly recognized in policy and planning. Several provinces have developed strategies to support aging in place (e.g., Manitoba Health [http://www.gov.mb.ca/health/aginginplace/] and the Ontario Ministry of Health and Long-Term Care [https://www.ontario.ca/page/aging-confidence-ontario-action-plan-seniors]), measures that are discussed

in Chapters 23 and 26. However, access to publicly funded home care varies from province to province, and for some older persons, the cost of purchasing needed home care services further limits their accessibility (Davies, Hirdes, & Mannell, 2017).

Nurses in the home setting provide comprehensive assessments; may provide and supervise care for older people who have a variety of care needs, including dementia care; and provide specific treatments such as wound care, catheter care, intravenous therapy, and tube feedings. Home care patients include persons with unstable medical conditions, persons with complex medication or care regimens, and persons receiving rehabilitation, supportive, or palliative care services. Advances in technology for remote monitoring of health status and safety show promise in improving outcomes for older people who want to age in place. These technologies present exciting opportunities for nurses in the management and evaluation of care (see Chapter 15). Gerontological nurses have opportunities to create practices in community-based settings with a focus not only on care for those who are ill but also on promoting health and addressing determinants of health.

Long-Term Care

Formal settings for long-term care include chronic-care hospitals, complex continuing care facilities, inpatient rehabilitation facilities, and LTC homes (also referred to as nursing homes). About 7% of older Canadians live in LTC homes where most of the residents are older persons (Statistics Canada, 2012). As the health care system evolved to support aging at home, the complexity and acuity of residents in LTC settings has increased considerably (Ontario Long Term Care Association, 2016).

Today, LTC homes are a complex mix of hospital, rehabilitation facility, hospice, and dementia support unit. For many older people, they are a final home. However, as previously noted, the LTC system is changing and providing more care for older persons requiring episodic or acute care. In addition, stringent regulations governing care practices, the interprofessional and cross-functional team models, the expanded use of nurses and health care aides, the innovative use of APNs and NPs, and the limited presence of physicians on site influence the role of professional nursing in these settings. Thus, excellent assessment skills; the ability to work in partnership with other team members and families; skills in acute, rehabilitative, and palliative care; and leadership, advocacy, management, collaboration, and delegation skills are essential.

Professional nurses in LTC homes must be highly skilled in order to practice independently and collaboratively. This setting provides significant opportunities for independent decision making, nursing leadership, optimized integrated team models of care, and evaluation of resident and family outcomes, including well-being. Nursing roles may include those of administrator, manager, supervisor, coordinator, educator, **minimum data set** coordinator, case manager, quality improvement coordinator, and clinical nurse.

LTC homes care for people who need skilled comprehensive nursing care but who may not need the intense care that is provided in complex continuing care hospitals. Such people include those who have had severe stroke, who have Alzheimer's disease and related dementias, who have Parkinson's disease, and who receive comfort care. Just over half of LTC home residents are aged 85 years or older (Statistics Canada, 2010). Residents of LTC homes represent the frailest of the older person population; their needs for 24-hour care cannot be met in the home or residential care setting or may have exceeded their families' abilities to provide care. A survey of Ontario LTC homes found that about two thirds of residents had dementia, 97% had two or more chronic conditions, and 33% were highly dependent on staff (Ontario Long Term Care Association, 2016). Payment for LTC homes is subsidized by provincial governments. Residents pay for basic accommodations and for medications that are not covered by provincial drug plans.

In 2014, there were 1,519 LTC homes in Canada, with 149,488 residents (Statistics Canada, 2015). Due to the aging population, the number of LTC homes is predicted to significantly increase. Adequate and competent staff continues to be of critical importance in these settings, especially in view of the acuity and complex needs of the residents. Provincial standards set staffing requirements by numbers of hours of care per resident, not by staff-to-resident ratios. Staffing levels have often been criticized as inadequate (Ontario Association of Non-Profit Homes and Services for Seniors, 2014), and many LTC homes do not consistently meet staffing requirements (Pemberton, 2016). More time spent by RNs providing direct care to each resident in LTC is associated with better resident outcomes as related to fall prevention, urinary tract infection, and hospitalization (Dellefield et al., 2015). Despite increases in the acuity level of LTC home residents' conditions and the positive relationship between nurse staffing and quality of care, relatively few RNs work in LTC homes.

There are several new initiatives in LTC that nurses can be involved with to improve professional nursing practice and resident quality outcomes, including the Registered Nurses Association of Ontario Spotlight Organization program for LTC and Sigma Theta Tau's Center for Nursing Excellence in Long Term Care. The culture change movement, discussed in Chapter 26, provides many exciting opportunities for nurses to lead the change from an institution-centred culture to a person-centred culture in LTC.

Health Care Aides

Although it is important to promote professional nursing care for older persons, **health care aides (HCAs)** provide the majority of care and services in LTC and home care settings (Berta et al., 2013), contributing significantly to the quality of life for LTC home residents and home care patients. Results of several studies confirm the deep commitment and passion that HCAs bring to their jobs and to the residents with whom they work (Berta et al., 2013). The significance and importance of close personal relationships between HCAs and residents (often described as "like family") form a central dimension of quality of care and positive outcomes (Carpenter & Thompson, 2008; Chung, 2013; Walsh & Shutes, 2013).

However, Carpenter and Thompson (2008) found that "difficulty recruiting and retaining these long-term care workers continues to plague nursing homes, as turnover rates approach 100%" (p. 26). In a Canadian study, HCAs in LTC homes reported being rushed in their care and not having sufficient time to complete needed tasks (Knopp-Sihota et al., 2015). Several recent studies have investigated the relationship of factors such as turnover, work satisfaction, staffing, and power relations to the quality of care and to positive outcomes in LTC homes. The results support the importance of developing a culture of respect in which the work of HCAs is understood and valued at all levels of the organization (Chamberlain et al., 2017).

One of the most important components of the culture change movement is the creation of team models of care that value and honour the important work of HCAs, who are undervalued in society and the health care system (Hewko et al., 2015). Such models are consistent with the Priory Method pioneered by Vera McIver (see Box 2.3). Culture change is equally concerned about the needs of residents and the well-being of staff. According to Thomas and Johnson, "An organization that learns to give love, respect, dignity, tenderness, and tolerance to all members of the staff will soon find these same virtues being practiced by the staff" (Thomas & Johnson, 2003, p. 3). Until health care providers and society make a real commitment to providing adequate wages, providing individual supports (e.g., benefits, education, career ladders), and appreciating the significant contribution by HCAs to the quality of care in LTC homes, these workers cannot be expected to have the energy or incentive to extend themselves fully to their work with older people (Kash, Castle, & Phillips, 2007). Chapter 26 discusses the culture change movement in more depth.

GERONTOLOGICAL NURSING AND GERONTOLOGY ORGANIZATIONS

Gerontological nursing organizations in Canada include the nationwide Canadian Gerontological Nursing Association (CGNA) and provincial gerontological nursing associations in Newfoundland and Labrador, Nova Scotia, Prince Edward Island, New Brunswick, Ontario, Manitoba, Alberta, and British Columbia. The CGNA publishes a refereed journal, *Perspectives*, and holds a national biennial conference.

In 2003, the CGNA and the National Gerontological Nursing Association (NGNA) in the United States formed an alliance to exchange information and share mutual goals and opportunities for the advancement of both groups. Gerontological nursing associations in the United States include the NGNA, the Gerontological Advanced Practice Nurses Association, and the

National Association of Directors of Nursing Administration in Long Term Care. The NGNA publishes the journal *Geriatric Nursing*. The US Coalition of Geriatric Nursing Organizations represents more than 28,700 gerontological nurses from eight organizations.

The Canadian Association on Gerontology (CAG) supports interdisciplinary and interprofessional collaboration in research and practice. The divisions of Health and Biological Sciences, Social Policy and Practice, Educational Gerontology, Psychology, and Social Sciences include members from myriad backgrounds and many disciplines who affiliate with CAG on the basis of their particular role and function rather than just their educational or professional credentials. The Association publishes the *Canadian Journal on Aging*. The CAG Student Connections is a national network for students interested in aging issues (http://cagacg.ca/student-connection/). Some provinces have provincial gerontology associations.

The Canadian Geriatrics Society (CGS) is devoted to promoting excellence in the medical care of older Canadians. Membership is open to all physicians with an interest in geriatrics. Nurses and other health care providers can join the CGS as associate members. The Canadian Academy of Geriatric Psychiatry is an association of physicians who have completed training in geriatric psychiatry or are in training. It provides leadership in the field of geriatric psychiatry and promotes the mental health of older persons. British Columbia and Ontario also have geriatric mental health associations.

International gerontology associations such as the Gerontological Society of America, the American Medical Directors Association, the American Geriatrics Society, the International Federation on Ageing, and the International Association of Gerontology and Geriatrics have interprofessional and interdisciplinary membership and offer the opportunity to study aging internationally.

IMPLICATIONS FOR GERONTOLOGICAL NURSING AND HEALTHY AGING

Nursing is a vital aspect of the health care of older people, and the practice of gerontological nursing provides a unique vantage point from which to make an impact. Nurses attracted to this specialized field recognize that expertise in caring for older persons can make a significant difference in the quality of life of the older person. Because of the complex needs of older persons with health problems, gerontological nursing is intellectually challenging. In times of illness, rehabilitation, and end-of-life care, outcomes for the older person more often than not depend on the nursing care received. Through research, gerontological nurses have made substantial contributions to the body of knowledge of best practices in the care of older persons, and they are recognized as leaders in aging care.

Gerontological nurses have opportunities to provide care across the continuum of aging services, caring for everyone from the most ill and frail to those who are active and independent. As phrased by Mezey and Fulmer, the commitment of gerontological nurses is to "tackle difficult but exceptionally meaningful issues that impact profoundly on the health and quality of life for older adults" (Mezey and Fulmer, 2002, p. 440). Gerontological nursing may be the most needed specialty in nursing, both now and in the future (Ebersole & Touhy, 2006). As Mezey and Fulmer have also suggested, we need to ensure that in the future, every older person will be cared for by a nurse who has competence and expertise in gerontological nursing (Mezey and Fulmer, 2002).

KEY CONCEPTS

- Certification assures the public of nurses' commitment to specialized education and qualification for the care of older persons.
- All students graduating from nursing programs and all practising nurses working with older persons should have competence in gerontological nursing.
- Major changes in health care delivery and the increasing number of older persons have resulted in numerous revised, refined, and emergent roles for nurses in the field of gerontological nursing. There is a critical shortage of competent and compassionate gerontological nurses.
- Advanced-practice nurses may have nurse practitioner qualifications, clinical nurse specialist education, or both.
- Advanced-practice opportunities for nurses are numerous and offer more independence, are cost-effective, and facilitate more holistic health care and improved outcomes for patients.
- Nursing and interprofessional gerontological associations support scholarship, the advancement and dissemination of new knowledge and best practices, and networking (including student member networking).

ACTIVITIES AND DISCUSSION QUESTIONS

1. Identify factors that have influenced the progress of gerontological nursing as a specialty practice.
2. Consider and discuss with classmates the various gerontological nursing roles that you find most interesting and stimulating.
3. Discuss what you consider the most important elements of the 2010 Canadian Gerontological Nurses Association *Nursing Competencies and Standards of Practice* and the National Initiative for Care of the Elderly *Core Interprofessional Competencies for Gerontology*.
4. Discuss the gerontological organizations of today and their significance to the practising nurse.
5. Reflect on why more students do not choose gerontological nursing as a specialty. What would increase interest in this area of nursing?
6. Discuss what you think are the most important issues in gerontological nursing education.

RESOURCES

Canadian Association on Gerontology (CAG)
http://www.cagacg.ca

Canadian Gerontological Nursing Association (CGNA)
http://www.cgna.net

Canadian Nurses Association (CNA) certification program
https://cna-aiic.ca/en/certification

Hartford Institute for Geriatric Nursing
https://hign.org/

National Gerontological Nursing Association (NGNA)
http://www.ngna.org

National Initiative for Care of the Elderly (NICE)
http://www.nicenet.ca

For additional resources, please visit *http://evolve*
.elsevier.com/Canada/Ebersole/gerontological/

REFERENCES

American Association of Colleges of Nursing in collaboration with the Hartford Institute for Geriatric Nursing at New York University (2000). *Recommended baccalaureate competencies and curricular guidelines for the nursing care of older adults: A supplement to The Essentials of Baccalaureate Education for Professional Nursing Practice.* Washington, DC: Author.

Baumbusch, J., Dahlke, S., & Phinney, A. (2012). Nursing students' knowledge and beliefs about care of older adults in a shifting context of nursing education. *Journal of Advanced Nursing,* 68, 2550–2558. doi:10.1111/j.1365-2648.2012.05959.x.

Beckingham, A. C., & DuGas, B. W. (1993). *Promoting healthy aging: A nursing and community perspective.* Toronto, ON: Mosby.

Berta, W., Laporte, A., Deber, R., et al. (2013). The evolving role of health care aides in long-term care and home and community care sectors in Canada. *Human Resources for Health,* 11, doi:10.1186/1478-4491-11-25.

Black, J., Allen, D., Redfern, L., et al. (2008). Competencies in the context of entry-level registered nurse practice: A collaborative project in Canada. *International Nursing Review,* 55, 171–178. doi:10.1111/j.1466-7657.2007.00626.x.

Boscart, V., McCleary, L., Huson, K., et al. (2016). Integrating gerontological competencies in Canadian health and social service education: An overview of trends, enablers, and challenges. *Gerontology & Geriatrics Education,* 38(1), 17–46. doi: 10.1080/02701960.2016.1230738.

Burns, L., MacLeod, F., MacTavish, M., et al. (1986). Career selection: Planting the seed for gerontological nursing. *Perspectives,* 10(8), 8–10.

Canadian Gerontological Nursing Association (2010). *Gerontological nursing competencies and standards of practice.* Vancouver, BC: Author.

Canadian Gerontological Nursing Association & National Gerontological Nursing Association (2008). *Prescriptions for excellence in gerontological nursing education: A joint position statement.* Vancouver, BC: Authors. Retrieved from http://www.cgna.net/uploads/CGNANGNAJointPositionStatement.pdf.

Canadian Institutes of Health Information (CIHI) (2012). *All-cause readmission to acute care and return to the emergency department.* Ottawa, ON: Author. Retrieved from https://secure.cihi.ca/free_products/Readmission_to_acutecare_en.pdf.

Canadian Institutes for Health Research (CIHR) (2008). *Knowledge translation strategy 2004–2009.* Ottawa: Author. Retrieved from http://www.cihr-irsc.gc.ca/e/26574.html#defining.

Canadian Nurses Association (CNA) (2010a). *2010 workforce profile of registered nurses in Canada.* Ottawa, ON: Author. Retrieved from https://www.cna-aiic.ca/~/media/cna/page-content/pdf-en/2010_rn_snapshot_e.pdf.

Canadian Nurses Association (CNA) (2010b). *Number of valid CNA certifications by specialty/area of nursing practice and province/territory, 2010.* Ottawa, ON: Author. Retrieved from https://www.cna-aiic.ca/~/media/cna/page-content/pdf-en/cert_by_specialty_and_area_2010_e.pdf?la=en.

Capezuti, E., Boltz, M., Cline, D., et al. (2012). Nurses Improving Care for Healthsystem Elders – a model for optimizing the geriatric nursing practice environment. *Journal of Clinical Nursing,* 21-22, 3117–3125. doi:10.1111/j.1365-2702.2012.04259.x.

Carpenter, J., & Thompson, S. A. (2008). CNAs experience in the nursing home: "It's in my soul.". *Journal of Gerontological Nursing,* 34(9), 25–32. doi:10.3928/00989134-20080901-02.

Chamberlain, S. A., Gruneir, A., Hoben, M., et al. (2017). Influence of organizational context on nursing home staff burnout: A cross-sectional survey of care aides in western Canada. *International Journal of Nursing Studies,* 71, 60–69. doi:10.1016/j.ijnurstu.2017.02.024.

Chung, G. (2013). Understanding nursing home workers conceptualizations about good care. *The Gerontologist,* 53(2), 246–254. doi:10.1093/geront/gns117.

College of Registered Nurses of British Columbia (2015). *Competencies in the context of entry-level registered nurse practice in British Columbia.* Vancouver, BC: Author. Retrieved from https://crnbc.ca/Registration/Lists/RegistrationResources/375CompetenciesEntrylevelRN.pdf.

Crandall, L. G., White, D. L., Schuldheis, S., et al. (2007). Initiating person-centered care practices in long-term care facilities. *Journal of Gerontological Nursing,* 33(11), 47–56.

Dahlke, S. (2011). Examining nursing practice with older adults through a historical lens. *Journal of Gerontological Nursing,* 37(5), 41–48. doi:10.3928/00989134-20110106-06.

Davies, L. A., Hirdes, J. P., & Mannell, R. (2017). When healthcare is delivered in your home, will you need to make economic trade-offs? In G. Joseph (Ed.), *Diverse perspectives on aging in a changing world* (pp. 145–166). New York, NY: Routledge.

Davis, B. (1984). Nursing care of the aged: Historical evolution. In S. Fondmiller (Ed.), *Conference proceedings. Historical basis of clinical nursing practice in the United States.* Chicago, IL: American Association for the History of Nursing. New Orleans, LA, June 26, 1984.

Dellefield, M. E., Castle, N. G., McGilton, K. S., et al. (2015). The relationship between registered nurses and nursing home quality: An integrative review (2008–2014). *Nursing Economic$,* 33(2), 95–116.

Dock, L. (1908). The crusade for almshouse nursing. *American Journal of Nursing,* 8(7), 520. doi:10.1097/00000446-190804000-00003.

Ebersole, P., & Touhy, T. (2006). *Geriatric nursing: Growth of a specialty.* New York, NY: Springer.

Fox, M. T., Persaud, M., Maimets, I., et al. (2012). Effectiveness of acute geriatric unit care using acute care for elders components: A systematic review and meta-analysis. *Journal of the American Geriatrics Society,* 60, 2237–2245. doi:10.1111/jgs.12028.

Gerontological Nursing Association (Ontario) (1987). *Standards of gerontological nursing.* Toronto, ON: Author. Retrieved from http://www.gnaontario.org/Images/GNAStandards.pdf.

Hirst, S., King, T., & Church, J. (1996). The emergence of geronto-logical nursing education in Canada. *Geriatric Nursing*, 17(3), 120–122. doi:10.1016/S0197-4572(96)80093-0.

Hirst, S. P., Lane, A. M., & Stares, B. (2012). Gerontological content in Canadian nursing and social work programs. *Canadian Geriatrics Journal*, 15(1), 8–15. doi:10.5770/cgj.15.21.

Hewko, S. J., Cooper, S. L., Huynh, H., et al. (2015). Invisible no more: A scoping review of the health care aide workforce litera-ture. *BMC Nursing*, 14, doi:10.1186/s12912-015-0090-x.

Kaasalainen, S., Wickson-Griffiths, A., Akhtar-Danesh, N., et al. (2016). The effectiveness of a nurse practitioner-led pain man-agement team in long-term care: A mixed methods study. *International Journal of Nursing Studies*, 62, 156–167. doi:10.1016/j.ijnurstu.2016.07.022.

Kash, B., Castle, N., & Phillips, C. (2007). Nursing home spending, staffing and turnover. *Health Care Management Review*, 32(3), 253–262. doi:10.1016/j.gerinurse.2008.01.005.

Knopp-Sihota, J. A., Niehaus, L., Squires, J. E., et al. (2015). *Journal of Clinical Nursing*, 24, 2815–2825. doi:10.1111/jocn.12887.

Mantle, J. H., & Funke-Furber, J. (2003). *The forgotten revolution: The priory method*. Victoria, BC: Tafford Publishing.

Martin-Misener, R., Donald, F., Wickson-Griffiths, A., et al. (2015). Mixed methods study of the work patterns of full-time nurse practitioners in nursing homes. *Journal of Clinical Nursing*, 24, 1327–1337. doi:10.1111/jocn.12741.

McCleary, L. (2010). Wiki supports excellence in gerontological nursing education. *Perspectives*, 34(1), 14–16.

McCleary, L., Boscart, V., Donahue, P., et al. (2017). Readiness of Canadian educators to improve gerontological curricula in health and social service education. *Canadian Journal of Aging*, 36(4).

McCleary, L., McGilton, K., Boscart, V., et al. (2009). Improv-ing gerontology content in baccalaureate nursing education through knowledge transfer to nurse educators. *Nursing Leadership*, 22(3), 33–46. doi:10.12927/cjnl.2009.21153.

McCloskey, R., Jarrett, P., Stewart, C., et al. (2014). Alternate level of care patients in hospitals: What does dementia have to do with this? *Canadian Geriatrics Journal*, 17(3), 88–94. doi:10.5770/cgj.17.106.

Mezey, M. D., & Fulmer, T. T. (2002). The future history of geron-tological nursing. *Journal of Gerontology*, 57A(7), M438–M441. doi:10.1093/gerona/57.7.M438.

National Initiative for Care of the Elderly (NICE) and Geriatric Education and Recruitment Initiative (GERI) (2010). *Core interprofessional competencies for gerontology*. Toronto, ON: Authors. Retrieved from http://www.nicenet.ca/files/NICE_Competencies.pdf.

Newhouse, R. P., Stankik-Hutt, J., White, K. M., et al. (2011). Advanced practice nurse outcomes 1990-2008: A systematic review. *Nurse Economic*, 29, 230–250.

Newton, K., & Anderson, H. (1950). *Geriatric nursing*. St. Louis, MO: Mosby.

Ontario Association of Non-Profit Homes and Services for Seniors. (2014). *OANHSS 2015 provincial budget submission*. Retrieved from http://theonn.ca/wp-content/uploads/2015/04/Ontario-Association-of-Non-Profit-Homes-and-Services-for-Seniors-BUDGET-SUBMISSION.pdf.

Ontario Human Rights Commission. (2011). *Ageism and age dis-crimination*. Retrieved from http://www.ohrc.on.ca/en/ageism-and-age-discrimination-fact-sheet.

Ontario Long Term Care Association (2016). *This is long term care 2016*. Toronto, ON: Author. Retrieved from http://www.oltca.com/OLTCA/Documents/Reports/TILTC2016.pdf.

Pemberton, K. (2016). Most senior nursing homes miss Ministry of Health staffing guideline. *Vancouver Sun*. Retrieved from http://vancouversun.com/news/local-news/vast-majority-of-senior-nursing-homes-below-the-ministry-of-healths-staffing-guideline.

Potter, P. A., Perry, A. G., Ross-Kerr, J. C., et al. (Eds.), (2009). *Canadian Fundamentals of Nursing* (4th ed.). Toronto, ON: Mosby Elsevier.

Roberts, E. (2008). *Developing gerontological nursing in British Columbia: An oral history study*. Victoria, BC: The University of Victoria. Retrieved from https://circle.ubc.ca/bitstream/handle/2429/5116/ubc_2008_fall_roberts_erica.pdf?sequence=1 Unpublished master's thesis.

Safran, D. G., Miller, W., & Beckman, H. (2006). Organizational dimensions of relationship-centered care theory, evidence, and practice. *Journal of General Internal Medicine*, 21(S1), S9–S15. doi:10.111/j.1525-1497.2005.00303.x.

Senior Friendly Hospitals. (2014). *About Senior Friendly Hospitals*. Retrieved from http://seniorfriendlyhospitals.ca/about-sfh.

Statistics Canada (2010). *Residential care facilities—2007/2008*. Ottawa, ON: Author. Retrieved from http://dsp-psd.pwgsc.gc.ca/collections/collection_2010/statcan/83-237-X/83-237-x2010001-eng.pdf.

Statistics Canada. (2012). *2011 Census of Population: Families, households, marital status, structural type of dwelling, collec-tives*. Retrieved from http://www.statcan.gc.ca/daily-quotidien/120919/dq120919a-eng.pdf.

Statistics Canada. (2015). *Long-term care facilities survey, 2013*. Retrieved from http://www.statcan.gc.ca/daily-quotidien/150504/dq150504b-eng.htm.

Sutherland, J. M., & Crump, R. T. (2013). Alternative level of care: Canada's hospital beds, the evidence and options. *Health Care Policy*, 9(1), 26–34. doi:10.12927/hcpol.2013.23480.

Thomas, W., & Johnson, C. (2003). Elderhood in Eden. *Topics in Geriatric Rehabilitation*, 19(4), 282–289. doi:10.1097/00013614-200310000-00009.

Wagner, L., Dickson, V. V., Shuluk, J., et al. (2013). Nurses' knowl-edge of geriatric nursing care in Canadian NICHE hospitals. *Perspectives*, 36(3), 6–14.

Walsh, K., & Shutes, I. (2013). Care relationships, quality of care and migrant workers caring for older people. *Ageing & Society*, 33, 393–420. doi:10.1017/s01446886x110001309.

Wiersman, E., & Dupuis, S. L. (2007). Managing responsive behaviours: How caring and non-caring styles affect resident behaviours, quality of life and caregiver satisfaction. *Canadian Nursing Home*, 18(2), 17–22.

Wykle, M., & McDonald, P. (1997). The past, present, and future of gerontological nursing. In S. Klein (Ed.), *A national agenda for geriatric education*. New York, NY: Springer.

Communicating With Older Persons

LEARNING OBJECTIVES

Upon completion of this chapter, the reader will be able to:

- Describe the importance of communication to the lives of older persons.
- Discuss how ageist attitudes affect communication with older persons.
- Describe interventions that facilitate communication individually and in groups.
- Understand the significance of the life story of an older person.
- Discuss the modalities of reminiscence and life review.
- Identify effective communication strategies for older persons with speech, language, hearing, vision, and cognitive impairments.

GLOSSARY

Ageism   Ageism incorporates two concepts: "way[s] of thinking about older persons based on negative attitudes and stereotypes about aging; and a tendency to structure society based on an assumption that everyone is young, thereby failing to respond appropriately to the real needs of older persons" (Ontario Human Rights Commission, 2011, ¶1).

Aphasia   Loss of the ability to express and understand spoken and written language.

Apraxia   An impairment in the ability to manipulate objects or perform purposeful acts, including the ability to speak.

Dysarthria   A speech disorder caused by weakness or incoordination of the muscles used for speech.

Elderspeak   A common speech style used when talking to older people that presupposes their dependence, incompetence, and control by the speaker. Elderspeak includes baby talk, using terms like "honey" and "dear," and speaking louder and more slowly.

Life review   A critical analysis of a person's past life, with the goal of facilitating integrity.

THE LIVED EXPERIENCE

Listen to the aged for they will tell you about living and dying.

Listen to the aged for they will enlighten you about problem-solving, sexuality, grief, sensory deprivation, and survival.

Listen to the aged for they will teach you how to be courageous, loving, and generous.

They are a distinguished faculty without formal classrooms, tenure, sabbaticals. They teach not from books but from long experience in living.

From Burnside, I. M. (1975). Listen to the aged. *American Journal of Nursing*, 75(10), 1801.

Communication is the most important ability of human beings, the ability that gives humans a special place in the animal kingdom. Little is more dehumanizing than the inability to reach out to others verbally. Maslow's hierarchy places the human need for affiliation second only to the need for safety and survival (Maslow, 1943). The need to communicate, to be listened to, and to be heard does not change with age or impairment. Meaningful communication and active involvement in society both contribute to healthy aging and could improve older persons' chances of living longer, responding better to health care interventions, and maintaining optimal function (La Tourette & Meeks, 2000).

Older people may have fewer opportunities for social interaction, owing to loss of family and friends; illnesses; and hearing, vision, and cognitive impairments. The ageist attitudes of the public, as well as those of health care providers, also present barriers to communicating effectively with older people. Good verbal and nonverbal communication skills are the basis for accurate assessment, care planning, and the development of therapeutic relationships between the nurse and the older person.

This chapter discusses the effect of health care providers' attitudes toward aging on their communication with older people; verbal and nonverbal communication skills essential to interactions with older people; and adapting communication for older people with vision and hearing impairments, speech and language disorders, and cognitive impairment. The significance of life story, reminiscence, life review, and communication with groups of older people is also discussed in this chapter. A discussion of age-related changes in hearing and vision is presented in Chapter 6; assessment of hearing, vision, and cognition in Chapter 13; diseases of the eye and ear in Chapter 19; and care of older people with cognitive impairment in Chapter 21.

AGEISM AND COMMUNICATION

Ageist attitudes, myths, and stereotypical ideas about older people can interfere with the nurse's ability to communicate with them effectively. For example, if the nurse believes that all older people have memory problems or are unable to learn and process information, he or she will be less likely to engage in conversation, provide appropriate health information, or treat the person with respect and dignity. **Ageism** is a term used to express prejudice toward older persons through attitudes and behaviour (Ontario Human Rights Commission, 2011). Similar to other prejudices (e.g., racism, anti-Semitism, and sexism), ageism affects us all. Although ageism is cross-cultural, it is essentially prevalent in the Western world, where aging is viewed with depression, fear, and anxiety (Rittenour & Cohen, 2016). It is important for gerontological nurses to be aware of their own attitudes toward aging and to recognize how their beliefs may influence their verbal and nonverbal communication. The evaluation and enhancement of interpersonal communication skills form the foundation for therapeutic interactions with older people.

Elderspeak is a form of ageism in which younger people alter their speech on the assumption that all older people have difficulty comprehending what is said to them (Grimme, Buchanan, & Afflerbach, 2015). Lagacé et al. (2012) explored the linguistic aspects of interactions between health care providers and long-term care (LTC) home residents and noticed not only the use of simplified speech but also the frequent use of the patronizing "we" form, pet names, diminutives, and interjections (Box 3.1).

Nurses may not be aware that they are using elderspeak. It is nonetheless important to note such speech style, as research has shown that this form of speech is offensive and patronizing and conveys the belief that older persons are dependent, incompetent,

---

BOX 3.1	Characteristics of Elderspeak

- Speaking slowly or loudly or both
- Using a singsong voice
- Using the pronouns "we," "us," and "our" in place of "you"
- Using pet names such as "honey," "dearie," or "sweetheart"
- Answering questions for the older person (e.g., "You would like your dinner now, wouldn't you?")

Source: Adapted from *Elderspeak: Babytalk directed at older adults.* Retrieved from http://changingaging.org/elderhood/elderspeak-babytalk-directed-at-older-adults/.

and controlled (Keaton & Giles, 2016). There is also evidence that elderspeak has a negative effect on the care of patients with dementia (Page & Rowles, 2016). Other examples of communication that convey ageist attitudes are ignoring the older person, talking to family and friends as if the older person were not present, and limiting interaction to task-focused communication only (Page & Rowles, 2016).

Therapeutic verbal and nonverbal communication strategies that apply to all situations in nursing—listening attentively, having an authentic presence, having a nonjudgemental attitude, being culturally competent, clarifying, giving information, seeking validation of understanding, keeping focus, and using open-ended questions—are all applicable to communicating with older persons. Older people may need more time for giving information or answering questions, simply because they have a larger life experience from which to draw. Sorting through thoughts requires intervals of silence; therefore, listening to older persons carefully and without rushing is very important. Retrieving words, particularly nouns and names, may be slower for them.

Open-ended questions are useful but difficult for some older persons. Those who wish to please, especially when feeling vulnerable or somewhat dependent, may wonder what it is you want to hear and may tell you what they think you want to hear rather than what they would like to say. Communication that is most productive will initially focus on the issue of major concern to the older person regardless of the priority of the nursing assessment. When using closed questioning to obtain specific information, the nurse should be aware that the older person may feel pressured; thus, the appropriate information may not be immediately forthcoming. This is especially true when the nurse is asking questions to determine mental status. The older person may develop a mental block because of anxiety or feel threatened if questions are asked in a quiz-like or demeaning manner. Furthermore, older people may be reluctant to disclose information for fear of the consequences. For example, if older persons are having problems remembering things or are experiencing frequent falls, they may assume that sharing that information will result in their having to leave their home and move to a more protective place.

A substantial portion of our communication is nonverbal. Older people respond to nurses' behaviours and nonverbal cues, including posture, facial expression, eye gaze, gesture, and tone of voice. Nonverbal details can reveal nurses' feelings and attitudes and affect relationships with other persons (Registered Nurses Association of Ontario [RNAO], 2015).

When communicating with older persons who are in a bed or wheelchair, it is important to position oneself at their level rather than talking over a side rail or standing above them. Nurses should pay attention to older persons' gazes, gestures, and body language, as well as to the pitch, volume, and tone of their voices to understand what they are trying to communicate. Thoughts left unstated are often as important as those that are verbalized. A nurse may ask, "What are you thinking about right now?" Clarification is essential to ensure that the older person and the nurse have the same framework of understanding. Many generational, cultural, and regional differences in speech patterns and idioms exist. Thus, frequently seeking validation of what the nurse thinks he or she has heard is important.

IMPLICATIONS FOR GERONTOLOGICAL NURSING AND HEALTHY AGING

Every time nurses communicate with someone, their words and actions affect the relationship in positive or negative ways, depending on the nurses' attitudes and skills (RNAO, 2015). Enhancing verbal and nonverbal communication with older persons is an important skill in gerontological nursing and is rewarding for both the nurse and the older person. Communication with older persons provides the nurse with the opportunity to share in their wisdom and gain insight on life.

COMMUNICATION WITH OLDER PERSONS WITH SENSORY IMPAIRMENTS

Sensory impairments, such as hearing or vision deficits, place older persons at risk for communication difficulties. People rely on their senses to perceive the environment and to enjoy the pleasures of life. Sensory impairments, along with altered environmental stimuli, can contribute to delirium by causing sensory deprivation (see Chapter 21). Gerontological nurses need special knowledge and skills to promote effective communication with older people who have these deficits. This section describes adaptations that enhance verbal and nonverbal communication with older people who have hearing and vision impairments.

HEARING IMPAIRMENT

While both vision and hearing impairments significantly affect all aspects of life, Oliver Sacks (1989), in his book *Seeing Voices: A Journey Into the World of the Deaf*, presents the view that blindness may in fact be less serious than the loss of hearing (Sacks, 1989). Hearing loss interferes with communication with others. In addition, hearing loss limits a person's opportunity to be part of an interaction and this can lead to a sense of not being engaged or involved in conversations. Hearing loss is a prevalent, persistent condition in older Canadians and is the most common sensory impairment in Canadians over 60 years of age, affecting 47% of people in this age group (Statistics Canada, 2015). In all age groups, men are more likely than women to be hearing impaired.

Hearing loss diminishes quality of life and is associated with numerous negative outcomes, including decreased function, miscommunication, social isolation, depression, safety risks, and reduced income and employment opportunities (Manrique-Huarte et al., 2016; McMahon, 2016). Also, a hearing impairment may cause older people to become suspicious or distrustful or to display paranoid thoughts. Because older persons with hearing loss may not understand or respond appropriately to conversation, they may be inappropriately diagnosed with cognitive impairment. Older people may be initially unaware of hearing loss because of the gradual manner in which it develops (Box 3.2). The Try This Series from the Hartford Institute for Geriatric Nursing provides guidelines for screening hearing ability (http://consultgerirn.org/uploads/File/trythis/try_this_12.pdf). The Better Hearing Institute provides an online hearing test for older people who want to check their hearing (http://www.betterhearing.org/check-your-hearing). Additional information about hearing assessment can be found in Chapter 13.

BOX 3.2   Do I Have a Hearing Problem?

- Do I sometimes feel embarrassed when I meet new people because I struggle to hear?
- Do I feel frustrated when talking to members of my family because I have difficulty hearing them?
- Do I have difficulty hearing or understanding co-workers, clients, or customers?
- Do I feel restricted or limited by a hearing problem?
- Do I have difficulty hearing when visiting friends, relatives, or neighbours?
- Do I have difficulty hearing in the movies or in the theatre?
- Does a hearing problem cause me to argue with family members?
- Do I have trouble hearing the TV or radio at levels that are loud enough for others?
- Do I feel that any difficulty with my hearing limits my personal life or social life?
- Do I have trouble hearing family or friends when we are together in a restaurant?

Source: National Institute on Deafness and Other Communication Disorders. (2016). *Do you need a hearing test?* Retrieved from https://www.nidcd.nih.gov/health/do-you-need-hearing-test.

Hearing impairment is underdiagnosed and undertreated in older people. Although screening for hearing impairment and its appropriate treatment is considered an essential part of primary care for older people, it is rarely done. Screening rates for hearing impairment among older people are estimated to be as low as 13% (Ham et al., 2007). About 12% of persons with hearing impairments use a hearing aid (Feder et al., 2015). Research has shown that 90% of those with hearing loss can improve their communication with hearing aids that are fitted properly (Canadian Hearing Society, 2017). Financial aid for older persons purchasing hearing aids in Canada varies among the provinces. The Canadian Hard of Hearing Association provides information about coverage at http://chha.ca/documents/Hearing_Aid_Subsidies_Across_Canada.pdf.

Findings of a recent study (Box 3.3) indicate that hearing loss is "an overlooked geriatric syndrome in primary care settings—an assessment gap that can have significant negative consequences" (Wallhagen & Pettengill, 2008, p. 41). Lack of assessment and treatment of hearing loss in an LTC home is even more of

BOX 3.3   Research for Evidence-Informed Practice: Severity of Age-Related Hearing Loss Is Associated With Impaired Activities of Daily Living

Problem: This study explored the association between hearing impairment and activity limitations.

Method: A total of 1,952 persons aged 60 years or more participated in the study. Their hearing levels were measured, and they also participated in a survey that focused on functional status, activities of daily living (ADLs), and instrumental activities of daily living (IADLs).

Findings: A higher proportion of persons who were hearing impaired had more difficulties in performing three of the seven basic ADLs and six of seven IADLs. Researchers also found that increased severity of hearing loss was associated with impaired ADLs.

Application to Nursing Practice: Hearing loss is an overlooked geriatric syndrome; a gap in assessment can have significant negative consequences. Nurses should be aware of the association between hearing loss and low performing of ADLs and IADLs. As well, nurses have the opportunity to support those with hearing impairments by assessing their needs and collaborating with older people in developing strategies to assist them with everyday ADLs and IADLs.

Source: Gopinath, B., Schneider, J., McMahon C. M., et al. (2012). Severity of age-related hearing loss is associated with impaired activities of daily living. *Age Ageing, 41*(2), 195–200. doi:10.1093/ageing/afr155.

a concern because the majority of the residents have a hearing impairment. In a study of hearing aid use in American nursing homes, Cohen-Mansfield and Taylor (2004) reported that 65% of the residents had a serious hearing loss but that staff members were aware of fewer than 50% of the problems. Of the 279 residents who participated in the study, 39% had been treated for excessive cerumen, but 81% had neither cerumen removal nor a hearing test.

The two major forms of hearing loss are conductive hearing loss and sensorineural hearing loss. Conductive hearing loss usually involves external and middle-ear abnormalities that reduce the transmission of sound to the middle ear. Otosclerosis, infection, perforated eardrum, fluid in the middle ear, or cerumen accumulation can all cause conductive hearing loss. Sensorineural hearing loss results from damage to any part of the inner ear or the neural pathways to the brain. *Presbycusis* is a form of sensorineural hearing loss that is related to aging. It is the most common form of hearing loss in Canada (Canadian Hearing Association, 2015) (see Chapter 13). Sensorineural hearing loss is treated with hearing aids and, in some cases, cochlear implants. Cerumen impaction, hearing aids, cochlear implants, and assistive listening and adaptive devices are discussed further in the next sections.

Cerumen Impaction

Cerumen impaction is the most common and easily corrected of all interferences in the hearing of older people. Cerumen interferes with the conduction of sound through air in the eardrum. The reduction in the number and activity of cerumen-producing glands results in a tendency toward cerumen impaction. Longstanding impactions become hard, dry, and dark brown. At particular risk of impaction are people who wear hearing aids and older men with large amounts of ear canal tragi (hairs in the ear) that tend to become entangled with the cerumen. When hearing loss is suspected or a person with existing hearing loss experiences increasing difficulty, it is important to first check for cerumen impaction as a possible cause (Meador, 1995).

Hearing Aids

A hearing aid is a personal amplifying system that includes a microphone, an amplifier, and a loudspeaker. The appearance and effectiveness of hearing aids have greatly improved in recent years, and many can be programmed to meet specific needs. Most people can obtain some hearing enhancement with a hearing aid. While hearing aids generally improve hearing by about 50%, they do not correct hearing deficits. It is important that hearing-impaired persons understand that the goal of hearing aid use is to improve communication and quality of life, not to restore normal hearing.

Hearing aids necessitate a period of adjustment and training in their correct use. Most provinces and territories provide some financial assistance for purchasing a hearing aid. There are also organizations and services that provide financial assistance with purchasing a hearing aid (e.g., Veterans Affairs Canada, First Nations and Inuit Health Branch) (Canadian Hard of Hearing Association [CHHA], 2009). The investment in a good hearing aid is considerable, and a good fit is critical. A person must be assessed by an audiologist or a physician before being fitted for a hearing aid (College of Audiologists and Speech-Language Pathologists of Ontario, 2014). Prices of hearing aids are regulated by the Canadian government, and costs depend on an individual's degree of hearing loss as well as the brand and model prescribed. Batteries are changed every 1 to 2 weeks, adding to overall costs. It is important for nurses in hospitals, in LTC settings, and in the community to be knowledgeable about the care and maintenance of hearing aids. In provinces and territories where financial assistance is available, assistance with replacement costs is limited. Many older people experience unnecessary communication problems because their hearing aids are not inserted and working properly or are lost.

Cochlear Implants

Cochlear implants are increasingly being used for older people who are profoundly deaf as a result of sensorineural hearing loss. Unlike a hearing aid, which magnifies sounds, a cochlear implant converts sound waves into electrical impulses and transmits them to the inner ear. A cochlear implant is surgically implanted in the mastoid bone behind the ear and electrically stimulates the cochlea, setting the cilia in motion and transmitting impulses along the auditory nerve to the brain's hearing centre. For persons whose hearing loss is so severe that amplification is of little or no benefit, the use of a cochlear implant is a safe and effective method of auditory rehabilitation.

Financial coverage of the cochlear implant procedure varies among provinces and territories. (For more information on this, see http://chha.ca/documents/Hearing_Aid_Subsidies_Across_Canada.pdf.) The transplant procedure carries some risk because the surgery destroys any residual hearing that remains. Therefore, cochlear implant users can never revert to using a hearing aid.

Assistive Listening and Adaptive Devices

Assistive listening devices (also called personal listening systems) are considered as adjuncts to hearing aids or are used in place of hearing aids for people with hearing impairment. These devices are available commercially and can be used to enhance face-to-face communication, to understand speech better in large rooms such as theatres, to use the telephone, and to listen to television. Examples of assistive listening and adaptive devices are text messaging devices for telephones and closed-caption television (now required on all televisions with screens that measure 33 cm [13 inches] or more). Also available are alerting devices, such as vibrating alarm clocks (that shake the bed or activate a flashing light) and sound lamps that respond with lights to sounds such as those of doorbells and telephones. Assistive devices, such as pocket talkers, that amplify sound and send it to the user's ears through earphones, clips, or headphones are helpful in health care situations in which privacy and accurate communication are essential. Nurses should be able to obtain appropriate devices to improve communication with hearing-impaired persons. (See the Resources section and http://evolve.elsevier.com/Canada/Ebersole/gerontological/ for additional information.)

A program called Hearing Dogs of Canada, run by the Lions Foundation of Canada, provides hearing dog guides throughout Canada (https://www.dogguides.com/hearing.html). A hearing dog guide serves to warn the hearing-impaired person of impending danger and to alert the person to audible signals, ringing telephones, fire and smoke alarms, emergencies, and intruders. Although other electronic means are available for dealing with these concerns, persons who have hearing dogs consistently comment on the alleviation of the sense of isolation that often accompanies hearing impairment. With a hearing dog companion, older people may experience renewed courage, confidence, and freedom, as well as reduced tension, anxiety, and depression (Pikhartova, Bowling & Victor, 2014).

 ## IMPLICATIONS FOR GERONTOLOGICAL NURSING AND HEALTHY AGING

Hearing impairment is very common among older people and significantly affects communication, function, safety, and quality of life. Inadequate communication with an older person with a hearing impairment can also lead to misdiagnosis and affect the person's compliance with the medical regimen. Gerontological

BOX 3.4	Strategies for Communicating With Older Persons Who Have Hearing Impairments

- Do not shout when speaking to an older person, as shouting increases pitch and makes it more difficult for the person to hear.
- Never assume hearing loss is due to age until other causes (infection, cerumen buildup, etc.) are ruled out.
- Inappropriate responses, inattentiveness, and apathy may be symptoms of hearing loss.
- Face the person, stand or sit at the same level, and do not turn away to face a computer screen when using verbal and nonverbal approaches.
- Gain the person's attention before beginning to speak.
- Determine if the person's hearing is better in one ear than in the other, and position yourself appropriately.
- If a hearing aid is used, make sure it is in place and that the batteries are functioning.
- Ask the person or a family member what helps the person to hear best.
- Keep your hands away from your mouth, and project your voice through controlled diaphragmatic breathing.
- Avoid conversations in which the speaker's face is in glare or darkness; orient the light source so that the light is on the speaker's face.
- Careful articulation and a moderate speed of speech are helpful.
- Lower your tone of voice and articulate clearly.
- Label the person's chart, and inform all caregivers that the person has a hearing impairment.
- Use nonverbal approaches: gestures, demonstrations, visual aids, and written materials.
- Pause between sentences or phrases to confirm the person's understanding of the communication.
- Restate with different words when you are not understood.
- When changing topics, preface the change by stating the topic.
- Reduce background noise (e.g., turn off the television, close the door).
- Use assistive listening devices, such as a pocket talker.
- Share resources with the hearing-impaired person, and refer to them as is appropriate.

nurses must be able to assess hearing ability and use appropriate verbal and nonverbal communication skills and devices to help older persons minimize or even avoid problems. Box 3.4 presents communication strategies for older people with impaired hearing.

VISION IMPAIRMENT

While vision decline occurs normally with age (see Chapter 6), the major causes of visual impairment and blindness among older persons are cataracts, macular degeneration, glaucoma, and diabetic retinopathy (see Chapter 19). About a half million Canadians live with vision loss that affects their quality of life (Canadian National Institute for the Blind [CNIB], 2017a).

Visual impairment (low vision) is generally defined as a Snellen reading of worse than 20/40 but better than 20/200. The definition of legal blindness may vary between countries. In Canada, legal blindness is defined as a Snellen reading equal to or worse than 20/200 with best correction in the better eye or a visual extent of less than 20 degrees in diameter (CNIB, 2017b). A reading of 20/50 may keep a person from obtaining a provincial or territorial driver's license or may restrict his or her driving to the daytime (CNIB, 2017b). Vision loss is becoming a major public health problem and is projected to increase substantially with the aging of the population.

A study by Gopinath et al. (2011) found an association between hearing loss and increased difficulties in performing activities of daily living and instrumental activities of daily living (Box 3.5). White people have higher rates of overall vision loss than do members of visible minorities (Muzychka, 2009). However, older women of visible minorities have the highest prevalence of cataracts, and men of visible minorities have higher rates of glaucoma. In comparison with White Canadians, Chinese Canadians have double the rate of age-related macular degeneration (AMD) and diabetic retinopathy. Indigenous people have higher rates of diabetic retinopathy; Inuit people have higher rates of primary angle-closure glaucoma. These differences are attributable not only to genetic factors but also to differences in access to health care services (Muzychka, 2009). Two serious barriers to vision screening are the cost of ophthalmic care and access to eye care services for those living in rural areas. It is estimated that, globally, 80% of all visual impairment can be prevented or cured (World Health Organization [WHO], 2014).

The prevalence of visual impairment among residents of LTC homes is estimated to be 3 to 15 times higher than that among adults of the same age who live in the community (Dev et al., 2014). A

| BOX 3.5 | Research for Evidence-Informed Practice: Declining Visual Ability Associated With Social Isolation and Depressed Mood |

Problem: The prevalence of visual impairment increases with age. It is known to be associated with decreased quality of life and increased risk of mortality and institutionalization. However, visual problems are often ignored by health care providers. The study described here examined (1) the prevalence of visual impairment and visual decline (decreased visual ability in the last 90 days) and (2) the association between visual decline and changes in social activity, loss of instrumental activities of daily living (IADLs), and patients' reluctance to going outdoors due to fear of falling.

Methods: The study outlined here was a prospective, observational study of home care patients aged 65 years and over in Ontario ($n = 101,618$), Finland ($n = 1,103$), and 11 European countries ($n = 3,793$). In all settings, data from the Resident Assessment Interview for Home Care (RAI-HC) were compiled in a database. The researchers used data from the three databases. The RAI-HC includes an item for visual ability and an item indicating whether visual ability declined in the previous 90 days.

Findings: The prevalence of visual impairment was between 19.8% (in Norway) and 55.3% (in France). It was 28% in Ontario. Recent visual decline was reported in 5.9% of patients in Ontario and in up to 49.3% of patients in the Czech Republic. Recent visual decline was associated with change in social activity (experienced by 51% of those with visual decline), distress (44.4%), and decreased ability to perform IADLs. Patients with recent visual decline had worse depression symptoms than did clients who had a stable visual impairment. Patients with recent visual decline were more likely than those with stable visual impairment to limit going outdoors because of fear of falling. Other variables that were associated with limiting going outdoors were being of older age, being female, and having an unsteady gait.

Implications for Nursing Practice: Visual impairment and recent visual decline were common among older home care patients. The researchers concluded that depression symptoms, changes in social activity, changes in the ability to perform IADLs, and reluctance to go outside should trigger a vision assessment by a nurse or physician. "Most likely, many seniors with [recent visual decline] are unfamiliar with the actions necessary to improve visual function, avoid obstacles, or move around safely."

Source: Grue, E. V., Finne-Soveri, H., Stolee, P., et al. (2010). Recent visual decline—A health hazard with consequences for social life: A study of home care clients in 12 countries. *Current Gerontology and Geriatrics Research, 2010,* article ID 503817. doi:10.1155/2010/503817.

recent study examining the effect of visual impairment among LTC residents with Alzheimer's disease reported that one in three residents were not using or did not have eyeglasses that were strong enough to correct their vision; they had either lost or broken their glasses, had prescriptions that were no longer adequate, or were too cognitively impaired to ask for help (Koch, Datta, Makhdoom, et al., 2005). The lack of routine eye care in LTC settings may result in functional decline, decreased quality of life, and depression (Owsley et al., 2007).

Low-Vision Assistive Devices

Technological advances in the past decade have produced some low-vision devices that may be used successfully in the care of the visually impaired older person. Persons with severe visual impairment may qualify for disability and financial and social services assistance through government and private programs, including vision rehabilitation programs. An array of low-vision assistive devices are now available, including insulin delivery systems, talking clocks and watches, large-print books, books on CDs, podcasts, magnifiers, telescopes (handheld or mounted on eyeglasses), electronic magnification through closed-circuit television or computer software, and software that converts text into artificial voice output. The website of the Canadian National Institute for the Blind (http://www.cnib.ca) lists several resources that are specifically related to older people. Because each person's needs are unique, it is recommended that before investing in vision aids, the person should consult a low-vision centre or a low-vision specialist. (See the Resources section and http://evolve.elsevier.com/Canada/Ebersole/gerontological/ for additional information.)

BOX 3.6 Strategies for Communicating With Older Persons Who Have Visual Impairment

- Make sure you have the person's attention before you start talking.
- Always speak promptly, and clearly identify yourself and others with you. State when you are leaving, and make sure the person is aware of your departure.
- Get down to the person's level and face her or him when speaking.
- Speak normally but not from a distance. Do not raise or lower your voice, and continue to use gestures if doing so is natural to your communication.
- When others are present, address the visually impaired person by prefacing remarks with his or her name or a light touch on the arm.
- Use the analogy of a clock face to help locate objects (e.g., describe positions of food on a plate in relation to clock positions, such as meat at 3 o'clock, dessert at 6 o'clock).
- Ensure adequate lighting on your face, and eliminate glare.
- Select rich, intense colours (e.g., red, orange) for paint, furniture, and pictures.

- Use large, dark, evenly spaced printing.
- Use contrast in printed material (e.g., black marker on white paper).
- Do not change the room arrangement or the arrangement of personal items without explanation.
- Use some means to identify persons who are visually impaired, and include visual impairment in the plan of care.
- Screen for vision loss, and recommend annual eye examinations for older people.
- If a person is in a nursing home or a communal home, label their eyeglasses and have a spare pair, if possible.
- Be aware of low-vision assistive devices such as talking watches and books, and facilitate access to these resources.
- If the person is blind, offer your arm while walking. Pause before stairs or curbs and alert the person. When seating the person, place his or her hand on the back of the chair. Always let the person know his or her position in relation to objects. Never play with or distract a guide dog.

IMPLICATIONS FOR GERONTOLOGICAL NURSING AND HEALTHY AGING

Vision impairment is common among older people, occurring in connection with eye diseases and with changes resulting from aging. It can significantly affect communication, functional ability, safety, and quality of life. To promote healthy aging and quality of life, nurses who care for older people in all settings can improve outcomes for visually impaired older people by assessing for vision changes and providing appropriate health teaching and referrals for the prevention and treatment of visual impairment. Suggestions for improving communication with and care for visually impaired older people are presented in Box 3.6.

COMMUNICATION WITH OLDER PERSONS WITH NEUROLOGICAL DISORDERS

Three major categories of impaired verbal communication arise from neurological disturbances: (1) reception, (2) perception, and (3) articulation. Reception is impaired by anxiety or is related to a specific disorder,

hearing deficits, or altered levels of consciousness. Perception is distorted by stroke, dementia, and delirium. Articulation is hampered by mechanical difficulties such as dysarthria, respiratory disease, destruction of the larynx, or cerebral infarction with neuromuscular effects. Specific difficulties can include the following:

- *Anomia:* Difficulty in retrieving words during spontaneous speech and naming tasks.
- *Aphasia*: A communication disorder that can affect a person's ability to use and understand spoken or written words. It results from damage to the side of the brain dominant for language; for most people, this is the left side. Aphasia usually occurs suddenly and often results from a stroke or head injury, but it can also develop slowly from a brain tumour, an infection, or dementia.
- *Dysarthria:* Impairment in the ability to articulate words as the result of damage to the central or peripheral nervous system that affects the speech mechanism.

APHASIA

The most common language disorder that occurs following a cerebral vascular accident, or stroke, is

aphasia. Aphasia, in varying degrees, affects a person's ability to communicate in one or more ways, including speaking, understanding, reading, writing, and gesturing. Depending on the type and severity of the aphasia, there may be little or no speech, speech that is fragmented or broken, or speech that is fluent but empty in content. When a cerebral vascular accident damages the dominant half of the brain, some disruption will occur in the "word factory." Broca's and Wernicke's areas in the cerebral cortex are integral to the expression and understanding of language. The Canadian Stroke Best Practices (2016) categorizes two broad types of aphasia: expressive and receptive. Within these types, there are many subtypes. The following describes several types of aphasia that nurses may encounter when caring for older persons:

- *Wernicke's aphasia* is the result of a lesion in the superior temporal gyrus, an area adjacent to the primary auditory cortex (Wernicke's area). Persons with Wernicke's aphasia speak easily and with many long runs of words, but the content does not make sense. There are word-finding problems and errors of word and sound substitution. Unrelated words may be strung together or syllables repeated. People with this type of aphasia also have difficulty understanding spoken language and may be unaware of their speech difficulties.
- *Broca's aphasia* typically involves damage to the posteroinferior portions of the dominant frontal lobe (Broca's area). This type of aphasia is also called motor or anterior aphasia. Persons with Broca's aphasia usually understand others but speak very slowly and use a minimal number of words. They often struggle to articulate a word and seem to have lost the ability to voluntarily control the movements of speech. They experience difficulties in communicating orally and in writing.
- *Verbal apraxia* or *apraxia of speech* is a motor speech disorder that affects the ability to plan and sequence voluntary muscle movements. The muscles of speech are not paralyzed; instead, there is a disruption in the brain's transmission of signals to the muscles. When the person is thinking about what to say, she or he may struggle to say words or be unable to speak at all. In contrast, when not thinking about what to say, the person may be able to say many words or sentences correctly. **Apraxia** frequently occurs with aphasia.
- *Anomic* or *nominal aphasia* is associated with lesions of the dominant temporoparietal regions of the brain, although no single locus has been identified. Persons with anomic aphasia understand and speak readily but may have severe difficulty finding the words. They may be unable to remember crucial content words. This frequent form of aphasia is characterized by the inability to name objects. The individual struggles to come forth with the correct noun and often becomes frustrated at his or her inability to do so.
- *Global aphasia* is the result of large left-hemisphere lesions and affects most of the language areas of the brain. Persons with global aphasia cannot understand words or speak intelligibly. They may use meaningless syllables repetitiously.

A speech-language pathologist (SLP) should be consulted for each type of aphasia to develop appropriate rehabilitative plans as soon as the affected person is physiologically stabilized. SLPs bring expertise in all types of communication disorders and are an essential part of the interprofessional team. The SLP can identify the areas of language that remain relatively unimpaired and can capitalize on the remaining strengths. Much can be done in aggressive speech-retraining programs to regain intelligible conversational ability. For those who do not regain meaningful speech, assistive and augmentative communication devices can be most helpful. McGilton et al. (2012) have noted the importance of consulting with the SLP to create an appropriate care plan and have described a pilot test they developed with a SLP to enhance the communication of nursing staff caring for patients who had a stroke and were experiencing communication difficulties.

Alternative and Augmentative Speech Aids

Alternative or augmentative speech aid systems are frequently used, and communication tools exist for every imaginable type of language disability. These can be low- or high-tech systems. An example of a low-tech system is an alphabet or picture board that the individual uses to point to letters that spell out messages or to point to pictures of common objects and situations. High-tech systems include electronic boards and computers. Studies have shown that computer-assisted therapy can help people with aphasia improve speech. An example is speech-therapy software that displays a word or picture, speaks the word (using pre-recorded human speech), records the user speaking it, and plays back the user's speech. Harty, Griesel and van der Merwe (2011) described how using a "talking mat" with older persons was effective in enhancing communication. The "talking mat" is a visual framework that uses picture symbols to help the user express feelings about activities, the environment, people in the user's life, and the user's own personal views and interests.

For individuals with hemiplegic conditions, electronic devices and computers can be voice activated or have specially designed switches that can be activated by one finger or by slight contact with the ear, nose, or chin. Some experimental studies indicate that medications, in addition to speech therapy, may help manage aphasia in the acute phase of stroke and be of help following the acute situation and in persistent aphasia.

DYSARTHRIA

Dysarthria is a speech disorder caused by poor coordination or weakness of the speech muscles. It occurs as a result of central or peripheral neuromuscular disorders that interfere with pronunciation and with the clarity of speech. Dysarthria is second in incidence only to aphasia as a communication disorder in older persons and may be the result of stroke, head injury, Parkinson's disease, multiple sclerosis, or other neurological conditions. Dysarthria is characterized by weakness, slow movement, and a lack of coordination of the muscles associated with speech. Speech may be slow, jerky, slurred, quiet, lacking in expression, and difficult to understand. The disorder may involve several mechanisms of speech, such as respiration, phonation, resonance, articulation, and prosody (the metre or rhythm of speech). Weakness or a lack of coordination in any one of the speech-related systems can result in dysarthria. If the respiratory system is

weak, then speech may be too quiet and be produced one word at a time. If the laryngeal system is weak, speech may be breathy, quiet, and slow. If the articulatory system is affected, speech may sound slurred and be slow and laboured.

Treatment of dysarthria depends on the cause, type, and severity of the symptoms. An SLP works with the individual to improve communication abilities. Therapy for dysarthria focuses on maximizing the function of all systems. In cases of progressive neurological disease, it is important to begin treatment early and continue it throughout the course of the disease, the goal being to maintain speech for as long as possible.

 IMPLICATIONS FOR GERONTOLOGICAL NURSING AND HEALTHY AGING

Nurses are responsible for accurately observing and recording the speech and word recognition patterns of persons affected by aphasia or dysarthria and for consistently implementing the recommendations of the SLP. Communication with the older person experiencing aphasia or dysarthria can be frustrating for both the affected person and the nurse as they struggle to understand each other. It is important to remember that in most cases of aphasia and dysarthria, the affected person retains normal intellectual ability. Therefore, verbal and nonverbal communication must always occur at an adult level but with special modifications. Furthermore, nurses need to be aware of their body language and other nonverbal behaviours when communicating with older people. Hearing and vision losses can further contribute to communication difficulties for older persons with aphasia or dysarthria. Sensitivity and patience are essential to effective communication. It is most helpful if staff members caring for the person remain consistent, so that they can come to know and understand the needs of the person and communicate them to others. It is exhausting for older persons to have to continually try to communicate their needs and desires to any number of staff members. Plans of care should include specific helpful verbal and nonverbal communication strategies so that all staff members and patients' families and significant others know the

BOX 3.7   Communicating With Individuals Experiencing Aphasia

- Explain situations, treatments, and anything else that is pertinent to the person. Treat the person as an adult, and avoid patronizing and childish phrases. Talk as if the person understands what you are saying.
- Be patient, and allow plenty of time to communicate in a quiet environment.
- Speak naturally. Speak slowly, ask one question at a time, and wait for a response. Do not shout. Repeat and rephrase as needed.
- Include the person in social gatherings and conversations. If needed, ensure that hearing aids are in place and eyeglasses are being worn. Create an environment in which the person is encouraged to make decisions, offer comments, and communicate thoughts and desires.
- Ask questions in a way that can be answered with a nod or the blink of an eye; if the person cannot respond verbally, instruct him or her in nonverbal responses. Use closed-ended questions so they can be answered with "yes" or "no." Responses written on paper can be used so that the person can point to the correct response.
- Be honest. Let the person know if you cannot quite understand what he or she is telling you but that you will keep trying.
- When you have not understood what the person said, it helps to repeat the part that you did understand as a question so that the person only has to repeat the part

that you did not understand. For example, you hear, "I would like an XX." Rather than saying "Pardon?" and getting a repeat of what was said (which may sound the same), try asking, "You would like a … ?"
- Speak of things that are familiar and of interest to the person.
- Use visual cues, objects, pictures, gestures, and touch, as well as words. Have paper and pencil available so you can write down key words or even sketch a picture.
- If the person has Wernicke's aphasia, listen and watch for the bits of information that emerge from the words, facial expressions, and gestures. Ignore the nonwords.
- Encourage all speech. Allow the person to try to complete his or her thoughts and to struggle with words. Avoid being too quick to guess what the person is trying to express.
- Use augmentative communication devices such as picture boards. These are useful to fill in answers to requests such as "I need" or "I want"; the person merely points to the appropriate picture.
- Try to keep staff who are caring for the person with aphasia consistent, and make the care plan specific to the most helpful communication techniques.
- Turn off the television or radio when speaking with the person.

most effective way to enhance communication. Suggestions for communicating with persons who have aphasia are presented in Box 3.7.

The gerontological nurse needs to be familiar with techniques that facilitate communication with the person who has aphasia or dysarthria, as well as with strategies that can be taught to the person to improve communication. Boxes 3.8 and 3.9 present suggestions for improving communication between the person with dysarthria and the listener.

The nurse may encounter older people who are in the acute or long-term phase of an illness that affects communication. Although early intensive rehabilitation efforts are most effective, all older persons with communication deficits should have access to state-of-the-art techniques and devices that enhance communication, a basic human need. In addition to being knowledgeable about appropriate communication techniques, nurses must be aware of equipment and resources that are available to the person with

aphasia or dysarthria so that hope can be offered. Teaching families and significant others effective communication strategies is also an important nursing task. (Several resources for people with aphasia and dysarthria are presented at the end of the chapter.)

COMMUNICATION WITH OLDER PERSONS WITH COGNITIVE IMPAIRMENT

The experience of losing cognitive and expressive abilities is both frightening and frustrating. One type of cognitive impairment that affects memory, speech, and communication is dementia (see Chapter 21). Older people who are experiencing dementia have difficulty expressing their personhood in ways easily understood by others. However, the need to communicate and the need to be treated as a person remain despite memory and communication impairments. No group of people is more in need of supportive relationships with skilled, caring health care providers.

BOX 3.8   Tips for the Person With Dysarthria

- Explain to people that you have difficulty with your speech.
- Try to limit conversations when you feel tired.
- Speak slowly and loudly and in a quiet place.
- Pace out one word at a time while speaking.
- Take a deep breath before speaking, so that there is enough breath for speech.
- Speak out as soon as you breathe out, to make full use of the breaths.
- Open the mouth more when speaking. Exaggerate tongue movements.
- Make sure you are sitting or standing in an upright posture; this will improve your breathing and speech.
- If you become frustrated, try to use other methods (such as pointing, gesturing, or writing), or take a rest and try again later.
- Practise facial exercises (blowing kisses, frowning, smiling), and massage your facial muscles.

Source: Adapted from *Dysarthria.* Retrieved from: http://www.asha.org/public/speech/disorders/dysarthria/.

BOX 3.9   Tips for Communicating With Individuals Experiencing Dysarthria

- Pay attention to the speaker; watch the speaker as he or she talks.
- Allow more time for conversation, and conduct conversations in a quiet place.
- Be honest, and let the speaker know when you have difficulty understanding.
- If the person's speech is very difficult to understand, repeat back what the person has said to make sure you understand.
- Remember that dysarthria does not affect a person's intelligence.
- Check with the person for ways in which you can help, such as guessing, finishing sentences, or writing.

Source: Adapted from *Dysarthria and coping with dysarthria.* Retrieved from the Royal College of Speech & Language Therapists (http://www.rcslt.org) and the American Speech-Language-Hearing Association (http://www.asha.org).

People with cognitive and communication impairments "depend on their relationship with and trust of others to provide emotional support, solve problems, and coordinate complex activities" (Buckwalter et al., 1995, p. 15).

Communicating with older people who are experiencing cognitive impairment requires special skills and patience. Dementia affects both receptive and expressive communication components and alters the way in which people speak. Early in the disease, finding words is difficult (a condition termed *anomia*), and remembering the exact facts of a conversation is challenging. The following reflection from a man with dementia illustrates this:

I'm aware that I'm losing larger and larger chunks of memory. … I lose one word and then I can't come up with the rest of the sentence. I just stop talking and people think something is really wrong with me. For awhile, I'll search for a word and I can see it walking away from me. It just gets littler and littler. It always comes back, but at the wrong time. You just can't be spontaneous. (Snyder, 2001, pp. 8, 11, 16)

As the disease progresses, the person has difficulty expressing thoughts and emotions and understanding verbal messages. In later stages, verbalization may be limited. Williams and Tappen (2008) remind us that even in the later stages of dementia, the person may understand more than health care providers realize, and he or she still needs opportunities for interaction and caring communication, both verbal and nonverbal. Often, health care providers do not communicate with older persons who have cognitive impairment, or they communicate only task-focused information. To effectively communicate with a person experiencing cognitive impairment, one must believe that the person is trying to communicate something and that what the person is trying to communicate is important enough to make the effort to understand. As nurses, the best thing we can do is to treat everything the person says or tries to communicate in a nonverbal manner as important and as an attempt to tell us something. It is our responsibility to know how to understand and respond verbally or nonverbally. The person with cognitive impairment cannot change his or her communication; we must change ours.

Tappen et al. (1999) have provided insight into communication strategies that are helpful in creating and maintaining a therapeutic relationship with people in moderate to later stages of dementia. Their research has challenged some of the commonly held beliefs about communication with persons

BOX 3.10   Useful Strategies for Communicating With Individuals Experiencing Cognitive Impairment

Simplification Strategies (Useful With Activities of Daily Living)
- Give one-step directions.
- Speak slowly.
- Allow time for a response.
- Reduce distractions.
- Interact with one person at a time.
- Be aware of your nonverbal communication.
- Give clues and cues and use gestures or pantomime to demonstrate what you want the person to do—for example, if you want the person to sit, put the chair in front of the person, point to it, pat the seat, and say, "Sit here."

Facilitation Strategies (Useful in Encouraging Expression of Thoughts and Feelings)
- Establish commonalities.
- Share self.
- Allow the person to choose subjects to discuss.
- Speak as if to an equal.
- Use broad openings, such as "How are you today?"
- Employ an appropriate use of humour.
- Follow the person's lead.

Comprehension Strategies (Useful in Assisting With Understanding of Communication)
- Identify time confusion. (In what time frame is the person operating at the moment?)
- Find the theme. (What connection is there between apparently disparate topics?) Recognize an important theme such as fear, loss, or happiness.

- Recognize hidden meanings. (What did the person mean to say?)

Supportive Strategies (Useful in Encouraging Continued Communication and Supporting Personhood)
- Introduce yourself and explain why you are there. Reach out to shake hands, and note the response to touch.
- If the person does not want to talk, go away and return later. Do not push or force.
- Sit closely and face the person at eye level.
- Limit corrections.
- Use multiple ways of communicating (nonverbal communication, gestures, touch).
- Search for meaning.
- Know the person's past life history as well as daily life experiences and events.
- Recognize and respond to feelings.
- Treat the person with respect and dignity.
- Show interest through body posture, facial expression, nodding, and eye contact. Assume a pleasant, relaxed attitude.
- Attend to vision and hearing losses.
- Do not try to bring the person to the present or use reality orientation. Go to where the person is, and enjoy the conversation.
- When leaving, thank the person for his or her time and attention as well as for information.
- Remember that the quality of the interaction, rather than its content or quantity, is basic to therapeutic communication.

who have cognitive impairment. For example, one of those beliefs is that one should use closed-ended questions. Tappen et al (1999) offer suggestions for specific verbal and nonverbal communication strategies that are effective in various nursing situations, as well as hope for nurses trying to establish meaningful relationships that nurture the personhood of people who have cognitive impairments. Williams and Tappen (2008, p. 93) note that "approaches to communication must be adapted not only to the person's ability to understand but to the purpose of the interaction. What is appropriate for assessment may be a barrier to conversation that is designed to facilitate expression of concerns and feelings." To this end, the Hartford Institute for Geriatric Nursing *Try This* series (https://consultgeri.org/) has made available

an evidence-informed practice guide for assessing communication abilities and for matching communication strategies to the communication abilities and problems of older persons with dementia. Box 3.10 presents suggestions for communication with persons experiencing cognitive impairment.

 ## IMPLICATIONS FOR GERONTOLOGICAL NURSING AND HEALTHY AGING

Care and communication that values and shows respect for the dignity and worth of all cared-for persons, including those with cognitive impairment, and the use of research-based communication techniques will enhance communication and affirm the patient's personhood. Buckwalter et al. (1995, p. 15) underscored this message with the following:

Gerontological nurses who are sensitive to communication and interaction patterns can assist both formal and informal caregivers in using more personal verbal and nonverbal communication strategies which are humanizing and show respect for the person. Similarly, they can monitor and try to change object-oriented communication approaches, which are not only insensitive and dehumanizing, but also often lead to diminished self-image and angry, agitated responses on the part of the patient with cognitive impairment.

THE LIFE STORY

Older people bring us complex stories derived from long years of living. In caring for older people, listening to life stories is an important component of communication. The life story can tell us a great deal about the person and is an important part of the assessment process. Stories are "critical sources of information about etiology, diagnosis, treatment, and prognosis from the patient's point of view" (Sandelowski, 1994, p. 25). Listening to memories and life stories requires time and patience and a belief that the story and the person are valuable and meaningful. A memory is an incredible gift given to the nurse, a sharing of a part of the patient when she or he may have little else to give. Personal memories are saved for persons who will patiently wait for their unveiling and who will treasure them. Stories are important. As Robert Coles (1989, p. 7) states, "The people who come to see us bring us their stories. They hope they tell them well enough so that we understand the truth of their lives. They hope we know how to interpret their stories correctly."

The life story—as constructed through reminiscence, journalizing, life review, or guided autobiography—has held great fascination for gerontologists in the last quarter century. The universal appeal of the life story as a vehicle of culture, a demonstration of caring and generational continuity, and an easily stimulated activity has held allure for many care providers. The most exciting aspect of working with older persons is being a part of the emergence of the life story, the shifting and blending patterns. When one is young, looking forward and planning for the future are important for emotional health and growth. As one ages, it becomes more important to look back, talk over experiences, review and make sense of it all, and feel satisfied with one's life. This very important work, which Erik Erikson called ego integrity versus self-despair, is the major developmental task of older adulthood. Ego integrity is achieved when the person has accepted both the triumphs and disappointments of life and is at peace and satisfied with the life lived (Erikson, 1963).

REMINISCING

Reminiscing is an umbrella term that includes any recalling of the past. Reminiscing occurs from childhood onward, particularly at life's junctures and transitions. Reminiscing cultivates (1) a sense of security through the recounting of comforting memories, (2) a sense of belonging through sharing, and (3) self-esteem through the confirmation of uniqueness. Robert Butler (2002) pointed out that 50 years ago, reminiscing was thought to be a sign of senility or what we now call Alzheimer's disease. Older people who talked about the past and told the same stories again and again were said to be boring and living in the past. Butler's seminal research showed that reminiscence is the most important psychological task of older people (Butler, 1963). For the nurse, having the patient reminisce is a therapeutic intervention that is important for assessment and understanding.

Reminiscence can have many goals. It not only provides a pleasurable experience that improves quality of life but also increases socialization and connectedness with others, provides cognitive stimulation, improves communication, and can be an effective therapy for depressive symptoms (Haight & Burnside, 1993; Fletcher & Eckberg, 2014). The therapeutic implications of reminiscence are discussed in Box 3.11.

The process of reminiscence can occur in individual conversations with older people; can be structured, as in a nursing history; or can occur in a group in which each person shares his or her memories and listens to others sharing theirs, as discussed later in this chapter. The nurse can learn much about a person's history, communication style, relationships, coping mechanisms, strengths, fears, affect, and adaptive

BOX 3.11   Uses of Reminiscence as a Developmental and Therapeutic Strategy

- Maintain continuity
- Extract meaning
- Define and develop personal philosophy
- Identify cycles and themes
- Recapitulate learning and growth
- Enhance self-worth and feeling of accomplishment
- Evolve identity
- Provide insight and growth
- Integrate and accept regrets and disappointments
- Perceive universality

capacity by listening thoughtfully as the life story is constructed. Box 3.12 provides some suggestions for encouraging reminiscence.

LIFE REVIEW

Robert Butler (1963) first noted and brought to public attention the review process that normally occurs in the older person as the realization of his or her approaching death creates a resurgence of unresolved conflicts. Butler called this process **life review.** Life review occurs quite naturally for many persons during periods of crisis and transition. However, Butler (2002) also noted that in old age, the process of putting one's life in order increases in intensity and

BOX 3.12   Suggestions for Encouraging Reminiscence

- Listen without correction or criticism.
- Encourage older people to reminisce about various ages and stages. Ask questions such as "What was it like growing up on that farm?" "What did teenagers do for fun when you were young?" and "What was school like for you?"
- Be patient with repetition. Sometimes people need to tell the same story often in order to come to terms with the experience, especially if it was very meaningful to them. If they have a memory loss, it may be the only story they can remember, and it is important for them to be a member of the group and to contribute to it.
- Be attuned to signs of depression in conversation (e.g., dwelling on sad topics) or changes in physical status or behaviour, and provide appropriate assessment and intervention.
- If a topic arises that the person does not want to discuss, change to another topic.
- If people are reluctant to share because they do not feel their life has been interesting, reassure them that everyone's life is valuable and interesting, and tell them how important their memories are to you and others.
- Keep in mind that reminiscing is not an orderly process; one memory triggers another in a way that may not seem related. It is not important to keep things in order or verify accuracy.
- Keep the conversation focused on the person who is reminiscing, but do not hesitate to share some of your own memories that relate to the situation being discussed.
- Listen actively, maintain eye contact, and do not interrupt.
- Respond positively, and give feedback by making caring and appropriate comments that encourage the person to continue.
- Use props and triggers, such as photographs, memorabilia (e.g., a childhood toy or antique), short stories or poems about the past, and favourite foods.
- Use open-ended questions to encourage reminiscing. You can prepare questions ahead of time, or you can ask the person to pick a topic that interests him or her. One question or topic may be enough for an entire session. Consider asking questions such as the following:

  How did your parents meet?
  What do you remember most about your mother? Father? Grandmother? Grandfather?
  What are some of your favourite memories from childhood?
  What was the first house you remember?
  What were your favourite foods as a child?
  Did you have a pet as a child?
  What do you remember about your first job?
  How did you celebrate birthdays or other holidays?
  What do you remember about your wedding day?
  What is your greatest accomplishment or joy in your life?
  What advice did your parents give you? What advice did you give your children? What advice would you give to young people today?

emphasis. Life review occurs most frequently as an internal review of memories, an intensely private and soul-searching activity.

Life review is considered more of a formal therapy technique than is reminiscence and takes a person through his or her life in a structured and chronological order. Life-review therapy (Butler and Lewis, 1983), guided autobiography (Birren and Deutchman, 1991), and structured life review (Haight and Webster, 1995) are psychotherapeutic techniques based on the concept of life review. Gerontological nurses participate with older persons in both reminiscence and life review, and it is important to acquire the skills needed to be effective in achieving the purposes of both. Life review may be especially important for older people facing death. Life review should occur not only when one is old or facing death but also frequently throughout one's life. This process can help one examine where one is in life and in changing course or setting new goals. Butler (2002) commented that if life review were conducted throughout one's life, one might avoid the overwhelming feelings of despair that may surface when there is no time left to make changes.

 ## IMPLICATIONS FOR GERONTOLOGICAL NURSING AND HEALTHY AGING

One of the greatest privileges of nursing older people is to accompany them in the final journey of life. As each person confronts mortality, there is a need for that person to integrate events and then transcend the self. Human experience, one's contributions, and the poignant anecdotes within the life story bind generations together, validate the uniqueness of each brief journey in this level of awareness, and provide the assurance that one will not be forgotten. The nurse who takes the time to listen to an older person share memories and life stories communicates respect for the person and an appreciation of that person as an individual. What more can one ask for at the end of life than to know who one is and to know that what one has accomplished holds personal meaning and meaning for others as well? This is the essence of life's final tasks—achieving ego integrity and self-actualization.

COMMUNICATION WITH GROUPS OF OLDER PERSONS

Group work with older people has been used extensively to meet a great number of needs in an economical manner. Nurses have worked with groups of older people for a variety of therapeutic reasons, and Box 3.13 presents some of the benefits of group work. Many groups can be managed effectively by staff with clear goals and guidance and training. Cook (2004) enumerated skills that are important for effective group leadership (Box 3.14). Volunteers, nursing assistants, and recreation staff can be taught to conduct many types of groups, but groups with a psychotherapy focus require a trained and skilled leader.

Groups can be implemented in many settings, including adult day health programs, retirement communities, assisted-living homes, community settings, and LTC homes. Examples of groups are reminiscence groups, psychoeducational groups, caregiver support groups, and groups for people with memory

---

BOX 3.13   Benefits of Group Work With Older Persons

- Group experiences provide older persons with an opportunity to try new roles—those of teacher, expert, storyteller.
- Groups may improve communication skills for lonely, shy, or withdrawn older persons, as well as those with communication disorders or memory impairment.
- Groups provide peer support and opportunities to share common experiences, and they may foster the development of warm friendships that endure long after the group has ended.
- Active listening and interest in what older persons have to say may improve their self-esteem and help them feel like worthwhile persons whose wisdom is valued.
- Group work offers the opportunity for leaders to be creative and use many modalities, such as music, art, dance, poetry, exercise, and current events.
- Groups provide an opportunity for the leader to assess the person's mood, cognitive abilities, and functional level on a regular basis.

Source: Adapted from Burnside, I. M. (1994). Group work with older persons. *Journal of Gerontological Nursing, 20*(1), 43.

BOX 3.14 Group Leadership Skills

- Attend to group participants.
- Reflect group and members' feelings.
- Link members to each other.
- Guide group discussion.
  a. Use open-ended questions.
  b. Shift the focus as needed.
  c. Hold the focus to complete a discussion.
- Scan the group to pick up nonverbal communication.
- Assist the group in processing the group experience.

Source: Linton, A. D., & Lach, H. W. (2007). *Matteson & McConnell's gerontological nursing: Concepts and practice* (3rd ed., p. 753). Philadelphia: Saunders.

---

impairment or other conditions such as Parkinson's disease or stroke.

GROUP STRUCTURE AND SPECIAL CONSIDERATIONS FOR GROUPS OF OLDER PERSONS

Implementing a group intervention follows a thorough assessment of the environment, needs, and potential of various group strategies. Major decisions regarding goals will influence the strategy selected; for instance, several older persons with diabetes in an acute care setting may need health care teaching on diabetes.

The nurse sees the major goal of group work as education and the restoring of order (or control) in each person's lifestyle. The strategy best suited for that would be motivational or educational. People experiencing early-stage Alzheimer's disease may benefit from a support group in which to express feelings or a group that teaches memory-enhancing strategies. Successful group work depends on organization; attention to details; agency support; assessment and consideration of the older person's needs and status; and caring, sensitive, and skillful leadership. Group work with older people is different from that with people of a younger age; it requires special skills and training and extraordinary commitment on the part of the leader. However, these unique aspects may not apply to all types of older-adult groups. Some of the common differences and particularities of such group work are presented in Box 3.15.

REMINISCING AND STORYTELLING WITH INDIVIDUALS EXPERIENCING COGNITIVE IMPAIRMENT

Cognitive impairment does not necessarily preclude older people from participating in reminiscence or storytelling groups. Opportunities for telling their life stories, enjoying memories, and achieving ego integrity and self-actualization should not be denied to people on the basis of their cognitive status. Some modifications might be needed so that those with mild to moderate memory impairment can enjoy and benefit from group work focused on reminiscence and storytelling.

When the nurse is working with a group of cognitively impaired older people, the emphasis in reminiscence groups is on sharing memories, however they may be expressed. There should be no pressure to answer questions such as "Where were you born?" or "What was your first job?" Rather, discussions may centre on places where people have lived. Additional props, such as music, pictures, and familiar objects (e.g., a Canadian flag or an old coffee grinder), can prompt many recollections and sharing. Many resources are available to guide these groups, including books such as *I Remember When* (Thorsheim & Roberts, 2000) that offer numerous ways to adapt the reminiscing process for those with cognitive impairment. Other helpful resources are listed at http://evolve.elsevier.com/Canada/Ebersole/gerontological/.

George et al. (2011) described a storytelling modality called TimeSlips, which is designed for people with cognitive impairment (http://www.timeslips.org). Group members, looking at a picture, are encouraged to use their imagination and create a story about the picture. The pictures can be fantastical and funny (like greeting cards) or more nostalgic (like Norman Rockwell paintings). All contributions are encouraged and welcomed—there are no right or wrong answers—and everything that the individuals say is included in the story and written down by the scribe. The stories that emerge are full of creativity and often include discussions about memories and reminiscing. John Killick (1999, p. 49), a writer-in-residence at an LTC home in Scotland, stated the following:

Having their words written down is empowering for people with dementia. It affirms their dignity and

---

BOX 3.15   Special Considerations in Group Work With Older Persons

- The leader must pay special attention to sensory losses and compensate for them.
- Pacing is different, and group leaders must slow down physical and psychological actions.
- Group members often need assistance or transportation to the group, and adequate time must be allowed for assembling the members and helping them to return to their homes or rooms.
- The time of day that a group meeting is scheduled is important. The meeting should not conflict with other important activities, and evening groups may not be good for older people who may be tired by then. For community-based groups, transportation logistics may become complicated in the evening.
- A warm and friendly climate of acceptance of each member is important, as is the expression of appreciation and enjoyment of the group and each member's contribution. Because of ageist attitudes in society, the wisdom and contributions of older people are often not valued.
- Older people may need more stimulation and be less self-motivating.
- Groups generally should include people with similar levels of cognitive ability. Mixing very intact older persons with those who have memory and communication impairments

calls for special skills. Burnside (1994) suggested that in groups of people with varying abilities, alert persons tend to ask, "Will I become like them?" whereas those with memory and communication impairments may become anxious when they are aware that they cannot perform as well as the other members.
- Many older people who are likely to be in need of groups may be depressed or have experienced a number of losses (e.g., health, friends, or spouse).
- Leaders must be prepared for some members to become ill, deteriorate, and die. Plans regarding the recognition of missing members will need to be clear.
- Leaders are continually confronted with their own aging and attitudes toward it. Having co-leaders is ideal; they can support each other. It is important to share thoughts and feelings, recapitulate group sessions, and modify approaches as needed. If the group is led by one person, it is good to have someone with expertise in group work with older persons discuss the group's experiences with the leader and provide support and direction. Skills in developing and implementing groups for older people improve with experience. Burnside reminded us that "all new group leaders should have guidance from an experienced leader to help them weather the difficult times" (Burnside, 1994).

---

gives an assurance that their words still have value. … One woman said, "Anything you can tell people about how things are for me is important. It's a rum do, this growing ancient. … The brilliance of my brain has slipped away when I wasn't looking."

SUMMARY

This chapter aimed to show the potential for respectful communication regardless of the impairment the older person may be experiencing. Communicating with older people calls for special skills, patience, and respect. As nurses, we must break through the barriers and continue to reach toward the humanity of these persons in the belief that communication is the most vital service we offer. This is the heart of nursing.

KEY CONCEPTS

- Communication is a basic need regardless of age or communication or cognitive impairment. Respect

for the person and a knowledge of therapeutic communication techniques are essential for gerontological nurses.
- Nurses need to develop and demonstrate effective communication strategies for older people who have speech, language, hearing, vision, or cognitive impairment.
- Group work can meet many needs and can be valuable and rewarding for older people.
- In a rapidly changing society, the shared life histories of older people provide a sense of continuity among generations.
- The life history of a person is a story to be developed and treasured. This is particularly important toward the end of life.
- Gerontological nursing communication is mainly focused on using interpersonal communication techniques, providing necessary information, encouraging individuals to express personal interests and preferences, and, when function is

impeded, ensuring that all needs are recognized, discussed, and met to the greatest extent possible.

ACTIVITIES AND DISCUSSION QUESTIONS

1. Using ear plugs or eyeglasses with the lenses covered in Vaseline, try performing some of your daily activities or engaging in conversation with your peers.
2. Discuss how you might provide medication instructions to a person with hearing or vision loss.
3. Discuss adaptations to communication for individuals with aphasia or dysarthria.
4. Discuss ways in which you might respond to a person with cognitive impairment who has difficulty expressing thoughts and feelings.
5. Role-play in a simulated interaction with an older person who is experiencing communication or cognitive impairments such as aphasia, dysarthria, or memory loss.
6. With a partner, plan and discuss an activity that would be appropriate for an individual with cognitive impairment.
7. Watch the movie *Iris*, *The Notebook*, *Alice*, or *Away from Her*, and discuss the effective and ineffective communication strategies that nurses used to interact with persons who are experiencing cognitive impairment.
8. With your peers, form a small group and share memories about an event you have all experienced in your lives (e.g., first date, first day of school).
9. Interview an older person and ask to hear his or her life story.

RESOURCES

Alzheimer Society of Canada. Daily Living: Communication
http://www.alzheimer.ca/english/care/ dailyliving-communication.htm

Canadian Association of the Deaf
http://www.cad.ca

Canadian Hearing Society
http://www.chs.ca

Canadian National Institute for the Blind (CNIB)
http://www.cnib.ca

Public Health Agency of Canada. Age-friendly communication: Facts, tips, and ideas
https://www.canada.ca/en/public-health/services/health -promotion/aging-seniors/publications/publications -general-public/friendly-communication-facts-tips-ideas/ introduction.html

Speech-Language & Audiology Canada
http://www.sac-oac.ca/

The Hartford Institute for Geriatric Nursing Try This series (provides an evidence-informed practice guide for assessing communication abilities and matching communication strategies)
https://consultgeri.org/

The Heart and Stroke Foundation (provides information on communication changes that can occur after a stroke)
http://www.heartandstroke.com

Unfair Hearing Test
http://www.irrd.ca/education/presentation.asp?refname =e2c1

Vision Simulator (to experience visual impairments)
http://www.visionsimulations.com/

For additional resources, please visit *http://evolve .elsevier.com/Canada/Ebersole/gerontological/*

REFERENCES

Birren, J. E., & Deutchman, D. E. (1991). *Guiding autobiography groups for older adults: Exploring the fabric of life.* Baltimore: Johns Hopkins University Press.

Buckwalter, K. C., Gerdner, L. A., Hall, G. R., et al. (1995). Shining through: The humor and individuality of persons with Alzheimer's disease. *Journal of Gerontological Nursing, 21*(3), 11–16. doi:10.3928/0098-9134-19950301-04.

Burnside, I. M. (1975). Listen to the aged. *American Journal of Nursing, 75*(10), 1800–1803. doi:10.2307/3423569.

Burnside, I. M. (1994). Group work with older persons. *Journal of Gerontological Nursing, 20*(1), 43. doi:10.3928/0098-9134 -19940101-09.

Butler, R. (1963). The life review: An interpretation of reminiscence in the aged. *Psychiatry, 26,* 65–76. doi:10.1080/00332747.1963 .11023339.

Butler, R. (2002). *Age, death and life review.* Retrieved from http:// www.hospicefoundation.org.

Butler, R., & Lewis, M. (1983). *Aging and mental health: Positive psychosocial approaches* (3rd ed.). St. Louis, MO: Mosby.

Canadian Hard of Hearing Association (CHHA). (2009). *Funding for my aids and devices*. Retrieved from http://chha.ca/chha/projects-funding.php.

Canadian Hearing Association. (2015). *The six types of age-related hearing loss*. Retrieved from https://www.chs.ca/blog/six-types-age-related-hearing-loss.

Canadian Hearing Society. (2017). *Facts and figures*. Retrieved from https://www.chs.ca/facts-and-figures.

Canadian National Institute for the Blind (CNIB). (2017a). *Fast facts about vision loss*. Retrieved from http://www.cnib.ca/en/about/media/vision-loss/Pages/default.aspx.

Canadian National Institute for the Blind (CNIB). (2017b). *Glossary of AMD terms*. Retrieved from http://www.cnib.ca/en/your-eyes/eye-conditions/amd/resources/glossary/Pages/default.aspx.

Canadian Stroke Best Practices. (2016). *Rehabilitation to improve language and communication*. Retrieved from http://www.strokebestpractices.ca/index.php/stroke-rehabilitation/rehabilitation-to-improve-communication/.

Cohen-Mansfield, J., & Taylor, J. (2004). Hearing aid use in nursing homes. Part 1: Prevalence rates of hearing impairment and hearing aid use. *Journal of the American Medical Directors Association*, 5(5), 283–296. doi:10.1016/S1525-8610(04)70017-1.

Coles, R. (1989). *The call of stories*. Boston: Houghton Mifflin.

College of Audiologists and Speech-Language Pathologists of Ontario. (2014). *Preferred practice guideline for ear impressions*. Retrieved from http://www.caslpo.com/sites/default/uploads/files/PPG_EN_Ear_Impressions.pdf.

Cook, M. J. (2004). Learning for clinical leadership. *Journal of Nursing Management*, 12(6), 436–444. doi:10.1111/j.1365-2834.2004.00420.x.

Dev, M. K., Paudel, N., Joshi, N. D., et al. (2014). Impact of visual impairment on vision-specific quality of life among older adults living in nursing home. *Current Eye Research*, 39(3), 232–238. doi:10.3109/02713683.2013.838973.

Erikson, E. H. (1963). *Childhood and society* (2nd ed.). New York: W. W. Norton.

Feder, K., Michaud, D., Ramage-Morin, P., et al. (2015). *Prevalence of hearing loss among Canadians aged 20 to 79: Audiometric results from the 2012/2013 Canadian health measures survey*. Retrieved from http://www.statcan.gc.ca/pub/82-003-x/2015007/article/14206-eng.htm.

Fletcher, T. S., & Eckberg, J. D. (2014). The effects of creative reminiscing on individuals with dementia and their caregivers: A pilot study. *Physical & Occupational Therapy In Geriatrics*, 32(1), 68–84. doi:10.3109/02703181.2014.880863.

George, D. R., Stuckey, H. L., Dillon, C. F., et al. (2011). Impact of participation in TimeSlips, a creative group-based storytelling program, on medical student attitudes towards persons with dementia: A qualitative study. *The Gerontologist*, 51(5), 699–703. doi:10.1093/geront/gnr035.

Gopinath, B., Schneider, J., McMahon, C. M., et al. (2011). Severity of age-related hearing loss is associated with impaired activities of daily living. *Age and Ageing*, 41(2), 195–200. doi:10.1093/ageing/afr155.

Grimme, T. M., Buchanan, J., & Afflerbach, S. (2015). Understanding elderspeak from the perspective of certified nursing assistants. *Journal of Gerontological Nursing*, 41(11), 42–49. doi:10.3928/00989134-20151015-05.

Haight, B., & Burnside, I. M. (1993). Reminiscence and life review: Explaining the differences. *Archives of Psychiatric Nursing*, 7(2), 91–98. doi:10.1016/S0883-9417(09)90007-3.

Haight, B. K., & Webster, J. D. (1995). *The art and science of reminiscing: Theory, methods and applications*. Washington, DC: Taylor and Francis.

Ham, R., Sloane, P., Warshaw, G., et al. (2007). *Primary care geriatrics* (5th ed.). St. Louis, MO: Mosby.

Harty, M., Griesel, M., & van der Merwe, A. (2011). The ICF as a common language for rehabilitation goal-setting: Comparing client and professional priorities. *Health and Quality of Life Outcomes*, 9(87), doi:10.1186/1477-7525-9-87.

Keaton, S. A., & Giles, H. (2016). Subjective health: The roles of communication, language, aging, stereotypes, and culture. *International Journal of Society, Culture, and Language*, 4(2), 1–10.

Killick, J. (1999). "What are we like here?" Eliciting experiences of people with dementia. *Generations (San Francisco, Calif.)*, 13(3), 46–49.

Koch, J., Datta, G., Makhdoom, S., et al. (2005). Unmet visual needs of Alzheimer's patients in long-term care facilities. *Journal of the American Medical Directors Association*, 6(4), 233–237. doi:10.1016/j.jamda.2005.04.001.

Lagacé, M., Tanguay, A., Lavallée, M.-L., et al. (2012). The silent impact of ageist communication in long term care facilities: Elders' perspectives on quality of life and coping strategies. *Journal of Aging Studies*, 26(3), 335–342. doi:10.1016/j.jaging.2012.03.002.

La Tourette, T. R., & Meeks, S. (2000). Perceptions of patronizing speech by older women in nursing homes and in the community: Impact of cognitive ability and place of residence. *Journal of Language and Social Psychology*, 19, 463–473. doi:10.1177/0261927X00019004004.

Manrique-Huarte, R., Calavia, D., Huarte Irujo, A., et al. (2016). Treatment for hearing loss among the elderly: Auditory outcomes and impact on quality of life. *Audiology & Neurotology*, 21(1), 29–35. doi:10.1159/000448352.

Maslow, A. (1943). A theory of human motivation. *Psychological Review*, 50, 370–396. doi:10.1037/h0054346.

McGilton, K. S., Sorin-Peters, R., Sidani, S., et al. (2012). Patient-centred communication intervention study to evaluate nurse-patient interactions in complex continuing care. *BMC Geriatrics*, 12, 61. doi:10.1186/1471-2318-12-61.

McMahon, C. M. (2016). Hearing loss in older age and its effect on the individuals, their families and the community. *Genetics of Deafness*, 20, 9–18. doi:10.1159/000444561.

Meador, J. A. (1995). Cerumen impaction in the elderly. *Journal of Gerontological Nursing*, 21(12), 43–45. doi:10.3928/0098-9134-19951201-09.

Muzychka, M., for The National Coalition for Vision Health. (2009). *Environmental scan of vision health and vision loss in the provinces and territories of Canada*. Retrieved from http://www.eyesite.ca/resources/NCVH-environment-scan Sept2009.pdf.

Ontario Human Rights Commission. (2011). *Ageism and age discrimination (fact sheet)*. Retrieved from http://www.ohrc.on.ca/en/ageism-and-age-discrimination-fact-sheet.

Owsley, C., Ball, K., McGwin, G., et al. (2007). Effect of refractive error correction on health-related quality of life and depression in older nursing home residents. *Archives of Ophthalmology, 125*(11), 1471–1477. doi:10.1001/archopht.125.11.1471.

Page, C. G., & Rowles, G. D. (2016). "It doesn't require much effort once you get to know them": Certified nursing assistants' views of communication in long-term care. *Journal of Gerontological Nursing, 42*(4), 42–51. doi:10.3928/00989134-20160104-01.

Pikhartova, J., Bowling, A., & Victor, C. (2014). Does owning a pet protect older people against loneliness? *BMC Geriatrics, 14*(1), 106. doi:10.1186/1471-2318-14-106.

Registered Nurses Association of Ontario (RNAO). (2015). *Person- and family-centred care*. Retrieved from http://rnao.ca/sites/rnao-ca/files/FINAL_Web_Version_0.pdf.

Rittenour, C. E., & Cohen, E. L. (2016). Age progression simulations increase young adults' aging anxiety and negative stereotypes of older adults. *The International Journal of Aging and Human Development, 82*(4), 271–289. doi:10.1177/0091415016641690.

Sacks, O. (1989). *Seeing voices: A journey into the world of the deaf.* Berkeley, CA: University of California Press.

Sandelowski, M. (1994). We are the stories we tell. *Journal of Holistic Nursing, 12*(1), 23–33. doi:10.1177/089801019401200105.

Snyder, L. (2001). The lived experience of Alzheimer's— Understanding the feeling and subjective accounts of persons with the disease. *Alzheimer Care Quarterly, 2*(2), 8–22.

Statistics Canada (2015). *Hearing loss of Canadians, 2012-2013.* Retrieved from http://www.statcan.gc.ca/pub/82-625-x/2015001/article/14156-eng.htm.

Tappen, R. M., Williams, C., Fishman, S., et al. (1999). Persistence of self in advanced Alzheimer's disease. *Image: Journal of Nursing Scholarship, 31*(2), 121–125.

Thorsheim, H., & Roberts, B. (2000). *I remember when: Activity ideas to help people reminisce.* Forest Knolls, CA: Elder Books.

Wallhagen, M., & Pettengill, E. (2008). Hearing impairment significant but under-assessed in primary care settings. *Journal of Gerontological Nursing, 34*(2), 36–42.

Williams, C., & Tappen, R. (2008). Communicating with cognitively impaired persons. In C. Williams (Ed.), *Therapeutic interaction in nursing* (2nd ed.). Boston: Jones and Bartlett.

World Health Organization (WHO). (2014). *Visual impairment and blindness.* Retrieved from http://www.who.int/mediacentre/factsheets/fs282/en/.

Culture, Ethnicity, and Aging

LEARNING OBJECTIVES

Upon completion of this chapter, the reader will be able to:

- Identify factors contributing to the nurse's cultural sensitivity and cultural competence.
- Discuss approaches that facilitate an appreciation of diverse cultural and ethnic experiences.
- Explain the prominent health care belief systems.
- Identify nursing care interventions appropriate for ethnoculturally diverse older persons.
- Formulate a plan of care incorporating ethnoculturally sensitive interventions.

GLOSSARY

Culture "Learned and transmitted beliefs, as well as information and values that shape attitudes and generate meaning among members of a social group" (Registered Nurses' Association of Ontario [RNAO], 2007, p. 28).

Determinants of health Factors and conditions that influence the health status of individuals, communities, and populations.

Ethnicity The cultural, racial, religious, or linguistic traditions of a people or country.

Ethnocentrism The belief in the inherent superiority of one's ethnic group, accompanied by the devaluation of other groups.

Family Class immigrant A Canadian Citizenship and Immigration term referring to immigrants who are eligible for sponsorship by a family member. Canadian citizens and permanent residents can sponsor a spouse, a common-law partner, a conjugal partner, dependent children, parents, grandparents, and certain other eligible relatives. The sponsor must promise to provide financial support to the immigrating relative for between 3 and 10 years.

Folk medicine Healing methods originating among the people of a given culture and primarily transmitted from person to person.

Health disparities "[D]ifferences in health status that occur among population groups defined by specific characteristics. … The most prominent factors in Canada are socio-economic status, Aboriginal identity, gender, and geographic location" (Health Disparities Task Group, 2004, p. viii). Disparities result from inequalities in the underlying determinants of health among population groups.

Health literacy The degree to which individuals have the ability to obtain, process, and understand the basic information and services they need to make appropriate health decisions.

Interpreter A person who transmits the meaning of what is spoken in one language in another spoken language.

Stereotype A belief applied to a group of persons on the basis of actual or assumed knowledge of an individual member of the group.

Translator A person who converts written materials from one language to another.

Visible minority A term referring to "persons of colour." As defined in Canadian federal data collection and official statistics, it refers to Chinese, South Asian, Black, Filipino, Latin American, Southeast Asian, Arab, West Asian, Korean, and Japanese people.

The following are voices of people who immigrated to Canada from China in older age:
"I feel happy most of [the] time living in this country. I have my daughter and granddaughter here, and I live close to them. If I have time, I go to English classes. Sometimes, I talk to my friends over the phone. I am happy here." (A woman in her late sixties)

"One of the things I am dissatisfied with is lack of social life. I feel very isolated after I arrived here. There is a lack of programs and place that we [elderly] could go for socialization. Transportation is also a barrier for me to go out. The public transportation is not that convenient; I feel [the] ticket fare is expensive for us, even if we have discounted fares." (A man in his mid-seventies)

Source: Da, W-W, & Garcia, A. (2015). Later life immigration: Sociocultural adaptation and changes in quality of life at settlement among recent older Chinese immigrants in Canada. *Activities, Adaptation, & Aging, 39*(3), 230.

Attention to **culture** and health care is increasing. In the field of gerontology in Canada, interest in culture is stimulated to a great extent by three major issues: (1) the realization of a "gerontological explosion," (2) the impact of Canadian policies of multiculturalism that were established in 1971, and (3) the recognition of **health disparities** for members of ethnocultural minorities. *Gerontological explosion* refers both to the rapid increases in the total number of older persons, especially those over the age of 85 years, and to the relatively high proportion of older persons in most countries across the globe (see Chapter 1). *Health disparities* refers to the differences in disease burden between groups of people.

Nurses are expected to provide competent care to persons whose life experiences, cultural perspectives, values, languages, and styles of communication are different from their own. To competently assess and intervene, nurses must first develop cultural sensitivity through an awareness of their own **ethnocentrism**. Effective nurses develop cultural competence through knowing about **ethnicity**, culture, language, and health belief systems, and also develop the skills needed to optimize intercultural communication.

Knowing how to provide culturally competent care is especially important in gerontological nursing, because many older persons are immigrants to Canada. Some have had limited opportunities to develop English or French language skills, increasing the risk for limited **health literacy** (see Chapter 7). Language challenges can result in cultural conflict in the health care setting and limit access to health promotion and health care. This chapter provides an overview of culture and aging, as well as strategies that gerontological nurses can use to best respond to the changing face of aging and thus help reduce health disparities.

THE GERONTOLOGICAL EXPLOSION

Multiculturalism is part of the Canadian identity and is valued by the vast majority of Canadians (Kymlicka, 2010), and Canada is officially a multicultural society. Multicultural policies were implemented by the federal government in 1971; the 1982 *Canadian Charter of Rights and Freedoms* states that the Charter "shall be interpreted in a manner consistent with the preservation and enhancement of the multicultural heritage of Canadians" (cited in Dewing & Leman, 2006, p. 6). The population of Canada is rapidly becoming more diverse. It is projected that by 2031, between 25% and 28% of the Canadian population will be immigrants, between 29% and 32% of the population will be members of a **visible minority,** and the proportion of Canadians of the Christian religion will decline from about 75% (in 2006) to about 65% (Statistics Canada, 2010).

Currently, 14.2% of Canadians most often speak a language other than French or English, and 19.1% report a mother tongue that is other than English or French (Statistics Canada, 2015a, 2015b). The number is higher for older Canadians; about 23% have a mother tongue that is other than French or English (Statistics Canada, 2015b). More than 6 million Canadians (19.1% of the population) are members of a visible minority (Statistics Canada, 2016a), and an

TABLE 4.1	Population of Canada by Ethnic Origin and Age	
ETHNIC ORIGIN*	**TOTAL POPULATION**	**POPULATION AGED 65 YEARS AND OLDER**
	N = 32,852,320 (% of Total)[†]	N = 4,551,535 (% of Age Group)[†]
Canadian	10,697,880 (32.6%)	1,247,905 (27.4%)
British Isles origins	11,343,710 (34.5%)	1,679,860 (36.9%)
European (excluding French)	11,917,250 (36.3%)	1,444,325 (31.7%)
French	5,077,215 (15.4%)	680,300 (14.9%)
South Asian	1,615,925 (5.0%)	132,385 (2.9%)
West Central Asian, Middle Eastern	778,465 (2.3%)	51,945 (1.1%)
East Asian, Southeast Asian	2,650,000 (8.1%)	228,205 (5.0%)
Indigenous (First Nations, Métis, Inuit)[‡]	1,836,035 (5.6%)	101,030 (2.2%)
Caribbean	627,590 (1.9%)	53,555 (1.2%)
Australian, New Zealander, Pacific Islander	74,875 (0.2%)	4,665 (0.1%)
African	766,735 (2.3%)	32,465 (0.7%)
Latin, Central, and South American	544,380 (1.7%)	23,605 (0.5%)
American	372,575 (1.1%)	50,815 (1.1%)

*The census question was, "What were the ethnic or cultural origins of this person's ancestors?"
[†]Percentages add to more than 100% because people could specify as many origins as applicable.
[‡]Figures for Indigenous peoples are underestimates because they do not include data from one or more incompletely enumerated Indigenous reserves or settlements.
Source: Adapted from Statistics Canada. (2016). *Ethnic origin (264), single and multiple ethnic origin responses (3), generation status (4), age groups (10) and sex (3) for the population in private households of Canada, provinces, territories, Census Metropolitan Areas and Census Agglomerations, 2011 National Household Survey.* Retrieved from http://www12.statcan.gc.ca/nhs-enm/2011/dp-pd/dt-td/Rp-eng.cfm?LANG=E&APATH=3&DETAIL =0&DIM=0&FL=A&FREE=0&GC=0&GID=0&GK=0&GRP=0&PID=105396&PRID=0&PTYPE=105277&S=0&SHOWALL=0&SUB=0&Temporal =2013&THEME=95&VID=0&VNAMEE=&VNAMEF.

additional 1.4 million report being Indigenous people (First Nations, Métis, or Inuit) (Statistics Canada 2016b).

Among Canadians older than 65 years of age, the numbers of immigrants and members of ethnocultural minorities are not as dramatic, but growing numbers are being seen in all aspects of gerontological nursing. For example, 10.6% of Canadians over the age of 65 years are members of visible minorities, but the number is increasing; among Canadians who are now between the ages of 45 and 64 years, 15.1% are members of a visible minority (Statistics Canada, 2016a). About one-third of Canadians aged 65 years and older are immigrants. However, a large proportion of older Canadian immigrants moved to Canada as younger adults; 70% immigrated before 1976 (Ng, 2010). Most recent immigrants came to Canada as younger adults; only 3.3% of those who came to Canada between 2006 and 2011 were aged 65 years or older (Statistics Canada, 2016a). Table 4.1 shows the distribution of ethnic origins in the Canadian population and in subgroups of older or middle-aged Canadians.

HEALTH DISPARITIES

Significant health disparities exist in Canada and have been a concern in Canadian health policy for almost 40 years (Lalonde, 1974). The most important factors associated with health disparities in Canada are low socioeconomic status, Indigenous identity, female gender, and living in a rural or remote community (Health Disparities Task Group, 2004). Other vulnerable populations include "immigrants, refugees, the disabled, … the homeless, people with stigmatizing conditions, the elderly, children and youth in disadvantaged circumstances, people with poor literacy skills, and women in precarious circumstances" (Beiser & Stewart, 2005, p. S4).

Indigenous Canadians include Canadians of First Nations, Inuit, or Métis heritage. Addressing the health disparities experienced by Indigenous persons in Canada requires an understanding of the differences and variability of disparities and inequities among and between First Nations, Inuit, and Métis peoples. Compared to non-Indigenous Canadians, Indigenous Canadians experience more chronic health conditions, disability, and death from injury, as well as lower life expectancy (Health Disparities Task Group, 2004; Cameron, Plazas, Salas, et al., 2014). Indigenous peoples are more likely to experience disadvantages related to other key **determinants of health** (see Chapter 1), including housing quality, access to safe drinking water, educational attainment, employment, income, and access to health services (Cameron et al., 2014). According to Cameron and colleagues, the factors that underlie health disparities for Indigenous Canadians are "the social, political, and colonial history that Aboriginal people have experienced, the dominance of biomedical perspectives in the health care system, the power imbalances within health care services, and the limited access to health care services." Access to health services continues to be experienced as problematic, difficult, and limited (Cameron et al., 2014).

Health disparities persist for older Indigenous Canadians, who report having lower levels of health and more chronic health conditions than other older Canadians (Beatty & Berdahl, 2011). Many older Indigenous Canadians attended residential schools (Box 4.1). There are approximately 78,750 residential school survivors in Canada (Assembly of First Nations, 2016).

People who are members of a visible minority or who are immigrants tend to have worse health than the rest of the population (Prus, 2011). There is significant evidence for health disparities associated with ethnicity and race, particularly in the United States. However, the existence of historical differences between Canada and the United States and differences in immigration and health care policies means that some evidence from the United States may not apply to Canada (Gee, Kobayashi, & Prus, 2007; Prus, 2011). Gee et al. (2007) found that health and economic security were affected by a complex interaction between ethnicity, immigration status, and gender. People who are members of a visible minority tend to be economically disadvantaged; people of colour and Indigenous peoples fare worst. There is considerable variety among visible minority and ethnocultural groups with respect to economic security and health status.

Most older immigrants have lived in Canada for decades and are less likely than younger and more recent immigrants to be members of visible minorities (Statistics Canada, 2006, 2010). The ethnocultural composition of the older immigrant population reflects historical immigration policies. Thus, most older immigrants were born in Europe, and a significant minority were born in Asian countries. Older immigrants are more likely than nonimmigrants to live in urban areas. This is especially true for more recent immigrants and members of visible minorities, who are most likely to live in Toronto or Vancouver (Statistics Canada, 2006).

Older persons who are immigrants to Canada may experience worse health than their Canadian-born counterparts. In a phenomenon known as the "healthy migrant effect," recent immigrants tend to have better health than long-term immigrants or nonimmigrants because of Canadian immigration policies. Over time, the health status of immigrants becomes more like that of their Canadian-born counterparts. There is evidence that the health of long-term immigrants may be worse than that of their Canadian-born counterparts in regard to certain health conditions, such as diabetes, cancer, tuberculosis, cardiovascular disorder, and mental health illness (Kobayashi & Prus, 2012). Although recent immigrants tend to have better health, age plays a role. Older recent immigrants, especially those who are refugees or who enter as **Family Class immigrants** sponsored by children or grandchildren, tend to have poorer health (Setia et al., 2011; Koehn, 2009). Most recent immigrants are not

BOX 4.1 Residential Schools and Older Indigenous Persons in Canada

The residential school system in Canada existed from 1800 to 1990. The system peaked in 1930, when there were 80 schools. The schools were funded by the federal government and were operated mainly by churches. Residential schools were more common in the Prairies, British Columbia, and northern Canada, but they existed in all provinces except Newfoundland, Prince Edward Island, and New Brunswick. Indigenous children were often removed from their communities and separated from their families for 10 months of the year. The system was founded on the assumption that assimilation into mainstream culture would facilitate adaptation to a modernizing society. Students were not allowed to speak their first language or practise their traditions. The conditions in the schools and the skills taught there were substandard. Many students experienced emotional or physical abuse, and some experienced sexual abuse. Many students were ill-prepared for life in urban settings or in their home communities. Long-term negative effects include "lateral violence (when an oppressed group turns on itself and begins to violate each other), suicide, depression, poverty, alcoholism, lack of parenting skills,

lack of capacity to build and sustain healthy families and communities" (Aboriginal Healing Foundation, 2010, 2). "The negative effects of these schools have, in many cases, been passed from one generation to the next. As a result, even though the residential school system no longer exists, an intergenerational legacy remains, affecting many Aboriginal people and their communities" (Statistics Canada, 2004, p. 22). The Prime Minister of Canada apologized in Parliament to Indigenous Canadians in June 2008. The *Indian Residential School Agreement* is a settlement package negotiated between the federal government, churches, the Assembly of First Nations, and lawyers representing former students. It includes payments to former students and funding for healing funds, a truth and reconciliation commission, and commemoration. The Truth and Reconciliation Commission of Canada (2015) received statements from more than 6,750 people, including former students, families, and others. *The Survivors Speak* is a compilation of stories of residential school survivors, published as part of the Truth And Reconciliation Commission report.

Sources: CBC News. (2010). *A history of residential schools in Canada: FAQs on residential schools and compensation.* Retrieved from http://www. cbc.ca/canada/story/2008/05/16/f-faqs-residential-schools.html; Statistics Canada. (2004). *Aboriginal Peoples survey 2001: Initial findings: Well-being of the non-reserve Aboriginal population.* Ottawa, ON: Author. Retrieved from http://www.statcan.gc.ca/pub/89-589-x/pdf/4228565-eng.pdf; Truth and Reconciliation Commission of Canada. (2015). *The survivors speak.* Ottawa: Author. Retrieved from http://www.trc.ca/websites/trcinstitution/File/2015/ Findings/Survivors_Speak_2015_05_30_web_o.pdf; Aboriginal Healing Foundation. (2010). *FAQs.* Retrieved from http://www.ahf.ca/faqs.

eligible for social security benefits such as old age security until they have lived in Canada for at least 10 years. After 10 years of residence, immigrants who are aged 65 years or older are entitled to partial social security benefits (Government of Canada, 2017) (see Chapter 22).

Barriers to accessing health care that may be experienced by ethnic-minority older persons include language barriers, cultural values and beliefs that can influence the seeking of health care, the lack of interpretation services, the absence of ethno-specific programs, and the lack of health care providers who understand the culture (Guruge, Thomson, & Seifi, 2015; Koehn, 2009; Lai & Surood, 2013). A study in Calgary found that older South Asian immigrants who experienced more barriers to accessing health care had worse physical and mental health (Lai & Surood, 2013) (Box 4.2).

REDUCING HEALTH DISPARITIES

Policies and practices that improve access to health care are important. However, reducing health disparities requires action and attention to the underlying causes of health disparities and determinants of health. Policies and practices related to socioeconomic status and poverty can have significant impacts on health. For example, Canadian income protection and pension policies have resulted in a decrease in poverty among older Canadians, from 21% in 1980 to a low of 7% in 2003 (NACA, 2005). The poverty rate among older persons has been increasing and is currently 12.1%; the rate is higher (28%) among older persons who are living alone (Statistics Canada, 2014). Political will is required to address ethnocultural determinants of health and health inequities. A national strategy consistent with the principles

---

BOX 4.2   Research for Evidence-Informed Practice: Older Members of Ethnic Minorities Face Barriers to Accessing Health Care

Problem: While it is known that members of ethnic minorities face barriers to accessing health care, little is known about how older members of ethnic minorities in Canada access health care. These older persons face the double disadvantage of a having greater need for health services and facing more barriers to accessing those services than older persons of the majority population face.

Methods: This study was a telephone-administered survey of South Asian immigrants aged 55 years and older in Calgary, Alberta. Participants were randomly selected from a list of potential participants identified by surname in the telephone directory. Two hundred and twenty people took part in a 45-minute telephone interview. They completed a questionnaire about physical and mental health and were asked about their experiences with 21 possible barriers to accessing health services.

Findings: The average number of barriers encountered was 5.9. The most commonly encountered barriers were long waiting lists; lack of knowledge about existing health services; health care providers who were too busy;

administrative procedures that were too complicated; and health care providers who did not speak the person's language or understand their culture. Those who encountered more barriers reported having worse physical and mental health. When other variables were statistically controlled for using multiple regression analysis, personal attitudes such as "feeling ashamed, feeling uncomfortable with asking for help, and not believing that professionals can help" were independently associated with health and mental health.

Application to Nursing Practice: The findings indicated that barriers to accessing health services were common for older members of ethnic minorities. Personal attitudes and beliefs can be a barrier to using services and can have an impact on health. The authors describe these attitudes as being related to the older person's culture and to a lack of understanding of the services. Other barriers, such as linguistically and culturally incompatible services, may influence attitudes toward service use. Nurses should be aware of the barriers that older adult members of ethnic minorities face in accessing health care.

Source: Lai, D., & Surood, S. (2013). Effect of service barriers on health status of aging South Asian immigrants in Calgary, Canada. *Health and Social Work, 38*(1), 41–50. doi:10.1093/hsw/hls065.

---

of primary health care is being called for to address older persons' determinants of health (Alliance for a National Seniors Strategy, 2016).

Health care providers should be aware of barriers to accessing health care and should possess cultural competence. The objective is not just to become competent but to become culturally proficient—that is, able to move smoothly between the world of the nurse and the world of the older person being cared for. Moving toward culturally proficient gerontological nursing care is an important strategy to reduce health disparities and increase accessibility.

INCREASING CULTURAL COMPETENCE

As nurses move toward cultural competence, they increase their cultural awareness, knowledge, and skills. Nurses can become aware of their personal biases, prejudices, attitudes, and behaviours toward persons different from themselves in race, ethnicity, age, sex, gender, sexual orientation, social class, economic situation, and many other factors. Through

increased knowledge, nurses can better assess the strengths and weaknesses of older persons within the context of their culture and know when and how to effectively intervene to support rather than hinder cultural patterns that enhance wellness and coping. Cultural competence means having the skills to put cultural knowledge to use in assessment, communication, negotiation, and intervention.

CULTURAL AWARENESS

Increased awareness calls for openness and self-reflection. A White nurse needs to realize that this whiteness means having special privileges and freedoms in a predominantly White society. Older persons who are members of an ethnocultural or visible minority group may not have had the same advantages or experiences as the nurse. For example, many older Indigenous Canadians experienced the residential school system (see Box 4.1), and many older Canadians who are members of a visible minority group may have experienced racism and discrimination. Racism itself is an important determinant of health (Edge & Newbold, 2013). Immigrants and members of visible minority groups also experience racism in the current Canadian health care system (Edge & Newbold, 2013; Hyman & Meinhard, 2016). Many older gay and lesbian persons have also experienced lifelong stigmatization and discrimination, both of which were also experienced within the health care system (Brotman et al., 2015).

Being culturally aware means recognizing the presence of "isms," such as racism. It is imperative to understand how these "isms" affect not only the pursuing and receiving of health care but also the quality of life for older persons. Moreover, as older persons, they may have to face ageism in addition to racism, sexism, classism, and other forms of discrimination.

The term *ageism* refers to discrimination and negative **stereotypes** that are based solely on age. Ageism is not universal but is most often reflective of Euro-American culture. In many other cultures, older people are treated with special respect and honour. For example, in Indigenous cultures, older people are respected and have an important role in maintaining and transmitting cultural practices (see Chapter 23).

Some health care providers demonstrate ageism, undoubtedly in part because these providers tend to see many frail older persons and fewer older people who are healthy and active. Ageism has been described as commonplace in health care (Centre for Addiction and Mental Health, 2008) and limits access to health services for older people. The experience of age discrimination is associated with psychological distress (Ferraro, 2014).

Before the gerontological nurse provides quality care to older people from ethnic or cultural backgrounds that are different from his or her own, it is useful for the nurse to self-reflect and consider whether he or she holds any personal beliefs about such persons, how these beliefs affect the providing of care, and whether these beliefs are based on facts rather than anecdotes.

CULTURAL KNOWLEDGE

Cultural knowledge is both what the nurse brings to a caring situation and what the nurse learns about older persons, their families, their communities, their behaviours, and their expectations. Essential knowledge includes knowledge of the person's way of life (i.e., ways of thinking, believing, and acting). This knowledge is obtained formally and informally through the individual's professional experience of nursing.

Some nurses prefer what can be called an "encyclopedic" approach to the details of a particular culture or ethnic group, such details as proper name usage, touch, greeting, eye contact, gender roles, foods, and beliefs about relevant topics (e.g., health-promoting practices, expression of pain, end-of-life rituals, and caregiving). This information is available in many compendiums of cross-cultural information (see the Resources section at the end of this chapter and at http://evolve.elsevier.com/Canada/Ebersole/gerontological/). When the nurse works with older persons from specific cultures, it is especially important for the nurse to know about their attitudes toward caregiving, decision making, and end-of-life rituals.

Although cultural knowledge is helpful and essential, caution must be used with regard to the potential for stereotyping. In *stereotyping,* limited knowledge about one person with specific characteristics is applied to other persons with the same characteristics; negative characteristics are especially prone to this treatment. Stereotyping limits recognition of the heterogeneity of the group. Relying on a positive stereotype can be useful as a starting point in understanding, but it can also be used to limit understanding of the uniqueness of the individual and impose unrealistic expectations. For example, a common way to stereotype older members of ethnic minority groups is to assume that religious organizations are a source of support to them or that adult children will be responsible for providing care at home. The nurse's assumption can easily have a negative outcome, such as fewer referrals for other forms of support (e.g., home-delivered meals, home care services, or respite care) or inadequate discharge planning.

Persons from a specific ethnocultural group may share a common geographical origin, migratory status, race, language or dialect, or religion. Traditions, symbols, literature, folklore, food preferences, and dress are expressions of ethnicity that are often adopted. This may be particularly true for older persons who have had no need to leave their culture-specific neighbourhoods. Persons who identify with the same ethnic group may or may not be of the same race. For example, persons who consider themselves Latin Americans are members of a diverse ethnic group and may be of any race and from any one of a number of countries. However, those who consider themselves Latin Americans usually have in common the Catholic religion and the Spanish language.

Health beliefs and practices are usually a mixed expression of life experience and cultural knowledge. In most cultures, older persons are likely to treat themselves for familiar or chronic conditions in ways they have found successful in the past, practices that are referred to as domestic medicine, **folk medicine**, or folk healing. Much folk medicine is based on making the most of whatever is available.

The culture of nursing and health care in Canada advocates what is called the "Western" or "biomedical" system, which has its own set of beliefs about the cause of illness, the choice of treatments, and so on. In most settings, this belief system is considered superior to all others, an ethnocentric viewpoint. However, many of the world's people have different beliefs, such as belief in a personalistic (magico-religious) system or a naturalistic (holistic) system. Each system is complete, with beliefs about disease causation and with recommendations for prevention and treatment. Nurses who are familiar with the range of health beliefs and realize the importance of those beliefs to the followers will be able to provide more sensitive and appropriate care. In the absence of understanding lies a great potential for conflict. This is especially important to remember when working with "ethnic immigrants" or with those who have lived in culturally homogeneous communities.

Western or Biomedical System

In the Western or biomedical belief system, disease is thought to be the result of abnormalities in the structure and function of body organs and systems, often caused by an invasion of germs. The terms *disease* and *illness* are subjective; they are used by health care providers and are not always understood by others. In the biomedical system, assessment and diagnosis are directed at identifying the pathogen or the processes causing the abnormality, using laboratory and other investigative procedures. Treatment consists of removing or destroying the invading organism, or

repairing, modifying, or removing the affected body part. In this belief system, prevention involves the avoidance of pathogens, chemicals, activities, and dietary agents known to cause abnormalities. Health has traditionally been considered the absence of disease, but Western conceptions of health are now more holistic (see Chapter 1).

Personalistic or Magico-Religious System

Those who follow the tenets of a personalistic or magico-religious system believe that illness is caused by the actions of supernatural entities such as gods or deities or by nonhuman beings such as ghosts, ancestors, or spirits. Health is viewed as a blessing or reward from God, and illness is seen as a punishment for breaching rules, breaking a taboo, or displeasing or failing to please the source of power. These beliefs may be more prevalent in the explaining of altered mental states, such as psychosis and dementia, and may influence the seeking of care for older persons with dementia. Personalistic or magico-religious systems are more common in certain cultures (for example, those of rural India) (Jiloha & Kukreti, 2016). Belief that illness and disease are caused by the wrath of God is prevalent among members of the Fundamentalist Baptist, Holiness, and Pentecostal churches. Examples of magical causes to which illness can be attributed are voodoo, hexing, and the "evil eye." Treatments may include religious practices such as praying, meditating, fasting, wearing amulets, burning candles, and establishing family altars.

Making sure that social networks of fellow humans are in good working order is viewed as the essence of prevention. It is therefore important to avoid angering a person's family, friends, neighbours, ancestors, and gods. This belief system can be traced back thousands of years to the ancient Egyptians and persists in its entirety or in parts in many groups. Current practices include rituals such as prayer circles and the "laying on of hands." In this context, it is not uncommon to hear an older person pray for a cure or ask, "What did I do to cause this?"

Naturalistic or Holistic Health System

The naturalistic or holistic health belief system is based on the concept of balance and stems from the ancient civilizations of China, India, and Greece

(Wang & Paulanka, 2008). Many people throughout the world view health as a sign of balance—the right amount of exercise, food, sleep, evacuation, interpersonal relationships, or the balance of the geophysical and metaphysical forces in the universe (e.g., chi). Disturbances in this balance result in disharmony and subsequent illness. Diagnosis calls for the determination of the type and extent of imbalance. The appropriate interventions, therefore, are methods of restoring balance and harmony.

Traditional Chinese medicine is based on belief in the balance between yin and yang, darkness and light, and hot and cold. Older persons who were raised in one of the Pacific Rim countries (especially in Asia and the Pacific islands) or in a traditional Indigenous community frequently rely on these beliefs. The naturalistic system practised in India and some of its neighbouring countries is known as Ayurveda. Another such system is practised by those who follow hot-cold beliefs apart from traditional Chinese medicine; illness is believed to be the result of excess heat or cold that has entered the body and caused an imbalance. Hot and cold are generally metaphoric, although actual temperature is sometimes an aspect. Various foods, medicines, environmental conditions, emotions, and body conditions such as menopause may possess the characteristics of either hot or cold (Spector, 2004).

Selecting an appropriate treatment requires the identification of disease type—either hot or cold. Treatments are likewise divided, focused on using the opposite element; disease resulting from excess heat is treated with something that has cold properties, and vice versa. The treatments may take the form of teas, herbs, food, dietary restrictions, or medications (such as antibiotics) and therapies from Western medicine that have hot and cold properties, such as massage, poultices, cupping, or other therapies.

Naturalistic healers can be physicians, advanced-practice nurses, or herbalists who specialize in symptomatic treatment and know which medicines will restore the body's equilibrium. Provincial nursing regulatory bodies offer nurses guidance in providing complementary therapies (College & Association of Registered Nurses of Alberta, 2011). In Indigenous cultures, the healer is referred to as a medicine man or woman who combines naturalistic and magico-religious systems. Prevention is directed at protecting oneself from imbalance.

CULTURAL SKILLS

Skillful cross-cultural nursing entails mutual respect between the nurse and the older person; it means working *with* the patient rather than *on* the patient. Providing the highest quality of care for ethnically diverse older people and enhancing healthy aging calls for a refined set of knowledge and skills, including listening carefully to the person (especially for his or her perception of the situation) and attending not just to the words but also to the nonverbal communications and the meanings behind the stories. As well, the nurse needs to be able to hear the older person's desired goals and ideas for treatment. Cultural skills required in gerontological nursing include the nurse's ability to explain his or her perceptions clearly and without judgement, acknowledging that there are both similarities and differences between the nurse's perceptions and goals and those of the older person. Finally, cross-cultural skills include the ability to develop a plan of action that takes both perspectives into account and negotiates an outcome that is mutually acceptable (Berlin & Fowkes, 1983).

Working With Interpreters

Working with persons in a cross-cultural nursing situation often includes working with an **interpreter**. *Interpretation* is the process of rendering oral expressions made in one language system into another in a manner that preserves the meaning and tone of the original without adding or deleting anything. The job of the interpreter is to work with two different linguistic codes in a way that will produce equivalent messages. The interpreter tells the older person what the nurse has said and tells the nurse what the older person has said, without adding any extra meaning or opinion, in a way in which communication is as accurate as possible. This is often confused with *translation* (when interpreters are called **translators**), which instead deals with the written word.

Although called for at all times, respectful communication is essential when the nurse works with people with limited or no English proficiency and with older persons from cultures in which respectful communication is the norm. Respectful communication includes addressing the person in the appropriate manner (with surname unless otherwise instructed by the person) and using acceptable body language. For example, people from most cultures other than those of northern Europe (including European Americans) consider direct eye contact to be disrespectful. To press for eye contact with an older person may be particularly rude.

An interpreter is needed when the nurse and the older person speak different languages, when the person has limited English proficiency, or when cultural tradition prevents the person from speaking directly to the nurse (for example, as a result of the nurse's being of a specific gender). The more complex the decision to be made (such as when determining the person's wishes regarding life-prolonging measures or the family's plan for caregiving), the more important the skills of the interpreter are. Whenever possible, it is ideal to engage persons who are trained in medical interpretation and who are of the same age, gender, and social status as the older person. Unfortunately, it is usually necessary to call on younger interpreters; the effectiveness of the exchange may be hampered by intergenerational boundaries. Children and grandchildren are often called on to act as interpreters. In this situation, the nurse may realize that the child or the older person is "editing" comments because of cultural restrictions about the sharing of certain information (i.e., what is or is not considered appropriate to speak of to an older person or to a child).

When working with an interpreter, the nurse should first introduce herself or himself to the patient and the interpreter and set the guidelines for the interview. Sentences should be short, employ the active voice, and avoid metaphors, as they may be impossible to convert from one language to another. The nurse asks the interpreter to articulate exactly what is being said, and all conversation is addressed directly to the older person. For more information on the use of an interpreter, see Box 4.3.

IMPLICATIONS FOR GERONTOLOGICAL NURSING AND HEALTHY AGING

The contact between older persons and gerontological nurses often begins with a story and an assessment.

BOX 4.3	Working With Interpreters

- Meet with the interpreter before an interview or session with an older person, to explain the purpose of the session.
- Encourage the interpreter to meet with the older person before the session in order to determine the person's educational level and attitudes toward health and health care and to determine the depth and type of information and explanation needed.
- Look and speak directly to the older person, not to the interpreter.
- Be patient. Interpreted interviews take more time because long, explanatory phrases are often needed.
- Use short units of speech. Long, involved sentences or complex discussions create confusion.
- Use simple language. Avoid technical terms, professional jargon, slang, abbreviations, abstractions, metaphors, and idiomatic expressions.
- Encourage interpretation of the person's own words rather than paraphrased professional jargon to get a better sense of the patient's ideas and emotional state.
- Request that the interpreter avoid inserting his or her own ideas and avoid omitting information.
- Listen to the older person and be aware of nonverbal communications (facial expression, voice intonation, body movement) to learn about his or her emotions regarding a specific topic.
- Clarify the older person's understanding and the accuracy of the interpretation by asking the person to tell you what he or she understands, facilitated by the interpreter.

Source: Adapted from Enslein, J., Tripp-Reimer, T., Kelley, L. S., et al. (2002). Evidence-based protocol: Interpreter facilitation for individuals with limited English proficiency. *Journal of Gerontological Nursing, 28*(7), 5–13.

During this process, the nurse and older person have an opportunity to get to know each other. Listening is key to the assessment; the nurse needs to try to understand the meaning of the situation and the person's perception of it. A thorough assessment includes a cultural assessment. A comprehensive assessment takes time. Not all situations allow for this, but even if the assessment is done bit by bit over time, it will give the nurse a better understanding of how to work with and within the person's culture.

Several tools or instruments can assist the nurse in eliciting health care beliefs and help the nurse identify

---

BOX 4.4 **Explanatory Model for Culturally Sensitive Assessment**

1. How would you describe the problem that has brought you here? (*What do you call your problem? Does it have a name?*)
   a. Who is involved in your decision making about health concerns?
2. How long have you had this problem?
   a. When do you think it started?
   b. What do you think started it?
   c. Do you know anyone else with it?
   d. Tell me what happened to that person when dealing with this problem.
3. What do you think is wrong with you?
   a. How severe is it?
   b. How long do you think it will last?
4. Why do you think this happened to you?
   a. Why has it happened to the involved part?
   b. What do you fear most about your sickness?
5. What are the chief problems your sickness has caused you?
6. What do you think will help clear up this problem? (*What treatment should you receive? What are the most important results you hope to receive?*) (If specific tests or medications are listed, ask what they are and what they do.)
7. Apart from me, who else do you think can make you feel better?
   a. Are there therapies *(maybe in another discipline)* I do not know about that make you feel better?

Source: Adapted from Kleinman, A. (1980). *Patient and healers in the context of culture: An exploration of the borderland between anthropology, medicine, and psychiatry.* Berkeley, CA: University of California Press; Pfeifferling, J. H. (1981). A cultural prescription for mediocentrism. In Eisenberg, L., & Kleinman, A. (Eds.), *The relevance of social science for medicine.* Boston: Reidel.

BOX 4.5 **The LEARN Model**

L Listen carefully to what the older person is saying. Attend not just to the words but also to the nonverbal communication and to the meaning of the stories. Listen to the person's perception of the situation, desired goals, and ideas for treatment.
E Explain your perception of the situation and problems.
A Acknowledge and discuss both the similarities and the differences between your perceptions and goals and those of the older person.
R Recommend a plan of action that takes both perspectives into account.
N Negotiate a plan that is mutually acceptable.

Source: Adapted from Berlin, E. A., & Fowkes, W. C. (1983). A teaching framework for cross-cultural health care: Application in family practice. *Western Journal of Medicine, 139*(6), 934–938.

---

his or her own perceptions of alternative beliefs. Although Leininger's Sunrise Model (Shen, 2004; Schim et al., 2007) is often recommended, alternative models may be more useful in today's fast-paced health care situations. The explanatory model developed by Kleinman, Eisenberg, and Good (1978) has become a classic and has helped nurses and other health care providers obtain the basic information needed in a culturally sensitive manner. An adaptation of this model that is used to obtain a meaningful cultural health assessment appears in Box 4.4. Use of the LEARN Model (Berlin & Fowkes, 1983) can increase the effectiveness of nursing interventions. It is a helpful guide for nurses in the clinical setting. Through its use, the nurse can increase his or her cultural sensitivity and provide more culturally competent care, thus helping to reduce health disparities (Box 4.5).

With an understanding of basic cross-cultural communication and assessment, the nurse can reach a clear understanding of problems and solutions with the older person or the older person's identified support figure. The nurse may then need to include consultation or collaboration with traditional or alternative healers if the older person believes this is important. Religious leaders or Indigenous healers may provide essential consultation, support, and interventions of their own. Supporting cultural beliefs and practices conveys a sense of caring, and unbiased caring can surmount cultural differences.

Also critical to the cultural assessment is determining the person's health beliefs, as discussed earlier. Most people (nurses and patients alike) subscribe to more than one belief system, combining Western biomedical approaches with those that may be considered more culturally traditional. People choose among the health belief systems or include aspects of several of them in an attempt to make sense of health, illness, and treatment. To optimize the healthy aging of the person who depends on the nurse for care, the nurse must be sensitive to the possibility that the person may hold one or more of these beliefs. When a patient refuses biomedical treatment because the health problem is viewed as destiny or as God's will, it is often particularly difficult for the nurse and other health care providers. Finding out more about the person's beliefs about the cause of disease and the type of treatments he or she believes are appropriate will allow the nurse to navigate the cultures of the health care establishment and of the patient in order to promote better health.

Nurses should not attempt to change the person's beliefs. This is difficult, if not impossible, and usually counterproductive, particularly when working with older persons who carry a lifetime of beliefs and illness experience. However, negotiating health, treatment, or prevention options can be helpful. The nurse can attempt to preserve helpful beliefs and practices, accommodate beliefs that are neither helpful nor harmful, or help patients give up beliefs or practices that have been shown to be harmful. The nurse who has little or no knowledge of the specific belief or practice will need to study and evaluate the belief or practice to determine its helpfulness or potential harm. In this way, beliefs and practices can be preserved whenever possible. The nurse's respectfully explaining concern about potentially harmful practices, along with offering possible alternatives, may show the person that the nurse is considering the person's preferences. When care is provided in the home, nurses must adapt home care strategies to the beliefs and culture of the patient and family if they hope to promote healthy aging and wellness. Special attention should be given to caregivers who are conflicted about their acculturated beliefs in respect to long-term care homes, work-caregiver demands, and expectations of the role of the adult child. Nurses need to work with the person's family in attempting to find a solution to cross-cultural and intergenerational conflicts in caregiving and health care settings. The nurse must also focus on the older person's overall health and help the person and family gain access to needed services. To do this, the nurse needs to ascertain the following: (1) affordability, efficacy, accessibility, and availability of services; (2) satisfaction with services; (3) availability of information; (4) perspective on illness; and (5)

informal support systems. Respect for the person's health beliefs is paramount.

CROSS-CULTURAL CARING AND LONG-TERM CARE

Long-term care (LTC) refers to ongoing assistance to persons who are physically or mentally fragile and unable to independently meet their basic needs (see Chapter 26). In many cultures outside of North America and in some subcultures in Canada, families have traditionally been expected to take care of their older members. Thus, institutional LTC has been used less often with these families than with families of European descent. Institutional LTC takes place in hospices and LTC homes and through assisted living and respite care. The preference for where care is received is influenced by culture, economic resources, and the availability of ethnoculturally specific services. Furthermore, as recognized in the *Gerontological Nursing Competencies and Standards of Practice*, providing relationship care (Standard IV) requires that nurses appreciate the influence of culture on how families and health care providers provide care in LTC homes (Canadian Gerontological Nursing Association, 2010, Chapter 2).

Senior and community centres provide a type of ongoing LTC, most of it social in nature. Many centres attract primarily long-term community members; rarely do they provide a service or a setting that is welcoming to other groups, such as new immigrants. By contrast, the On Lok program in San Francisco is a model for the provision of LTC services to diverse older persons (see Chapter 26). Originally designed to meet the home care needs of Chinese and Italian immigrants, it now has the capacity to provide every level of short- and long-term care to the diverse population of San Francisco. Services are provided in the language of the older person and in a manner that optimizes each person's cultural heritage (Kornblatt, Eng, & Hansen, 2003). In Canada, some ethno-specific LTC homes are available in larger cities, but like most LTC homes, the number of beds available does not meet demand (Um, 2016). Ethno-specific LTC homes may also be less accessible in smaller communities, although ethno-specific health and social services for older persons are increasingly available in larger cities. Nurses can learn from the work of On Lok and other programs to enhance care and encourage the health of ethnically diverse older persons.

On Lok and other programs have found that the well-being of ethnically diverse older persons is enhanced by modifying existing LTC services through the following:

1. Ensuring that residents have access to professional interpreter services if needed
2. Developing programs that reflect the diversity of the residents and staff
3. Considering monocultural facilities or units when population demographics warrant
4. Attempting to employ staff that reflects the diversity of the residents or participants

The study of the uniqueness of each older person is one of the most complex and intriguing fields of the present day. Realistically, it is almost impossible for nurses to become familiar with the whole range of clinically relevant cultural differences that may be encountered among older persons. Nonetheless, caring for older persons holistically and sensitively can be the most challenging and potentially satisfying opportunity for nurses who work in a variety of settings.

KEY CONCEPTS

- Population diversity will continue to increase rapidly for many years. Thus, nurses will be caring for a greater number of ethnoculturally diverse older persons than in the past.
- Recent research has revealed significant and persistent disparities in the outcomes of health for persons from minority groups, and members of these groups will bear the burden of morbidity and mortality in most areas.
- Nurses can contribute to the reduction of health disparities through increasing their own cultural awareness, knowledge, and skills.
- Negative stereotyping is never appropriate.
- Cultural awareness, knowledge, and skills are necessary to increase cultural competence.
- Nurses caring for ethnoculturally diverse older persons must be aware of and let go of their own ethnocentrism before they can give effective care.
- Ethnoculturally diverse older persons may hold health beliefs different from those of the biomedical or Western medicine used by most health care providers in Canada.
- Lack of awareness of the older person's health beliefs can produce conflict in the nursing situation.
- The more complex the communication or decision-making needs in a given situation, the greater the need for skilled interpreter services for persons with limited English proficiency.
- Programs staffed by persons who reflect the ethnocultural background of the participants and speak their language may be preferred by older people.
- The explanatory model and the LEARN model provide a useful framework for working with older people of any ethnocultural background.

ACTIVITIES AND DISCUSSION QUESTIONS

1. Discuss your personal beliefs regarding health and illness and how they fit into the three major classifications of health systems. How can this knowledge affect culturally competent care for ethnoculturally diverse older persons?
2. Explain the types of questions that would be helpful in assessing an older person's health problems or challenges in a way that is respectful of the person and his or her cultural background and ethnic identity.
3. Propose strategies that would be helpful in planning care for older persons from different ethnocultural backgrounds.
4. Identify sensitive areas in which discussion is frequently needed with older persons, and suggest how these areas would be affected by differences in the cultural backgrounds of the patient and the nurse.
5. After speaking with some of your own older family members, discuss your familial and culturally determined views of aging.

RESOURCES

General

Canadian Nurses Association. *Position statement: Promoting cultural competence in nursing*
https://www.cna-aiic.ca/~/media/cna/page-content/pdf-en/ps114_cultural_competence_2010_e.pdf?la=en

Health Canada. *Reaching out: A guide to communicating with Aboriginal seniors*
http://publications.gc.ca/collections/Collection/H88-3-20-1998E.pdf

Registered Nurses Association of Ontario (RNAO). *Embracing cultural diversity in health care: Developing cultural competence*
http://rnao.ca/bpg/guidelines/embracing-cultural-diversity-health-care-developing-cultural-competence

Stanford Geriatric Education Center: A repository of reputable information related to cultural knowledge, including a core curriculum for ethnogeriatrics, online modules, and resources.
http://sgec.stanford.edu

University of Victoria. *Cultural safety learning modules*
http://web2.uvcs.uvic.ca/courses/csafety/mod1/index.htm

http://web2.uvcs.uvic.ca/courses/csafety/mod2/notes4.htm

http://web2.uvcs.uvic.ca/courses/csafety/mod3/

Winnipeg Regional Health Authority. *Guide to health and social services for Aboriginal people in Manitoba*
http://www.wrha.mb.ca/aboriginalhealth/services/files/AHSGuide.pdf

Residential Schools
Aboriginal Healing Foundation
http://www.ahf.ca/about-us

The survivors speak: A report of the Truth and Reconciliation Commission of Canada
http://www.trc.ca/websites/trcinstitution/File/2015/Findings/Survivors_Speak_2015_05_30_web_o.pdf

Where are the children: Healing the legacy of residential schools. Multimedia resource
http://www.wherearethechildren.ca/en/

For additional resources, please visit *http://evolve.elsevier.com/Canada/Ebersole/gerontological/*

REFERENCES

Aboriginal Healing Foundation. (2010). *FAQs*. Retrieved from http://www.ahf.ca/faqs.

Alliance for a National Seniors Strategy. (2016). *An evidence-informed national seniors strategy for Canada* (2nd ed.). Toronto, ON: Author. Retrieved from: http://www.nationalseniorsstrategy.ca/wp-content/uploads/2015/01/National-Seniors-Strategy-Second-Edition.pdf.

Assembly of First Nations. (2016). *Indian residential schools annual report*. Retrieved from http://www.afn.ca/en/policy-areas/indian-residential-schools.

Beatty, B. B., & Berdahl, L. (2011). Health care and Aboriginal seniors in urban Canada: Helping a neglected class. *International Indigenous Policy Journal, 2*(1), article 10. doi:10.18584/iipj.2011.2.1.10.

Beiser, M., & Stewart, M. (2005). Reducing health disparities: A priority for Canada. *Canadian Journal of Public Health, 96*(Suppl. 2), S4–S5. Retrieved from http://ir.lib.uwo.ca/iipj/.

Berlin, E. A., & Fowkes, W. C. (1983). A teaching framework for cross-cultural health care: Application in family practice. *Western Journal of Medicine, 139*(6), 934–938.

Brotman, S., Ferrer, I., Sussman, T., et al. (2015). Access and equity in the design and delivery of health and social care to LGBTQ older adults: A Canadian perspective. In N. A. Orel & C. A. Fruhauf (Eds.), *The lives of LGBT older adults: Understanding challenges and resilience* (pp. 111–140). Washington, DC: American Psychological Association.

Cameron, B. L., Plazas, M. P. C., Salas, A. S., et al. (2014). Understanding inequalities in access to health care services for Aboriginal people: A call for nursing action. *Advances in Nursing Science, 37*(3), E1–E16. doi:10.1097/ANS.0000000000000039.

Canadian Gerontological Nursing Association (2010). *Gerontological nursing competencies and standards of practice*. Vancouver, BC: Author.

Centre for Addiction and Mental Health. (2008). *Improving our response to older adults with substance use, mental health and gambling problems: A guide for supervisors, managers and clinical staff*. Toronto, ON: Author.

College & Association of Registered Nurses of Alberta. (2011). *Complementary and/or alternative therapy and natural health products: Standards for Registered Nurses*. Edmonton, AB: Author. Retrieved from http://www.nurses.ab.ca/content/dam/carna/pdfs/DocumentList/Standards/RN_CompAltTherapy_Jan2011.pdf.

Dewing, M., & Leman, M. (2006). *Current issue review: Canadian multiculturalism*. Ottawa, ON: Library of Parliament, Parliamentary Research Branch. Retrieved from http://www2.parl.gc.ca/content/lop/researchpublications/936-e.pdf.

Edge, S., & Newbold, B. (2013). Discrimination and the health of immigrants and refugees: Exploring Canada's evidence base and directions for future research in newcomer receiving countries. *Immigrant Minority Health, 15*, 141–148. doi:10.1007/s10903-012-9640-4.

Ferraro, F. R. (2014). Ageism in US and Canadian samples. *International Journal of Psychology Research, 9*(2), 85–90. https://www.novapublishers.com/catalog/product_info.php?products_id=4634.

Gee, E. M., Kobayashi, K. M., & Prus, S. (2007). *Ethnic inequality in Canada: Economic and health dimension*. Hamilton, ON: Social and Economic Dimensions of an Aging Population (SEDAP). Retrieved from http://socserv.mcmaster.ca/sedap/p/sedap182.pdf.

Government of Canada. (2017). *Support for senior citizens*. Retrieved from http://www.cic.gc.ca/english/newcomers/before-rights -seniors.asp.

Guruge, S., Thomson, M. S., & Seifi, S. G. (2015). Mental health and service issues faced by older immigrants in Canada: A scoping review. *Canadian Journal on Aging, 34*, 431–444. doi:10.1017/ S0714980815000379.

Health Disparities Task Group of the Federal/Provincial/Territorial Advisory Committee on Populations Health and Health Security. (2004). *Reducing health disparities—Roles of the health sector: Discussion paper*. Ottawa: Public Health Agency of Canada. Retrieved from http://www.phac-aspc.gc.ca/ph-sp/ disparities/ddp-eng.php.

Hyman, I., & Meinhard, A. (2016). Public policy, immigrant experiences, and health outcomes in Canada. In D. Raphael (Ed.), *Immigration, public policy, and health: Newcomer experiences in developed nations* (pp. 97–132). Toronto, ON: Canadian Scholars' Press.

Jiloha, R. C., & Kukreti, P. (2016). Caregivers as the fulcrum of care for mentally ill in the community: The urban rural divide among caregivers and care facilities. *Indian Journal of Social Psychiatry, 32*(1), 35–39. doi:10.4103/0971-9962 .176765.

Kleinman, A., Eisenberg, L., & Good, B. (1978). Culture, illness, and care: Clinical lessons from anthropologic and cross-cultural research. *Annals of Internal Medicine, 88*(2), 251–258. doi:10 .7326/0003-4819-88-2-251.

Kobayashi, K. M., & Prus, S. G. (2012). Examining the gender, ethnicity, and age dimensions of the healthy immigrant effect: Factors in the development of equitable health policy. *International Journal for Equity in Health, 11*, 8. Retrieved from http:// www.equityhealthj.com/content/11/1/8.

Koehn, S. (2009). Negotiating candidacy: Ethnic minority seniors' access to care. *Ageing & Society, 29*, 585–608. doi:10.1017/ S0144686X08007952.

Kornblatt, S., Eng, C., & Hansen, J. C. (2003). Cultural awareness in health and social services: The experience of On Lok. *Generations (San Francisco, Calif.), 26*(3), 46–53.

Kymlicka, W. (2010). *The current state of multiculturalism in Canada*. Ottawa: Minister of Public Works and Government Services Canada. Retrieved from http://www.cic.gc.ca/english/ pdf/pub/multi-state.pdf.

Lai, D. W. L., & Surood, S. (2013). Effect of service barriers on health status of aging South Asian immigrants in Calgary, Canada. *Health & Social Work, 38*(1), 41–50. doi:10.1093/hsw/ hls065.

Lalonde, M. (1974). *A new perspective on the health of Canadians*. Ottawa, ON: Minister of Supply and Services Canada. Retrieved from http://www.phac-aspc.gc.ca/ph-sp/pdf/perspect-eng.pdf.

National Advisory Council on Aging (NACA). (2005). *Seniors on the margins: Aging in poverty in Canada*. Ottawa, ON: Public Health Agency of Canada. Retrieved from http:// dsp-psd.pwgsc.gc.ca/Collection/H88-5-3-2005E.pdf.

Ng, E. (2010). *Demographic and socio-economic profile of immigrant seniors in Canada*. Presentation at the Metropolis Policy-Research Seminar on Immigrant and Refugee Families, Children and Youth, and Seniors. Retrieved from http://canada.metropolis.net/events/metropolis_presents/ priority_seminar/presentations/ng_panel4_e.pdf.

Prus, S. G. (2011). Comparing social determinants of self-rated health across the United States and Canada. *Social Science & Medicine, 73*, 50–59. doi:10.1016/j.socscimed.2011.04.010.

Registered Nurses' Association of Ontario (RNAO). (2007). *Embracing cultural diversity in health care: Developing cultural competence*. Toronto, ON: Author. Retrieved from http:// www.rnao.org/Storage/29/2336_BPG_Embracing_Cultural _Diversity.pdf.

Schim, S. N., Doorenbos, A., Benkert, R., et al. (2007). Culturally congruent care: Putting the pieces together. *Journal of Transcultural Nursing, 18*(2), 57–62. doi:10.1177/1043659606298613.

Setia, M. S., Lynch, J., Abrahamowicz, M., et al. (2011). Self-rated health in Canadian immigrants: Analysis of the Longitudinal Survey of Immigrants to Canada. *Health and Place, 17*, 658–670. doi:10.1016/j.healthplace.2011.01.006.

Shen, Z. (2004). Cultural competence models in nursing: A selected annotated bibliography. *Journal of Transcultural Nursing, 15*(4), 317–322. doi:10.1177/1043659604268964.

Spector, R. E. (2004). *Cultural diversity in health and illness* (6th ed.). Upper Saddle River, NJ: Prentice-Hall Health.

Statistics Canada. (2004). *Aboriginal Peoples survey 2001: Initial findings: Well-being of the non-reserve Aboriginal population*. Ottawa, ON: Author. Retrieved from http://www.statcan.gc.ca/ pub/89-589-x/pdf/4228565-eng.pdf.

Statistics Canada. (2006). *A portrait of seniors in Canada 2006*. Ottawa, ON: Author. Retrieved from http://www.statcan.gc.ca/ pub/89-519-x/89-519-x2006001-eng.pdf.

Statistics Canada. (2010). Study: Projections of the diversity of the Canadian populations 2006 to 2031. *The Daily*, March 9. Retrieved from http://www.statcan.gc.ca/daily-quotidien/ 100309/dq100309a-eng.htm.

Statistics Canada. (2014). Canadian income survey, 2012. *The Daily*. Retrieved from http://www.statcan.gc.ca/daily-quotidien/ 141210/dq141210a-eng.pdf.

Statistics Canada. (2015a). *Linguistic characteristics of Canadians*. Retrieved from https://www12.statcan.gc.ca/census -recensement/2011/as-sa/98-314-x/98-314-x2011001-eng.cfm.

Statistics Canada. (2015b). *Detailed mother tongue (192), single and multiple language responses (3), age groups (7) and sex (3) for the population excluding institutional residents of Canada, provinces, territories, Census Divisions and Census Subdivisions, 2011 Census* (Catalogue number 98-314-XCB2011016). Retrieved from https://www12.statcan.gc.ca/census-recensement/2011/dp -pd/tbt-tt/Rp-eng.cfm?LANG=E&APATH=5&DETAIL=0 &DIM=0&FL=A&FREE=0&GC=4811061&GID=0&GK =3&GRP=0&PID=103251&PRID=0&PTYPE =101955&S=0&SHOWALL=0&SUB=0&Temporal =2011&THEME=90&VID=0&VNAMEE=&VNAMEF=.

Statistics Canada. (2016a). *Immigration and ethnocultural diversity in Canada*. Retrieved from http://www12.statcan.gc.ca/ nhs-enm/2011/as-sa/99-010-x/99-010-x2011001-eng.cfm#a4.

Statistics Canada. (2016b). *Aboriginal Peoples in Canada: First Nations People, Métis and Inuit*. Retrieved from http://

www12.statcan.gc.ca/nhs-enm/2011/as-sa/99-011-x/99-011-x2011001-eng.cfm.

Truth and Reconciliation Commission of Canada. (2015). *The survivors speak: A report of the Truth and Reconciliation Commission of Canada*. Ottawa, ON: Author. Retrieved from http://www.trc.ca/websites/trcinstitution/File/2015/Findings/Survivors_Speak_2015_05_30_web_o.pdf.

Um, S.-G. (2016). *Serving seniors better through equity and diversity in long-term care*. Retrieved from http://www.wellesleyinstitute.com/health/serving-seniors-better-through-equity-and-diversity-in-long-term-care/.

Wang, Y., & Paulanka, B. J. (2008). People of Chinese culture. In L. Purnell & B. J. Paulanka (Eds.), *Transcultural health care: A culturally competent approach* (pp. 129–144). Philadelphia, PA: FA Davis.

Nursing Documentation

LEARNING OBJECTIVES

Upon completion of this chapter, the reader will be able to:

- Describe the reasons for accurate and thorough documentation in gerontological nursing.
- Compare the major documentation methods used in acute care, residential and long-term care, and home care.
- Identify potential problems in documentation.
- Describe the responsibilities of the nurse in protecting the privacy of older people.
- Identify ways in which errors in documentation and communication are dangerous when older persons are being cared for.
- Identify ways to reduce the possibility of errors by making appropriate use of documentation when caring for older persons.

GLOSSARY

Activities of daily living (ADLs) Routine activities that people tend to do every day without needing assistance. There are six basic ADLs: eating, bathing, dressing, toileting, transferring (walking), and continence.

Minimum data set (MDS) The smallest number of a standardized data set that can be collected to identify essential, common, and core data elements of patients receiving nursing care.

Personal Health Information Protection Act (PHIPA) The *Personal Health Information Protection Act* of 2004 (revised in 2016), which legislates the handling of confidential patient information.

Resident Assessment Instrument (RAI) A standardized approach to examining quality of care and to improving regulation.

Resident Assessment Protocol (RAP) A reference to documents that form part of the Resident Assessment Instrument. The Resident Assessment Protocol provides a statement about the health problem; on the basis of that information, the minimum data set then triggers care planning.

THE LIVED EXPERIENCE

I was so happy to be able to make a big difference in Mrs. Jones's life. She was 97 and had grown slowly confused over the years. She was also profoundly hard of hearing. She spent the majority of time calling for "Mary," her deceased sister. We really could not communicate effectively with her; we could only show her that we cared and kept her safe. Eventually she became acutely ill, and a decision had to be made about CPR [cardiopulmonary resuscitation]. When we tried to find out what her wishes were, we could not immediately find any record of them, and she had no living relatives or friends, just an attorney. I searched and searched and finally found documentation about her wishes. We were able to provide her the comfort she wanted because of a nurse's careful documentation years before.

Kathleen, a gerontological nurse

DOCUMENTATION

Nursing documentation is a mandatory practice of making a permanent record of nursing actions, the patient's conditions, and the patient's responses to nursing actions or the actions of others (Canadian Nurses Association [CNA], 2010). All nurse-regulating bodies in Canada consider nursing documentation as a mandatory practice. If nurses perform a specific nursing act but fail to document the action, it will appear that the act was not performed.

Clinical documentation chronicles, supports, and communicates the condition of the person receiving care at all times. Appropriate and correct documentation will help the nurse identify, implement, monitor, and evaluate treatments or interventions. The recorded assessment provides the information needed for the careful development of individualized care plans and the tracking and evaluation of outcomes. Documentation also ensures that the patient continues to receive the care needed regardless of shifts, health care providers, and care settings. At the same time, documentation is the major means by which nurses demonstrate the quality of care they provide (Kelley, Brandon, & Docherty, 2011).

Detailed and accurate documentation is especially important in gerontological nursing. In the acute care setting, an older person is often seriously ill and at special risk for accidents, iatrogenic problems, and adverse reactions to interventions and treatments, because the normal changes of aging are superimposed on acute and complex health problems. Furthermore, most older persons will require care across care settings at some point. Continuity of care within care facilities and from one setting to another (e.g., hospital to home) is especially important and is possible only with careful documentation. In long-term care (LTC) homes, residential facilities, and home care, health care aides or unregulated workers supervised by registered nurses and by registered or licensed practical nurses provide most of the care. In these settings, documentation often serves as a basis for calculating the overall quality of care and for justifying funding for care resources.

In Canada, advance directives—collectively known as advanced care planning—fall under provincial and territorial jurisdictions (Fowler & Hammer, 2013) and

are documented in the health record (see Chapter 25). They are put in place for the benefit of a substitute decision maker from whom nurses have to receive consent if an older person cannot give his or her own consent. On June 17, 2016, the federal government passed Bill C-14, which outlines requirements that all patients must meet to be eligible to receive medical assistance in dying. Bill C-14 also "establishes safeguards that a doctor or nurse practitioner must follow to legally provide medical assistance in dying" (Ministry of Health and Long-Term Care [MOHLTC], 2017). Nursing records supplement this documentation with more details about patients' wishes, including who they want involved in their care and who they want to have access to their records, as well as the use of cardiopulmonary resuscitation (CPR) and the handling of their bodies after death. Older persons often discuss these wishes with nurses during conversations while receiving care. By recording these conversations in the nursing records, nurses are making sure that this important information can be shared with other members of the care team and that the older person's wishes are respected.

DOCUMENTATION ACROSS CARE SETTINGS

Documentation begins as soon as a person enters the health care system. Ongoing documentation provides not only the basis for care and the evaluation of any interventions and treatments but also the basis for providing care continuity when a person moves from one care setting to another (including the home). This chapter provides an overview of nursing documentation to optimize the care of vulnerable older people in a variety of care settings. A description of standardized assessment tools can be found in Chapter 13.

ACUTE CARE SETTING

Documentation in the acute care setting has undergone significant change in recent years. Computers and tables can be found at the bedside, in nurses' pockets, and at strategic locations on the unit. Individual patient and nurse bar codes are scanned both for access to records and for the administration of treatments and medications. The use of electronic checklists, flow sheets, and standardized tools has become the norm (see Chapter 13). In some settings, "lower-tech" approaches may still be used, and some documentation is manually completed in the form of notes in the clinical record.

Mandatory nursing documentation includes findings from the patient's assessment (usually with a checklist), identified nursing diagnoses, and care plans. When the nurse needs to document a particular event in the course of a patient's stay, a SOAP (Subjective, Objective, Assessment, Plan) note may be used. The subjective section of the note (also called the chief complaint) represents the patient's own words in regard to how he or she is feeling. The objective section includes data (related to the chief complaint) on what the nurse can measure, observe, see, feel, touch, or smell. The assessment is the result of the nurse's analysis of the patient's condition, considering both subjective and objective data. The care plan then includes those nursing interventions that have been completed or will be carried out to address the chief complaint. The education section includes the patient and family teaching that took place or is needed (Box 5.1). The SOAP approach is very useful for the succinct communication of information related to a specific problem. However, if the patient has multiple problems, as do many older persons, this form of documentation can be complicated and lengthy.

Other approaches to nursing documentation include the DARE (document Data, Action, Response,

and Evaluation) approach; FOCUS charting (which integrates narrative notes with the care plan and records relevant patient information in a systematic, accessible fashion) (College of Registered Nurses of British Columbia [CRNBC], 2017); the SBAR (Situation, Background, Assessment and Recommendation) approach; the IDRAW (Identify patient, Diagnosis, Recent changes, Anticipated changes, and What to watch for) approach; and narrative charting (nursing interventions and the impact of these interventions on patient outcomes, recorded in chronological order and covering a specific time frame) (CRNBC, 2017).

RESIDENTIAL CARE SETTINGS

In LTC homes, assisted living facilities, and retirement homes, documentation is generally done only if a nurse has been providing care to the older person. In retirement homes, nursing services are optional and are usually limited to the administration of medications and treatments or to assistance with **activities of daily living (ADLs)** by health care aides. Some health care aides are not allowed to document their care in the nursing record, as this is beyond their scope of practice; however, the level and type of documentation required varies by setting and by province or territory. If nurses chart on the health care aides' behalf, it is important that they follow their provincial professional regulatory organization's documentation guidelines for second-hand charting.

When older persons move to LTC homes, they often face challenges that are functional, cognitive, or both, and they may experience the onset or exacerbation of an acute or chronic problem. They are dependent on assistance for their ADLs (see Chapter 13).

Documentation in LTC homes encompasses the recording of day-to-day ADL care as well as vital signs, periodic assessment, medication and treatment administration, assessment of any unusual event or change in condition, and quarterly mandated comprehensive assessments. Documentation includes narrative progress notes, flow sheets, checklists, and mandated standardized and comprehensive instruments. Timely and correct documentation is a requirement for all registered and health care aides providing care. The nurse is ultimately responsible for the quality of care provided and for the completeness and accuracy of the documentation.

BOX 5.1 Example of a Subjective, Objective, Assessment, and Plan (SOAP) Note

S "I have to go to the toilet a lot, and when I urinate, it burns. ... It started last week and is getting worse." Denies history of urinary-tract infections.
O 72-year-old White female. Temp 99, pulse 94, blood pressure 140/86, respirations 18. Urine is dark yellow with strong foul odour, skin slightly damp, face flushed, abdomen tender.
A Altered elimination, elevated temperature, mild distress, possible infection.
P Call nurse practitioner with report. Provide treatment as prescribed. Ask patient to increase fluid intake, hourly. Check vital signs every 4 hours until resolved.

Resident Assessment Instrument

The **Resident Assessment Instrument (RAI)** is a standardized approach used to gather comprehensive assessment information on a person's functioning. The RAI consists of different **minimum data sets (MDS)**, each of which is specific to a care setting (e.g., LTC, home care, mental health). As of 2010, eight Canadian provinces and territories were using RAI-MDS version 2.0 in LTC homes (Hirdes et al., 2011). The core component of the MDS 2.0 enables the care team to assess multiple key domains such as function, health, social support, and service use. **Resident Assessment Protocols (RAPs)** are additional assessments that are completed depending on the information gleaned from the initial MDS 2.0 assessment. RAPs are structured, problem-oriented frameworks for the organization and direction of care. The RAP provides a statement about the health problem; on the basis of that information, the minimum data set then triggers care planning.

In most provinces and territories, nurses are responsible for the coordination of the MDS 2.0 within 14 days of a resident's admission, at quarterly intervals, and any time there is a significant change in the resident's status. The reassessments allow the care team to document and track the progress toward the resolution of identified problems and to make changes to the care plan as necessary. This type and level of documentation facilitates reliable and measurable communication and, when used properly, improves outcomes for residents (Hirdes et al., 2011). The resulting picture of the resident is as clear as possible. For persons who will benefit from active rehabilitation, the outcomes include discharge to a lower level of care. For persons whose condition is one of progressive decline, the RAI can lead to increased comfort and appropriate care. Although the MDS is completed in collaboration with all members of the care team, the nurse is responsible for verifying its accuracy and completion.

In Canada, MDS 2.0 data is subsequently submitted to the Continuing Care Reporting System database for ease of analysis and communication of patient profiles. This information is then shared with the Canadian Institute for Health Information to become part of an aggregate national database to conduct research to better respond to the needs of residents in Canadian LTC homes. This thorough assessment and documentation requirement in LTC is an attempt to improve and standardize the quality of care provided and to help LTC residents achieve the highest level of functioning and the highest quality of life possible.

HOME CARE

Personal care at home is often provided informally by family and friends (see Chapters 23 and 26); yet, the requisite professional care is provided through home visits from nurses, health care aides, occupational therapists, physiotherapists, or others. These services are delivered by provincial and territorial governments and, in some instances, by municipal governments (Coyte & McKeever, 2016). For example, Ontario's Local Health Integration Networks (LHINs) coordinate these services through Ontario's Ministry of Health and Long-Term Care (MOHLTC), while home care in Alberta is organized through Alberta Health Services.

Home care services utilize the RAI system to collect an MDS for home care clients and determine the care required. Clinical Assessment Protocols (CAPs), used for documenting assessments, inform and guide comprehensive care and service planning in the home care setting. These CAPs are intended as a companion resource for RAI-Home Care (R.A.I. Home Care, 2008). Family and other care partners often develop documentation systems of their own to track appointments, medication administration, and instruction from health care providers. This system increases the continuity of care. Nurses may need to assist the family in developing and using effective systems.

As with all other documentation systems, home care documentation is used to improve both quality of care and the communications about the older person. In addition, the RAI system serves as a guide for quality care, resource allocation, and reimbursement. The documentation is completed in the person's home, recorded directly on portable or hand-held computers, and later transferred to a central database.

IMPLICATIONS FOR GERONTOLOGICAL NURSING AND HEALTHY AGING

Health care documentation, whether written or electronic, contains highly personal and private information about patients or residents. For many years, the confidentiality of health and medical information was protected through professional codes of ethics (CNA, 2008; Prater, 2014). The expectation has always been that nurses and other health care providers would be able to access only information that relates to a specific person in their care. Nursing students are taught to avoid talking about their patients or residents in any public space or with persons outside their clinical groups, such as friends and family members. The nurse who notes that a friend or neighbour has been admitted to a care setting cannot review that person's health and medical information unless the nurse is assigned to provide care or services to that person.

However, not all health care providers are as respectful of people's privacy as they should be. The use of social media, coupled with the electronic exchange of personal health information, has significantly increased the risk for breaches of confidentiality. While the influence of social media on professional practice varies depending on the user and the context of his or her practice, the central concern for all nurses is patient confidentiality and privacy (CNA, 2012).

The *Personal Health Information Protection Act* **(PHIPA)**, 2004 and 2016, outlines the rules for the collection, use, and disclosure of personal health information. The PHIPA also requires that all personal health information be kept confidential and secure. The Office of the Information and Privacy Commissioner of Canada has the responsibility to ensure this protection. Patients and residents may request that all reasonable steps be taken to ensure that their verbal communications are confidential and that they have complete control as to who has access to their information. In the case of guardianship or in the case of a person who is not capable of making health care decisions, information can be shared with the guardian or with whoever has power of attorney, respecting the PHIPA rules. It is expected that nursing actions to protect privacy include closing the patient's or resident's door before having health-related conversations and not discussing a patient's or resident's needs or condition in a location where the discussion could be overheard, such as hallways or some nurses' stations.

Communication through documentation has become critical to ensuring patients' rights and adequate care and to providing data for policy and funding decisions. It is the responsibility of the nurse to make sure that communication and documentation are of the highest quality so as to provide error-free and appropriate care and continuity and to maximize both patient and resident outcomes and accurate reimbursement.

KEY CONCEPTS

- Excellence in documentation sets the stage for excellence in care.
- Standardized instruments for care outcomes and evaluation are integral to the consistent determination of the needs and the health and wellness status of older people, as well as appropriate funding.
- Documenting the patient's status and needs is a key responsibility of the nurse.
- Nurses have a responsibility to protect patient confidentiality at all times, both in spoken communication and in the clinical record.

ACTIVITIES AND DISCUSSION QUESTIONS

1. Discuss the origins and purpose of the development of standardized documentation systems.
2. Discuss incomplete data or poor documentation problems you have experienced in a health care setting.
3. Discuss the potential uses of the RAI-MDS.
4. Discuss the ways in which patient confidentiality is breached and what the nurse can do to prevent such breaches.
5. Explain why documentation is critical to care.

RESOURCES

Canadian Nurses Association. Code of Ethics, 2008: *https://www.cna-aiic.ca/~/media/cna/files/en/codeofethics .pdf*

Personal Health Information Protection Act (PHIPA), 2004, 2016 (Office of the Information and Privacy Commissioner of Canada) *http://www.priv.gc.ca/* and *https://www.ontario.ca/laws/ statute/04p03#BK43*

RAI-MDS 2.0 and RAPs, Canadian Version: User's Manual, Canadian Version, Addendum-Original Resident Assessment Protocols (RAPs)
https://secure.cihi.ca/estore/productSeries.htm?pc =PCC585

Documentation Standards by Province and Territory
Alberta:
http://www.nurses.ab.ca/content/dam/carna/pdfs/ DocumentList/Standards/DocumentationStandards _Jan2013.pdf

British Columbia:
https://www.crnbc.ca/standards/lists/standardresources/ 151nursingdocumentation.pdf

Manitoba:
https://www.crnm.mb.ca/support/practice-and-standards -consultation/documentation

New Brunswick:
http://www.nanb.nb.ca/practice/standards

Newfoundland and Labrador:
https://www.arnnl.ca/sites/default/files/ID_Documentation _Standards_for_Registered_Nurses.pdf

Northwest Territories and Nunavut:
http://www.rnantnu.ca/professional-practice/standards -practice/documentation-guidelines

Nova Scotia:
https://crnns.ca/practice-standards/standards-of-practice/

Ontario:
http://www.cno.org/globalassets/docs/prac/41001 _documentation.pdf

Prince Edward Island:
http://www.arnpei.ca/Registration/Continuing-Competence -Program/ARNPEI-Standards-For-Nursing-Practice/

Saskatchewan:
http://www.srna.org/images/stories/pdfs/nurse_resources/ documentation_guidelines_for_registered_nurses_22_11 _2011.pdf

Yukon:
http://yukonnurses.ca/images/YRNA/Documents/ Standards2013.pdf

Quebec:
http://www.oiiq.org/sites/default/files/uploads/pdf/ pratique_infirmiere/pti/document_explicatif_en.pdf

For additional resources, please visit *http://evolve .elsevier.com/Canada/Ebersole/gerontological/*

REFERENCES

Canadian Nurses Association (CNA). (2008). *Code of Ethics for Registered Nurses.* Retrieved from https://www.cna-aiic.ca/~/ media/cna/files/en/codeofethics.pdf.

Canadian Nurses Association (CNA). (2010). *Canadian Registered Nurse Examination Competencies.* Retrieved from http:// www.cna-nurses.ca/CNA/nursing/rnexam/competencies/ default_e.aspx.

Canadian Nurses' Association. (2012). *Ethics in practice for registered nurses: When private becomes public: The ethical challenges and opportunities of social media.* Retrieved from https:// www.cna-aiic.ca/~/media/cna/page-content/pdf-en/ethics_in_ practice_feb_2012_e.pdf?la=en.

College of Registered Nurses of British Columbia (CRNBC). (2017). *Nursing documentation.* Retrieved from https://www .crnbc.ca/standards/lists/standardresources/151nursing documentation.pdf.

Coyte, P. C., & McKeever, P. (2016). Home care in Canada: Passing the buck. *Canadian Journal of Nursing Research Archive, 33*(2), 11–25.

Fowler, R., & Hammer, M. (2013). End-of-life care in Canada. *Clinical & Investigative Medicine, 36*(3), 127–132. doi:10.1186/ s12904-016-0133-4.

Hirdes, J. P., Mitchell, L., Maxwell, C. J., et al. (2011). Beyond the 'iron lungs of gerontology': using evidence to shape the future of nursing homes in Canada. *Canadian Journal on Aging, 30*(03), 371–390. doi:10.1017/S0714980811000304.

Kelley, T. F., Brandon, D. H., & Docherty, S. L. (2011). Electronic nursing documentation as a strategy to improve quality of patient care. *Journal of Nursing Scholarship, 43*(2), 154–162. doi:10.1111/j.1547-5069.2011.01397.x.

Ministry of Health and Long-Term Care (MOHLTC). (2017). *Medical assistance in dying.* Retrieved from http://health.gov .on.ca/en/pro/programs/maid/.

Prater, V. S. (2014). *Confidentiality, privacy and security of health information: Balancing interests.* Retrieved from http:// healthinformatics.uic.edu/resources/articles/confidentiality -privacy-and-security-of-health-information-balancing -interests/.

R.A.I. Home Care. (2008). *Introducing the InterRAI Home Care.* Retrieved from http://www.interrai-au.org/downloads/interRAI _HC_overview.pdf.

Biological Theories and Physical Changes of Aging

CHAPTER 6

LEARNING OBJECTIVES

Upon completion of this chapter, the reader will be able to:

- Identify the physical changes that are associated with normal aging.
- Begin to differentiate normal age-related changes from those that are potentially pathological.
- Incorporate prevention and health promotion in a plan of care for an older person.

GLOSSARY

Glomerular filtration rate The rate at which the kidneys filter blood.

Hypercapnia High levels of carbon dioxide in the blood.

Hypoxia Low levels of oxygen supply to body tissues.

Kyphosis C-shaped curvature of the cervical vertebrae.

Presbycusis Progressive, bilateral, and symmetrical age-related hearing loss.

Presbyopia Reduced near vision occurring normally with age, usually resulting in improved distance vision.

Proprioception The sense, independent of vision, of movements and position of the body in space.

Xerostomia Excessive mouth dryness.

THE LIVED EXPERIENCE

Strange how these things creep up on you. I really was surprised and upset when I first realized it was not the headlights on my car that were dim but only my aging night vision. Then I remembered other bits of awareness that forced me to recognize that I, that 16-year-old inside me, was experiencing changes that go along with getting older.

   Sally, 60 years old

Later life is a time of opportunities and challenges. Among the challenges are those related to age-related physical changes. Some changes are considered a normal part of aging; others are the result of pathological conditions that are mistakenly considered to be an expected part of the aging process.

Aging consists of a series of complex changes and occurs in all living organisms. Most of these changes are intrinsic, coming from within; others are a result of extrinsic environmental factors, such as exposure to smoke or other pollutants. Just why the changes occur has been of interest to scientists for decades. It is known that the triggers of aging are influenced by genetics as well as by injury to the body earlier in life.

This chapter discusses the prominent biological theories of aging and some of the major physical changes associated with normal aging. This chapter also addresses some changes that indicate pathological conditions commonly seen in older persons. With this knowledge, the nurse can begin to differentiate

69

normal aging from health problems that require treatment and to help facilitate prompt intervention that in turn promotes healthy aging.

BIOLOGICAL THEORIES OF AGING

A *theory* is an explanation that makes sense of some phenomenon. A theory remains a reasonable explanation until someone finds it to be incorrect. Most theories can be neither proved nor disproved, but they are useful as points of reference. Theories of aging provide clues to the aging process. However, many unanswered questions remain.

The biological theories of aging today evolved from the early study of changes over the lifespan of the organism. Two related viewpoints form the foundation of the biological theories: (1) error (stochastic) theories and (2) predetermined or programmed aging (nonstochastic) theories. Both viewpoints agree that in the end, the cells in the body become disorganized, the cells are no longer able to replicate, and cellular death occurs. When enough cells die, so does the organism. In recent years, research on the biological theories of aging has focused on cells, genes, and other cell components. A short description of emerging theories is provided in Box 6.1.

ERROR (STOCHASTIC) THEORIES

Error theories explain aging as being the result of an accumulation of errors in the synthesis of cellular deoxyribonucleic acid (DNA) and ribonucleic acid (RNA), the basic building blocks of the cell (Short et al., 2005). With each replication, more errors occur, until the cell is no longer able to function. The visible signs of aging, such as grey hair, are thought to be the result of the accumulation of these cellular errors. Three of the most common theories of error are the wear-and-tear, cross-link, and oxidative stress theories.

Wear-and-Tear Theory

One of the earliest theories of aging is known as the wear-and-tear theory. According to this theory, cell errors are the result of a "wearing out" over time due to trauma and continued use. Internal and external stressors (e.g., in the shoulder joints of baseball pitchers or the knees of runners) increase the number of

---

| BOX 6.1 | Emerging Biological Theories of Aging |

Neuroendocrine or Pacemaker Theory
The neuroendocrine system regulates many essential activities related to an organism's growth and development. The neuroendocrine or pacemaker theory focuses on changes in the neuroendocrine system over time. Common neurons in the higher brain centres may act as pacemakers—regulators of the biological clock during development and aging—that slow down and eventually shut off at a predetermined time. Much of the current research in this area is on the influence of hormones (especially dehydroepiandrosterone and melatonin) on neuroendocrine functioning over time.

Genetic Research
As the human genome is being mapped, scientists are examining the roles played by genetics and ribonucleic acid (RNA) in both random and programmed aging. Among the findings are that telomeres (which cap the ends of chromosomes) shorten with each cellular reproduction until eventually the telomeres disappear and the cell can no longer reproduce and dies. Abnormal cells (such as cancer cells) produce an enzyme called *telomerase* that lengthens the telomeres, enabling the cells to continue to reproduce. The manipulation of telomerase may have implications for the control of both cellular reproduction and aging.

Progerin and Telomeres
Some of the latest research in this field has found an association between telomeres and a toxic protein called progerin. As long as a telomere is securely bound to the chromosome, the cell is able to replicate and essentially live forever. With aging, however, telomeres wear away at the same time the cell produces more and more progerin. Progerin, a mutated version of normal cell protein, interferes with the stability of the telomeres and ultimately the length of the cell's life (Cao et al., 2011).

---

errors and the speed with which they occur. These errors may cause a progressive decline in cellular function.

Cross-Link Theory

The cross-link theory explains aging in terms of the accumulation of errors by *cross-linking,* or the stiffening of proteins in the cell. Proteins link with glucose and other sugars in the presence of oxygen and become stiff and thick (Marin-Garcia, 2008). Cross-linking is most easily seen with collagens because they are the most plentiful proteins in the body. Skin that was once smooth, silky, firm, and soft becomes drier and less elastic with age. Collagen is also a key component of the lungs, the arteries, and the tendons, and similar changes can be seen in these body parts (e.g., stiffened joints).

Oxidative Stress (Free-Radical) Theory)

The oxidative stress theory, also known as the free-radical theory of aging, is among the theories that are most understood and accepted. *Free radicals* are natural by-products of cellular activity and are always present to some extent. It is believed that cellular errors are the result of random damage from molecules (free radicals) in the cells. Exposure to environmental pollutants increases the production of free radicals and increases the rate of damage. The best-known pollutants include smog and ozone, pesticides, and radiation (Hodjat et al., 2015). Other environmental sources thought to cause increases in free radicals are gasoline, by-products of the plastics industry, and drying linseed oil paints. In youth, naturally occurring vitamins, hormones, enzymes, and antioxidants neutralize the free radicals as needed (Valko et al., 2005). However, with aging, the damage caused by free radicals occurs faster than the rate at which the cells can repair themselves, and cell death occurs (Marin-Garcia, 2008).

PROGRAMMED AGING (NONSTOCHASTIC) THEORIES

The nonstochastic theories attribute aging to a process thought to be predetermined or "programmed" at the cellular level; this means that each cell has a natural life expectancy. As more and more cells cease to replicate, the signs of aging appear, and ultimately the person dies at a "predetermined" age. These theories evolved from the groundbreaking work of Hayflick and Moorehead (1981), who referred to this process as the inner "biological clock." In other words, each cell is "born" with a limited number of replications and then stops replicating and dies.

Neuroendocrine-Immunological Theory

The neuroendocrine-immunological theory of aging attributes aging to changes in the integrated neuroendocrine and immune systems. The emphasis is on the programmed deaths of the immune cells due to damage caused by the increase of free radicals as aging progresses (Effros et al., 2005; Marin-Garcia, 2008). The immune system is a complex network of cells, tissues, and organs that function separately and together to protect the body from outside substances such as bacteria. The immune system is highly dependent on the release of hormones. In the simplest terms, the specialized B lymphocytes (humoral) and T lymphocytes (cellular) protect the body against infection or from other matter that is considered foreign, such as tissue or organ transplants. Animal studies have shown that the cells of the immune system become progressively more diversified with age and (in a somewhat predictable fashion) lose some of their ability to self-regulate. T lymphocytes show more signs of "aging" than do B lymphocytes. The reduced T cells are thought to be responsible for hastening the age-related changes caused by autoimmune reactions as the body battles itself; healthy cells are mistaken for foreign substances and are attacked.

In summary, it is important for the nurse to understand that the exact cause of aging is unknown. There is considerable variation in the aging process. There is variation between persons and between the systems within any one person. Aging is a wholly unique and individual experience.

PHYSICAL CHANGES OF AGING

INTEGUMENT

The skin is composed of the epidermis, the dermis, and the hypodermis. It the largest and most visible organ of the body. The various layers of the skin meld and model the individual, providing much of his or her personal and sexual identity. The skin is important both in health and in illness; it provides clues to hereditary, racial, dietary, physical, and emotional conditions. Hair, also a part of the integument, provides recognizable characteristics.

Many age-related changes in the skin are functionally inconsequential. Others have implications for organs throughout the body and a more far-reaching impact. Changes in the skin are due to both genetic (intrinsic) factors and environmental (extrinsic) factors such as wind, sun, and pollution. Cigarette smoking causes coarse wrinkles, and photo-damage from the sun is evidenced by rough, leathery texture; itching; and mottled pigmentation, among other signs. Signs of skin changes that may be genetic or environmental or both include dryness, thinning, decreased elasticity, and the development of prominent small blood vessels. Skin tears, purpura (large purple spots), and xerosis (excessive dryness) are common but not normal aspects of physical aging. Visible changes of the skin—colour, firmness, elasticity, and texture—affirm aging.

Epidermis

The *epidermis* is the tough outer layer of skin, composed primarily of *keratinocytes,* which are stratified, squamous, epithelial cells. With age, the epidermis thins, which makes blood vessels and bruises much more visible. T-cell function declines, and there may be a reactivation of a latent condition such as herpes zoster (shingles) or herpes simplex (see Chapter 11). The shingles vaccine, covered by some provincial health plans, is recommended for most people aged 60 years or more.

Cell renewal time increases by up to one-third after 50 years of age; 30 or more days may be necessary for epithelial replacement (Gosain & DiPietro, 2004). This change significantly affects wound healing. If a younger adult's skin is injured (e.g., cut or scraped), the surrounding tissue becomes erythematous almost immediately. This inflammatory response is the first step in the natural healing process. For an older person, this inflammatory first step may take 48 to 72 hours. A laceration that becomes pink several days after the event may be misinterpreted by the nurse as being infected; in reality, the healing process will have only just started. Evidence of a true skin infection in older persons is no different from such evidence in younger adults—namely, increasing redness, pain, swelling, and purulent drainage.

Melanocytes produce melanin, which gives the skin colour. The number of melanocytes in the epidermis decreases with aging. Fewer melanocytes means a lightening of overall skin tone (regardless of the original skin colour) and a decrease in the amount of protection from ultraviolet (UV) rays. Thus, the importance of sunscreen use significantly increases

(see Chapter 12). In some body areas, however, melanin synthesis is increased. Pigment spots (freckles and nevi) enlarge and become more numerous with increased exposure to light. Lentigines (commonly referred to as "age spots" or "liver spots") appear; they are frequently found on the backs of the hands and the wrists and on the faces of light-skinned persons older than 50 years. Thick, brown, raised lesions with a "stuck-on" appearance (seborrheic keratoses) are more common in men; they are not clinically significant but can become cosmetically disfiguring if severe (see Chapter 11).

Dermis

The *dermis,* lying beneath the epidermis, is a supportive layer of connective tissue composed of a matrix of yellow elastic fibres that provide stretch and recoil, and white fibrous collagen fibres that provide tensile strength. The dermis supports hair follicles, sweat and sebaceous glands, nerve fibres, muscle cells, and blood vessels (which provide nourishment to the epidermis). Sun exposure accelerates skin tissue changes by hastening collagen fibre alterations.

Many of the visible signs of aging skin are reflections of changes in the dermis (McCann & Huether, 2015). The dermis thins, causing older skin to look more transparent and fragile. Dermal blood vessels are reduced, resulting in skin pallor and cooler skin temperature. Collagen synthesis decreases, causing the skin to "give" less under stress and tear more easily. Elastin fibres thicken and fragment, leading to the loss of stretch and resilience and to a "sagging" appearance. Loss of elasticity accentuates jowls and elongated ears and contributes to the formation of a "double" chin. Breasts begin to sag and become pendulous. Melanocytes decrease, increasing the risk of UV damage from exposure to the sun.

Hypodermis

The *hypodermis* is the subcutaneous, innermost layer of the skin and contains connective tissues, blood vessels, and nerves. Its major component is subcutaneous fat, called adipose tissue. The primary purposes of adipose tissue are to store calories and provide thermal regulation. It also provides shape and form to the body and acts as a shock absorber against trauma. With age, some areas of the hypodermis atrophy.

As the natural insulation of fat decreases, a person becomes more sensitive to cold.

Changes in the hypodermis also increase the chance for hyperthermia as a result of the reduced efficiency of the sweat (eccrine) glands. Sweat glands are located all over the body and respond to thermostimulation and neurostimulation in response to internal changes (e.g., fever, menopausal "hot flashes") or increases in environmental temperatures. The usual body response to heat is to produce moisture or sweat from these glands and thus cool the skin by evaporation. With aging, the glands become fibrotic, and the surrounding connective tissue becomes avascular, leading to a decline in the efficiency with which the body cools down. It is not uncommon for older persons to complain of being either too hot or too cold in environments that are comfortable to others. Older persons are at significant risk for both hyperthermia and hypothermia. When caring for frail older persons, gerontological nurses can help them avoid extremes of temperature, prevent drying of the skin, and prevent exposure to toxic products (see Chapter 11).

Sebaceous glands, which secrete sebum (oil), also atrophy. Sebum protects the skin by preventing the evaporation of water from the epidermis; it possesses bactericidal properties and contains a precursor of vitamin D. When the skin is exposed to sunlight, vitamin D is produced and absorbed into the skin. Producing vitamin D is especially important because it is essential for calcium absorption and the prevention of osteoporosis (see Chapters 12 and 18). Vitamin D deficiency is linked to higher risks for cancer, cardiovascular disease, diabetes, multiple sclerosis, falls, fractures, influenza, and septicemia (Grant et al., 2010). All people need sunshine or vitamin D supplementation every day (Hanley et al., 2010), including those living in residential care settings. In Canada, where direct sunlight is limited in the winter months, supplementation is recommended. Osteoporosis Canada (2017) recommends daily supplements of at least 800 IU per day for people over 50 years of age.

Hair and Nails

As part of the integument, hair has biological, psychological, and cosmetic value. Hair is composed of tightly fused horny cells that arise from the dermal layer of the skin and obtain colouration from melanocytes. Genetics, race, sex, and testosterone and estrogen hormones influence hair distribution in both men and women.

Race, sex, and hormones also determine the maximum amount of body and scalp hair and the changes that occur in hair throughout life. Men and women of all races have less hair as they age. Hair on the head thins. Scalp hair loss is prominent in men, beginning as early as their twenties. The hair in the ears, nose, and eyebrows of older men increases and stiffens. Women have a less pronounced loss of scalp hair (Luggen, 2005). For some older people, the accustomed hair colour remains; for most, however, there is a gradual loss of pigmentation (melanin), and the scalp hair becomes dryer and coarser. Older women develop chin and facial hair because of the decreased estrogen-to-testosterone ratio. Leg, axillary, and pubic hair lessens and in some instances disappears in postmenopausal women. This normal absence of leg hair can be misinterpreted as a sign of peripheral vascular disease in older persons. People of the various races have distinctive hair characteristics, which the nurse should keep in mind when caring for older persons.

The nails become harder and thicker, more brittle, dull, and opaque. They change shape, becoming flat or concave instead of convex. Vertical ridges appear because of decreasing water, calcium, and lipid content. The blood supply, as well as the rate of growth, decreases. The half moon (lunule) of the fingernail may disappear, and the colour of the nails may vary from yellow to grey.

Fungal infection of the nails (onychomycosis) is not the result of aging but is quite common. Fungus invades the space between the layers of the nails, leaving a thick and unsightly appearance. The slowness of growth and the reduced circulation in the nails of older persons make treatment very difficult (see Chapter 11). Actions older persons can take to keep skin healthy while aging are presented in Box 6.2.

MUSCULO-SKELETAL SYSTEM

A functioning musculo-skeletal system is necessary for movement, gross responses to environmental forces, and maintenance of posture. This complex

---

BOX 6.2   Promoting Healthy Skin While Aging

- Avoid excessive exposure to ultraviolet (UV) light. In Canada, the highest sunlight UV levels occur from 1100 hours to 1600 hours, between May and August.
- Apply moisturizer to damp skin after bathing.
- Avoid the use of drying soaps; use low-pH cleansers.
- Always use sunscreens, paying special attention to the face, ears, neck, and hands.
- Wear a broad-brimmed hat when in sunshine.
- Keep well hydrated. Drink >1.5 L of water per day. Use a humidifier in the winter.

Sources: Canadian Dermatology Association. (2017). *Photoaging.* Retrieved from http://www.dermatology.ca/skin-hair-nails/skin/photoaging/#!/skin-hair-nails/skin/photoaging/what-is-photoaging/; van der Horst, M. (2007). Myth busting: The skin care issue. *BP Blogger, 2*(5). Retrieved from http://www.the-ria.ca/wp/wp-content/uploads/2014/01/BP_Skin-Care-May-2007.pdf.

BOX 6.3   Promoting Healthy Bones and Muscles

- Ensure regular intake of vitamin D and calcium (Osteoporosis Canada, 2017).
- Engage in regular weight-bearing exercise (e.g., tai chi).
- Engage in regular flexibility and balance exercises (e.g., yoga).
- Consider preventive pharmacotherapeutics if you are a woman.

---

system comprises bones, joints, tendons, ligaments, and muscles.

As seen with the skin, changes in the musculo-skeletal system are influenced by many factors, such as age, sex, race, and environment. Although none of the age-related changes to the musculo-skeletal system are life threatening, any of them could affect a person's ability to function and therefore affect his or her quality of life. Some of the changes are visible to others and have the potential to affect the individual's self-esteem.

The musculo-skeletal changes that have the most effect on function are in the ligaments, tendons, and joints. Over time, these become dry, hardened, more rigid, and less flexible. In joints subjected to trauma earlier in life (e.g., from injuries or repetitive movement), these changes can be seen earlier and in more severe forms. If joint space is reduced, arthritis is diagnosed.

Bone mass decreases with age; the bones lose strength and become increasingly brittle. Bone loss is related to genetics; decreased hormone levels; decreased bone formation; deficiencies of vitamin D, magnesium, and calcium; and lifestyle (smoking, alcohol use, and physical inactivity) (Crowther-Radulewicz, 2015). Age-related changes to muscles are known as *sarcopenia* and are seen almost exclusively in skeletal muscle. Muscle mass can continue to build until the person is in their fifties. However, between 30% and 40% of the skeletal muscle mass of a 30-year-old may be lost by the time the person reaches their nineties (Crowther-Radulewicz, 2015). Disuse of the muscles accelerates the loss of strength. In key areas, muscle tissue mass decreases (atrophies), whereas adipose tissue increases. Replacement of lean muscle by adipose tissue is most noticeable in men in the area of the waist and in women between the umbilicus and the symphysis pubis. Nurses can encourage older persons to exercise, especially through weight-bearing exercises, to help maintain healthy bones and muscles and flexibility (Box 6.3). Chapter 10 discusses the importance of exercise.

Structure, Posture, and Body Composition

Changes in stature and posture are two of the more obvious signs of aging and are associated with factors that involve skeletal, muscular, subcutaneous, and fat tissue. Vertebral disks become thin as a result of dehydration, causing a shortening of the trunk. These changes may begin to be seen as early as the fifties (Crowther-Radulewicz, 2015). The trunk shortens as a result of gravity and dehydration of the vertebral disks. The person may have a stooped appearance from **kyphosis,** a curvature of the cervical vertebrae that results from reduced bone mineral density (BMD). Some loss of BMD in women is associated with the reduction of estrogen levels after menopause; with the shortened appearance, the bones of the arms and the legs may appear disproportionate in size. If a person's BMD is very low, osteoporosis is diagnosed; a loss of 5–8 cm (2–3 inches) in height is not uncommon (see Chapter 18).

Alteration in body shape and weight occurs as lean body mass declines and body water is lost (54 to 60%

Proportion of Body Weight Represented by Water

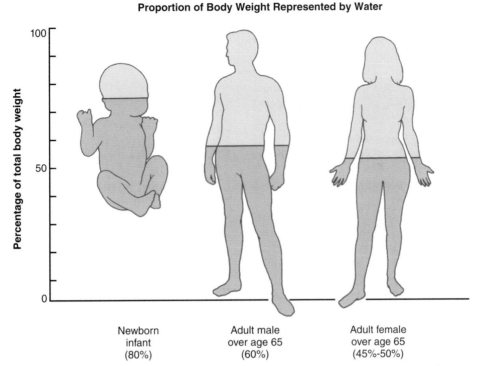

FIGURE 6.1 Changes in body water distribution. From Thibodeau, G. A., & Patton, K. T. (2004). *Structure and function of the body* (12th ed.). St. Louis, MO: Mosby.

in men; 46 to 52% in women) (Kee et al, 2009). Fat tissue increases until 60 years of age. Therefore, body density is higher in youth because of the density of muscle compared to the lightness of fat. From 25 to 75 years of age, the fat content of the body increases by 16%. Changes in water distribution have significant implications for dramatically increased risk for dehydration (Fig. 6.1).

CARDIOVASCULAR SYSTEM

The cardiovascular (CV) system is responsible for the transport of oxygen and nutrient-rich blood to the organs and the transport of metabolic waste products to the kidneys and bowels. The most relevant age-related changes are myocardial and blood vessel stiffening and a decreased responsiveness to sudden changes in demand (Cunningham et al., 2015). Changes in the CV system are progressive and cumulative.

Cardiac Changes

The age-related changes of the heart (called *presbycardia*) are structural, electrical, and functional. The size of the heart remains relatively unchanged in healthy older persons. However, the left ventricle wall thickens by as much as 50% by 80 years of age, and the left atrium increases slightly in size—an adaptation that enhances ventricular filling (Cunningham et al., 2015). Maximum coronary-artery blood flow, stroke volumes, and cardiac output are decreased. The changes have little or no effect on the heart's ability to function in day-to-day life. The changes only become significant when there are environmental, physical, or psychological stresses. With sudden demands for more oxygen, the heart may not be able to respond adequately (Marin-Garcia, 2008); it takes longer for the heart to accelerate and then return to a resting state. For the gerontological nurse, this means that the increased heart rate one might expect to see when a person is anxious, febrile, hemorrhaging, or in pain may not be present or will be delayed in an older person. Similarly, the older heart may not be able to respond to other calls for increased cardiac demand, such as infection, anemia, pneumonia, cardiac dysrhythmias, surgery, diarrhea, hypoglycemia, malnutrition, and medication-induced and noncardiac illnesses such as renal disease and prostatic obstruction. Instead, the nurse must depend on other signs of distress in the older patient and be alert to signs of rapid decompensation in both a previously well older person and a person who is already frail.

Heart disease is the number one cause of nonaccidental death worldwide. Often the changes associated with disease are thought to be a part of normal aging, but they are not. The gerontological nurse can promote healthy aging with recommendations for heart-healthy life choices and support the older person in obtaining excellent health care.

Blood Vessels

Several age-related changes in the skin and muscles affect the lining *(intima)* of the blood vessels, especially the arteries. As in the skin, the most significant change is decreased elasticity and recoil. The blood supply to various organs decreases, and peripheral resistance increases. Change in flow to the coronary arteries and the brain is minimal, but decreased perfusion of other organs, especially the liver and kidneys, has potentially serious implications for medication use (see Chapter 14). When a person already has or develops arteriosclerosis or hypertension, the age-related changes can have serious consequences.

Less dramatic changes are found in the veins, although the veins do become somewhat stretched and the valves less efficient. This means that lower-extremity edema develops more quickly and that the older person is at greater risk for deep vein thrombosis because of the increased sluggishness of the venous circulation. The normal changes, when combined with a longstanding but unknown weakness of the vessels, may become visible in marked varicosities and can lead to an increased rate of stroke and aneurysms. However, the promotion, and attainment, of a healthier heart is possible (Box 6.4).

BOX 6.4   Promoting a Healthy Heart

- Do not smoke.
- Keep cholesterol, blood pressure, and blood sugar levels normal.
- Engage in at least 30 minutes of physical activity most days.
- Maintain a healthy weight.
- Eat a wide variety of foods, following *Canada's Food Guide*. Eat seven servings of vegetables and fruits each day.
- Learn how to cope with stress in a healthy way.
- Avoid trans-fat, and limit saturated fats.
- Limit sodium intake.

Source: Adapted from Government of Canada. (2016). *Heart disease – heart health.* Retrieved from http://healthycanadians.gc.ca/diseases-conditions-maladies-affections/disease-maladie/heart-disease-eng.php.

RESPIRATORY SYSTEM

The respiratory system is the vehicle for ventilation and gas exchange, particularly the transfer of oxygen into and the release of carbon dioxide from the blood. The respiratory structures depend on the full functioning of the musculo-skeletal and nervous systems. The respiratory system matures by the age of 20 years and then begins to decline. Subtle and mostly insignificant changes occur in the lungs, the thoracic cage, the respiratory muscles, and the respiratory centres in the central nervous system. The more specific changes include loss of elastic recoil, stiffening of the chest wall, inefficiency in gas exchange, and increased air flow resistance (Fig. 6.2). Respiratory problems are common but almost always result from exposure to environmental toxins (e.g., pollution, cigarette smoke) and not the aging process (Sheahan & Musialowski, 2001).

As in the cardiovascular system, the biggest change is in efficiency. Under usual conditions, this has little or no effect on the performance of customary life activities. However, when an individual is confronted with a sudden demand for increased oxygen, a respiratory deficit may become evident. Chemoreceptor function is altered or blunted at the peripheral and central chemoreceptor sites in the central nervous system, reducing the ability to respond to **hypoxia** or **hypercapnia**.

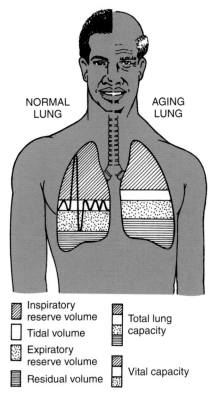

NORMAL
LUNG

AGING
LUNG

Inspiratory reserve volume

Tidal volume

Expiratory reserve volume

Residual volume

Total lung capacity

Vital capacity

FIGURE 6.2 Changes in lung volumes with aging. From McCance, K. L., & Huether, S. E. (Eds.). (2006). *Pathophysiology: The biologic basis for disease in adults and children* (5th ed.). St. Louis, MO: Mosby.

The changes that occur in the anatomical structures of the chest and the alterations in muscle strength can significantly affect one's ability to cough forcefully enough to quickly expel materials that accumulate in or obstruct airways. In addition, respiratory cilia are less effective. The reduced effectiveness of the cough response and cough reflex increases the risk of potentially life-threatening infections and aspiration, especially when the person has swallowing or gastrointestinal impairments such as dysphagia or decreased esophageal motility. The lack of basilar inflation, an ineffective cough response, and a less efficient immune system pose potential problems for older persons who are sedentary, bedridden, or limited in activity. All of these risks and conditions make the administration of annual influenza immunizations and a single pneumococcal vaccine of the

---

BOX 6.5   Promoting Healthy Lungs

- Obtain pneumonia immunization.
- Obtain annual influenza immunization.
- Avoid exposure to pollutants inside. Vent moisture to the outside, maintain home appliances, clean surfaces, control dust, and ventilate.
- Do not smoke, and avoid second-hand smoke.
- Avoid persons with respiratory illnesses.
- Seek prompt treatment of respiratory infections.
- Wash hands frequently with soap and water.
- Practice thorough regular oral hygiene.

Sources: Canadian Lung Association. (2016). *Prevent lung disease.* Retrieved from https://www.lung.ca/lung-health/prevent-lung-disease; Public Health Agency of Canada. (2008). *How can I keep my lungs healthy?* Retrieved from http://www.phac-aspc.gc.ca/cd-mc/crd-mrc/ healthy_lungs-poumons_en_sante-eng.php.

highest importance. In promoting the appropriate immunizations, the nurse is promoting healthy aging (Box 6.5).

RENAL SYSTEM

The renal system is responsible for regulating water and salts in the body and for maintaining the acid–base balance in the blood. Blood passes through the nephrons in the kidneys for filtering. The glomerulus is the key structure that controls the rate of filtering (**glomerular filtration rate).** Kidney function is measured indirectly by means of the plasma creatinine through the calculation of the creatinine clearance rate.

Among the many changes to the kidneys are changes of blood flow and the ability to regulate body fluids. Blood flow through the kidneys decreases by about 10% per decade, from about 1,200 mL/min in young adults to about 600 mL/min by the age of 80 years as a result of vascular and fixed anatomical and structural changes (MacAas-Naaez & Cameron, 2008; Wiggins & Patel, 2009). The kidneys lose as many as 50% of the nephrons, with little change in the body's ability to regulate body fluids. The age-related decrease in size and function occurs primarily in the kidney cortex, begins in a person's thirties, and becomes significant by his or her seventies (MacAas-Naaez & Cameron, 2008). However, renal reserve is lost, and the ability to respond to either a salt or water load or deficit is compromised.

Whereas plasma creatinine is constant throughout life, urine creatinine declines even in healthy aging because of the reduced lean muscle mass. Creatinine clearance, a measurement of glomerular filtration rate, is decreased to 100 mL/min by the age of 80 years. Urine creatinine clearance is an important indicator for appropriate medication therapy, reflecting the ability to handle medications passing through and metabolized by the kidneys (see Chapter 14). Persons with a reduced creatinine clearance usually need lower doses of medications to prevent potential toxicity, and caution must be used in the administration of fluids (see Chapter 9).

Age-related changes in the renal system are significant because of resultant heightened susceptibility to fluid and electrolyte imbalance, as well as structural damage from medications and from the contrast media of diagnostic tests. Under normal circumstances, renal function is sufficient to meet the regulation and excretion demands of the body (MacAas-Naaez & Cameron, 2008). However, with the stress of disease, surgery, or fever, the kidneys have a reduced capacity to respond and are therefore at greater risk for renal insufficiency and failure.

ENDOCRINE SYSTEM

The endocrine system, working in tandem with the neurological system, regulates and controls the integration of body activities by secreting hormones from glands throughout the body. As the body ages, most glands atrophy and decrease their rate of secretion. However, other than the decrease in estrogen, which causes menopause, the impact of the changes is not clear.

Pancreas Function

The endocrine pancreas secretes insulin, glucagon, somatostatin, and pancreatic polypeptides. The secretion of these substances does not appear to decrease to any level of clinical significance in older persons. However, for unknown reasons, the tissues of the body often develop a decreased sensitivity to insulin. When combined with increased needs for insulin in the presence of obesity, the result is often the development of type 2 diabetes. Older persons have the highest rate of type 2 diabetes of any age group, with significant variation by ethnicity and region (see Chapter 17). When

the pancreas is stressed with sudden concentrations of glucose, blood levels remain high longer. These temporary levels of increased blood glucose make the diagnosis of diabetes or glucose intolerance difficult.

Thyroid Function

With aging, slight changes occur in the structure and function of the thyroid gland, which may explain the increased incidence of hypothyroidism in older persons (Brashers et al., 2015). Some atrophy, fibrosis, and inflammation occur. Although other evidence of change is inconclusive at this time, diminished secretion of thyroid-stimulating hormone (TSH) and thyroxine (T_4) and decreased plasma triiodothyronine (T_3) appear to be age related. Serum T_3 decreases with age, perhaps as a result of decreased secretion of TSH by the pituitary gland. When thyroid hormone replacement therapy is needed, lower doses are necessary. The required dose of thyroxine may change over time, and monitoring is required. Collective signs, such as a slowed basal metabolic rate, thinning hair, and dry skin, are characteristic of hypothyroidism in the young but are normal manifestations in older persons who have no history of thyroid deficiencies, making the recognition of thyroid disturbances difficult.

REPRODUCTIVE SYSTEM

The reproductive systems in men and women serve the same physiological purpose—human procreation. Although aging men and women both undergo age-related changes, the changes affect women significantly more than men. Women lose the ability to procreate after menopause (cessation of ovulation), whereas men remain fertile their entire lives. Regardless of the physical changes, sexual needs remain (see Chapter 23).

Female Reproductive System

As menopause signals the end of the reproductive phase in a woman's life, several other age-related changes occur, particularly in breast tissue and urogenital structures. The breasts of older women are smaller, pendulous, and less firm. The labia majora and minora become less prominent, and the pubic hair thins. The ovaries, cervix, and uterus slowly atrophy. The vagina shortens, narrows, and loses some of its elasticity. Vaginal walls lose their ability to lubricate quickly, especially if the woman is not sexually active, and more stimulation is needed to achieve orgasm. The vaginal epithelium changes considerably; the pH rises from 4.0 to 6.0 before menopause to 6.5 to 8.0 afterward (Tufts et al., 2015). The vaginal changes result in the potential for dyspareunia (painful intercourse), trauma during intercourse, and higher susceptibility to infection.

Male Reproductive System

Although men continue to have the ability to produce sperm in late life, changes in the functioning of the reproductive and urogenital organs occur. The changes are usually more subtle and are noticed only as they accumulate, beginning when men are in their fifties. The testes atrophy and soften, the seminiferous tubules thicken, and obstruction caused by sclerosis and fibrosis can occur. Although the sperm count does not decrease, fertility may be reduced because of sperm that lack motility or because of structural abnormalities. Erectile changes are also seen; more stimulation is needed to achieve a full erection, ejaculation is slower and less forceful, and refractory periods are longer (Tufts et al., 2015). As with women, alterations in hormone balance may play a part in the age-related changes in men. Testosterone level is reduced in all men but only rarely to a level that would be considered a true deficiency.

By the age of 50 years, up to 50% of men have some degree of prostatic enlargement, and the prevalence of this is higher with increasing age (Kim et al., 2016). The condition, known as *benign prostatic hypertrophy*, is so common that it is considered normal with aging. It is considered problematic only when the enlargement causes compression of the urethra. As a result, the older man may experience urinary retention leading to repeated urinary tract infections and overflow incontinence. Medications or surgical interventions are pursued only when the symptoms of benign prostatic hypertrophy interfere with quality of life (Kim et al., 2016). Annual prostate examination by a primary health care provider is important.

GASTROINTESTINAL SYSTEM

The digestive system includes the gastrointestinal tract and the accessory organs that aid digestion. As with the endocrine system, few age-related changes affect function. However, a number of common health problems can have a great effect on the digestive system. Changes in other systems can also affect gastrointestinal structure and function (Doig & Huether, 2015).

Mouth

Age-related changes affect both the teeth and the mouth. With the wear and tear of years of use, the teeth eventually lose enamel and dentin and then become more vulnerable to decay (the development of caries). The roots become more brittle and break more easily. For unknown reasons, the gums are also more susceptible to periodontal disease. Without good mouth care, teeth may be lost. Taste buds decline in number, reducing the sense of taste, and salivary secretion lessens. A very dry mouth (**xerostomia**) is common. In 2009, up to 22.3% of Canadians aged 65 years and older had all of their teeth removed (i.e., became edentulous) (Statistics Canada, 2015). When dentures are used, it is important to ensure their fit and cleanliness and the appropriate diet.

Even in health, the changes described here, when combined, have the potential to decrease the pleasure and comfort in eating and increase the risk of poor nutrition, anorexia, and weight loss (Ramage-Morin & Garriguet, 2013). A number of medications taken for common health problems can quickly exacerbate oral problems, especially xerostomia. When the gerontological nurse administers medications or teaches about medication, the older person should be warned about this effect (see Chapter 14).

Esophagus

In youth, food passes quickly through the esophagus to the stomach because of the strong and coordinated contractions of associated muscle and peristalsis. In aging people, the contractions increase in frequency but are more disordered; thus, propulsion is less effective. This is called *presbyesophagus*. The sluggish emptying of the esophagus forces its lower end to dilate, creating greater stress in this area and possibly causing digestive discomfort. Pathological processes that are more common with advanced age include gastroesophageal reflux disease (GERD) and hiatal hernias.

Stomach

Decreased gastric motility and volume as well as reduced secretion of bicarbonate and gastric mucus are also associated with aging (Doig & Huether, 2015). These reductions are caused by gastric atrophy and result in hypochlorhydria (insufficient hydrochloric acid). Decreased production of intrinsic factor can lead to pernicious anemia if the stomach is not able to utilize ingested B_{12} vitamins. The protective alkaline viscous mucus of the stomach is lost because of the increase in stomach pH, which makes the stomach more susceptible to peptic ulcer disease, particularly if nonsteroidal anti-inflammatory drugs such as aspirin and ibuprofen are taken. The loss of smooth muscle in the stomach delays emptying time, which may lead to anorexia or weight loss (as a result of distension), meal-induced fullness, and a feeling of satiety (Price & Wilson, 2002).

Intestines

Age-related changes in the small intestine include those noted earlier that involve smooth muscle and those related to the villi, the anatomical structures in the intestinal walls that are essential for the absorption of nutrients. The villi become broader, shorter, and less functional. Nutrient absorption is affected; proteins, fats, minerals (including calcium), vitamins (especially B_{12}), and carbohydrates (especially lactose) are absorbed more slowly and in lesser amounts (Doig & Huether, 2015). Changes in motility, epithelial membranes, vascular perfusion, and gastrointestinal membrane transport may affect the absorption of lipids, amino acids, glucose, calcium, and iron.

Peristalsis slows with aging, and the response to rectal filling is blunted; the extent of the change should not be sufficient to cause problems with defecation. In other words, constipation, often thought of as a normal part of aging, is not a normal part of aging. Constipation is often a side effect of medications, life habits, immobility, inadequate fluid intake, and lack of attention to the gastrocolic reflex and the postprandial urge to defecate (see Chapter 8). Suggestions for promoting healthy digestion are found in Box 6.6.

Accessory Organs

The accessory organs of the digestive system are the liver and the gallbladder. The liver continues to

---

BOX 6.6   Promoting Healthy Digestion

- Practice good oral hygiene.
- Wear properly fitting dentures.
- Seek prompt treatment of dental caries and periodontal disease.
- Eat meals in a relaxed atmosphere.
- Maintain adequate intake of fluids.
- Provide time for response to gastrocolic reflex.
- Respond promptly to the urge to defecate.
- Eat a balanced diet.
- Avoid prolonged periods of immobility.
- Avoid tobacco products.

---

function throughout life despite a decrease in volume and weight (mass) and a concomitant decrease in liver blood flow of 30 to 40% by a person's late nineties (Hall, 2009). These decreases carry implications for impaired metabolism of medications and are associated with an increased half-life of fat-soluble medications (see Chapter 14). Liver regeneration, although slow, is not greatly impaired, and liver function test results remain unaltered with age.

There does not seem to be a specific change in the gallbladder with aging; however, the incidence of gallstones increases (Doig & Huether, 2015), possibly due to the increased lipogenic composition of bile from biliary cholesterol. The decrease in bile salt synthesis increases the incidence of cholelithiasis and cholecystitis (Hall, 2009). In addition, the decrease in bile acid synthesis causes a reduction in hydroxylation of cholesterol. This, in conjunction with a decrease in hepatic extraction of low-density lipoprotein cholesterol from the blood, increases the level of serum cholesterol in the older person. In women, the increase in cholesterol begins to be seen after menopause.

NEUROLOGICAL SYSTEM

Contrary to popular belief, the older person's nervous system, including the brain, is remarkably resilient, and changes in cognitive functioning are not a normal part of aging. Neither the older person nor the nurse should accept an assessment of "confusion" without making sure the cause is identified and treated if possible. Although many neurophysiological changes occur with aging, they do not occur in all older persons and do not affect everyone the same

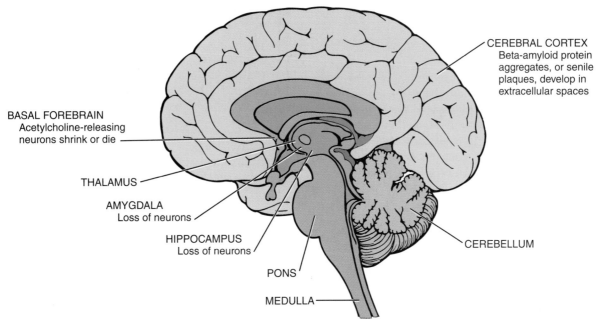

BASAL FOREBRAIN
Acetylcholine-releasing
neurons shrink or die

THALAMUS

AMYGDALA
Loss of neurons

HIPPOCAMPUS
Loss of neurons

PONS

MEDULLA

CEREBRAL CORTEX
Beta-amyloid protein
aggregates, or senile
plaques, develop in
extracellular spaces

CEREBELLUM

FIGURE 6.3 Changes in the brain with aging. Courtesy Carole Donner, Tucson, AZ.

way. For example, neurofibrillary tangles are a classic sign of dementia and are present in the brains of all persons with Alzheimer's disease, but they are also found in the brains of persons without dementia. Although it is difficult to show the true causes and effects of age-related changes in the nervous system, some changes appear to be consistent.

Central Nervous System

The major changes in the aging nervous system are found in the central nervous system. With aging, the dendrites appear to "wear out," and the number of neurons decreases with a corresponding decrease in brain weight and size (Fig. 6.3). This change in size is primarily in the frontal lobe and appears as atrophy on computed tomography scans and magnetic resonance imaging; it is considered to be clinically insignificant. Decreased adherence of the dura mater to the skull, fibrosis, thickening of the meninges, narrowing of the gyri, widening of the sulcus, and increased subarachnoid space also occur (Sugarman, 2015).

Sleep changes resulting from changes in the reticular formation may also be a normal part of aging. The reticular formation is a set of neurons that extend from the spinal cord through the brainstem and into the cerebral cortex. With aging, there may be a loss of deep sleep (stages 3 and 4). Compared with younger people, older people spend more time in bed to get the same amount of "sleep," because the time they spend in light sleep increases in proportion to the time they spend in deep sleep (Huether et al., 2015). However, excessive daytime drowsiness is not typical and should lead to a thorough assessment of causative factors, especially depression and the side effects of medication (see Chapters 14 and 24).

Subtle changes in cognitive functioning (thinking) and motor functioning (movement) occur in very old people. Mild memory impairment and difficulties with balance may be seen as normal age-related changes in neurodegeneration and neurochemistry (see Chapters 7 and 21). Intellectual performance without brain dysfunction remains constant. However, the performance of tasks may take longer, an indication that central processing is slowed. There are also decreasing levels of the neurotransmitters acetylcholine, serotonin, dopamine, and catecholamine. Other enzymes, such as monoamine oxidase, increase. Redundancy of brain cells may forestall the effects of these changes;

the exact number of cells required for certain functions is unknown.

Peripheral Nervous System

The most important effect of normal changes in the aging peripheral nervous system is the increased risk for injury. Vibratory sense in the lower extremities may be nonexistent. Somesthesia, or tactile sensitivity, decreases in connection with the loss of nerve endings in the skin; this is most notable in the fingertips, the palms of the hands, and the lower extremities. This decreased sensitivity is translated into delayed reactions to things such as hot surfaces, significantly increasing the risk for burns and the extent of any burns. (The presence of a functioning smoke detector in the home is particularly important.)

Kinesthetic sense, or **proprioception**, is altered because of changes in both the peripheral and central nervous systems. If one is less aware of body position and has less tactile awareness, one's risk of falling is dramatically increased. With reduced proprioception, it takes a little longer to realize that the surface is uneven and a little longer still to realize that one has tripped (changed position in space). This slight delay can result in an older person falling, whereas younger people are able to immediately balance themselves and prevent a fall. Conditions such as arthritis, stroke, some cardiac disorders, or damage to the structures of the inner ear may also affect peripheral and central mechanisms of mobility. A further discussion of sensory alterations appears in Chapter 19.

Sensory Changes

A number of changes (some loss of smell, sight, sound, and touch) occur in the sensory organs as a result of a combination of intrinsic and extrinsic factors. The gerontological nurse can make a big difference in the quality of life for the person with sensory changes (Box 6.7). Chapter 3 discussed communication with older persons who have vision and hearing impairments.

Eyes and Vision. Changes in vision and the eyes begin very early and are both functional and structural. All changes affect visual acuity and accommodation (the ability of the eyes to adjust to changes in the environment).

BOX 6.7 Promoting Healthy Eyes

- Have eyes examined regularly.
- Use bright lighting.
- See a health professional if there are changes in your vision.
- Do not smoke.
- Reduce glare as much as possible.
- Wear sunglasses that provide 99 to 100% UV-A and UV-B protection.
- Protect eyes from accidents and injury (e.g., use grease shields, safety glasses).

Source: Public Health Agency of Canada. (2006). *Vision care—Info sheet for seniors.* Retrieved from http://giic.rgps.on.ca/files/Falls_pc_ip _PHACVisionCareInfoSeniors.pdf.

Presbyopia is an age-related decrease in near vision that begins to become noticeable in midlife. Nearly 95% of adults older than 65 years wear eyeglasses for close vision (Burke & Laramie, 2000), and 18% also use a magnifying glass for reading and close work. Although presbyopia is first seen in people who are between 45 and 55 years of age, 80% of those older than 65 years have fair to adequate far vision past 90 years of age. Pathological conditions that are more common in aging include glaucoma, cataracts, and macular degeneration (see Chapter 19).

Extraocular Changes. Age-related changes affect both the form and function of the eyes. The eyelids lose elasticity, resulting in drooping (*senile ptosis*). In most cases, only the appearance is affected; in extreme cases, the lids sag enough to block vision. Spasms of the orbicular muscle may cause the lower lid to turn inward; the prolonged turning inward of the lower lid is called *entropion*. The lower lashes that curl inward irritate and scratch the cornea, and surgery may be needed to prevent permanent injury. Decreases in orbicular muscle strength may result in *ectropion*, the turning outward of the lower lid. Without the integrity of the trough of the lower lid, tears run down the cheek instead of bathing the cornea. Ectropion and an inability to close the lid completely lead to excessively dry eyes and the need for artificial tears. Exacerbating this problem is a decrease in the number of goblet cells that provide mucin, which is essential for eye lubrication and movement. A severe deficiency of lubrication is known as *dry eye syndrome.*

Ocular Changes. The cornea is the avascular transparent outer surface of the eye globe that refracts (bends) light rays entering the eye through the pupil. With aging, the cornea becomes flatter, less smooth, thicker, and duller in appearance. The result is increased far-sightedness (hyperopia). For a person who was nearsighted (myopic) earlier in life, this change may actually improve vision.

Arcus senilis, a ring or partial ring that is grey-white to silver in colour, may be observed 1 to 2 mm inside the limbus at the juncture of the iris and cornea. It is composed of deposits of calcium and cholesterol salts. It does not appear to have any clinical significance.

The anterior chamber is the space between the cornea and the lens. The edges of the chamber include canals that control the volume and movement of aqueous fluid within the space. With aging, the chamber decreases slightly in size and capacity because of thickening of the lens. Resorption of the intraocular fluid becomes less efficient with age; a significant decrease can lead to increased intraocular pressure and glaucoma (Huether et al., 2015). Any eye pain or acute changes in vision should be considered medical emergencies and be responded to accordingly.

The ability to adjust to changes in light and the need for higher levels of lighting are the result of reduced responsiveness of the pupils and changes in the lens. The lens—a small, flexible, biconvex, crystal-like structure just behind the iris—is most responsible for visual acuity; it adjusts the light entering the pupil and focuses it on the retina. Age-related changes in the lens begin in a person's forties. The origins of these changes are not fully understood, although ultraviolet rays of the sun contribute to the problem, and cross-linkage of collagen creates a more rigid and thickened lens structure.

With age, light scattering increases and colour perception decreases. As a result, glare is a problem not only when created by sunlight outdoors but also when created by the reflection of light from any shiny object, such as a polished floor or surface (Meisami et al., 2007). Eventually, people require three times as much light to see things as they required when they were younger. It is more effective to place high-intensity light on the object or surface to be observed than to increase the intensity of the light in the entire room (for example, focusing a light directly on the newspaper a person is reading instead of adding more light sources to the room).

Intraocular Changes. The retina, which lines the inside of the eye, has less-distinct margins and is duller in appearance in older persons than in younger adults. Colour clarity diminishes by 25% in the sixth decade and by 59% in the eighth decade, especially the clarity of blues, violets, and greens; light colours such as reds, oranges, and yellows are more easily seen. Some of this difficulty is linked to the yellowing of the lens and impaired transmission of light to the retina. Finally, the number of rods and associated nerves at the periphery of the retina is reduced, resulting in peripheral vision that is not as clear as previously or is absent (Meisami et al., 2007). Arteries in the back of the eye may show atherosclerosis and slight narrowing. If a person has a long history of hypertension, veins may show indentations (nicking) as they pass over the arteries. As long as these changes are not accompanied by distortion of objects or a significant decrease in vision, they are not clinically significant.

Ears and Hearing. Similar to the way it affects the eyes, aging affects both the structure and the function of the ears. Hearing loss that affects the ability to hear normal speech is more common in older persons, affecting 38% of Canadians between 60 and 69 years of age and 65% between 70 and 79 years of age (Feder et al., 2015). The most common kind of hearing loss in older persons is a high-frequency, sensorineural loss known as **presbycusis**. Hearing loss can lead to social withdrawal and increase the risk for depression and falls (Canadian Hearing Society, 2017).

Several age-related changes in the ear's appearance occur, especially in men. The auricle loses flexibility and becomes longer and wider as a result of diminished elasticity. The lobe sags, elongates, and wrinkles. Together, these changes make the ear appear larger. In addition, coarse, wiry, stiff hairs grow at the periphery of the auricle. In men, the tragus enlarges.

The auditory canal narrows through inward collapse, and stiffer and coarser hairs line the canal. Cerumen glands atrophy, producing a thicker and dryer wax that is more difficult to remove; this is a substantial cause for temporary, reversible obstructive hearing loss. The gerontological nurse should be sensitive to this possibility and be skilled at safe cerumen removal.

On otoscopic examination, the tympanic membrane appears dull and grey. Structurally, the ossicle joints between the malleus and the stapes become calcified, causing reduced vibration of these bones and a mechanical reduction in the amount of sound transmitted to the auditory nerve.

With presbycusis, there is a decrease in vestibular sensitivity as a result of otic nerve loss and the degeneration of the organ of Corti in the cochlea. The transmission of sound waves to the brain is thereby impaired. Genetically influenced change in the electrophysiological function of the organ of Corti is the basis of metabolic hearing loss. Hearing loss develops slowly. Whereas obstructive causes are reversible, sensorineural ones are not.

Presbycusis is primarily the loss of the ability to hear high-frequency sounds, such as consonants, the chirping of birds, and the rustling of leaves. "The Cat in the Hat" may be heard as "e at in e at." Although the person may be able to decipher what is said if it is in context, this processing takes longer than usual, or language is processed incorrectly. It is important to note that with normal age-related hearing loss, the person can still hear but may not be able to make sense of the partially heard words. Inaccurate responses too often lead to the incorrect suspicion of cognitive impairment when in fact the problem is hearing loss.

IMMUNE SYSTEM

The immune system protects the host from invasions by foreign substances and organisms. To do so, it must be able to differentiate the self from the nonself (Shames & Kishiyama, 2009). The immune system includes elements of many other systems, including white blood cells, bone marrow, thymus, lymph nodes, and spleen.

A number of age-related changes have been implicated in the increased risk for infection in the older person. For example, the skin is thinner and therefore less resistant to bacterial invasion. The reduced number of cilia in the lungs leads to the increased risk for pneumonia. The friability of the urethra increases the risk for urinary tract infections, especially in women. But perhaps most important of all is the reduced immunity at the cellular level, which is now understood to have a significant genetic underpinning.

In late life, a decrease in innate immunity, adaptive immunity, and self-tolerance brings a decrease in T-cell function. The response to foreign antigens decreases, but immunoglobulins increase, creating an autoimmune response not associated with autoimmune diseases that may have developed earlier (Michel & Proust, 2000). Older persons are thus likely to experience infections in the absence of characteristic symptoms such as fever. For example, in older adults, urinary tract infections may present with symptoms suggestive of respiratory infection or with changes only in mental status (Wordsworth & Dunn-Walters, 2011). Being alert for atypical signs and symptoms of infection is especially important to gerontological nursing, as is the responsibility to promote disease prevention and protection from infection. A pneumococcal vaccine is recommended for persons aged 65 years and older, and annual influenza vaccines are recommended for all adults. A target of a 70% influenza and pneumonia vaccination rate among adults aged 65 years and older was set in 1993 and was increased to 80% in 2005. In 2013, 64% of older Canadians received the influenza vaccine, a decrease from 67% in 2003. These rates differ by province; levels are lower in Saskatchewan and in Newfoundland and Labrador than in other provinces (Gionet, 2015). Rates are also lower for pneumococcal vaccination (Krueger et al., 2010). Older persons are also at increased risk for serious health effects from foodborne illnesses (Box 6.8).

The changes in immune function affect the older person's response to illness. Early studies by Stengel (1983) found significantly lower oral temperature norms in healthy older persons. Thus, a febrile response suggestive of infection is not restricted to a temperature higher than 37°C. Instead, an older person may have a core temperature elevation at much lower numbers. Very old persons may have an average normal temperature of 35.5°C and an average range of 35.0°C to 36.1°C (Hogstel, 1994).

These findings emphasize the need to carefully evaluate the basal temperature of older persons and to recognize that even low-grade fevers (e.g., 37°C) may signify serious illness. When such temperature changes are combined with the age-related delay in the increases in white blood cell count as compared with that of younger adults, early detection of serious

---

BOX 6.8   Reducing Risk for Foodborne Illness

- Follow Health Canada recommendations for safer choices among deli meats.
- Do not eat hot dogs straight from the package; heat to an internal temperature of 74°C.
- Avoid raw sprouts; refrigerated patés; raw or lightly cooked eggs; raw or undercooked meat; and unpasteurized dairy products, fruit juice, or cider.
- Take the following four steps for safe food handling, storage, and preparation:
  - Separate raw foods from cooked foods.
  - Wash your hands, kitchen surfaces, utensils, and reusable shopping bags with warm soapy water.
  - Promptly refrigerate food leftovers at 4°C or below.
  - Cook meat to recommended safe internal temperatures.

Source: Health Canada. (2015). *Food safety for older persons.* Retrieved from http://healthycanadians.gc.ca/eating-nutrition/healthy-eating-saine -alimentation/safety-salubrite/vulnerable-populations/older-adults -adultes-agees-eng.php.

---

illness can be difficult. *A lack of fever (a temperature greater than 37°C) or a normal white blood cell count does not rule out an infection.* Instead, the whole person must be considered, including mood, level of consciousness, and other factors, such as a recent fall or a change in cognitive abilities.

EVIDENCE-INFORMED PRACTICE: SMOKING CESSATION

The common health advice to older persons is to stop smoking or not smoke at all, to promote oral health, heart health, and healthy eyes, lungs, digestion, and brain function. Cessation of smoking results in health benefits at any age, even in older age. According to the Centre for Addiction and Mental Health (2008), there is no evidence that smoking-cessation interventions tested in younger adults do not work with older persons (Box 6.9). The Registered Nurses' Association of Ontario (RNAO) has a website (http:// www.tobaccofreernao.ca) that helps nurses integrate smoking cessation into daily practice. The site includes a link to the relevant RNAO Best Practice Guideline.

BOX 6.9   Research for Evidence-Informed Practice: Telephone Support and Nicotine Replacement Therapy Support Smoking Cessation Among Older Smokers

Problem: Older persons who quit smoking enjoy significant health benefits, but health professionals are less likely to promote smoking cessation with older patients.

Methods: Australian researchers tested the effect of a combination of telephone support plus nicotine replacement among 215 community-dwelling smokers aged ≥68 years. Participants who indicated they were considering quitting ($n = 165$) received regular ongoing individualized counselling and education by telephone and were provided with nicotine replacement therapy (NRT).

Findings: At 6-month follow-up, 88.5% had made an attempt to quit; 25% had abstained from smoking for at least 30 days; and 20% had abstained for 6 months. There was a statistically significant reduction in median daily cigarette consumption among those who did not quit. Those who accepted and used NRT were more likely to succeed. The results were consistent across age subgroups.

Application to Nursing Practice: Older smokers can successfully quit or reduce cigarette consumption. Nurses should assess their older patients' interest in quitting and help them to quit or reduce smoking.

Source: Tait, R. J., Hulse, G. K., Waterreus, A. et al. (2007). Effectiveness of a smoking cessation intervention in older persons. *Addiction, 102,* 148–155. doi:10.1111/j.1360-0443.2006.01647.x

---

SUMMARY

With the current biological theories of aging, supported by clinical evidence, it can be concluded that complex functions of the body decline more than do simple body processes; that coordinated activity (which relies on interacting systems such as nerves, muscles, and glands) shows a greater decremental loss than single-system activity shows; and that a uniform and predictable loss of cell function occurs in all vital organs. Yet, the older person is able to function effectively within the physical dictates of his or her body and continues to live to a healthy and satisfactory old age, capable of wisdom, judgement, and accomplishments.

The physical changes that accompany aging affect every body system, and the theories of why they occur are many. Although there are numerous ways and interventions by which nurses can promote healthy aging in the presence of these changes, the positive effect of these interventions is multiplied when nurses differentiate between normal changes and the signs and symptoms of potential health problems.

KEY CONCEPTS

- Many physical changes accompany aging; however, some of them are relatively insignificant in the absence of disease or unusual stress.
- Physiological aging begins at birth and is universal, progressive, and intrinsic.
- There are enormous individual variations in the rate of aging of body systems and functions.
- Many of the normal changes that occur with aging may be misinterpreted as pathological, and some pathological conditions may be mistaken for normal changes of aging.
- Careful assessment of lifestyle, desires, and individual age-related changes is fundamental to providing quality nursing care to older persons.

ACTIVITIES AND DISCUSSION QUESTIONS

1. Identify for each body system at least two normal changes that accompany aging.
2. Identify for each body system two abnormal physical, physiological, or both physical and physiological changes commonly seen in older persons.
3. Discuss the changes of aging you would find most difficult to accept.
4. Develop a nursing care plan for promoting the health of the older person's cardiac system.
5. Describe some nursing interventions to maintain healthy skin for older persons.
6. Interview an older person about his or her health practices and views on healthy aging. Discuss what you learned from the older person with your classmates.
7. Search for images of healthy aging (e.g., on the websites of the Hartford Institute for Geriatric Nursing or at http://www.bandwidthonline.org). Discuss how these images compare with the images of aging shown in popular media.

RESOURCES

Canadian Nurses Association. Aging and seniors care
https://www.cna-aiic.ca/en/policy-advocacy/ aging-and-seniors-care

Health Canada. Seniors
https://www.canada.ca/en/health-canada/services/healthy -living/seniors.html

Immunize Canada
https://www.immunize.ca/

Osteoporosis Canada
http://www.osteoporosis.ca/

Public Health Agency of Canada. Aging and seniors–Publications
https://www.canada.ca/en/public-health/services/health -promotion/aging-seniors/aging-seniors-publications.html

Registered Nurses' Association of Ontario. Integrating tobacco interventions into daily practice
http://rnao.ca/bpg/guidelines/integrating-tobacco -interventions-daily-practice

For additional resources, please visit *http://evolve .elsevier.com/Canada/Ebersole/gerontological/*

REFERENCES

Brashers, V. L., Jones, R. E., & Huether, S. E. (2015). Mechanisms of hormonal regulation. In K. L. McCance, S. E. Huether, V. L. Brashers, et al. (Eds.), *Pathophysiology: The biologic basis for disease in adults and children* (7th ed., pp. 689–716). St. Louis, MO: Mosby.

Burke, M., & Laramie, J. A. (2000). *Primary care of the older adult: A multidisciplinary approach* (2nd ed.). St. Louis, MO: Mosby.

Canadian Hearing Society. (2017). *Facts and figures*. Retrieved from http://www.chs.ca/facts-and-figures.

Cao, K., Blair, C. D., Faddah, D. A., et al. (2011). Progerin and telomere dysfunction collaborate to trigger cellular senescence in normal human fibroblasts. *The Journal of Clinical Investigation, 121*, 2833–2844. doi:10.1172/JCI43578.

Centre for Addiction and Mental Health (2008). *Improving our response to older adults with substance use, mental health and gambling problems: A guide for supervisors, managers and clinical staff*. Toronto, ON: Author.

Crowther-Radulewicz, C. L. (2015). Structure and function of the musculoskeletal system. In K. L. McCance, S. E. Huether, V. L. Brashers, et al. (Eds.), *Pathophysiology: The biologic basis for disease in adults and children* (7th ed., pp. 1510–1539). St. Louis, MO: Mosby.

Cunningham, S. G., Brashers, V. L., & McCance, K. L. (2015). Structure and function of the cardiovascular and lymphatic systems. In K. L. McCance, S. E. Huether, V. L. Brashers, et al. (Eds.), *Pathophysiology: The biologic basis for disease in adults and children* (7th ed., pp. 1083–1128). St. Louis, MO: Mosby.

Doig, X. K., & Huether, S. E. (2015). Structure and function of the digestive system. In K. L. McCance, S. E. Huether, V. L. Brashers, et al. (Eds.), *Pathophysiology: The biologic basis for disease in adults and children* (7th ed., pp. 1393–1422). St. Louis, MO: Mosby.

Effros, R. B., Dagarag, M., Spaulding, C., et al. (2005). The role of CD8+ T-cell replicative senescence in human aging. *Immunologic Review, 205,* 147–157. doi:10.1111/j.0105-2896.2005.00259.x.

Feder, K., Michaud, D., Ramage-Morin, P., et al. (2015). Prevalence of hearing loss among Canadians aged 20 to 79: Audiometric results from the 2012/2013 Canadian Health Measures Survey. *Health Reports, 26*(7), 18–25. Retrieved from http://www.statcan.gc.ca/pub/82-003-x/2015007/article/14206-eng.pdf.

Gionet, L. (2015). Flu vaccination rates in Canada. *Health at a Glance* (Catalogue no: 82-624-X). Ottawa, ON: Statistics Canada. Retrieved from http://www.statcan.gc.ca/pub/82-624-x/2015001/article/14218-eng.pdf.

Gosain, A., & DiPietro, L. A. (2004). Aging and wound healing. *World Journal of Surgery, 28*(3), 321–326.

Grant, W. B., Schwalfenberg, G. K., Genuis, S. J., et al. (2010). An estimate of the economic burden and premature deaths due to vitamin D deficiency in Canada. *Molecular Nutrition and Food Research, 54,* 1172–1181. doi:10.1002/mnfr.200900420.

Hall, K. E. (2009). Effect of aging on gastrointestinal function. In J. B. Halter, J. G. Ouslander, M. Tinetti, et al. (Eds.), *Hazzard's geriatric medicine and gerontology* (6th ed., pp. 1059–1064). New York, NY: McGraw-Hill.

Hanley, D. A., Cranney, A., Jones, G., et al. (2010). Vitamin D in adult health and disease: A review and guideline statement from Osteoporosis Canada. *Canadian Medical Association Journal, 182*(12), E610–E618. doi:10.1503/cmaj.091062.

Hayflick, L., & Moorehead, P. S. (1981). The serial cultivation of human diploid cell strains. *Experimental Cell Research, 25,* 585. doi:10.1016/0014-4827(61)90192-6.

Hodjat, M., Rezvanfar, M. A., & Abdollahi, M. (2015). A systematic review on the role of environmental toxicants in stem cells aging. *Food and Chemical Toxicology : An International Journal Published for the British Industrial Biological Research Association, 86,* 298–308. doi:10.1016/j.fct.2015.11.002.

Hogstel, M. O. (1994). Vital signs are really vital in the old-old. *Geriatric Nursing, 15*(5), 253. doi:10.1016/S0197-4572(09)90079-9.

Huether, S. E., Rodway, G., & DeFriez, C. B. (2015). Pain, temperature regulation, sleep, and sensory function. In K. L. McCance, S. E. Huether, V. L. Brashers, et al. (Eds.), *Pathophysiology: The biologic basis for disease in adults and children* (7th ed., pp. 484–526). St. Louis, MO: Mosby.

Kee, J. L., Paulanka, B. J., & Polek, C. (2009). Fluids and their influence on the body. In J. L. Kee, B. J. Paulanka, & C. Polek (Eds.), *Handbook of fluids, electrolytes and acid–base imbalances* (pp. 1–48). Albany, NY: Delmar.

Kim, E. H., Larson, J. A., & Andriole, G. L. (2016). Management of benign prostatic hyperplasia. *Annual Review of Medicine, 67,* 137–151. doi:10.1146/annurev-med-063014-123902.

Krueger, P., St. Amant, O., & Loeb, M. (2010). Predictors of pneumococcal vaccination among older adults with pneumonia: Findings from the Community Acquired Pneumonia Impact Study. *BMC Geriatrics, 10,* 44. doi:10.1186/1471-2318-10-44.

Luggen, A. S. (2005). Rapunzel no more: Hair loss in older women. *Advance for Nurse Practitioners, 13*(10), 28–33.

MacAas-Naaez, J. F., & Cameron, J. S. (2008). The ageing kidney. In A. M. Davison, J. S. Cameron, J. P. Grünfeld, et al. (Eds.), *Oxford textbook of clinical nephrology* (3rd ed., pp. 33–87). New York, NY: Oxford University Press.

Marin-Garcia, J. (2008). *Aging and the heart: A post genomic view.* New York, NY: Springer.

McCann, S. A., & Huether, S. E. (2015). Structure, function, and disorders of the integument. In K. L. McCance, S. E. Huether, V. L. Brashers, et al. (Eds.), *Pathophysiology: The biologic basis for disease in adults and children* (7th ed., pp. 1616–1652). St. Louis, MO: Mosby.

Meisami, E., Brown, C. M., & Emerle, H. F. (2007). Sensory systems: Normal aging, disorders, and treatments of vision and hearing in humans. In P. S. Timiras (Ed.), *Physiological basis of aging and geriatrics* (4th ed., pp. 109–137). New York, NY: CRC Press.

Michel, J., & Proust, J. (2000). Aging and the immune system. In M. H. Beers & R. Berkow (Eds.), *The Merck manual of geriatrics* (3rd ed.). Whitehouse Station, NJ: Merck Research Laboratories.

Osteoporosis Canada. (2017). *Vitamin D: An important nutrient that protects you against falls and fractures.* Retrieved from http://www.osteoporosis.ca/osteoporosis-and-you/nutrition/vitamin-d/.

Price, S., & Wilson, L. (2002). *Pathophysiology: Clinical concepts of disease processes* (6th ed.). St. Louis, MO: Mosby.

Ramage-Morin, P., & Garriguet, D. (2013). Nutritional risk among older Canadians. *Health Reports, 24*(3), 3–13. Retrieved from http://www.statcan.gc.ca/pub/82-003-x/2013003/article/11773-eng.htm.

Shames, R. S., & Kishiyama, J. L. (2009). Disorders of the immune system. In S. J. McPhee & G. D. Hammer (Eds.), *Pathophysiology of disease: An introduction to clinical medicine* (6th ed., pp. 28–49). New York, NY: McGraw Hill Medical.

Sheahan, S. L., & Musialowski, R. (2001). Clinical implications of respiratory system changes in aging. *Journal of Gerontological Nursing, 27*(5), 26–34. doi:10.3928/0098-9134-20010501-08.

Short, K. R., Bigelow, M. L., Kahl, J., et al. (2005). Decline in skeletal muscle mitochondrial function with aging in humans. *Proceedings of the National Academy of Sciences of the United States of America, 102*(15), 5618–5623. doi:10.1073/pnas.0501559102.

Statistics Canada. (2015). *Oral health: Edentulous people in Canada 2007-2009.* Retrieved from: http://www.statcan.gc.ca/pub/82-625-x/2010001/article/11087-eng.htm.

Stengel, G. B. (1983). Oral temperature in the elderly. *The Gerontologist, 23*(special issue), 306.

Sugarman, R. A. (2015). Structure and function of the neurologic system. In K. L. McCance, S. E. Huether, V. L. Brashers, et al.

(Eds.), *Pathophysiology: The biologic basis for disease in adults and children* (7th ed., pp. 447–483). St. Louis, MO: Mosby.

Tufts, G., Rodway, G., Heuther, S. E., et al. (2015). Structure and function of the reproductive systems. In K. L. McCance, S. E. Huether, V. L. Brashers, et al. (Eds.), *Pathophysiology: The biologic basis for disease in adults and children* (7th ed., pp. 768–799). St. Louis, MO: Mosby.

Valko, M., Morris, H., & Cronin, M. (2005). Metals, toxicity and oxidative stress. *Current Medical Chemistry*, *12*(10), 1161–1208.

Wiggins, J., & Patel, S. (2009). Changes in kidney function. In J. B. Halter, J. G. Ouslander, M. Tinetti, et al. (Eds.), *Hazzard's geriatric medicine and gerontology* (6th ed., pp. 1009–1016). New York, NY: McGraw-Hill.

Wordsworth, D. T. H. J., & Dunn-Walters, D. K. (2011). The ageing immune system and its clinical implications. *Reviews in Clinical Gerontology*, *21*, 110–124. doi:10.1017/S0959259810000407.

Social, Psychological, Spiritual, and Cognitive Aspects of Aging

LEARNING OBJECTIVES

Upon completion of this chapter, the reader will be able to:

- Explain the major cognitive, psychological, and sociological theories of aging.
- Discuss the influence of culture and cohort on psychological and social adaptation.
- Discuss the importance of spirituality to healthy aging.
- Explain several normal cognitive changes of aging.
- Discuss factors influencing learning in late life and appropriate teaching and learning strategies.

GLOSSARY

Cognition The mental process characterized by knowing, thinking, learning, and judging.

Cross-sectional A study design in which data are collected at one time on several variables such as age, gender, education, and health status.

Eurocentric Viewing the world from a European perspective, in the conscious or unconscious belief in the pre-eminence of European (and more generally, Western) culture, concerns, and values over those of non-Europeans.

Face validity "The extent to which a measuring instrument looks as though it is measuring what it purports to measure" (Polit & Beck, 2006, p. 500).

Geragogy The application of the principles of adult learning theory to teaching older persons.

Health literacy The ability to access, understand, and act on information concerning health.

Longitudinal research A study that repeatedly and at predetermined intervals assesses the experiences, states, or situations of a group of research participants.

THE LIVED EXPERIENCE

Accounts of Aging Well

Bassett et al. (2008) asked older persons, "What do you think makes people live long and keep well?" They shared the following:

Take things as they come, don't worry, accept life as it is handed out. (p. 116)

If you can't do that (retain autonomy), it's the beginning of the end. (p. 116)

Don't complain, take care of yourself, don't take risks, don't lose your temper, be a little contrary and don't take yourself too seriously. (p. 120)

Keep busy, work hard. (p. 120)

Good health; poor health leads to too many problems. (p. 121)

If you're lucky, you'll keep well, the good Lord governs that. (p. 121)

You have to have some social activity; don't be afraid to meet and speak to people. (p. 121)

You've got to get out of your house. (p. 121)

Think the best of everyone: Hate affects your health. (p. 122)

Don't be envious of others, it's harder. (p. 122)

SOCIAL, PSYCHOLOGICAL, SPIRITUAL, AND COGNITIVE ASPECTS OF AGING

Each individual has unique life experiences. Thus, each person must be seen holistically, through the lens of his or her time, place, culture, gender, and personal history. The close relationship between biological, social, and psychological development that exists through childhood and adolescence varies more in adulthood because of the greater variations in life experiences and demands as one matures. This chapter discusses the psychological, social, cognitive, and spiritual aspects of aging. Also discussed are factors that influence learning later in life, as well as appropriate teaching and learning strategies for older persons.

LIFESPAN DEVELOPMENT AND LIFE-COURSE APPROACHES

Human development is a lifelong process of adaptation. *Lifespan development* is an individual's progress through time and the expected patterns of change, biologically, sociologically, and psychologically. The lifespan theory of development is a psychological theory. The key principles of this theory, which is based on the work of Baltes and colleagues (Baltes, 1987; Baltes et al., 1998), have been summarized by Papalia et al. (2002). The principles include the following:

- Development is a lifelong process. Each part of the lifespan is influenced by the past and will affect the future. Each period of the lifespan has unique characteristics and value; no one period is more important than any other.
- Development depends on history and on social and cultural context. Each person develops under a certain set of circumstances and conditions that are defined by time and place.

- Development within each lifespan is multidimensional and multidirectional and involves a balance of growth and decline. Whereas children usually grow consistently in size and abilities, the balance gradually shifts in adulthood. Some abilities, such as acquiring a vocabulary, continue to increase, whereas others, such as speed of information retrieval, may decrease. New abilities, such as those involving wisdom and expertise, may emerge with age.
- Development is malleable and influenced by external conditions. With training and practice, a person's functioning and performance can improve throughout his or her lifespan. However, there are limits to how much performance can improve at any age.

Life-course theory is closely related to sociological theory; lifespan theory, social relations, age, and the timing of events in the course of life are integrated (Elder, 1998, as cited in Lerner, 2002). As in lifespan theory, historical times and places experienced during a lifetime affect the course of a person's life (Lerner, 2002). Furthermore, the impact of an event or transition depends on when it occurs during the life course. Social roles and interdependent social relationships are viewed as having an important influence on the life course. Finally, "individuals construct their own life course through the choices and actions they take within the constraints and opportunities of history and social circumstances" (Elder, 1998, as cited in Lerner, 2002, pp. 235–236).

TYPES OF AGING

People age in a number of ways. Aging can be viewed in terms of *chronological age, biological age, psychological age,* and *social age.* Chronological age is measured by the number of years lived. Biological age is predicted by the person's physical condition and by how well vital organ systems are functioning. Psychological age is indicated by the person's ability and control in regard to memory, learning capacity, skills, emotions, and judgement. Maturity and capacity direct the manner in which a person is able to adapt psychologically over time to the requirements of the environment. Social age is measured by age-graded behaviours that conform to an expected social status and social roles within a particular culture or society.

These different types of the aging of a person do not necessarily have to match. A person may have a chronological age of 80 years but a biological age of 60 years because he or she has remained fit by maintaining a healthy lifestyle. Conversely, a person with a persistent, chronic illness may have a biological age of 70 years but a much younger psychological age, due to an active and involved lifestyle.

There are several psychological and sociological theories of aging. Most adopt a **Eurocentric** perspective and may thus be less useful for describing the aging process in other cultures, especially those that are collective rather than individualistic (see Chapter 4); the importance of opportunity, ethnicity, gender, and social status is largely ignored. As current generations of older people move through later life, many of the current ideas and theories about this period of life development will continue to be redefined.

SOCIOLOGICAL THEORIES OF AGING

Sociological theories of aging attempt to explain and predict changes in roles and relationships in middle and late life, with an emphasis on adjustment. The basic theories were developed in the 1960s and 1970s and must be viewed within the context of the historical period from which they emerged. Some of the theories, such as modernization and social exchange theories, continue to generate interest and thought, while others, such as disengagement theory, are no longer accepted as explaining a normative experience of aging.

DISENGAGEMENT THEORY

According to the criticized theory of disengagement (Cumming & Henry, 1961), old age is "a time when both the older person and society engage in mutual separation, as in the case of retirement" (Moody, 2010, p. 9). The theory was developed in the early 1960s, and disengagement was viewed as natural and functional for the aging person and society. However, it is now recognized that although some people do disengage—for example, when they are unable to participate in certain activities—disengagement is not a natural pattern nor is it inevitable. Older persons who experience disability (for example, problems with activities of daily living) may need to disengage or to adjust their goals and activities. Canadian researchers found that people who were able to adjust their goals experienced better mental health (Dunne et al., 2011).

ACTIVITY THEORY

Activity theory is based on the belief that remaining as active as possible contributes to successful aging (Maddox, 1963). Evidence from gerontological research connects continued physical activity, social engagement, and productive roles to better outcomes (Gilmour, 2012; Moody, 2010). However, other research indicates that the meaning of an activity to the person may be more important than the activity per se (Moody, 2010, p. 11; Pushkar et al., 2010). Many older Canadians judge successful aging partly in terms of physical, mental, and social activity (Tate et al., 2013). Older people tend to remain active in retirement and may do so through the "productive activity" of paid and unpaid work. A Canadian survey (Vézina & Crompton, 2012) found that 40% of those aged 65 years and older volunteer. Furthermore, older people spend more time volunteering (an average of 223 hours per year) than younger Canadians do. Accessibility and opportunities to participate in society have an important influence on activity. The federal government's Age-Friendly Communities Initiative, based on the World Health Organization's Global Age-Friendly Cities Project, is an example of the application of this theory to policy. In age-friendly communities, "policies, services and structures related to the physical and social environment are designed to support and enable older people to 'age actively' … to continue to participate fully in society" (Public Health Agency of Canada [PHAC], 2016, ¶2). Older people and their communities work together, for example, to reduce ageist attitudes in businesses, to lobby for accessible public transportation, or to make parks accessible and safe.

CONTINUITY THEORY

According to continuity theory, people use continuity strategies to adapt to the changes of normal aging; people are "motivated toward inner psychological continuity as well as outward continuity of social behaviour and circumstances" (Atchley, 2000, p. 47). Inner continuity is "a remembered inner structure such as the persistence of a psychic structure of ideas, temperament, affect, experiences, preferences, dispositions, and skills" (Atchley, 2000, p. 49). Inner continuity provides a foundation for decision making, is a means of meeting important needs, and supports a sense of self, identity, and self-esteem. External continuity is "a remembered structure of physical and social environments, role relationships, and activities [that] result from being and doing in familiar environments, practicing familiar skills, and interacting with familiar people" (Atchley, 2000, p. 50). Too little or too much continuity feels uncomfortable to the person.

Continuity is a fluid concept and does not imply that people do not change; rather, there is coherence and consistency of patterns over time. For example, an older person who enjoys decorating is more likely to take up a new activity in the same domain (such as painting) than a new activity in another domain (such as a sport). Continuity theory is supported by research on retirement. When people take on new volunteer roles after retirement, they tend to select volunteer roles in which they can continue to use skills from their work roles (Cook, 2013). Furthermore, research supports the continuity theory's prediction that retirement and the resultant relief from work pressure will bring increased psychological well-being (Latif, 2011).

AGE-STRATIFICATION THEORY

Age-stratification theory (Marshall, 1996) goes beyond the individual to the age structure of society. Social institutions such as workplaces or families are partly organized by age; within these institutions, older people are segregated from younger people (Street, 2007). According to age-stratification theory, older people can be understood as belonging to specific "birth cohorts" (e.g., "baby boomers") whose members have shared specific historical periods in their lives, thus sharing the effect of having lived through similar conditions. They have been exposed to similar events and conditions; have lived under common global, environmental, and political circumstances (Street, 2007); and have had similar racial and cultural experiences (Hooks, 2000). Age norms are socially and culturally based ideas about what is appropriate at a certain age. The cohort effect can be a powerful tool for understanding the life experiences of people from different cultures and different parts of the world. Structural lag, another concept of the age-stratification theory, "occurs when social structures (e.g., incentives for early retirement) are out of synch with population dynamics (fewer younger workers) and individual lives (increasing life expectancy, later onset of disabilities or frailty)" (Street, 2007, p. 156). This example of structural lag is currently relevant in North America. Age-stratification theory may be particularly useful for examining aging in a global context.

SOCIAL EXCHANGE THEORY

Social exchange theory challenges both disengagement theory and activity theory. It is based on the consideration of the cost–benefit model of social participation (Dowd, 1980). In social exchange theory, withdrawal or social isolation is the result of an imbalance in the social exchanges between older persons and younger members of society. The balance determines the older person's personal satisfaction and social support at any point.

Older persons are often viewed as unequal partners in the exchange, and they may need to depend on metaphorical reserves of contributions to the pool of reciprocity. For example, this theory has been used to explain social support in families. In some cultures, there is an expectation that older persons should be cared for in return for their having provided care to others earlier in their lives (Jett, 2006). It has been noted that "although older individuals may have fewer economic and material resources, they often have nonmaterial resources such as respect, approval, love, wisdom, and time for civic engagement and giving back to society" (Hooyman & Kiyak, 2008, p. 317). Some older people care for their young grandchildren so that the parents can work; in return, they may receive other support (i.e., room, board, and income). Although this exchange may appear uneven, it can also be viewed from the more holistic perspective of a lifetime of exchanges and contributions. Intergenerational programs in which older and younger people interact, such as older persons volunteering in classrooms, are an example of the value of social exchange between generations.

MODERNIZATION THEORY

Modernization theory focuses on the social changes that have resulted in the devaluation of the contributions of older people as well as older people themselves. Before about 1900, according to this theory, materials and political resources were controlled by the older members of society (Street, 2007). These resources included time, knowledge, skills, and experience. Modernization theory assumes "that there was a gold age of the aged: preindustrial societies where elderly people were revered for their wisdom" (Street, 2007, p. 156). But this assumption may be faulty. According to this theory, the status and thus the value of older people are lost to society when their labour is no longer considered useful. Kinship networks are dispersed, the information they hold is no longer useful to the society in which they live, and the culture to which they belong no longer reveres them. It has been proposed that these changes are the result of health technology, industrial technology, urbanization, and mass education.

The treatment of older people in modern Japan was long considered evidence of the inaccuracy of the theory. Historically, older people in Japan were given the highest status and held the greatest power. This did not seem to change with the industrial advances after World War II. Today, however, Japan is not only a highly modern country from an industrial standpoint; it is also a country showing signs of "modernization" in social relations with regard to older persons. Researchers have also found support for the modernization theory in other countries, such as India and Taiwan (Dandekar, 1996; Silverman et al., 2000).

SYMBOLIC INTERACTION THEORIES

Symbolic interaction theories propose that the aging process a person experiences is a result of interactions between the environment, the person, and the meaning the person attributes to his or her activities (Gubrium, 1973; Hooyman & Kiyak, 2008). "Whether a new activity increases or decreases life satisfaction depends on an older individual's resources (health, socioeconomic status, and social support), along with the environmental norms for interpreting activities" (Hooyman & Kiyak, 2008, p. 313). With this perspective, one has to examine how the individual's resources and activities, as well as the environmental demands, can be altered to enhance satisfaction and self-concept. For example, if an older person needs to move to a long-term care home, it is useful to determine how the new environment can be structured to support the person's resources and lifestyle so that he or she can continue to maintain a positive self-concept and to experience life satisfaction and well-being.

IMPLICATIONS FOR GERONTOLOGICAL NURSING AND HEALTHY AGING

Sociological theories of aging give the gerontological nurse useful information and a background for enhancing healthy aging and adaptation (Box 7.1). Although these theories have been neither proven nor disproven, many of the ideas discussed have withstood the test of time. The theories have been adapted and applied to contemporary approaches to aging in many ways, from the concept of seniors' centres (activity theory) to nursing assessments of social support (social exchange theory). Unfortunately, the disengagement theory is incorrectly applied any time that depression and isolation are assumed to be normal parts of aging. Further research is needed to explore how culture, ethnicity, and gender influence aging and adaptation. Such research is particularly important in light of the expected growth of the diverse aging population in Canada.

PSYCHOLOGICAL THEORIES OF AGING

Psychological theories of aging presuppose that aging is one of many developmental processes experienced between birth and death. Life, then, is a dynamic process. These theories are widely accepted because of their **face validity.** Like the sociological theories, however, they are not well suited to testing or

- Currently held roles, role satisfaction, and emerging roles *(activity, continuity)*.
- Individual's and family's expectations of age norms and the effects of these expectations on self-esteem *(age stratification)*.
- Current level of activity and satisfaction with it *(activity)*.
- Effect of changes in health on usual roles and activity *(activity, continuity)*.
- Cultural beliefs and expectations related to roles and activity, and related engagement and disengagement *(activity, disengagement)*.
- Usual life patterns and personality as they influence adaptation to change *(continuity)*.
- Historical context of the individual and its potential influence on perception and responses *(age stratification)*.
- Complexity of social support and network *(social exchange)*.
- Opportunities to contribute knowledge to society *(modernization)*.
- Sense of self and self-worth *(continuity, modernization)*.

measurement and do not address the influence of culture, gender, and ethnicity.

JUNG'S THEORIES OF PERSONALITY

Psychologist Carl Jung, a contemporary of Sigmund Freud, proposed a theory about the development of a personality from childhood to old age (Jung, 1971). Jung was one of the first psychologists to regard the last half of life as having a purpose of its own. He noted that the last half of life is often a time of inner discovery, as opposed to the great amount of outward attention demanded by biological and social issues during the first half of life. Ideally, the last half of life is less intensely demanding and allows more time for inner growth, self-awareness, and reflectiveness.

According to this theory, an individual's personality is either extroverted and oriented toward the external world or introverted and oriented toward the subjective inner world. Jung suggested that aging results in a movement from extraversion to introversion. Beginning perhaps in midlife, individuals begin to question their own dreams, values, and priorities.

The potentially resulting crisis or emotional upheaval is a step in the process of personality development. Jung proposed that with chronological age and personality development, a person is able to move from a focus on outward achievement to an acceptance of the self and to an awareness that both the accomplishments and challenges of one's lifetime can be found within oneself. The development of the psyche and the inner person is accomplished by a search for personal meaning and the spiritual self. This personality of later life can easily be compared to Erikson's notion of ego integrity and Maslow's theory of self-actualization (Erikson, 1963; Maslow, 1968).

DEVELOPMENTAL THEORIES

The psychologist Erik Erikson is well known for articulating the developmental stages and tasks of life from early childhood to later "elderhood" (Erikson, 1963). Erikson theorized a predetermined order of development and specific tasks that were associated with specific periods in the course of life. He proposed that one needed to successfully accomplish one task before complete mastery of the next was possible, and he originally articulated these developmental tasks in "either-or" language. He proposed that all persons would return again and again to a task that had been poorly resolved in the past. Erikson's task of middle age is generativity; contributing to the future and to future generations in meaningful ways. Failure to accomplish this task results in stagnation. Erikson saw the last stage of life as a vantage point from which one could look back with ego integrity or despair in one's life. *Ego integrity* implies a sense of the completeness and cohesion of the self. In achieving this final task, people can look back over their lives—at the joys, sorrows, mistakes, and successes—and feel satisfied with the way they lived.

In later years, as octogenarians, Erikson and his wife reconsidered his earlier work from the perspective of their own aging. They changed their "either-or" stance of the developmental tasks to the recognition of the balance of each of the tasks. Thus, ego integrity is tinged with some regrets, wisdom is balanced with frivolity, and letting go is balanced with hanging on (Erikson et al., 1986).

Peck (1968), expanding on the work of Erikson, identified the specific tasks of old age that must be addressed in order to establish ego integrity. The following lists Peck's tasks, which represent the process or movement toward Erikson's final stage:

- *Ego differentiation* versus *work role preoccupation*. The individual is no longer defined by his or her work.
- *Body transcendence* versus *body preoccupation*. The body is cared for but does not consume the interest and attention of the individual.
- *Ego transcendence* versus *ego preoccupation*. The self becomes less central, and the person feels a part of the mass of humanity, sharing its struggles and its destiny.

Peck's theoretical model states that to achieve ego integrity, one must develop the ability to redefine the self, to let go of occupational identity in order to rise above bodily discomforts, and to establish meanings that go beyond the scope of self-centredness. Although these are admirable and idealistic goals, they place a considerable burden on the older person. Not everyone may have the courage or the energy to laugh in the face of adversity or surmount all of the assaults of old age. The wisdom of old age involves a crisis of understanding in which ordinary structures are shaken and the meaning of life is re-examined; it may or may not include the wisdom of questioning assumptions in the search for meaning in the last stage of life.

Havighurst (1971) is another developmental theorist who has proposed specific tasks to be accomplished in middle age and later maturity. Havighurst's developmental tasks are presented in Box 7.2.

THEORY OF GEROTRANSCENDENCE

Tornstam (1994, 1996, 2005) theorized that human aging brings about a general potential for *gerotranscendence* (a gradual and ongoing shift in perspective from the material world to the cosmic world) along with an increasing satisfaction with life. Gerotranscendence is generated by the normal processes of living, sometimes hastened by serious personal disruptions. As are Erikson's concept of integrity and Maslow's self-actualization, it is associated with wisdom and spiritual growth. The characteristics of gerotranscendence include the following:

- High degree of satisfaction with life
- Prime motivators other than midlife patterns and ideals

BOX 7.2   Havighurst's Developmental Tasks

Middle Age
- Assisting teenage children to become responsible and happy adults.
- Achieving adult social and civic responsibility.
- Reaching and maintaining satisfactory performance in one's occupational career.
- Developing adult leisure-time activities.
- Relating to one's spouse as a person.
- Accepting and adjusting to the physiological changes of middle age.
- Adjusting to aging parents.

Later Maturity
- Adjusting to decreasing physical strength and health.
- Adjusting to retirement and reduced income.
- Adjusting to the death of a spouse.
- Establishing an explicit affiliation with one's age group.
- Adopting and adapting social roles in a flexible way.
- Establishing satisfactory living arrangements.

Source: Havighurst, R. (1971). *Developmental tasks and education* (3rd ed.). New York: Longman.

- Complex and active coping patterns
- Greater need for solitary philosophizing, meditation, and solitude
- Realization that social activities are not essential to well-being
- Satisfaction with self-selected social activities
- Less concern with body image and material possessions
- Decreased fear of death
- Affinity with past and future generations
- Decreased self-centredness and increased altruism

IMPLICATIONS FOR GERONTOLOGICAL NURSING AND HEALTHY AGING

Knowledge about lifespan development and the various ways people experience aging can help gerontological nurses understand the meaning of healthy aging for each person. Future generations of older persons will redefine what are now considered the norms for aging. People can expect to spend 30 or more years in "late life," and there are many important tasks to accomplish during this period.

SPIRITUALITY AND AGING

Spirituality has been defined as a "quality of a person derived from the social and cultural environment that involves faith, a search for meaning, a sense of connection with others, and a transcendence of self, resulting in a sense of inner peace and well-being" (Delgado, 2007, p. 230). The spiritual aspect of people's lives transcends the physical and psychosocial realms and reaches the deepest capacity for love, hope, and meaning. Erickson's concept of ego integrity and Maslow's concept of self-actualization seem closely related to the development of a spiritual self.

Although religious needs are important for many older people, spirituality is much broader and more personal. Spirituality is a significant factor in understanding healthy aging. The model of successful aging proposed by Rowe and Kahn (1998) includes active engagement in life, minimal risk and disability, and high cognitive and physical function. Crowther et al. (2002) maintained that spirituality is the fourth integrated element of this model. This conclusion is supported by research that has found that spirituality is associated with life satisfaction, over and above other factors that influence healthy aging (Thomás et al., 2016).

Spirituality and the religious practices of older persons are linked to positive health outcomes in regard to life expectancy, cardiovascular conditions, chronic conditions, disability, and mental health (Zimmer et al., 2016). The effects of religious practice on health outcomes may be partly related to social support obtained through religious communities. Canadian researchers interviewed religious leaders and older churchgoers to understand findings that showed that older persons who attend religious services are less likely to have cardiovascular disease or diabetes. The researchers found that attending religious services has a direct effect on a person's mental health and also provides social connections, social activity, and social support (Banerjee et al., 2014).

Spirituality and religious practice may be particularly important to healthy aging in historically disadvantaged populations (Hooyman & Kiyak, 2008, p. 213). Declining physical health, loss of loved ones, and a realization that life's end may be near often challenge older people to reflect on the meaning of their lives, and spirituality may become more important (Harrington, 2016) (Fig. 7.1). Older Canadians are more likely than younger Canadians to report a religious affiliation (92% versus 76%) (Statistics Canada,

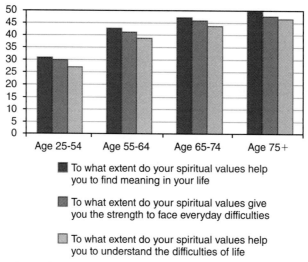

■ To what extent do your spiritual values help you to find meaning in your life

■ To what extent do your spiritual values give you the strength to face everyday difficulties

☐ To what extent do your spiritual values help you to understand the difficulties of life

FIGURE 7.1 Importance of spirituality in the lives of older Canadians. Rates indicate percentage responding "a lot" to three spirituality items on the Canadian Community Health Survey, by age. *Source:* Statistics Canada. (2002). *Canadian community health survey.* Retrieved from http://www.statcan.gc.ca/pub/89-519-x/2006001/t/4122073-eng.htm.

2016). Canadian researchers have found that spirituality and religion are important for older persons who are caring for a relative who has dementia (Jacklin et al., 2015; Damianakis et al., 2016).

IMPLICATIONS FOR GERONTOLOGICAL NURSING AND HEALTHY AGING

Gerontological nurses have many opportunities to help older persons reflect on the meaning and purpose of life and achieve spiritual well-being (Box 7.3). Spiritual well-being can be considered the ability to experience and integrate meaning and purpose in life through connectedness with self, others, art, music, literature, nature, or a power greater than oneself (Gaskamp et al., 2006).

BOX 7.3	Brief Assessment of Spiritual Resources and Concerns

Instructions: Use the following questions as a guide to interview the older adult (or caregiver):

- Does your religion or spirituality provide comfort or serve as a cause of stress? (*Ask to explain in what ways spirituality is a comfort or stressor.*)
- Do you have any religious or spiritual beliefs that might conflict with health care or affect health care decisions? (*Ask to identify any conflicts.*)
- Do you belong to a supportive church, congregation, or faith community? (*Ask how the faith community is supportive.*)
- Do you have any practices or rituals that help you express your spiritual or religious beliefs? (*Ask to identify or describe practices.*)
- Do you have any spiritual needs you would like someone to address? (*Ask what those needs are and if referral to a spiritual professional is desired.*)
- How can we (health care providers) help you with your spiritual needs or concerns?

Sources: Extracted from: Gaskamp, C., Sutter, R., Meraviglia, M., et al. (2006). Evidence-based practice guideline: Promoting spirituality in the older adult. *Journal of Gerontological Nursing, 32*(11), 8–11, p. 10, adapted from Meyer, C. L. (2003). *Dissertation Abstracts International, 55*(6), 2158B, UMI No 9428614; Koenig, H. G., & Brooks, R. G. (2002). Religion, health, and aging: Implications for practice and public policy. *Public Policy & Aging Report, 12*(4), 13.

ASSESSMENT

Older persons welcome a discussion of spiritual matters and want health care providers to consider their spiritual needs. The older person may have a pressing need to talk about philosophy and spiritual development. Private time for prayer, meditation, and reflection may be needed. Nurses may neglect exploring this issue with older persons because religion and spirituality may not seem a high priority. The patient should be assured that religious longings and rituals are important and that opportunities to fulfill longings or practice rituals will be made available as desired. Nurses must be knowledgeable about and respectful of various cultural beliefs, values, and religious rites and rituals; they must also understand age-related or generational differences in religious practices. It is important for the nurse to avoid imposing his or her own beliefs and to respect the patient's privacy in matters of spirituality and religion (Touhy & Zerwekh, 2006).

A comprehensive, evidence-informed guideline for promoting spirituality in the older person provides a framework for spiritual assessments and interventions (Gaskamp et al., 2006). Its use identifies older persons who may be at risk of spiritual distress and who might be most likely to benefit from the guideline (Box 7.4). Spiritual distress is "an individual's perception of hurt or suffering associated with that part of his or her

---

BOX 7.4	Indications of Risk of Spiritual Distress in Older People

- Experiences of events or conditions that affect the ability to participate in spiritual rituals.
- Diagnosis and treatment of a life-threatening, chronic, or terminal illness.
- Expressions of interpersonal or emotional suffering, loss of hope, lack of meaning, and the need to find meaning in suffering.
- Evidence of depression.
- Cognitive impairment.
- Verbalized questioning or loss of faith.
- Loss of interpersonal support.

Source: Adapted from Gaskamp, C., Sutter, R., Meraviglia, M., et al. (2006). Evidence-based practice guideline: Promoting spirituality in the older adult. *Journal of Gerontological Nursing, 32*(11), 8–11.

person that seeks to transcend the realm of the material. Spiritual distress is manifested by a deep sense of hurt stemming from feelings of loss or separation from one's God or deity, a sense of personal inadequacy or sinfulness before God and man, or a pervasive condition of loneliness" (Gaskamp et al., 2006, p. 9). The person experiencing spiritual distress is unable to experience hope, connectedness, and transcendence. Spiritual distress may be manifested by anger, guilt, blame, hatred, expressions of alienation, turning away from family and friends, an inability to enjoy, and an inability to participate in religious and spiritual activities and rituals that have provided comfort.

INTERVENTIONS

Religious and spiritual resources, such as pastoral visits, should be available in all settings where older people reside. In focus groups conducted as part of a Canadian study of mental health in late life, older Canadians identified the following ideas that nurture spiritual well-being (Seniors to Seniors, n.d., pp. 22–25):

- The natural world can nurture the spirit.
- Self-reflection can refresh the spirit.
- Religious beliefs can be comforting.
- Positive attitudes promote well-being.
- Being useful can be fulfilling.
- Good relationships can promote well-being.

Caring relationships between the nurse and the older person being cared for are at the heart of nursing that touches and supports the spirit. Knowing a person in their complexity, responding to that which matters most to the person, identifying and nurturing connections, listening, using presence and silence, and fostering connections to that which is sacred to the person are spiritual nursing responses that arise from a caring, connected relationship (Touhy, 2001). Suggestions for spiritual nursing responses are presented in Box 7.5.

COGNITION AND AGING

Cognition is both a biological and a psychological factor that must be considered in caring for the older person. This chapter discusses processes of normal cognition and learning in late life. Care of

---

BOX 7.5 Spiritual Nursing Responses

- Relieving physical discomfort, thus permitting focus on the spiritual.
- Touching in a comforting manner, which fosters the nurse–patient connection.
- Being authentically present.
- Listening attentively.
- Knowing the person behind the disease.
- Listening to life stories.
- Sharing fears and listening to expression of self-doubts or guilt.
- Fostering forgiveness and reconciliation.
- Sharing caring words and love.
- Fostering connections to that which is held sacred by the person.
- Respecting religious traditions, and providing for access to religious objects and rituals.
- Referring the person to a spiritual counsellor.

Sources: Gaskamp, C., Sutter, R., Meraviglia, M., et al. (2006). Evidence-based practice guideline: Promoting spirituality in the older adult. *Journal of Gerontological Nursing, 32*(11), 8–11; Touhy, T., Brown, C., & Smith, C. (2004). Spiritual caring: End of life in a nursing home. *Journal of Gerontological Nursing, 31*(9), 27–35; Touhy, T., & Zerwekh, H. (2006). Spiritual caring. In Zerwekh, J. (Ed.), *Nursing care at the end of life: Palliative care for patients and families*. Philadelphia: FA Davis.

---

older persons with impaired cognition is discussed in Chapter 21.

Cognition is the process of acquiring, storing, sharing, and using information. Cognitive function includes language, thought, memory, executive function, judgement, attention, and perception (Desai et al., 2010).

Early studies about cognition and aging were based on **cross-sectional** rather than **longitudinal research** and were often conducted with older persons who were in an institution or who had coexisting illnesses. It has been generally believed that cognitive function declines in old age because of a decreased number of neurons, decreased brain size, and diminished brain weight. Although these losses are features of aging, they are not consistent with deteriorating mental function (Sugarman, 2014), nor do they interfere with everyday routines. Neuron loss occurs mainly in the brain and spinal cord and is most pronounced in the cerebral cortex. The neuronal dendrites atrophy with aging, resulting in impairment of the synapses and changes in the transmission of the chemical neurotransmitters dopamine, serotonin, and acetylcholine. This process causes the slowing of many neural processes. However, cognitive abilities remain intact.

The determination of intellectual capacity and performance has been the focus of gerontological research. Specific cognitive functions may remain stable or may decline with increasing age. The cognitive functions that remain stable include attention span, language skills, communication skills, comprehension and discourse, and visual perception. The cognitive skills that tend to decline are verbal fluency, logical analysis, selective attention, object naming, and complex visuospatial skills (Hooyman & Kiyak, 2008).

The aging brain maintains resiliency (the ability to compensate for age-related changes). The old adage "use it or lose it" applies to cognitive as well as physical health. Stimulating the brain increases brain tissue formation, enhances the synaptic regulation of messages, and enhances the development of *cognitive reserve*. Cognitive reserve is based on the concept of neuroplasticity, which is the capacity of the brain to change in response to various stimuli, such as daily stressors and activities. Neuroplasticity was once thought to decrease with age, but current literature suggests that cognitive performance can be enhanced with mental stimulation. Maximizing the potential benefits of brain plasticity and cognitive reserve requires engaging in challenging cognitive, sensory, and motor activities, as well as meaningful social interactions, on a regular basis throughout life.

Many myths about aging and the brain may be believed by both health care providers and older persons. It is important to understand late-life cognition, memory, and learning and to dispel myths that can have a negative effect on wellness and that may in fact contribute to unnecessary cognitive decline.

Late adulthood is no longer seen as a period when growth has ceased and cognitive development has halted; rather, it is seen as a life stage programmed for plasticity and the development of unique capacities. Older people do maintain their ability to understand situations and learn from new experiences. These findings are significant to satisfaction in later life, because the capacity for effective lifestyle management and one's cognitive resources contribute to adaptation and enjoyment. Brain function that becomes impaired in old age is a result of disease or illness, not aging.

FLUID AND CRYSTALLIZED INTELLIGENCE

Fluid intelligence (often called *native intelligence*) is biologically determined, independent of experience or learning. It is associated with flexibility in thinking, inductive reasoning, abstract thinking, and integration; it helps people identify and draw conclusions about complex relationships. Fluid intelligence is related to learning and problem solving in novel situations. *Crystallized intelligence* comprises knowledge and abilities that a person acquires through education and life. Measures of crystallized intelligence include verbal meaning, word association, social judgement, and number skills. Older people perform more poorly on performance scales (fluid intelligence), but scores on verbal scales (crystallized intelligence) remain stable. This phenomenon is known as the *classic aging pattern* (Hooyman & Kiyak, 2008). The tendency to do poorly on performance tasks may be related to age-related changes in sensory and perceptual abilities as well as psychomotor skills. Lower cognitive processing speed and slower reaction time also affect performance.

MEMORY

Memory is the ability to retain or store information and to retrieve it when needed. Memory is a complex set of processes and storage systems. Three components characterize memory: immediate recall, short-term memory (ranging from minutes to days), and remote or long-term memory (Gallo et al., 2003). Biological, functional, environmental, and psychosocial influences affect memory development throughout adulthood. *Immediate recall* of newly encountered information seems to decrease with age, and declines in memory are noted in connection with complex tasks and strategies. Even though some older persons show decrements in reaction time, perception, the capacity for attentional tasks, and the ability to process information, most functioning remains intact and sufficient. *Recall of long-term events*, familiarity, previous learning, and life experience compensate for the minor loss of efficiency in the basic neurological processes. In unfamiliar, stressful, or demanding situations, however, these changes may be more marked.

Age-associated decline in memory is a major focus of research on aging and dementia. Healthy older persons may complain of memory problems, but their symptoms do not meet the criteria for mild cognitive impairment or dementia (see Chapter 21). *Age-associated memory impairment* is memory loss that is considered normal in light of a person's age and education level.

Many medical or psychiatric difficulties, such as depression and anxiety, also influence memory and concentration. Thus, it is important for older persons with memory complaints to have a comprehensive geriatric evaluation. In many cases, memory impairment is related to reversible and treatable conditions such as delirium, thyroid disease, injury, infection, depression, untreated diabetes, vitamin B_{12} deficiency, and anxiety. The assessment of cognitive function is discussed in Chapter 21.

IMPLICATIONS FOR GERONTOLOGICAL NURSING AND HEALTHY AGING

Nurses can educate people of all ages about effective strategies to enhance cognitive health and vitality and to promote cognitive reserve and brain plasticity. Suggested strategies include preventing and managing chronic conditions, maintaining a healthy weight, avoiding excess caloric intake, limiting sodium and fat intake, increasing antioxidant defence by consuming fresh fruits and vegetables, being physically active, participating in mentally stimulating activity, and engaging in social contact (Yevchak et al., 2008).

Older persons should remain active and engaged in activities that stimulate the mind as well as the body. Cognitive stimulation and memory training may be helpful for cognitively intact older persons, as well as for those with cognitive impairment (Naqvi et al., 2013; Yevchak et al., 2008). Cognitive stimulation and memory training techniques include mnemonics (strategies to enhance coding, storage, and recall), internal and external aids, reasoning and speed-of-processing training, cognitive games (e.g., Scrabble, chess, crossword puzzles), and spaced retrieval techniques (in which information is recalled over increasing lengths of time, such as 1 minute, 2 minutes, 4 minutes, and longer).

LEARNING IN LATE LIFE

Basic intelligence remains unchanged with increasing years, and older persons should be given opportunities for continued learning. **Geragogy** is the application of the principles of adult learning theory to teaching for older persons. Teaching for older persons should be relevant; new learning should be related to what is already known and should emphasize concrete and practical information. Box 7.6 presents additional strategies for enhancing the learning of older persons.

Opportunities for older people to learn are available in many formal and informal modes: self-teaching, college and university classes, seminars and conferences, public broadcasting television programs, DVDs, web-based courses, and countless other modes. Older persons are able to learn and to reap the benefits of learning—improved health, life satisfaction, coping abilities, friendships, joy, and satisfaction from learning (Narushima, 2008; Narushima et al., 2016) (Box 7.7). The benefits of engaging in life-long learning are greater for vulnerable older persons (Narushima et al., 2016).

The Internet has become one of the major vehicles of learning for older persons, and older persons make up the fastest growing group using social networking sites such as Facebook. Two-thirds of Canadians aged between 65 and 74 years use the Internet (Allen, 2013). Increasingly, older people are taking charge of their own learning and are scanning the Internet for information about health and lifestyles. Many reliable Internet resources related to health and aging are available. Examples include the websites of Health Canada (https://www.canada.ca/en/health-canada/services/healthy-living/seniors.html), the Public Health Agency of Canada (https://www.canada.ca/en/public-health/services/health-promotion/aging-seniors.html), the Government of Canada Seniors Canada Online (http://www.seniors.gc.ca/eng/index.shtml), and the US National Institute on Aging (NIA) (http://www.nia.nih.gov/health/). The Canadian Public Health Association website provides tips for evaluating the credibility of online health information (http://www.cpha.ca/en/programs/portals/h-l/web.aspx).

HEALTH LITERACY

Health literacy is the ability to access, understand, and act on information concerning health. Health literacy

---

BOX 7.6   Strategies to Enhance the Learning of Older Persons

- Make sure the person is ready to learn before trying to teach him or her. Watch for cues that may indicate that the person is preoccupied or too anxious to comprehend the material.
- Be sensitive to cultural, language, and other differences among the older persons you serve. Some suggestions may not be appropriate for everyone.
- Provide adequate time for learning, and use self-pacing techniques.
- Create a shame-free environment in which older persons feel free to ask questions and stay informed.
- Provide regular positive feedback.
- Avoid distractions, and present one idea at a time.
- Present pertinent, specific, practical, and individualized information. Emphasize concrete rather than abstract material.
- Use past experience; connect new learning to what has already been learned.
- Use written material to supplement verbal instruction. Use a list format; a low literacy level vocabulary; and large, readable font (e.g., 14- to 16-point Arial).
- Use high-contrast (e.g., black print on white paper) visual materials and handouts.
- Consider using Braille and digitally recorded material whenever necessary.
- Pay attention to reading ability. Use tools other than printed material, such as drawings, pictures, and discussion.
- Use bullets or lists to highlight pertinent information.
- Sit facing the person so he or she can watch your lip movements and facial expressions.
- Speak slowly.
- Keep the pitch of your voice low. Older people hear low-frequency sounds better than they hear high-frequency sounds.
- Encourage the learner to develop various mediators or mnemonic devices (e.g., visual images, rhymes, acronyms, and self-designed coding schemes).
- Have shorter, more frequent sessions with appropriate breaks. Pay attention to fatigue and physical discomfort.

Sources: Adapted from *Bridging principles of older adult learning: Reconnaissance phase final report.* (1999). Washington, DC: SPRY Foundation; Hayes, K. (2005). Designing written medication instructions: Effective ways to help older adults self-medicate. *Journal of Gerontological Nursing, 32*(5), 5–10.

BOX 7.7   Research for Evidence-Informed Practice: Lifelong Learning Is a Health Promotion Strategy

Problem: Older persons who participate in lifelong learning experience psychosocial benefits. It is important to understand how these benefits translate into health effects, especially in light of decreased funding for learning opportunities for older persons.

Methods: A qualitative case study of the Toronto District School Board Seniors' Daytime Program, including document analysis, observation of five classes, and interviews with 15 older students (64 to 83 years old) and four key informants.

Findings: All but one participant had a chronic health condition, and some participants were described as frail. They attended the program once or twice a week. They were motivated by health benefits (e.g., keeping the brain active) and by the pleasure of studying something that was interesting, often a subject that had interested them since youth. Learning was a pleasure and was meaningful. Participants described gaining a sense of confidence and control, and the social benefits were equally important. The older persons developed friendships and enhanced their social networks, and a sense of community developed in the classroom. Participants "forcefully articulated their wish that the school board continue providing affordable and accessible learning opportunities by talking of the 'entitlement' of 'taxpayers'" (Narushima, 2008, p. 686). Several participants worked collectively to lobby for continued program funding, an empowering experience.

Application to Nursing Practice: The major benefits of learning identified in this study are all factors that promote psychosocial health. The researchers critiqued funding and policies that tended to be based on the potential for education to train or qualify citizens as workers. "Non-vocational general interest programs for the post-work generation are every bit as important, and as cost-effective, as investing in younger people through vocational training" (Narushima, 2008, p. 688). Even though lifelong learning is funded through the education sector, it has health benefits, which indicates the importance of intersectoral collaboration. Nurses should support affordable, accessible public continuing education programs that meet the needs of older learners.

Source: Narushima, M. (2008). More than nickels and dimes: The health benefits of a community-based lifelong learning programme for older adults. *International Journal of Lifelong Education, 27*(6), 673–692.

is more than the ability to read and write. It includes listening skills, the ability to speak and communicate health needs, and the ability to act on written health information and instructions from health care providers. Factors influencing health literacy include the person's basic literacy skills and culture, the situations encountered in the health care system, and the cultural competence and communication skills of health care providers.

Six of ten adult Canadians do not have proficient health literacy. Literacy levels are lower for older persons, persons who do not speak English or French, and immigrants (Murray et al., 2007). Average health literacy varies among provinces and territories; the highest level is in Yukon and the lowest level is in Nunavut. Especially in the older population, lower literacy levels are found among those with less than a high-school education. Chronic health conditions and vision and hearing impairments may further limit health literacy.

Limited literacy skills influence the learning and understanding of health-related information, such as prescription directions, consent documents, and health education materials. The consequences of limited literacy include poorer health, less importance given to health-related information, poorer compliance with instructions, increased hospitalizations, and increased health care costs (Cho et al., 2008; Hayes, 2000). Many health education materials and information on websites are written at reading levels above the recommended fifth-grade reading level. The *Quick Guide to Health Literacy and Older Adults* (https://health.gov/communication/literacy/olderadults/literacy.htm) provides information for health care providers and strategies for communicating effectively.

Health literacy experts recommend the "teach-back" method of health education, which results in better understanding and retention of information by older people (White et al., 2013). Using this method, the nurse breaks down the teaching into small chunks and then verifies the patient's understanding by asking the patient to explain what he or she needs to do. It must be emphasized that it is the nurse's responsibility to explain the material clearly; the checking of the patient's understanding is not a test of the patient. If needed, the nurse follows up

| BOX 7.8 | Ten Elements of the Teach-Back Method of Health Education |

1. Use a caring tone of voice and attitude.
2. Display comfortable body language and make eye contact.
3. Use plain language.
4. Ask the patient to explain back, using their own words.
5. Use nonshaming, open-ended questions.
6. Avoid asking questions that can be answered with a simple "yes" or "no."
7. Emphasize that the responsibility to explain clearly is on you, the provider.
8. If the patient is not able to teach back correctly, explain again and re-check.
9. Use reader-friendly print materials to support learning.
10. Document use of and patient's response to teach-back.

Source: Adapted from Iowa Health System, Picker Institute, Des Moines University, & Health Literacy Iowa. (n.d.). *Always Use Teach-Back! Ten Elements of Competence for Using Teach-back Effectively.* Retrieved from http://www.teachbacktraining.org/assets/files/PDFS/Teach%20Back%20-%2010%20Elements%20of%20Competence.pdf.

by explaining again and checking understanding again. The ten principles of the teach-back method are presented in Box 7.8. The Agency for Healthcare Research and Quality health literacy toolkit website has links to excellent online information about the teach-back method (https://www.ahrq.gov/professionals/quality-patient-safety/quality-resources/tools/literacy-toolkit/healthlittoolkit2-tool5.html).

 IMPLICATIONS FOR GERONTOLOGICAL NURSING AND HEALTHY AGING

Caring for older persons means caring for body, mind, and spirit—holistic nursing at its finest. Understanding and appreciating the social, psychological, spiritual, and cognitive aspects of aging provides a foundation for nursing assessments and interventions that enhance lifelong growth, development, health, and well-being. A rich and stimulating environment should be available to all older persons in all care settings so that they can thrive, not merely survive, in old age.

KEY CONCEPTS

- Normal aging involves a gradual process of biopsychosocial change over time.
- Lifespan development theorists tend to study the total life course of cohort groups to determine the influence of major historical events on their development.
- The impact of gender, ethnicity, culture, and cohort must always be considered when the validity of biopsychosocial theories are discussed.
- Spirituality must be considered a significant factor in healthy aging.
- Late adulthood is no longer seen as the period when growth ceases and cognitive development halts; rather, it is seen as a life stage programmed for plasticity and the development of unique capacities.
- Cognitive stimulation and attention to brain health is just as important as attention to physical health.
- Learning in late life can be enhanced by using principles of geragogy and adapting teaching strategies to minimize barriers such as hearing and vision impairment and low literacy levels.

ACTIVITIES AND DISCUSSION QUESTIONS

1. Identify and discuss the major flaws in the sociological theories of aging.
2. How well do the psychological and sociological theories of aging fit within your own cultural perspective?
3. Discuss the variables that must constantly be considered when the psychosocial aspects of the aging experience are assessed. Identify and discuss those that seem most significant.
4. Discuss some of the problems of adequately testing the cognitive function of older persons.
5. How would you respond to the following myth of aging: "You can't teach an old dog new tricks"?
6. Complete a "Myths of Aging" quiz (e.g., at http://faculty.webster.edu/woolflm/myth.html). Identify and discuss strategies you can use to dispel myths about older persons' adaptability, intelligence, activity, social relationships, and productivity.
7. Discuss some ways that nurses can respond to the spiritual needs and concerns of older persons.
8. Practice using the teach-back method with classmates.

RESOURCES

Agency for Healthcare Research and Quality. *Use the teach-back method*
https://www.ahrq.gov/professionals/quality-patient-safety/quality-resources/tools/literacy-toolkit/healthlittoolkit2-tool5.html

Alzheimer Society of Canada. *Brain Health*
http://www.alzheimer.ca/en/About-dementia/Brain-health

Government of British Columbia. *Active aging*
http://www2.gov.bc.ca/gov/content/family-social-supports/seniors/health-safety/active-aging

National Institute on Aging. Health information (senior health: age pages and convenient one-page information sheets on health and aging)
https://www.nia.nih.gov/health

Public Health Agency of Canada. *Age-Friendly Communities Initiative*
https://www.canada.ca/en/public-health/services/health-promotion/aging-seniors/friendly-communities.html

U.S. Department of Health and Human Services. *Quick guide to health literacy and older adults*
http://www.health.gov/communication/literacy/olderadults/default.htm

The Hartford Institute for Geriatric Nursing. FICA spiritual history tool
https://consultgeri.org/try-this/specialty-practice/issue-sp5

World Health Organization. Age-friendly world
https://extranet.who.int/agefriendlyworld/

For additional resources, please visit *http://evolve.elsevier.com/Canada/Ebersole/gerontological/*

REFERENCES

Allen, M. K. (2013). *Consumption of culture by older Canadians on the internet* (Catalogue no. 75-006-X). Ottawa, ON: Statistics Canada. Retrieved from http://www.statcan.gc.ca/pub/75-006-x/2013001/article/11768-eng.htm.

Atchley, R. C. (2000). A continuity theory of normal aging. In J. F. Gubrium & J. A. Holstein (Eds.), *Aging and everyday life*. Malden, MA: Blackwell Publishers.

Baltes, P. B. (1987). Theoretical propositions on life-span developmental theory: On the dynamics between growth and decline. *Developmental Psychology, 23*(5), 611–626. doi:10.1037/0012 -1649.23.5.611.

Baltes, P. B., Lindenberger, U., & Staudinger, U. (1998). Life-span theory in developmental psychology. In R. Lerner (Ed.), *Handbook of child psychology (Vol. 1). Theoretical models of human development*. New York, NY: Wiley.

Banerjee, A. T., Strachan, P. H., Boyle, M. H., et al. (2014). Attending religious services and its relationship with coronary heart disease and related risk factors in older adults: A qualitative study of church pastors' and parishioners' perspectives. *Journal of Religion and Health, 53*, 1770–1785. doi:10.1007/s10943 -9783-1.

Bassett, R., Bourbonnais, V., & McDowell, I. (2008). Living long and keeping well: Elderly Canadians account for success in aging. *Canadian Journal on Aging, 26*(2), 113–126. doi:10.3138/ cja.26.2.113.

Cho, Y., Lee, S., Arozullah, A., et al. (2008). Effects of health literacy on health status and health service utilization amongst the elderly. *Social Science & Medicine, 66*, 1809–1816. doi:10.1016/j. socscimed.2008.01.003.

Cook, S. L. (2013). Redirection: An extension of career during retirement. *The Gerontologist, 55*(3), 360–373. doi:10.1093/ geront/gnt105.

Crowther, M., Parker, M., Achenbaum, W., et al. (2002). Rowe and Kahn's model of successful aging revisited: positive spirituality—the forgotten factor. *The Gerontologist, 42*(5), 613–620. doi:10.1093/geront/42.5.613.

Cumming, E., & Henry, W. (1961). *Growing old*. New York, NY: Basic Books.

Damianakis, T., Wilson, K., & Marziali, E. (2016). Family caregiver support groups: Spiritual reflections' impact on stress management. *Aging & Mental Health*. doi:10.1080/13607863.2016.1231 169. epub ahead of print.

Dandekar, K. (1996). *The elderly in India*. Thousand Oaks, CA: Sage.

Delgado, C. (2007). Sense of coherence, spirituality, stress and quality of life in chronic illness. *Journal of Nursing Scholarship, 39*(3), 229–234. doi:10.1111/j.1547-5069.2007.00173.x.

Desai, A., Grossberg, G., & Chibnall, J. (2010). Healthy brain aging: A road map. *Clinics in Geriatric Medicine, 26*(1), 1–16. doi:10.1016/j.cger.2009.12.002.

Dowd, J. J. (1980). *Stratification among the aged*. Monterey, CA: Brooks Cole.

Dunne, E., Wrosch, C., & Miller, G. E. (2011). Goal disengagement, functional disability, and depressive symptoms in old age. *Health Psychology, 30*, 763–770. doi:10.1037/10024019.

Erikson, E. H. (1963). *Childhood and society* (2nd ed.). New York, NY: WW Norton.

Erikson, E. H., Erikson, J. M., & Kivnick, H. Q. (1986). *Vital involvement in old age: The experience of old age in our time*. New York, NY: WW Norton.

Gallo, J. J., Fulmer, T., & Paveza, G. (2003). *Handbook of geriatric assessment* (3rd ed.). Boston, MA: Jones & Bartlett.

Gaskamp, C., Sutter, R., Meraviglia, M., et al. (2006). Promoting spirituality in the older adult. *Journal of Gerontological Nursing, 32*(11), 8–11. Retrieved from http://www.healio.com/ geriatric-medicine/journals/jgn/2006-11-32-11/%7B3acbab2f -ccde-4f2b-9e94-540f0a782a90%7D/promoting-spirituality-in -the-older-adult.

Gilmour, H. (2012). *Social participation and the health and well-being of Canadian seniors* (Catalogue no. 82-003-X). Ottawa, ON: Statistics Canada. Retrieved from http://www.statcan.gc.ca/ pub/82-003-x/2012004/article/11720-eng.pdf.

Gubrium, J. F. (1973). *The myth of the golden years*. Springfield, IL: Charles C. Thomas.

Harrington, A. (2016). The importance of spiritual assessment when caring for older adults. *Ageing & Society, 36*, 1–16. doi:10.1017/ S0144688X14001007.

Havighurst, R. (1971). *Developmental tasks and education* (3rd ed.). New York, NY: Longman.

Hayes, K. (2000). Literacy for health information of adult patients and caregivers in the rural emergency department. *Clinical Excellence for Nurse Practitioners, 4*(1), 35–40.

Hooks, B. (2000). *Feminist theory: From margin to center*. Cambridge, MA: South End Press.

Hooyman, N., & Kiyak, H. (2008). *Social gerontology* (8th ed.). Boston, MA: Pearson.

Jacklin, K., Pace, J. E., & Warry, W. (2015). Informal dementia caregiving among indigenous communities in Ontario, Canada. *Care Management Journals, 16*(2), 106–120. doi:10.1891/1521 -0987.16.2.106.

Jett, K. R. (2006). Mind loss in the African-American community: Dementia as a normal part of aging. *Journal of Aging Studies, 20*(1), 1–10. doi:10.1016/j.jaging.2005.05.002.

Jung, C. (1971). The stages of life. In J. Campbell (Ed.), *The portable Jung*. New York, NY: Viking Press. translated by R. F. C. Hull.

Latif, E. (2011). The impact of retirement on psychological well-being in Canada. *The Journal of Socio-Economics, 40*, 373–380. doi:10.1016/j.socec.2010.12.011.

Lerner, R. M. (2002). *Concepts and theories of human development* (3rd ed.). Mahwah, NJ: Lawrence Erlbaum Associates.

Maddox, G. (1963). Activity and morale: A longitudinal study of selected elderly subjects. *Social Forces, 42*(2), 195–204. doi: 10.1093/sf/42.2.195.

Marshall, V. (1996). The state of theory in aging and the social sciences. In R. H. Binstock & L. K. Geroge (Eds.), *Handbook of aging and the social sciences* (4th ed., pp. 12–30). San Diego, CA: Academic Press.

Maslow, A. H. (1968). *Toward a psychology of being*. Princeton, NJ: Van Nostrands.

Moody, H. R. (2010). *Aging: Concepts and controversies*. Thousand Oaks, CA: Pine Forge Press.

Murray, S., Rudd, R., Kirsch, I., et al. (2007). *Health literacy in Canada: Initial results from the International Adult Literacy and Skills Survey, 2007*. Ottawa, ON: Canadian Council on Learning.

Narushima, M. (2008). More than nickels and dimes: The health benefits of a community-based lifelong learning programme for older adults. *International Journal of Lifelong Education, 27*(6), 673–692. doi:10.1080/02601370802408332.

Narushima, M., Liu, J., & Diestelkamp, N. (2016). Lifelong learning in active ageing discourse: Its conserving effect on well-being, health and vulnerability. *Ageing & Society.* doi:10.1017/S0144686X16001136.

Naqvi, R., Liberman, D., Rosenberg, J., et al. (2013). Preventing cognitive decline in healthy older adults. *CMAJ, 185*, 881–885. doi:10.1503/cmaj.121448.

Papalia, D., Sterns, H., Feldman, R., et al. (2002). *Adult development and aging.* Boston, MA: McGraw-Hill.

Peck, R. (1968). Psychological developments in the second half of life. In B. Neugarten (Ed.), *Middle age and aging.* Chicago, IL: University of Chicago Press.

Polit, D., & Beck, C. (2006). *Essentials of nursing research: Methods, appraisal and utilization* (6th ed.). Philadelphia: Lippincott Williams & Wilkins.

Public Health Agency of Canada (PHAC). (2016). *Age-friendly communities initiative.* Retrieved from http://www.phac-aspc.gc.ca/seniors-aines/afc-caa-eng.php.

Pushkar, D., Chaikelson, J., Conway, M., et al. (2010). Testing continuity and activity variables as predictors of positive and negative affect in retirement. *Journal of Gerontology: Psychological Sciences, 65B*(1), 42–49. doi:10.1093/geronb/gbp079.

Rowe, J. W., & Kahn, R. L. (1998). *Successful aging.* New York, NY: Pantheon-Random House.

Seniors to Seniors. (n.d.). *Psychosocial Approaches to the Mental Health Challenges of Late Life Project.* Retrieved from http://www.seniorsmentalhealth.ca/Seniors2SeniorsENG_17_06.pdf.

Silverman, P., Hecht, L., & McMillin, J. (2000). Modeling life satisfaction among the aged: A comparison of Chinese and Americans. *Journal of Cross-cultural Gerontology, 15*(4), 289. doi:10.1023/A:1006793304508.

Statistics Canada. (2016). *Religion (108), Immigrant Status and Period of Immigration (11), Age Groups (10) and Sex (3) for the Population in Private Households of Canada, Provinces, Territories, Census Metropolitan Areas and Census Agglomerations, 2011 National Household Survey.* Catalogue no. 99-010-X2011032. Retrieved from http://www12.statcan.ca/nhs-enm/2011/dp-pd/dt-td/Rp-eng.cfm?TABID=2&LANG=E&A=R&APATH=3&DETAIL=0&DIM=3&FL=A&FREE=0&GC=01&GL=-1&GID=1118296&GK=1&GRP=0&O=D&PID=105399&PRID=0&PTYPE=105277&S=0&SHOWALL=0&SUB=0&Temporal=2013&THEME=95&VID=21289&VNAMEE=&VNAMEF=&D1=0&D2=0&D3=0&D4=0&D5=0&D6=0.

Street, D. A. (2007). Sociological approaches to understanding age and aging. In J. A. Blackburn & C. N. Dulmus (Eds.), *Handbook of gerontology: Evidence based approaches to theory, practice, and policy* (pp. 143–168). Hoboken, NJ: John Wiley & Sons.

Sugarman, R. A. (2014). Structure and function of the nervous system. In K. L. McCance & S. E. Huether (Eds.), *Pathophysiology: The biologic basis for disease in adults and children* (7th ed., pp. 447–483). St. Louis, MO: Mosby.

Tate, R. B., Swift, A. U., & Bayomi, D. J. (2013). Older men's lay definitions of successful aging over time: The Manitoba follow-up study. *International Journal of Aging and Human Development, 76*, 297–322. doi:1-.2190/AG.76.4.b.

Thomás, J. M., Sancho, P., Galiana, L., et al. (2016). A double test of the importance of spirituality, the "forgotten factor", in successful aging. *Social Indicators Research, 127*, 1377–1389. doi:10.1007/s11205-015-1014-6.

Tornstam, L. (1994). Gerotranscendence: A theoretical and empirical exploration. In L. E. Thomas & S. A. Eisenhandler (Eds.), *Aging and the religious dimension* (pp. 203–225). Westport, CT: Greenwood Publishing Group.

Tornstam, L. (1996). Gerotranscendence: A theory about maturing into old age. *Journal of Aging & Identity, 1*(1), 37–50.

Tornstam, L. (2005). *Gerotranscendence: A developmental theory of positive aging.* New York, NY: Springer.

Touhy, T. (2001). Nurturing hope and spirituality in the nursing home. *Holistic Nursing Practice, 15*(4), 45–56. doi:10.1097/00004650-200107000-00008.

Touhy, T., & Zerwekh, J. (2006). Spiritual caring. In J. C. Zerwekh (Ed.), *Nursing care at the end of life: Palliative care for patients and families.* Philadelphia, PA: FA Davis.

Vézina, M., & Crompton, S. (2012). Volunteering in Canada. *Canadian Social Trends, 93*, 37–55. Retrieved from http://www.statcan.gc.ca/pub/11-008-x/2012001/article/11638-eng.htm.

White, M., Garbez, R., Carroll, M., et al. (2013). Is 'teach-back' associated with knowledge retention and hospital readmission in hospitalized heart failure patients? *Journal of Cardiovascular Nursing, 28*(2), 137–146. doi:10.1097/JCN.0b013e31824987bd.

Yevchak, A., Loeb, S., & Fick, D. (2008). Promoting cognitive health and vitality: A review of clinical implications. *Geriatric Nursing, 29*(5), 302–330. doi:10.1016/j.gerinurse.2007.10.017.

Zimmer, Z., Jagger, C., Chiu, C., et al. (2016). Spirituality, religiosity, aging and health in global perspective: A review. *SSM-Population Health, 2*, 373–381. doi:10.1016/j.ssmph.2016.04.009.

Nutritional Needs

LEARNING OBJECTIVES

Upon completion of this chapter, the reader will be able to:

- Assess nutritional requirements.
- Identify factors affecting nutrition.
- Discuss nursing interventions to promote nutrition.
- Discuss assessment and interventions for older persons with dysphagia.
- Identify strategies to promote adequate nutrition for older persons who are experiencing physical and cognitive impairments or are in an institution or hospital.
- Discuss nursing interventions that promote good oral hygiene.
- Discuss nursing interventions to promote healthy bowel function.
- Discuss assessments and interventions for older persons with malnutrition.

GLOSSARY

Dysphagia The sensation of impaired passage of food from the mouth to the esophagus and stomach; difficulty swallowing.

Gastro-esophageal reflux disease The backward flow of stomach contents into the esophagus.

Xerostomia Excessive mouth dryness.

THE LIVED EXPERIENCE

If I do reach the point when I can no longer feed myself, I hope that the hands holding my fork belong to someone who has a feeling for who I am. I hope my helper will remember what she learns about me. If she would talk to me, if we could laugh together, I might even forget the chagrin of my useless hands. We could have a conversation rather than a feeding.

From Lustbader, W. (1999). Thoughts on the meaning of frailty. *Generations, 13*(4), 21–22.

NUTRITION

Nutrition is a leading indicator of the health status among Canadians (Health Canada, 2012a). Proper nutrition means that all of the essential nutrients (carbohydrates, fat, protein, vitamins, minerals, and water) are adequately supplied and used to maintain optimal health and well-being. Adequate nutrition is critical to preserving the health of older people and is an integral part of health, happiness, independence, quality of life, and physical, social, and mental functioning. This chapter discusses the dietary needs of older persons, risk factors contributing to inadequate nutrition, bowel function, malnutrition, dental health concerns, the effects of disease and functional impairment on nutrition, age-related changes that affect

My Food Guide

As a man aged 71 years or older, this is how many Food Guide Servings you need from each food group every day.

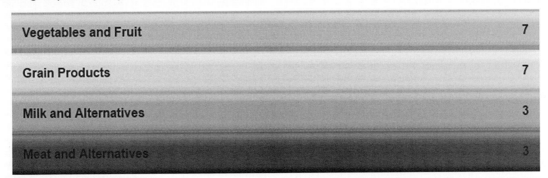

Vegetables and Fruit	7
Grain Products	7
Milk and Alternatives	3
Meat and Alternatives	3

My Food Guide

As a woman aged 71 years or older, this is how many Food Guide Servings you need from each food group every day.

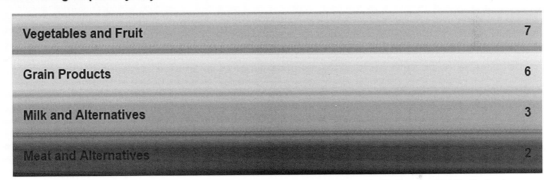

Vegetables and Fruit	7
Grain Products	6
Milk and Alternatives	3
Meat and Alternatives	2

FIGURE 8.1 *My Food Guide* for adults aged 71 years and older. From Health Canada. (2013). *My food guide*. Retrieved from https://www.canada.ca/en/health-canada/services/canada-food-guides.html. [Reproduced with permission of the Minister of Public Works and Government Services Canada, 2017.]

nutrition, and special considerations for older persons with cognitive and physical impairments.

NUTRITION-RELATED CONCERNS FOR OLDER PERSONS

While the fulfillment of an older person's nutritional needs can be affected by age-related changes, it is more often affected by numerous other factors, including lifelong eating habits, ethnicity, socialization, income, transportation, housing, food knowledge, health, and dentition.

My Food Guide for adults 71 years of age and older, adapted from *Eating Well with Canada's Food Guide* (Health Canada, 2011a), indicates the types and amounts of food that should be eaten to optimize nutrient intake (Fig. 8.1). The adapted food guide emphasizes increased servings of vegetables, fruits, and grain products. With proper instruction, this guide can be an easy and systematic way for a person to evaluate his or her own nutritional intake and independently make corrective adjustments. Health Canada also provides culturally relevant food guides for First Nations, Inuit, and Métis peoples (Health Canada, 2010). There is also a wide variety of recommended diets, such as diets for persons with diabetes and the Mediterranean diet for heart health (World Health Organization, 2017).

Age-Related Concerns

A number of age-related factors can contribute to poor nutrition for the older person, including changes in taste, smell, the digestive system, and appetite.

Taste. The sense of taste primarily depends on receptor cells in the taste buds, which are scattered on the surface of the tongue, the cheek, the soft palate, the upper tip of the esophagus, and other parts of the mouth and throat. Individuals have varied levels of taste sensitivity that seem predetermined by genetics and constitution as well as by age. Research findings suggest that the number of taste buds decreases as a person ages and that the remaining taste cells shrink (National Institutes of Health, 2014).

Age-related changes do not affect all taste sensations equally; with age, the ability to detect sweet taste seems to remain intact, whereas the ability to detect sour, salty, and bitter tastes declines. Many denture wearers say they lose some of their satisfaction with food, possibly because dentures cover the palate and because texture is a very important element in food enjoyment. The addition of flavour enhancers (e.g., bouillon cubes), concentrated flavours (e.g., jellies or sauces), and fresh herbs and spices can amplify both taste and smell and may increase enjoyment and interest in eating. The bland diets often found in hospitals and long-term care (LTC) homes contribute to decreased appetite.

Smell. Smell occurs when nerve receptors in the nose send messages to the brain. The oral and nasal senses interact to give the impression of a certain food, combining to heighten the sensory perceptions received. Smells also create positive or negative emotional responses to food, because emotions and smell sensations overlap in the brain.

Studies have shown that the sense of smell declines as a person ages. A decreased sense of smell may be related to many factors, including nasal sinus disease, repeated injury to olfactory receptors through viral infections, age-related changes in central nervous system functioning, cigarette smoking, medications, and periodontal disease or other dentition problems. Changes in the sense of smell are also associated with Parkinson's disease (Haehner et al., 2014) and Alzheimer's disease (Zou et al., 2016).

Many older people, particularly those who are in LTC settings, no longer cook and never have the experience of smelling food as it is cooking, an important appetite stimulant. As a way of increasing residents' interest and enjoyment in food, some LTC settings have adapted kitchens and dining rooms so that residents can smell the food cooking and even participate in the preparation of food.

Digestive System. Age-related changes in the oral cavity, esophagus, stomach, liver, pancreas, gallbladder, and small and large intestines may influence nutritional status.. A study found that edentulous persons generally eat fewer servings of fruit and vegetables (De Marchi et al., 2011).

Regulation of Appetite. Appetite in persons of all ages is regulated by a combination of a peripheral satiation system and a central feeding drive and is influenced by physical activity, functional limitations, smell, taste, mood, socialization, and comfort. With aging, the physiological basis for appetite regulation begins to differ from that of younger adults. Although the specifics await further research, changes in energy regulation mechanisms and neurotransmitter regulators of appetite have been implicated in impaired appetite and decreased intake associated with aging (de Boer et al., 2013).

Disease states also increase cytokine levels as a result of releasing diseased tissues, thereby decreasing appetite. There is some suggestion that alterations in endogenous opioid peptides are involved in food cravings, further contributing to decreased appetite (de Boer et al., 2013). Nogueiras et al. (2012) found that the blockade of opioid receptors diminishes patients' food intake, which could have implications for older persons who take opioids.

Nutritional Needs

Several considerations are important when nutrition for older people is addressed (Box 8.1). Increased amounts of calcium and vitamins D and B_{12} are needed in later life. Total caloric intake should decline in response to corresponding changes in metabolic rate and a general decrease in physical activity. The

BOX 8.1 Nutritional Goals: Key Recommendations for Older Persons

- Consume adequate nutrients within calorie needs.
- Consume a variety of nutrient-dense foods and drinks among the basic food groups. Eliminate saturated and trans fats, cholesterol, added sugar, salt, and alcohol from the diet.
- Meet energy needs by adopting a balanced eating pattern.
- Consume two to three servings of meat and alternatives (good sources of B vitamins) per day.
- Adults over 50 years of age should take 400 IU of vitamin D supplement daily.
- Maintain body weight in a healthy range, balancing calories from foods and beverages with calories expended.
- Prevent or delay onset of hypertension; increase potassium intake, reduce salt intake, eat a healthy diet, and engage in regular physical activity to achieve a healthy weight.
- If hypertensive, aim to consume no more than 1,500 mg of sodium per day, and meet the recommended potassium intake of 4,700 mg/day with food.
- To prevent or delay the onset of heart disease, eat less saturated or trans fat. Consume 30–45 mL of unsaturated fats per day. Wise fat choices include fish, nuts, oil-based salad dressings, nonhydrogenated margarine, and vegetable oils.
- If the level of low-density lipoproteins (the dangerous lipids) is elevated, decrease the amount of saturated fat calories to fewer than 7% of total calories.
- If alcoholic beverages are consumed, limit intake to one drink a day.
- Do not eat or drink raw, unpasteurized milk or any products made from raw milk. Do not eat raw or partially cooked eggs; foods containing raw eggs; raw or undercooked meat and poultry; raw or undercooked fish or shellfish; unpasteurized juices; or raw sprouts.
- Eat sufficient fibre-rich foods to maintain a fibre intake of 20–30 g per day.

Source: Dietitians of Canada. (2013). Planning meals using *Eating Well with Canada's Food Guide.* Planning meals: Variety and balance; Planning meals: Fibre facts. Retrieved from http://www.dietitians.ca/Downloads/Public/Senior-Friendly-collection.aspx.

Sodium Reduction Strategy for Canada reduces the recommended daily value for sodium to 1,500 mg and even lower for older persons (https://www.canada.ca/en/health-canada/services/food-nutrition/healthy-eating/sodium/related-information/reduction-strategy/recommendations-sodium-working-group.html). The intake of fluid is emphasized because thirst mechanisms may be less responsive in older people.

The major nutrition-related concerns with older persons are obesity and malnutrition. In 2004, 62.8% of females aged 65 years or older were overweight or obese. In 2008, this percentage crept up to nearly 70% (Statistics Canada, 2016). The percentage of males who were overweight or obese was 73.5% in 2004 and crept up to 76.6% in 2008 (Statistics Canada, 2016). Obesity in later life can further exacerbate the seriousness of a number of age-related health problems, depending on weight gain patterns and the health history of the obese person. Obesity is also connected with hypertension and with kidney and cardiovascular disease. Intervention trials indicate clinically significant benefits of weight reduction with regard to lower blood pressure, cholesterol, and blood sugar (Centers for Disease Control and Prevention, 2015). Maintaining a healthy weight is important for people of all ages.

Malnutrition is the other major nutrition-related concern. Malnutrition often goes unrecognized and affects morbidity, mortality, and quality of life. Furthermore, malnutrition is a precursor to frailty in older persons (Boulos et al., 2016). It is important to note that obese older persons are also at risk for malnutrition, particularly if they are losing weight because of the onset of an acute or chronic illness (White et al., 2012).

Lifelong Eating Habits

The nutritional state of a person often reflects his or her dietary history and present eating practices. Lifelong eating habits develop from tradition, ethnicity, religion, and societal influences (e.g., the availability of fast food), all of which can be collectively called "culture" and influence the food intake of older persons.

Members of a particular ethnic or religious group can have unique eating patterns, so individual assessment is important. Culturally and religiously appropriate diets should be available in any facility or congregate dining program.

For healthy older persons, essential nutrients should be obtained from food sources rather than dietary supplements. Recent studies have shown that diet can affect longevity and, combined with lifestyle changes, reduce disease risk. A diet consisting of nutrient- and fibre-rich fruits, brightly coloured vegetables, whole grains, legumes, lean proteins, and healthy fats—as well as unrefined, unprocessed foods—is beneficial (Cecchini et al., 2010). By following the recommendations in *Eating Well with Canada's Food Guide,* older persons may lower their risk of chronic disease and ensure health-protective nutrition.

Socialization

The social aspect of eating involves sharing with others and a feeling of belonging. People use food as a means of giving and receiving love, friendship, or a sense of belonging. Often, older persons may be isolated from the mainstream of life because of chronic illness, depression, and other functional limitations. When the older person has to prepare his or her own meals and eat alone, the outcome sometimes is either overindulgence or disinterest in eating. The presence of others during meals is a significant predictor of caloric intake (Higgs & Thomas, 2016).

Disinterest in food may also result from the effects of medications or disease processes. Over-the-counter and prescribed medications have the potential to cause adverse effects that can affect dietary intake (Peterson, 2015). A number of medications also interact with food (in what are called drug-nutrient interactions), resulting in the reduced absorption of nutrients. Both of these problems can adversely affect nutritional status (Carlo & Alpert, 2016).

The misuse of alcohol is prevalent among older persons and is a growing public health concern. Excessive consumption of alcohol interferes with nutrition; alcohol depletes the body of necessary nutrients and often replaces meals, thus making the person more susceptible to malnutrition (see Chapter 24).

Most cities and rural areas throughout Canada support a wide range of nutrition services for older persons, including home-delivered meals, congregate dining sites, and home visits by registered dietitians.

Congregate dining programs and home-delivered meal services have been shown to improve or help maintain nutritional status in older persons, thereby enabling them to avoid or delay costly institutionalization and allowing them to stay in their homes and communities. Many of these programs are funded by municipal or provincial governments (sometimes by both), by charitable organizations such as the United Way, and by private donations.

Income

There is a strong relationship between poor nutrition and low income. In Canada, the most accepted measure of poverty is what is known as the low income cut-off (LICO). Statistics Canada measures the number of families that are below the LICO—families that spend 20 percentage points or more of their gross income on food, shelter, and clothing. According to Statistics Canada, up to 8.4% of males and 13.9% of females 65 years of age or older are living below the LICO (Statistics Canada, 2013). Poverty rates among older Indigenous persons and recent immigrants are much higher, as these persons are more vulnerable to low income and unemployment than are other Canadians (Statistics Canada, 2015a).

Older persons with low incomes may need to choose among several essential needs, such as food, heat, telephone bills, medications, and health care visits, all of which affect overall health. Some older people eat only once per day in an attempt to make their income last through the month. Free food programs and donated commodities are available at distribution centres (e.g., food banks) for those with limited incomes. Although this is a valuable option for older people, the use of such programs is not always feasible. The types of food available any particular day or week can vary, and the quantities distributed are frequently too large for an older person to use or even carry from the distribution site. Some food sources do not support the dietary recommendations to prevent or manage certain disease conditions (e.g., processed canned food is high in sodium and sugar). The distribution site may be too far away or difficult to reach, and the time of distribution may be inconvenient. Although some restaurants provide special meal prices for older people, they often increase their prices as food costs rise.

Transportation

Available and easily accessible transportation to where food is sold or served is often limited for older people. Many small, longstanding neighbourhood food stores have been closed in the wake of the expansion of larger supermarkets that are located in areas that serve a greater segment of the population. It may become difficult for an older person to walk to the supermarket, reach it by public transportation, or carry a bag of groceries while using a cane or walker.

Functional impairments also make the use of public transportation difficult for some older people. For a person whose income is limited, transportation by taxicab is often unrealistic, but sharing a taxicab with others who also need to shop may enable the older person to purchase food. Organizations for older persons in many parts of Canada have been helpful in providing older persons with "van service" to shopping areas. In housing complexes, it may be possible to schedule group trips to the supermarket. Most communities have multiple sources of transportation available, but the older person may be unaware of them. It is important for nurses to be knowledgeable about community resources that are available to older people.

Many older persons, particularly widowed men, may never have learned how to shop for and prepare food. Older persons often have to rely on others to shop for them, and this may be a cause of concern, depending on the availability of support. The older person may also be reluctant to be dependent on others, particularly family members. For older people who own a computer, shopping on the Internet and having groceries delivered offer advantages, although prices may be higher than store prices. A new option is home delivery of nutritious meals made without additives or preservatives. Costs can vary from $6.50 to $37.00 per meal. The meals and are prepared and delivered by private companies and can be eaten immediately or stored for future use. An example of such a service can be found at https://mamaluv.com.

Housing

Older people who are poor or near-poor are likely to reside in substandard housing (International Housing Coalition, 2006). Some older persons who live in single rooms lack a stove for cooking, a means of refrigeration, and storage space for food. During the colder months, some single-room dwellers use window ledges and fire escapes to keep perishables cool for several days' use, which causes a high risk of spoiled food and food poisoning.

MALNUTRITION

Malnutrition among older adults has been documented in acute care, in LTC homes, and in the community. Protein-calorie malnutrition (PCM) is the most common form of malnutrition among older persons. It is characterized by clinical (muscle wasting, low body mass index) and biochemical signs (decreased albumin or other serum protein) indicative of insufficient intake. Many of the factors discussed previously contribute to malnutrition in older persons (Box 8.2).

The prevalence of PCM varies with the population observed and the definition of malnutrition. The prevalence of malnutrition in older persons depends on their health and functional capacity (Esmayel et al.,

---

BOX 8.2 Risk Factors for Malnutrition in Older Persons

Psychosocial Risk Factors
Limited income
Misuse of alcohol and other central nervous system depressants
Bereavement, loneliness, isolation, or living alone
Removal from usual cultural patterns
Memory loss
Depression

Mechanical Risk Factors
Decreased or limited strength and mobility
Neurological deficits, arthritis, impairment of hand-arm coordination, loss of tongue strength, dysphagia
Blindness or decreased or diminished vision
Inability to shop, prepare food, or feed self, and lack of adequate assistance with these activities
Pressure ulcers
Loss of teeth, poor-fitting dentures, or chewing problems
Difficulty breathing
Polypharmacy
Surgery, nothing by mouth (NPO) orders for extended periods of time, and fluid restriction

2013). As health and functional capacity deteriorate, the prevalence of malnutrition increases dramatically, reaching up to 60% in LTC or hospital settings (Sauer et al., 2016). Malnutrition has serious consequences, including infections, pressure ulcers, anemia, hypotension, impaired cognition, hip fractures, and increased mortality and morbidity. Most pathological causes of weight loss are considered to be reversible. A study by Neyens et al. (2012) found that malnutrition is associated with an increased risk of falling and impaired activity in older persons who reside in LTC homes. Malnutrition can be assessed with standardized tools such as the Mini Nutritional Assessment or the Nutritional Risk Screening tool (Deer et al., 2017).

Depression, frequent in older persons, is a common and reversible cause of weight loss. Screening for depression with validated tools such as the Geriatric Depression Scale and the Cornell Scale for Depression in Dementia should be included in the assessment of older people who are experiencing weight loss (see Chapter 24). A thorough medication review is important when nutritional concerns are assessed, since many medications affect appetite and can affect nutritional status. Medications that are most frequently associated with malnutrition include digoxin, theophylline, nonsteroidal anti-inflammatory drugs, iron supplements, and psychoactive medications.

ORAL HEALTH

Dental health is a basic need for older persons that is increasingly neglected. Oral and dental health is integral to general health (Health Canada, 2015). Poor oral health is recognized as a risk factor for dehydration and malnutrition as well as a number of systemic diseases, including aspiration pneumonia, joint dysfunctions, cardiovascular disease, and poor glycemic control (Berkey & Scannapieco, 2013). Furthermore, poor oral health—which leads to missing teeth, teeth in ill repair, and oral pain—contributes to chewing and swallowing problems that affect adequate nutritional intake (Berkey & Scannapieco, 2013). Health Canada's *Report on the Findings of the Oral Health Component of the Canadian Health Measures Survey 2007–2009* can be obtained by visiting the Federal, Provincial and Territorial Dental Working Group website

(http://www.fptdwg.ca/assets/PDF/CHMS/CHMS-E -summ.pdf).

The percentage of people aged 60 to 79 years who are without natural teeth is 22.3% for men and 21.1% for women (Statistics Canada, 2015b). The prevalence of periodontitis, which is the main cause of the loss of natural teeth, is decreasing as knowledge about it increases and more people use fluorides, improve their nutrition, engage in oral hygiene practices, and take advantage of improved dental health care. However, older people may not have had the advantages of preventive treatment, and those with functional and cognitive limitations may be unable to perform oral hygiene. Decades ago, dental care was extremely painful, and fear of the dentist still exists (Borreani et al., 2010). Access to dental care for older people may be limited as well as cost prohibitive. Also, some Canadian cities, such as Calgary and Windsor, choose not to fluoridate the water, which further affects residents' oral health (Rugg-Gunn & Do, 2012).

The low priority of dental care in the existing health care system is reflected by the absence or inadequacy of third-party reimbursement for the type of dental care needed by older persons. The *Canada Health Act* has designated dental surgery in hospitals as a "medically necessary" health service, resulting in the coverage of this service by provincial health insurance. However, this health insurance does not cover regular dental services in a dentist's office. Canadians rely on their employers, individual private insurance, or their own financial resources for paying for dental treatments. In some jurisdictions, public health units have been involved in providing targeted programs to address the needs of older persons or those who receive social assistance. The Canadian Association of Public Health Dentistry tracks those programs and has been advocating for the extension of coverage to persons who are currently unable to pay for dental care (Canadian Association for Public Health Dentistry, 2017).

Older people have fewer dentist visits than members of any other age group have. Older Canadians with the poorest oral health are those who are economically disadvantaged, lack insurance, and are members of racial and ethnic minorities. Furthermore, in hospitals and LTC homes, oral care is often overlooked (Coker et al., 2016). Some of the

BOX 8.3	Age-Related Changes of the Buccal Cavity

- Decrease in the cellular compartment
- Loss of submucosal elastin in oral mucosa
- Loss of connective tissue (collagen)
- Increase in thickness of collagen fibres
- Decrease in function of minor salivary glands
- Decrease in number and quality of blood vessels and nerves
- Attrition on occlusal contact surfaces
- Decrease of enamel permeability (teeth more brittle)
- Change of tooth colour
- Formation of excessive secondary dentin
- Decrease at the cement/enamel junction
- Decrease in size of pulp chamber and root canals
- Decrease in size and volume of tooth pulp
- Increase in pulp stones and dystrophic mineralization

BOX 8.4	Signs and Symptoms of Oral and Throat Cancer

- Swelling or thickening, lumps or bumps, or rough spots or eroded areas on the lips, gums, or other areas inside the mouth
- Velvety white, red, or speckled patches in the mouth
- Persistent sores on the face, neck, or mouth that bleed easily
- Unexplained bleeding in the mouth
- Unexplained numbness, pain, or tenderness in any area of the face, mouth, neck, or tongue
- Soreness in the back of the throat; a persistent feeling that something is caught in the throat
- Difficulty chewing or swallowing, speaking, or moving the jaw or tongue
- Hoarseness, chronic sore throat, or changes in the voice
- Dramatic weight loss
- Lump or swelling in the neck
- Severe pain in one ear (with a normal eardrum)
- Pain around the teeth; loosening of the teeth
- Swelling or pain in the jaw; difficulty moving the jaw

age-related physiological changes and common problems associated with oral care are discussed later in this chapter.

AGE-RELATED CHANGES OF THE BUCCAL CAVITY

Aging teeth become worn and darker and tend to yellow over time (Haralur, 2015). In addition to years of exposure of the teeth and related structures to microbial assault, the oral cavity shows evidence of wear and tear as a result of normal use (chewing and talking) and destructive oral habits such as bruxism (habitual grinding of the teeth). People who are edentulous and are using complete dentures continue to have oral health care needs. Ill-fitting dentures affect chewing and hence nutritional intake. Age-related changes in the buccal cavity also predispose older people to oral and dental problems (Box 8.3).

XEROSTOMIA

A common oral problem among older persons is dry mouth (**xerostomia**). Prevalence of xerostomia increases with age and affects approximately 35% of the population aged 65 years and older (Liu et al., 2012). Reduced salivary flow is a side effect of more than 500 medications. A reduction in saliva and a dry mouth make eating, swallowing, and speaking difficult. It can also lead to significant problems of the

teeth and their supporting structure. Artificial-saliva preparations are available (those containing sorbitol should be avoided), and adequate fluid intake is also important when xerostomia occurs. Chewing gum with xylitol stimulates saliva flow and promotes oral hygiene (Karami-Nogurani et al., 2011). Medication review is also indicated in order to eliminate, if possible, the use of medications that contribute to xerostomia.

ORAL CANCER

Oral cancers occur more frequently in late life, and men are affected twice as often as are women. For all stages combined, the 5-year survival rate is 63%, compared to the survival rates for cervical cancer (75%), melanoma cancers (89%), and prostate cancer (95%) (Health Canada, 2009). Oral examinations are important as they can assist in the early detection and treatment of oral cancers and other oral and dental problems. Box 8.4 presents the common signs and symptoms of oral cancer.

Risk factors for oral cancer are tobacco use, alcohol use, and exposure to ultraviolet light (especially for cancer of the lips). Pipe, cigar, and cigarette smoking

TABLE 8.1	Oral Signs and Symptoms Associated With Patient Stressors in the Critical Care Unit Setting	
STRESSOR	**SIGNS**	**SYMPTOMS**
Mechanical Ventilation and Oxygen Therapy		
Dry mouth	• Dry, red mucosa and depapillated, lobulated, or fissured tongue • Dry, cracked lips • Buildup of debris in mouth	• Burning sensation • Dryness • Difficulty swallowing
Medication Therapy		
Immunosuppression, change in flora	• White plaques and inflammation associated with *Candida albicans*, herpetic ulcers, and halitosis	• Pain or discomfort • Halitosis
Xerostomia	• Decreased salivary flow • Dry, red mucosa and depapillated, lobulated, or fissured tongue • Dry, cracked lips • Buildup of debris in mouth	• Burning sensation • Dryness • Difficulty swallowing
Therapeutic Dehydration		
Xerostomia	• See above	• See above

Source: Registered Nurses' Association of Ontario (RNAO). (2008). *Oral health: Nursing assessment and interventions.* Toronto: Author. Retrieved from http://rnao.ca/sites/rnao-ca/files/Oral_Health_-_Nursing_Assessment_and_Interventions.pdf. Based on Jones, H., Newton, J., Bower, E. (2004). A survey of the oral care practices of intensive care nurses. *Intensive and Critical Care Nursing, 20*(2), 69–76. doi:10.1016/j.iccn.2004.01.004.

are all implicated. Other risk factors are age, sex, local tissue irritation, poor nutrition, use of mouthwash with a high alcohol content, human papillomavirus (HPV) infection, and immunosuppressant medications. Therapy options are based on diagnosis and staging and include surgery, radiation, and chemotherapy. If detected early, these cancers can often be treated successfully.

IMPLICATIONS FOR GERONTOLOGICAL NURSING AND HEALTHY AGING

ASSESSMENT

Good oral hygiene and assessment of oral health are essentials of nursing care. In addition to identifying oral health problems, an examination of the mouth can lead to early diagnosis and treatment for some diseases. All persons, especially those over 50 years of age, with or without dentures, should have oral examinations on a regular basis. Although an oral examination is best performed by a dentist, nurses can perform basic screening examinations. A list of instruments and signs and symptoms are also

provided by the Registered Nurses' Association of Ontario as part of its Best Practice Guidelines (Registered Nurses' Association of Ontario [RNAO], 2008) (Table 8.1). Gil-Montoya et al. (2006) developed an oral clinical assessment appropriate for residents of LTC homes (Fig. 8.2).

INTERVENTIONS

The prescribed oral hygiene regimen for a person with teeth consists of brushing and flossing twice a day and using a fluoride dentifrice and nonalcoholic mouthwash. There is evidence that cleaning the teeth with a toothbrush after meals lowers the risk for aspiration pneumonia (Li et al., 2016).

Impaired manual dexterity may make it difficult for older persons to adequately maintain their dental routine and remove plaque adequately. The handgrip of a manual toothbrush is often too small to grasp and manipulate easily. Using a child's toothbrush or enlarging the handle of an adult-sized toothbrush by adding a foam grip or wrapping it with gauze has been effective in facilitating grasp. The ultrasonic toothbrush is an effective tool that older people or their caregivers can use. Occupational therapists can be

Oral Clinical History
Date of examination:
Name:
Room No:
1. Does he/she have any natural teeth? ( ) No ( ) Yes, Upper ( ) Yes, Lower
2. Does he/she use a removable dental prosthesis? ( ) No ( ) Yes, Upper ( ) Yes, Lower
3. Are his/her gums inflamed (reddened or bleeding)? ( ) No ( ) Yes
4. Does he/she have bacterial plaque or tartar on teeth or prosthesis? ( ) No ( ) Medium amount ( ) A lot
5. Does his/her mouth show signs of dryness? ( ) No ( ) Yes
6. He/she carries out hygiene ( ) on his/her own ( ) with some help ( ) someone has to do it for him/her

7. ( ) Immediate dental care by the dental service is required.	Reason

Recommendations for care of teeth and prostheses	
	Encourage/supervise tooth and/or prosthesis brushing
	Remove prostheses at bedtime
	Clean teeth with electric toothbrush
	Clean prostheses with electric toothbrush
	Clean oral mucosa with gauze - 0.12% CLX
	Rinse with 0.12% Chlorhexidine solution
	Moisten/coat lips with Vaseline or lip balm
	Transfer for immediate dental care

Dates	Incidences

FIGURE 8.2 Oral history. Data from Registered Nurses' Association of Ontario (RNAO). (2008). *Oral health: Nursing assessment and interventions.* Retrieved from http://rnao.ca/sites/rnao-ca/files/Oral_Health_-_Nursing_Assessment_and_Interventions.pdf.

helpful in the assessment of functional impairments and the provision of adaptive equipment for oral care.

Therapeutic rinses contain an agent that is beneficial to the surface of the teeth and to the oral environment. Some therapeutic rinses (such as chlorhexidine [Peridex], which contains alcohol but is also a broad-spectrum antimicrobial agent that helps control plaque) require a prescription. Original formula Listerine, a commercial over-the-counter product, should not be used by persons who have severe oral mucositis, because it contains a high quantity of alcohol (26.9% by volume). Listerine and generic equivalents that contain alcohol may be mixed with water but should always be used in conjunction with, not instead of, brushing.

Enteral feeding of older persons is associated with significant pathological colonization of the mouth, greater than that observed in people who receive oral

BOX 8.5   Instructions for Caregivers Providing Dental Care

1. If the person is in bed, elevate his or her head by raising the bed or propping up the patient's head and neck with pillows, and have the person turn his or her head to face you. Place a clean towel across the chest and under the chin, and place a basin under the chin.
2. If the person is sitting in a chair or a wheelchair, stand behind the person and stabilize the head by placing one hand under the chin and resting the head against your body. Place a towel across the chest and over the shoulders. The basin can be kept handy in the person's lap or on a table placed at the front or side. A wheelchair may be positioned in front of the sink.
3. Brush and floss the person's teeth (use an electric toothbrush if possible). It may be helpful to retract the person's lips and cheek with a tongue blade or with the fingers in order to see the area that is being cleaned. Use a mouth prop as needed. If manual flossing is too difficult, use a floss holder or interproximal brush to clean the proximal surfaces between the teeth.
4. If the person's lips are dry or cracked, apply a light coating of petroleum jelly or lip balm.
5. Provide a conscious person with fluoride rinses or other rinses as indicated.

feeding. Therefore, oral care should be undertaken every 4 hours for people with gastrostomy tubes, and teeth should be brushed after each feeding, to decrease the risk for aspiration pneumonia (Li et al., 2016). The oral mucosa of unconscious or severely cognitively impaired patients should be hydrated by using gauze soaked in physiological saline, and the lips should be coated with petroleum jelly or lip balm (Kobayashi et al., 2017).

When the person is unable to carry out his or her own dental or oral regimen, it is the responsibility of the caregiver to provide oral care (Box 8.5). Oral care is an often-neglected part of daily nursing care. Poor oral health and a lack of attention to oral hygiene are major concerns in residential settings and contribute significantly to poor nutrition and other negative outcomes such as aspiration pneumonia. There are many reasons for this deficit, including inadequate knowledge of how to assess and provide care, difficulty in providing oral care to dependent and cognitively impaired older persons, inadequate training and staffing, and the lack of appropriate supplies.

Many LTC homes have implemented specific programs, such as staff training or dental care teams, mobile dentistry units, or oral screening and teeth cleaning done by dental students. Evidence-informed protocols combined with educational training sessions have been shown to have a positive impact on the oral health status of older persons (RNAO, 2008). An oral health protocol for older persons residing in institutions has been provided by Gil-Montoya et al. (2006).

Dentures

Older persons with dentures should be taught the proper care of their dentures and oral tissue to prevent odour, staining, plaque buildup, and oral infections. Care should include the removal of debris under dentures in order to prevent pressure and shrinkage of underlying support structures. Dentures and other dental appliances, such as bridges, should be rinsed after each meal and brushed thoroughly once a day, preferably at night (Box 8.6). To allow relief from compression on the gums, dentures should not be worn at night.

Dentures are very personal and expensive possessions; in LTC homes, hospitals, and other care centres, patients' dentures are often misplaced or mixed up with those of others. The utmost care should be taken when handling, cleaning, and storing dentures. Dentures should incorporate some means of identifying the patient who owns them. Broken or damaged dentures and dentures that no longer fit because of the wearer's weight loss are a common problem for older persons. Relining (adding material to the acrylic surface of the denture) can be used to improve the fit of dentures. Ill-fitting dentures or dentures that are not cleaned contribute to oral problems as well as to poor nutrition and reduced enjoyment of food. Daily removal and cleaning of dentures and brushing of teeth should be a part of the care routines in every facility.

All staff need to be knowledgeable about oral hygiene and techniques for the care of teeth and dentures. Oral hygiene protocols and appropriate oral care equipment should be available. Older persons and families also need to be educated about the

BOX 8.6 Instructions for Cleaning Dentures

1. Rinse the denture after each meal to remove soft debris.
2. Once a day, preferably before the person retires, remove the denture and brush it thoroughly.
   a. Although an ordinary soft toothbrush is adequate, a specially designed denture brush may clean more effectively.
   b. Brush the denture over a sink lined with a facecloth and half filled with water, to prevent the denture from breaking if it is dropped.
   c. Hold the denture securely in one hand but do not squeeze; hold the brush in the other hand. It is not essential to use a denture paste, particularly if the dentures are soaked to soften debris before being brushed. Plain water, mild soap, or sodium bicarbonate may be used.
   d. When a removable partial denture is being cleaned, great care must be taken to remove plaque from the curved metal clasps that hook around the teeth, either with a regular toothbrush or with a specially designed clasp brush.
3. After brushing, rinse the denture thoroughly, then place it in a denture-cleaning solution and allow it to soak overnight. In the morning, remove the denture from the cleaning solution, rinse it thoroughly, and then insert it into the mouth. Use denture paste if necessary to secure dentures.

importance of oral health and taught the techniques of adequate oral care.

HEALTH CONDITIONS AFFECTING NUTRITION

CHRONIC DISEASES

Chronic diseases and their sequelae that pose nutritional challenges to older persons include osteoporosis, gastrointestinal disorders, obesity, diabetes, cardiovascular and respiratory diseases, cancer, dysphagia, and dementia. Functional impairments associated with chronic disease interfere with the person's ability to shop, cook, and eat independently. For example, heart failure and chronic obstructive pulmonary disease are associated with fatigue, increased energy expenditure, and decreased appetite. Alzheimer's disease and other dementias affect adequate nutritional intake. Depression can cause changes in appetite (resulting in loss or gain of weight), and the side effects of antidepressant medications affect appetite and nutrition (see Chapters 14 and 24). A number of prevalent disorders of the gastrointestinal tract—including **gastro-esophageal reflux disease,** ulcers, constipation, diverticulosis, and colon cancer—are associated with nutritional problems.

The following section discusses nutritional concerns and nursing interventions related to dementia, dysphagia, constipation, and fecal impaction. (For more detailed information on health conditions and chronic diseases in older persons, see Chapters 15, 17, 18, 20, and 21.)

Dementia

Dementia affects adequate nutritional intake, and weight loss and malnutrition become considerable concerns in late dementia. The loss of weight may be the result of physiological changes, cognitive deficits, unawareness of the need to eat, loss of independence for self-feeding, ill-fitting dentures, depression, or increased energy output caused by pacing or wandering (Alzheimer Disease International, 2014).

One of the best strategies for managing poor food intake for a person with dementia is to find foods that the person enjoys. Nutrient-dense foods are preferred. Attention to mealtime ambience is important, and the person should be able to take as much time as needed to eat. Food should be available 24 hours a day, and the person should be allowed to follow his or her accustomed eating schedule (e.g., late breakfast, early dinner). Finger foods may be a good choice when utensils are too difficult to manage. Serving one dish and using only one utensil at a time may assist in promoting adequate intake. Demonstrate eating motions that the person can imitate; use verbal cueing and prompting (e.g., take a bite, chew, swallow) and the hand-over-hand guiding technique to support self-feeding. Offer small amounts of fluid between bites of food and throughout the day. Refreshment stations with easy access to juices, water, and healthy snacks also promote adequate food intake.

Dysphagia

Dysphagia is difficulty in swallowing. Dysphagia may occur as a result of neurological diseases such as stroke, Parkinson's disease, multiple sclerosis, and dementia. Dysphagia can be classified as oropharyngeal or esophageal. *Oropharyngeal dysphagia* refers to difficulty in the passage from the mouth to the esophagus. *Esophageal dysphagia* refers to disordered passage of food through the esophagus. The two types can be distinguished on the basis of the person's medical history, specific signs and symptoms on physical examination, and diagnostic tests.

Dysphagia is a serious problem; its consequences include malnutrition, dehydration aspiration, and pneumonia (Sura et al., 2012). For the older person, dysphagia is superimposed on the slowed swallowing rate associated with normal aging, creating an even greater risk of complications.

The exact prevalence of dysphagia is unknown, but a systematic review by Madhavan et al. (2016) indicates that it may be present in 15% of community-dwelling older persons.

BOX 8.7	Symptoms of Dysphagia or Possible Aspiration

- Difficult, laboured swallowing
- Drooling
- Copious oral secretions
- Coughing or choking while eating
- Holding or pocketing food in the mouth
- Difficulty moving food or liquid from mouth to throat
- Difficulty chewing
- Nasal voice or hoarseness
- Wet or gurgling voice
- Excessive throat clearing
- Sensation of something stuck in the throat during swallowing
- Reflux of food or liquid into the throat, mouth, or nose
- Heartburn
- Chest pain
- Hiccups
- Weight loss
- Frequent respiratory infections, pneumonia

IMPLICATIONS FOR GERONTOLOGICAL NURSING AND HEALTHY AGING

ASSESSMENT

It is important to obtain a careful history of the older person's response to dysphagia and to observe the person during mealtime. Symptoms that will alert the nurse to possible swallowing problems and aspiration are presented in Box 8.7. When any of these symptoms are present, it is important to contact a speech-language pathologist (SLP), who will conduct specific tests to identify the cause of the person's swallowing problem and restore swallowing function to as normal a level as possible.

INTERVENTIONS

The most profound and dangerous problem for older persons experiencing dysphagia is aspiration, in which oral or gastric contents (food, saliva, or nasal secretions) enter the bronchial tree. Aspiration during swallowing is best detected by procedures such as videofluoroscopy or fibre-optic endoscopy, but clinical observations and evaluation by an SLP are important as well.

Aspiration pneumonia (i.e., a bronchopneumonia as a result of aspiration) is underdiagnosed in older persons, and its signs and symptoms manifest themselves differently in members of this age group as compared to other age groups. Small-volume aspirations that produce few overt symptoms are common and are often not discovered until the condition has progressed to a more serious condition such as aspiration pneumonia (Hollaar et al., 2016). An elevated respiratory rate and alterations in mental status may be early symptoms of aspiration pneumonia.

It is important to have suctioning equipment available at the bedside or in the dining room in institutional settings. In the home setting, a call for emergency help should be immediate if the person is having trouble breathing, is choking, or has stopped breathing. Perform first aid and cardiopulmonary resuscitation (CPR) if consented to and necessary. People with dysphagia should have supervision at all mealtimes, and observation of persons who are at high risk for aspiration pneumonia should be ongoing.

The gerontological nurse must work closely with other members of the interprofessional team, such as the SLP, in implementing suggested interventions to prevent aspiration. Research on the appropriate management of swallowing disorders in older people, particularly during acute illness and in LTC, is limited.

BOX 8.8	Preventing Aspiration in Older Persons With Dysphagia

- Provide a 30-minute rest period before feeding; a rested person will likely have less difficulty swallowing.
- The person should sit at 90 degrees during all oral (PO) intake.
- Maintain the 90-degree positioning for at least 1 hour after PO intake.
- Avoid mixed-consistency food items (e.g., fruit cups, soup).
- Adjust the rate of feeding and the size of bites to the person's tolerance; avoid rushed or forced feeding.
- Alternate solid and liquid boluses.
- Follow the speech-language pathologist's recommendation for safe swallowing techniques and modified food consistency (thickened liquids, pureed foods).
- Place food on the unimpaired side of the mouth.
- Avoid sedatives and hypnotics that may impair the cough reflex and swallowing ability.
- Keep suction equipment ready at all times.
- Supervise all meals.
- Visually check the mouth for pocketing of food in cheeks.

Source: Adapted from Metheny, N. A. (2012). Preventing aspiration in older adults with dysphagia. *The Hartford Institute for Geriatric Nursing, 20.*

A comprehensive protocol for preventing aspiration in older persons with dysphagia is available from https://consultgeri.org/try-this/general-assessment/issue-20.pdf. Interventions that are helpful in preventing aspiration during hand feeding are presented in Box 8.8.

Constipation

Bowel function in the older person, although normally only slightly altered by physiological changes of age, can be a source of concern and a potentially serious problem, especially for the older person who is functionally impaired. Normal elimination is the easy passage of feces without undue straining or a feeling of incomplete evacuation or defecation. Constipation is a common gastro-intestinal complaint; an estimated 30 to 50% of older persons living in the community regularly use laxatives (RNAO, 2011). The percentage is higher for the population of older persons who are living in LTC homes (RNAO, 2011).

It is important that nurses realize that constipation is a symptom. It is often a reflection of poor habits, postponed passage of stool, and many chronic physical and psychological illnesses. It is also a common side effect of medication. Constipation can also signal more serious underlying problems, such as colonic dysmotility or mass lesions. Poor diet and lack of activity play significant roles in constipation. Numerous precipitating factors or conditions can cause or worsen constipation (Table 8.2).

Fecal Impaction. Fecal impaction is a major complication of unrecognized or unattended constipation. Fecal impaction is especially common in older people who are cognitively impaired and living in institutions and is a serious and often dangerous problem. The symptoms of fecal impaction include malaise, urinary retention, elevated temperature, incontinence of bladder or bowel or both, alterations in cognitive status, fissures, hemorrhoids, and intestinal obstruction. Leakage of liquid stool from around the impaction can be seen. Continued obstruction by a fecal mass may eventually impair sensation, leading to the need for larger stool volume to stimulate the urge to defecate, which contributes to megacolon (Hussain et al., 2014). Valsalva's manoeuvre with straining during stool defecation can cause transient ischemic attacks and syncope, especially in frail older persons.

Removal of a fecal impaction is at times worse than the misery of the condition. The management of fecal impaction requires the digital removal of the hard, compacted stool from the rectum with the use of a lubricant containing lidocaine jelly. Generally, this is preceded by an oil-retention enema to soften the feces in preparation for manual removal. Suppositories are not effective, because their action is blocked by the amount and size of the stool in the rectum.

Several sessions or days may be necessary to totally clear the sigmoid colon and rectum of impacted feces. Once this is achieved, attention should be directed to planning a regimen that includes adequate fluid intake, increased dietary fibre, administration of stool softeners if needed, and many of the suggestions presented here for the prevention of constipation. For persons who are in hospital or residing in LTC settings, accurate bowel records are essential; unfortunately, they are often overlooked or inaccurately completed. All direct care providers should be

TABLE 8.2   Precipitating Factors for Constipation and Recommended Best Practice for Prevention

PRECIPITATING FACTORS	PREVENTION	PRECIPITATING FACTORS	PREVENTION
Physiological • Dehydration • Insufficient fibre intake • Poor dietary habits	Encourage fluid intake of 1,500–2,000 mL per day and fibre intake of 25–30 g per day	**Systemic** • Diabetic neuropathy • Hypercalcemia • Hyperparathyroidism • Hypothyroidism • Hypokalemia • Porphyria • Uremia • Parkinson's disease • Cerebro-vascular disease • Defective electrolyte transfer	Assess and obtain information and dietary history on systemic factors related to constipation.
Functional • Decreased physical activity • Inadequate toileting • Irregular defecation habits • Irritable bowel disease • Weakness	Encourage physical activity tailored to the person; promote regular and consistent toileting daily, based on the person's triggering meal; assess and obtain information about functional factors related to constipation.		
Mechanical • Abscess or ulcer • Fissures • Hemorrhoids • Megacolon • Pelvic floor dysfunction • Postsurgical obstruction • Prostate enlargement • Rectal prolapse • Rectocele • Spinal cord injury • Strictures	Assess and obtain information about mechanical factors related to constipation, and complete a physical assessment.	**Pharmacological** • ACE inhibitors • Antacids: calcium carbonate, aluminum hydroxide • Antiarrhythmics • Anticholinergics • Anticonvulsants • Antidepressants • Anti–Parkinson's disease medications • Calcium channel blockers • Calcium supplements • Diuretics • Iron supplements • Overuse of laxatives • Nonsteroidal anti-inflammatory drugs • Opiates • Phenothiazines • Sedatives	Review medications and identify those associated with increased risk for constipation (e.g., long-term laxative use).
Other • Lack of abdominal muscle tone • Obesity • Recent environmental changes • Poor dentition	Assess and obtain information related to constipation, and complete a physical assessment.		
Psychological • Avoidance of urge to defecate • Confusion • Depression • Emotional stress	Assess and obtain information on psychological factors related to constipation.		

ACE, angiotensin-converting enzyme
Adapted from Registered Nurses' Association of Ontario (RNAO). (2011). *Prevention of constipation in the older adult population.* Toronto, ON: Author.

educated about the importance of bowel function and the accurate reporting of the size and consistency of stools and the frequency of bowel movements.

IMPLICATIONS FOR GERONTOLOGICAL NURSING AND HEALTHY AGING

ASSESSMENT

The precipitants and causes of constipation must be included in the evaluation of the older person. A review of these factors will also determine if the person is at risk for altered bowel function. Older people at high risk for constipation and subsequent fecal impaction are those who have hypotonic colon function, who are immobilized and cognitively impaired, or who have central nervous system lesions. It is important to note that incontinence, increased temperature, poor appetite, unexplained falls, or altered cognitive status may be the only clinical symptom of constipation in a cognitively impaired or frail older person.

Recognizing constipation can be a challenge because there may be a significant difference between a patient's definition of constipation and that of the clinician. Assessment begins with the clarification of what the older person means by "constipation." It is also important to obtain a bowel history that includes the person's usual patterns of elimination; the frequency, size, and consistency of bowel movements; and any changes that have occurred. Many clinicians think of bowel movement infrequency as the main indicator of constipation, but people with chronic constipation are more likely to report straining, a sense of incomplete or ineffective defecation, and hard or lumpy stools (RNAO, 2011).

A physical examination is needed to rule out systemic causes of constipation such as neurological, endocrine, or metabolic disorders. Symptoms that may indicate an underlying gastro-intestinal disorder are abdominal pain, nausea, cramping, vomiting, weight loss, melena, rectal bleeding, rectal pain, and fever. A review of food and fluid intake may be necessary to determine the amount of fibre and fluid ingested. The nurse should ask questions about the level of physical activity and the use of medications. A psychosocial history with attention to depression, anxiety, and stress management is also indicated.

The abdomen should be examined for masses, distension, tenderness, and high-pitched or absent bowel sounds. A rectal examination is important for revealing painful anal disorders such as hemorrhoids or fissures, which impede the evacuation of stool, and for evaluating sphincter tone, stool presence, and anal reflex, as well as the presence of an enlarged prostate, rectal prolapse, strictures, and masses. Biochemical tests should include a complete blood count, fasting glucose, chemistry panel, and thyroid studies. Other diagnostic studies such as flexible sigmoidoscopy, colonoscopy, a computed tomography scan of the abdomen, or an abdominal X-ray study may also be indicated.

INTERVENTIONS

The first steps in treating constipation are to examine the medications the person is taking, eliminate any that cause constipation, and change the regimen to medications that do not cause constipation. Medications that affect the central nervous system, nerve conduction, and smooth muscle function are associated with the highest frequency of constipation. Anticholinergics, pain opiates, and many psychoactive medications can be especially problematic.

Nonpharmacological interventions for constipation can be grouped into four areas: (1) fluid- and fibre-related interventions, (2) exercise, (3) environmental manipulation, and (4) a combination of these. Adequate hydration, mainly with water, is the cornerstone of constipation therapy (RNAO, 2011).

A low-fibre diet and insufficient fluid intake contribute to constipation. Fibre is an important dietary component that many older people do not consume in sufficient quantities. Fibre is abundant in raw fruits and vegetables and in unrefined grains and cereals. It facilitates the absorption of water, increases bulk, and improves intestinal motility. Fibre helps prevent or reduce the incidence of constipation by increasing the weight of the stool and shortening transit time.

Individuals who can chew foods well can benefit from eating increased amounts of fresh fruits and vegetables daily or combining unsweetened bran with other types of food. People who have difficulty chewing can sprinkle bran on cereals or use it in soups and casseroles. The quantity of bran depends on the individual, but generally 1 to 2 tablespoons (15–30 mL) daily is sufficient. Individuals who have not used bran previously should begin with 1 teaspoon (5 mL) and progressively increase the amount until the quantity of fibre intake is enough to accomplish its purpose. Adequate fluid intake is also important. If megacolon or colonic dilation from bowel obstruction is suspected, fibre supplements are not advised.

Exercise

Exercise is important as an intervention to stimulate colon motility and bowel evacuation. Daily walking for 20 to 30 minutes is helpful, especially after a meal. Pelvic-tilt and range-of-motion exercises (passive or active) are beneficial for those who are less mobile or who are bedridden (see Chapter 10).

Positioning

A squatting or sitting position, if the person is able to assume it, facilitates bowel function. A similar position may be obtained by leaning forward and applying firm pressure to the lower abdomen or placing the feet on a stool. Massaging the abdomen may help stimulate the bowel.

Regularity

Establishing a toileting routine promotes or normalizes (retrains) bowel function. The gastro-colic reflex occurs after breakfast or supper and may be enhanced by a warm drink. Given privacy and sufficient time (a minimum of 10 minutes), many people will have a daily bowel movement. Any urge to defecate should be followed by a trip to the toilet. Older people who depend on others to meet toileting needs should be assisted in maintaining normal routines and be provided with opportunities for routine toilet use. (Additional information on bowel management programs can be found in Chapter 9.)

Laxatives

When changes in diet and lifestyle are not effective in treating constipation, the use of laxatives can be considered. Older persons receiving opiates need to have a constipation-prevention program in place, because these medications delay gastric emptying and decrease peristalsis. The correction of constipation associated with opiate use calls for a senna or osmotic laxative to overcome the strong opioid effect; stool softeners and bulking agents alone are inadequate. Commonly used laxatives for chronic constipation include the following:

- Bulking agents (e.g., psyllium, methylcellulose)
- Stool softeners (e.g., docusate sodium)
- Osmotic laxatives (e.g., lactulose, sorbitol)
- Stimulant laxatives (e.g., senna, bisacodyl)
- Saline laxatives (e.g., milk of magnesia)

Because of their safety, bulk laxatives are often the first laxatives prescribed. Bulk laxatives absorb water from the intestinal lumen and increase stool mass; adequate fluid intake is essential. The use of these laxatives is contraindicated in the presence of obstruction or compromised peristaltic activity. A saline or osmotic laxative can be added if the bulk laxative is not effective, but saline laxatives should be avoided in people with poor renal function or heart failure, because they may cause electrolyte imbalances. Stimulant laxatives should be used when other laxatives are ineffective. An emollient laxative, such as mineral oil, should be avoided because of the risk for lipoid aspiration pneumonia. Stool softeners have shown little effect when given to older persons with limited mobility, and their use should be limited to people who experience excessive straining or painful defecation or to people who are at a high risk for developing constipation (Emmanuel et al., 2017).

Combinations of natural fibre, fruit juices, and natural laxative mixtures (raisins, pitted prunes, figs, dates, currants, and prune concentrate) are often recommended in clinical practice. Some studies have found an increase in bowel frequency and a decrease in laxative use when these mixtures are used (Emmanuel et al., 2017) (Box 8.9).

Enemas

An enema is a procedure for introducing liquids into the rectum and colon via the anus. Enemas should not be used on a regular basis and should be used only when other methods produce no response or when there is an impaction. A normal saline or tap-water enema (500 to 1,000 mL) at 40.5°C is the best choice. Soap suds (a mixture of mild soap and warm water) and phosphate enemas irritate the rectal mucosa and should not be used. Oil-retention enemas such as bisacodyl (Dulcolax) are used to increase the motility of the bowel (Lilley et al., 2011).

BOX 8.9 Research for Evidence-Informed Practice: Fibre Is As Effective As Laxatives for Relieving Constipation

Purpose: To determine whether the use of fibre can be as effective as taking laxatives in relieving constipation in older persons.

Study Design: The authors reviewed two randomized controlled trials and one intervention trial investigating the effectiveness of supplemental fibre in managing constipation in older persons. Participants included residents or patients of a long-term care home or hospital, and interventions consisted of an additional natural fibre laxative mixture during meals over an 8-week trial, the addition of 7–8 g of an oat bran fibre product during meals over the course of 12 weeks, and the introduction of a porridge containing 7.5 g of fibre per serving at breakfast over a 2-week period. Intervention outcomes were measured by discomfort level, ease of bowel movement, undesired effects of laxative use, and frequency of defecation.

Results: All three studies demonstrated that the use of dietary fibre can be an effective alternative to using laxatives in a geriatric population. Outcomes indicated a reduction in laxative use, high compliance with the recommended fibre intake, improved bowel movement and comfort, and less abdominal discomfort.

Implications: Dietary fibre can be used as an effective alternative to laxatives in managing constipation in older people.

Source: Batunkyi, S. (2012). Will the use of fiber be as effective as laxatives in relieving constipation in the geriatric population? *PCOM Physician Assistant Studies Student Scholarship*, 94. Retrieved from http://digitalcommons.pcom.edu/pa_systematic_reviews/94.

A constipation prevention and treatment program that includes a high-fibre diet, liberal fluid intake, daily exercise, and environmental modifications that promote a regular pattern of bowel elimination must be developed for each older person.

OLDER PERSONS IN HOSPITALS AND INSTITUTIONS

Older persons in hospitals and LTC settings are more likely to experience a number of problems that contribute to inadequate nutrition. In addition to the risk factors mentioned above, isolation, severely restricted diets, long periods of nothing-by-mouth (NPO) status, and insufficient time and support staff for meals contribute to inadequate nutrition. Malnutrition can cause prolonged hospital stays, increased risk of poor health status, institutionalization, and mortality (Vandewee et al., 2010). Assessing the patient's nutritional status to identify malnutrition and the risk factors for malnutrition is important. Sufficient time, care, and attention should be given to helping dependent older people with meals.

About 97% of residents of LTC homes require some assistance with activities such as eating (Ontario Long Term Care Association, 2016). Inadequate staffing in LTC homes is associated with inadequate organizational support, which may lead to poor nutrition in residents (Watkins et al., 2017). Keller and colleagues found that residents significantly increased their oral food and fluid intake when they received one-on-one eating assistance (Keller et al., 2017).

Family members (and volunteers in some settings) are often able to assist at mealtimes and provide a familiar social context for the older person. Nurses need to provide guidance and support families about meal assistance and nutritional intake.

The use of restrictive therapeutic diets (e.g., low cholesterol, low salt, no concentrated sweets) for frail older people in LTC homes often reduces their food intake without significantly helping their clinical status (Darmon et al., 2010). If caloric supplements are used (e.g., Ensure, Boost, Sustacal), they should be administered at least 1 hour before meals, or they will interfere with food intake. These products are widely used, can be expensive, and are often not dispensed or consumed as ordered. More research related to their effectiveness is needed (Gammack & Sanford, 2015).

Dispensing a small amount (2 calories/mL) of calorically dense oral nutritional supplement during the routine medication pass may have a greater effect on weight gain than that of a traditional supplement (1.06 calories/mL) with or between meals. Small volumes of nutrient-dense supplement may also have less of an effect on appetite and will increase food intake during meals and snacks. This method of dispensing supplements allows nurses to observe and document consumption. A study of the effect of a nutrient-dense supplement given while medication was being given to residents who were at high nutritional risk found

---

BOX 8.10   Suggestions for Improving Older Persons' Nutritional Intake

- Serve meals with the person in a chair rather than in bed when possible.
- Provide analgesics and antiemetics on a schedule that provides comfort at mealtime.
- Determine the person's food preferences; include culturally appropriate food.
- Have food available 24 hours per day; provide snacks between meals and at night.
- Do not interrupt meals to administer medication if possible.
- Walk around the dining area or the rooms at mealtime to determine if food is being eaten or assistance is needed.
- Encourage family members to be present during mealtimes to provide an enhanced social situation.
- Offer caloric supplements, if used, between meals or with the medication pass.
- Recommend an exercise program that may increase appetite.
- Ensure proper fit of dentures and proper denture use.
- Provide oral hygiene, and allow the person to wash his or her hands.
- Allow the person to wear his or her eyeglasses if the person is vision impaired.
- Sit while assisting the person with the meal, use touch, and carry on a social conversation.
- Provide soft music during the meal.
- Use small round tables seating six to eight people; consider using tablecloths and centrepieces.
- Seat people with similar interests and abilities together, and encourage socialization.
- Use restorative dining programs and the use of adaptive equipment.
- Make diets as liberal as possible, especially for frail older persons who are not consuming adequate amounts.
- Consider a referral to a speech-language pathologist for a person experiencing difficulties with eating, a referral to an occupational therapist for adaptive equipment, or a referral to both.

---

that their weight and albumin levels were maintained or improved (Harding et al., 2016).

Attention to the environment in which meals are served is also important. Assisting older people who have difficulty eating independently can become mechanical and devoid of feeling. The assistance process becomes a task, and even if the older person requires additional time, the meal may be ended abruptly, depending on the time the caregiver has allotted for assistance. Any pleasure derived through socialization and eating and any dignity that could be maintained are often lost. Older persons who are accustomed to certain table manners may feel ashamed at their inability to behave in a way that they feel is appropriate.

In addition to having competent and adequate staff, LTC homes can use innovative and evidence-informed strategies to improve their residents' nutritional intake. The many suggestions in the literature include the following:

- Restorative dining programs
- Home-like dining rooms
- Individualized menu choices that include ethnic foods
- Cafeteria-style service
- Kitchens on the units or wards
- Availability of food around the clock
- Choice of mealtimes
- Liberal diets
- Finger foods
- Visually appealing puréed foods (with texture and shape)
- Music
- Touch
- Verbal cueing
- Hand-over-hand guiding
- The nurse's sitting (instead of standing) while assisting the person to eat

Other suggestions can be found in Box 8.10.

In light of current population projections, the number of older persons requiring hospital care, rehabilitative care, and LTC will dramatically increase, leading to increased hospital stays, increased costs, and considerable mortality (McElhaney et al., 2011). Since the risk for malnutrition rises as soon as a person is put under one of these three types of care, malnutrition is a serious challenge for health care providers in all settings.

IMPLICATIONS FOR GERONTOLOGICAL NURSING AND HEALTHY AGING

ASSESSMENT

Older people are less likely than younger people to show the signs of malnutrition and nutrient malabsorption. Although the evaluation of nutritional health can be difficult in the absence of severe malnutrition, a comprehensive assessment and physical examination can reveal deficits (Touhy & Jett, 2013).

A nutritional assessment that provides the most conclusive data about a person's actual nutritional state consists of the following steps: interview, physical examination, anthropometrical measurements, and biochemical analysis. The collective result can provide the gerontological nurse with the data needed to identify immediate and potential nutritional problems. The nurse can then begin to establish plans for supervising, assisting, and educating the person, the goal being adequate nutrition.

The Mini Nutritional Assessment, developed by Nestlé of Geneva, Switzerland, is intended for use by health care providers who are screening patients for malnutrition (http://www.hartfordign.org). More information on nutrition and older persons can be found at https://consultgeri.org/geriatric-topics/nutrition-elderly.

The Minimum Data Set (MDS) includes assessment information that can be used to identify potential nutritional problems, risk factors, and potential for improved function. The nutrition and dehydration Resident Assessment Protocols (RAPs) guide staff in the assessment of nutritionally related problems. Triggers for more thorough investigation include weight loss, alterations in taste, medical therapies, prescription medications, hunger, parenteral or intravenous feedings, mechanically altered or therapeutic diets, percentage of food left uneaten, pressure ulcers, and edema. Chapters 5 and 13 provide further information on the MDS and RAPs. An evidence-informed guideline on nutritional management in LTC is available at http://www.rnao.org.

Interview

The interview provides background information and clues to the older person's nutritional state and to the actual and potential problems of the older person. The nurse should ask questions about state of health, social activities, normal patterns, and changes that have occurred. The nurse should also explore the person's needs, how the person obtains food, and the person's ability to prepare food.

Information about the relationship of food to daily events will provide clues to the meaning and significance of food. The older person who eats alone is considered a candidate for malnutrition. Information about occupation and daily activities will suggest the degree of energy expenditure and caloric intake most appropriate for the overall activity. A person's economic status will have a direct bearing on nutrition. It is therefore important to explore the person's financial resources to determine how much income is available for purchasing food.

The nutrition history should include data on the medications being taken. Additional medical information about visual difficulty, bowel and bladder function, and the presence or absence of mouth pain or discomfort should be obtained, as well as a history of illness.

Diet Histories. A 24-hour diet recall compared with the age- and gender-specific recommendations in *Eating Well with Canada's Food Guide* can provide an estimate of nutritional adequacy. When the older person cannot supply all of the information requested, it may be possible to obtain it from a family member or another source. There will be times, however, when the information is not as complete as one would like or when the older person, too proud to admit that he or she is not eating well, furnishes erroneous information. Even so, the nurse will be able to obtain additional data from other areas of the nutritional assessment, as discussed later in this chapter.

Keeping a dietary record for 3 days is another assessment tool. What food was eaten, when it was eaten, and the amount eaten must be carefully recorded. Analysis of the dietary records provides information on energy, vitamin, and mineral intake. The accuracy of dietary records in hospitals and LTC homes can be problematic, and intake may be either underestimated or overestimated. Standardized observational protocols can improve the accuracy of oral intake documentation as well as the quality of feeding assistance. Nurses should ensure that direct caregivers are educated in the proper observation and documentation of intake.

Physical Examination

The physical examination furnishes clinically observable evidence of the existing state of nutrition. Data such as height and weight; vital signs; condition of the tongue, lips, and gums; skin turgor, texture, and colour; and functional ability are assessed, and the overall general appearance is scrutinized for evidence of wasting. Height should be measured and not estimated or self-reported. If the person cannot stand, an alternative way of measuring standing height is to use knee-height calipers (Froehlich-Grobe et al., 2011). The body mass index (BMI) should be calculated to determine whether weight for height is within the normal range of 18.5 to 24.9. A BMI below 18.5 is a sign of undernutrition (Health Canada, 2011b).

A detailed weight history should be taken along with a measurement of current weight. This history should include information about the person's history of weight loss, the period during which the weight loss occurred, and whether the weight loss was intentional or unintentional. How to determine the appropriate weight charts for an older person is still under debate. Although weight alone does not indicate the adequacy of diet, unplanned fluctuations in weight are significant and should be evaluated.

Weight changes may be the result of fluid retention, edema, or ascites and thus merit investigation. An unintentional weight loss of more than 5% of body weight in 1 month, more than 7.5% in 3 months, or more than 10% in 6 months is considered a significant indicator of poor nutrition as well as an MDS trigger.

Anthropometrical Measurements

Obtained with simple procedures, anthropometrical measurements include measurements of height, weight, midarm circumference, and triceps skinfold thickness. They offer information about the status of the older person's muscle mass and body fat in relation to height and weight. Muscle mass is found by measuring the circumference of the nondominant upper arm. Body fat and lean muscle mass are assessed by measuring specific skinfolds with Lange or Harpenden calipers at the midpoint of the upper arm. If there is a neuropathological condition or hemiplegia

following a stroke, the unaffected arm should be used for measurements.

Biochemical Examination

The final step in a nutritional assessment is the biochemical examination. Suggested biochemical parameters include serum albumin, cholesterol, and serum transferrin. Although these parameters may also be abnormal in several conditions not associated with malnutrition, they are useful as guides to interventions (Ahmed & Haboubi, 2010). Serum albumin of more than 40 g/L (4 g/dL) is desirable; less than 35 g/L (3.5 g/dL) is an indicator of a poor nutritional state. Prealbumin level may be a better indicator of protein loss, because it changes rapidly in the presence of malnutrition. Transferrin, an iron transport protein, is diminished in protein malnutrition. However, it increases in iron deficiency anemia, which is common in older persons, so it is not a sensitive indicator of protein-caloric malnutrition. Laboratory test results, although not definitive for malnutrition, provide important clues to nutritional status but should be evaluated in relation to the person's overall health status.

INTERVENTIONS

Interventions are often formulated around the identified nutritional problem. Nursing interventions are centred on techniques to increase food intake and enhance and manage the environment to promote increased food intake (DiMaria-Ghalili, 2012). Collaboration with the interprofessional team (which may include a dietitian, pharmacist, social worker, occupational therapist, or SLP) is important in planning interventions. For the community-dwelling older person, nutrition education and working together with the person and their family members on how to best resolve the potential or actual nutritional deficit are important.

The causes of poor nutrition are complex. It is important to assess all of the factors emphasized in this chapter when individualized interventions to ensure adequate nutrition are being planned.

Pharmacological Therapy

Medications that stimulate the appetite (*orexigenic medications*) should be considered for reversing resistant anorexia after all other interventions have been tried (see Chapter 25). Older persons taking these medications must be monitored closely for side effects, as these medications have not been evaluated well in frail older people. Their benefits are restricted to small weight gains without indication of decreased morbidity, mortality, or improved quality of life or functional ability. Megestrol acetate (Megace) may be effective at a dosage of 800 mg daily for 3 months. Older persons should be monitored closely for adrenocortical insufficiency, and megestrol should not be given to bedridden older persons because of the risk for deep venous thrombosis. Dronabinol (Marinol), although not adequately tested with older people, has shown some potential benefits because it stimulates appetite, has antinausea properties, decreases pain, and enhances general well-being. Weight gain from the use of these two medications comes primarily from increased adipose tissue and not lean body mass (Bodenner et al., 2007).

For older persons who are depressed and have weight loss or a poor appetite, mirtazapine (Remeron), an antidepressant, has been shown to increase appetite and weight gain as well as improve depressed mood (Watanabe et al., 2011).

Patient and Family Education

Patients and families need to be educated in how to read nutritional information on labels. In 2016, the Food and Drug Regulations were modified to mandate nutritional labelling on most food labels (Government of Canada, 2016). The choice of nutrients was based on evidence that eating too much or too little of these substances has the greatest impact on health. Health Canada defines a "good source" as a food that contains 5 to 15% of the recommended daily value per serving (Health Canada, 2012b). Balance is the key to a healthy diet.

Enteral Feeding

When all the interventions discussed above fail and problems with nutritional intake in older people persist, the decision is sometimes made to insert a feeding tube into the patient to provide an enteral feeding route. A comprehensive assessment of swallowing problems and other factors that influence intake must be conducted before initiating severely restricted diet modifications or considering the use of feeding tubes, particularly for older people with advanced dementia. The use of enteral feeding routes for people with advanced dementia to prevent aspiration, pneumonia, malnutrition, and infections provides few long-term benefits and may in fact contribute to further decline. Enteral feeding has never been shown to reduce a person's risk of regurgitating gastric contents and cannot be expected to prevent the aspiration of oral secretions (Ahmed & Haboubi, 2010).

The use of percutaneous endoscopic gastrostomy (PEG) feeding tubes in older persons has increased at an astonishing rate in recent years. Few complications occur with the insertion of a PEG tube; however, numerous complications occur from having one (American Geriatrics Society [AGS], 2006). Aspiration pneumonia, diarrhea, metabolic problems, and cellulitis are just a few of these complications. Persons who aspirate oral feedings are also likely to aspirate enteral feedings, be they by way of either nasogastric tubes or gastrostomy tubes (Ahmed & Haboubi, 2010).

As discussed earlier, food and eating are closely tied to socialization, comfort, pleasure, love, and basic biological needs. Decisions about enteral feeding are some of the most challenging of the many decisions that face families, health care providers, and facilities that care for older persons with dementia. Decisions to provide or not provide enteral feeding must be made carefully. Health care providers must take the time to listen to the wishes and concerns of the person and his or her family. Individuals have the right to refuse or accept enteral feeding but should be given accurate information about both the risks and the benefits of enteral feeding in late-stage dementia (AGS, 2005).

Discussion about advance directives and feeding support should begin early in the course of the illness rather than being delayed until a crisis develops. The best advice is to allow individuals to state their preferences regarding enteral feeding in a written advance directive. Surrogate decision makers should use advance directives and previously expressed wishes to decide what a person with advanced dementia who is not eating would want in the particular circumstance.

Hospitals, LTC homes, and other care settings must promote choice and honour patient preferences in regard to enteral feeding and should not exert pressure on patients or on medical care providers to institute artificial feeding. LTC homes should have policies in place to ensure that patients with remediable causes of weight loss are appropriately evaluated and treated and that enteral feeding is not regarded as the only treatment of choice (Hanson et al., 2016).

Everyone involved in the care of the older person must be informed about the potential benefits and risks of enteral feeding. Whether enteral feeding provides any benefit to the person is uncertain. However, the question should never be whether enteral feeding is or is not to be used. No family members should be made to feel that they are starving their loved one to death if it is decided not to institute enteral feeding. Comprehensive attempts to continue to provide nutrition should always be made. Excellent information about enteral feeding, both for patients and their families, can be found at http://www.chcr.brown.edu/dying/consumerfeedingtube.htm.

Short-term enteral feeding may be indicated for some conditions (e.g., after a hip fracture when serum albumin is low), but evidence supporting the effectiveness of enteral feeding for older people with dementia is scant. When enteral feeding is indicated, the nurse and dietitian must work closely together to determine the appropriate formula and rate of administration, as well as the patient's tolerance, weight, and hydration status. The head of the bed should be elevated at least 30 degrees for patients receiving continuous enteral feedings. When patients receive nutrition by bolus, the head of the bed should be elevated at least 30 degrees during feeding and for 1 hour after feeding. Gavi et al. (2008) have provided a guide for the management of LTC residents' enteral feeding complications.

SUMMARY

The maintenance of adequate nutritional health as a person ages is extremely complex. A knowledge of normal nutrition in later years and the many factors contributing to inadequate nutrition is essential for the gerontological nurse, and the consideration of these matters should be a part of every assessment of the older person. Whether in a community, hospital, or LTC setting, nurses must work with members of the interprofessional team to conduct appropriate assessments and develop therapeutic interventions. The use of evidence-informed practice protocols is important for determining nursing interventions to support and enhance nutritional status and promote adequate bowel function. The prevention of undernutrition and malnutrition and the maintenance of dietary needs and food enjoyment until the end of the patient's life are also ethical responsibilities of gerontological nurses. No older person should be hungry or thirsty because he or she cannot shop, cook, or buy food, nor should any older person have to suffer because of a lack of assistance with these activities, regardless of the setting in which they reside.

KEY CONCEPTS

- Recommended dietary patterns for the older person are similar to those for younger persons but incorporate some reduction in caloric intake, based on decreased caloric requirements.
- Many factors affect adequate nutrition in later life, including income, chronic illness, dentition, mood disorders, capacity for food preparation, functional limitations, and lifetime eating habits.
- Protein-caloric malnutrition is the most common form of malnutrition in older persons. Estimates are that 50% of residents of LTC homes, 50% of patients in hospital, and 44% of home care patients over the age of 65 years are malnourished.
- A comprehensive nutritional assessment is an essential component of the assessment of older persons.
- Making mealtime pleasant and attractive for the older adult who is unable to eat unassisted is a nursing priority, and adequate assistance must be provided.
- Dental health is a basic need of older persons that is increasingly neglected. Poor oral health is a risk factor for dehydration, malnutrition, and aspiration pneumonia.
- Bowel function in older persons is minimally affected by the physiological changes of aging. Constipation is a common complaint, and non-pharmacological interventions, such as exercise and increased fluid and fibre intake, are important to maintain normal bowel function.

ACTIVITIES AND DISCUSSION QUESTIONS

1. What factors affect nutrition in the older person?
2. How can the nurse intervene to provide better nutrition for older people in the community, acute care, and LTC settings?
3. What are the causes of malnutrition?
4. What is included in the nutritional assessment of an older person?
5. What factors contribute to changes in bowel function as a person ages?
6. What proactive measures can the nurse take to promote adequate bowel function for older persons in the community, acute care, and LTC settings?
7. How is dysphagia assessed, and what interventions may be helpful in preventing aspiration?
8. Develop a nursing care plan for an older person at risk for malnutrition.

RESOURCES

Nutrition

Alzheimer Society of Canada. *Meal times*
http://www.alzheimer.ca/default/files/Files/national/brochures-day-to-day/day_to_day_meal_times_e.pdf

American Geriatrics Society Health in Aging Foundation
http://www.healthinaging.org/

An approach to the management of unintentional weight loss in elderly people
http://www.cmaj.ca/content/cmaj/172/6/773.full.pdf

Assessing nutrition in older adults
https://consultgeri.org/try-this/general-assessment/issue-9.pdf

Eating and feeding issues in older adults with dementia: Part I: Assessment
https://consultgeri.org/try-this/dementia/issue-d11.1

Eating and feeding issues in older adults with dementia: Part II: Interventions
https://consultgeri.org/try-this/dementia/issue-d11.2.pdf

EatRightOntario. Older adults eating well
https://www.eatrightontario.ca/en/Articles/Seniors-nutrition/Older-adults-eating-well

Government of Canada. *Canada's food guides*
https://www.canada.ca/en/health-canada/services/canada-food-guides.html

Preventing aspiration in older adults with dysphagia
https://consultgeri.org/try-this/general-assessment/issue-20.pdf

Province of British Columbia. *Healthy Eating for Seniors Handbook*
http://www2.gov.bc.ca/gov/content/family-social-supports/seniors/health-safety/active-aging/healthy-eating/healthy-eating-for-seniors-handbook

Oral Health

Oral health; preventing cavities, gum disease, tooth loss, and oral cancers: At a glance 2011
https://stacks.cdc.gov/view/cdc/11862

Registered Nurses' Association of Ontario (RNAO). Oral health: Nursing assessment and intervention
http://rnao.ca/bpg/guidelines/oral-health-nursing-assessment-and-intervention

Report on the findings of the Oral Health Component of the Canadian Health Measures Survey 2007–2009
http://www.fptdwg.ca/assets/PDF/CHMS/CHMS-E-summ.pdf

Constipation

Registered Nurses' Association of Ontario (RNAO): Prevention of constipation in the older adult population
http://rnao.ca/sites/rnao-ca/files/Prevention_of_Constipation_in_the_Older_Adult_Population.pdf

For additional resources, please visit *http://evolve.elsevier.com/Canada/Ebersole/gerontological/*

REFERENCES

Ahmed, T., & Haboubi, N. (2010). Assessment and management of nutrition in older people and its importance to health. *Clinical Intervention in Aging, 5*(1), 207–216. Retrieved from https://pdfs.semanticscholar.org/7b2c/54265b18b549f2030f6cc2888c276aaf17ca.pdf.

Alzheimer's Disease International. (2014). *Nutrition and dementia: A review of available research.* Retrieved from http://www.alzheimer.ca/~/media/Files/national/Breaking-news/ADI-nutrition-and-dementia.pdf.

American Geriatrics Society (AGS) (2005). *Feeding tube placement in elderly patients with advanced dementia.* Retrieved from http://www.americangeriatrics.org/products/positionpapers/feeding_tube_placement.pdf.

American Geriatrics Society (AGS) (2006). *Geriatric review syllabus*. New York: Author.

Berkey, D. B., & Scannapieco, F. A. (2013). Medical considerations relating to the oral health of older adults. *Special Care in Dentistry, 33*(4), 164–176. doi:10.1111/scd.12027.

Bodenner, D., Spencer, T., Riggs, A. T., et al. (2007). A retrospective study of the association between megestrol acetate administration and mortality among nursing home residents with clinically significant weight loss. *American Journal of Geriatric Pharmacotherapy, 5*(2), 137–146. doi:10.1016/j.amjopharm.2007.06.004.

Borreani, E., Jones, K., Scambler, S., et al. (2010). Informing the debate on oral health care for older people: a qualitative study of older people's views on oral health and oral health care. *Gerodontology, 27*(1), 11–18. doi:10.1111/j.1741-2358.2009.00274.x.

Boulos, C., Salameh, P., & Bargerger-Gateau, P. (2016). Malnutrition and frailty in community dwelling older adults living in a rural setting. *Clinical Nutrition: Official Journal of the European Society of Parenteral and Enteral Nutrition, 35*(1), 138–143. doi:10.1016/j.clnu.2015.01.008.

Canadian Association of Public Health Dentistry. (2017). *Position statements*. Retrieved from http://www.caphd.ca/advocacy/position-statements.

Carlo, A. D., & Alpert, J. E. (2016). Clinically relevant complications of drug-food interactions in psychopharmacology. *Psychiatric Annals, 46*(8), 448–455. doi:10.3928/00485713-20160613-01.

Cecchini, M., Sassi, F., Lauer, J. A., et al. (2010). Tackling of unhealthy diets, physical inactivity, and obesity: health effects and cost-effectiveness. *The Lancet, 376*(9754), 1775–1784. doi:10.1016/S0140-6736(10)61514-0.

Centers for Disease Control and Prevention. (2015). *Losing weight*. Retrieved from https://www.cdc.gov/healthyweight/losing_weight/.

Coker, E., Ploeg, J., Kaasalainen, S., et al. (2016). Observations of oral hygiene care interventions provided by nurses to hospitalized older people. *Geriatric Nursing, 38*(1), 17–21. doi:10.1016/j.gerinurse.2016.06.018.

Darmon, P., Kaiser, M. J., Bauer, J. M., et al. (2010). Restrictive diets in the elderly: never say never again? *Clinical Nutrition: Official Journal of the European Society of Parenteral and Enteral Nutrition, 29*(2), 170–174. doi:10.1016/j.clnu.2009.11.002.

de Boer, A., Ter Horst, G. J., & Lorist, M. M. (2013). Physiological and psychosocial age-related changes associated with reduced food intake in older persons. *Ageing Research Reviews, 12*(1), 316–328. doi:10.1016/j.arr.2012.08.002.

De Marchi, R. J., Hugo, F. N., Padilha, D. M. P., et al. (2011). Edentulism, use of dentures and consumption of fruit and vegetables in south Brazilian community-dwelling elderly. *Journal of Oral Rehabilitation, 38*(7), 533–540. doi:10.1111/j.1365-2842.2010.02189.x.

Deer, R. R., Goodlett, S., & Volpi, E. (2017). Comparison of four malnutrition screening tools to the Subjective Global Assessment (SGA) in a Cohort of Acutely Ill Older adults. *The FASEB Journal, 31*(1 Suppl.), 151–154. Retrieved from http://www.fasebj.org/content/31/1_Supplement/151.4.short.

DiMaria-Ghalili, R. (2012). *Nutrition in the elderly*. New York: The Hartford Institute for Geriatric Nursing. Retrieved from https://consultgeri.org/geriatric-topics/nutrition-elderly.

Emmanuel, A., Mattace-Raso, F., Neri, M. C., et al. (2017). Constipation in older people: A consensus statement. *International Journal of Clinical Practice, 71*(1), e12920. doi:10.1111/ijcp.12920.

Esmayel, E. M., Eldarawy, M. M., Hassan, M. M., et al. (2013). Nutritional and functional assessment of hospitalized elderly: impact of sociodemographic variables. *Journal of Aging Research, 2013*(101725), 1–7. doi:10.1155/2013/101725.

Froehlich-Grobe, K., Nary, D. E., Van Sciver, A., et al. (2011). Measuring height without a stadiometer: empirical investigation of four height estimates among wheelchair users. *American Journal of Physical Medicine & Rehabilitation/Association of Academic Physiatrists, 90*(8), 658. doi:10.1097/PHM.0b013e31821f6eb2.

Gammack, J. K., & Sanford, A. M. (2015). Caloric supplements for the elderly. *Current Opinion in Clinical Nutrition & Metabolic Care, 18*(1), 32–36. doi:10.1097/MCO.0000000000000125.

Gavi, S., Hensley, J., Cervo, F., et al. (2008). Management of feeding tube complications in the long-term care resident. *Annals of Long-Term Care, 16*(4), 28–32.

Gil-Montoya, J., Ferreira, A., & Lopez, I. (2006). Oral health protocol for the dependent institutionalized elderly. *Geriatric Nursing, 27*(2), 95–101. doi:10.1016/j.gerinurse.2005.12.003.

Government of Canada. (2016). *Food labelling changes*. Retrieved from: http://www.healthycanadians.gc.ca/eating-nutrition/label-etiquetage/changes-modifications.php.

Hanson, E., Hellström, A., Sandvide, A., et al. (2016). The extended palliative phase of dementia—an integrative literature review. *Dementia (Basel, Switzerland)*, 1471301216659797. doi:10.1177/1471301216659797.

Haralur, S. B. (2015). Effect of age on tooth shade, skin color and skin-tooth color interrelationship in Saudi Arabian subpopulation. *Journal of International Oral Health, 7*(8), 33–36.

Haehner, A., Hummer, T., & Reichmann, H. (2014). A clinical approach towards smell loss in Parkinson's Disease. *Journal of Parkinson's Disease, 4*(2), 189–195. doi:10.3233/JPD-130278.

Harding, K. M., Dyo, M., Goebel, J. R., et al. (2016). Early malnutrition screening and low cost protein supplementation in elderly patients admitted to a skilled nursing facility. *Applied Nursing Research, 31*, 29–33. doi:10.1016/j.apnr.2015.12.001.

Health Canada. (2009). *Oral cancer*. Retrieved from http://www.hc-sc.gc.ca/hl-vs/oral-bucco/disease-maladie/cancer-eng.php.

Health Canada. (2010). *Eating well with Canada's food guide—First Nations, Inuit and Métis*. Retrieved from https://www.canada.ca/en/health-canada/services/food-nutrition/canada-food-guide/eating-well-with-canada-food-guide-first-nations-inuit-metis.html.

Health Canada. (2011b). *Canadian guidelines for body weight classification in adults*. Retrieved from https://www.canada.ca/en/health-canada/services/food-nutrition/healthy-eating/healthy-weights/canadian-guidelines-body-weight-classification-adults/questions-answers-public.html.

Health Canada. (2012a). *Household food insecurity in Canada: Overview*. Retrieved from https://www.canada.ca/en/health-canada/

services/food-nutrition/food-nutrition-surveillance/health
-nutrition-surveys/canadian-community-health-survey-cchs/
household-food-insecurity-canada-overview.html.

Health Canada. (2012b). *How do you use the % DV?* Retrieved
from https://www.canada.ca/en/health-canada/services/food
-nutrition/food-labelling/nutrition-labelling/educators.html.

Health Canada. (2015). *The effects of oral health on overall health.*
Retrieved from https://www.canada.ca/en/health-canada/
services/healthy-living/your-health/lifestyles/effects-oral
-health-overall-health.html.

Higgs, S., & Thomas, J. (2016). Social influences on eating.
Current Opinion in Behavioral Sciences, 9, 1–6. doi:10.1016/
j.cobeha.2015.10.005.

Hollaar, V., van der Maarel-Wierink, C., van der Putten, G. J.,
et al. (2016). Defining characteristics and risk indicators for
diagnosing nursing home-acquired pneumonia and aspiration pneumonia in nursing home residents, using the
electronically-modified Delphi Method. *BMC Geriatrics, 16,* 60.
doi:10.1186/s12877-016-0231-4.

Hussain, Z. H., Whitehead, D. A., & Lacy, B. E. (2014). Fecal impaction. *Current Gastroenterology Reports, 16*(9), 1–7. doi:10.1007/
s11894-014-0404-2.

International Housing Coalition (IHC). (2006). *Case study 3:
Aboriginal housing in Canada: Building on promising practices.*
Prepared for presentation at the World Urban Forum III, June
2006.

Karami-Nogourani, M., Kowsari-Isfahan, R., & Hosseini-Beheshti,
M. (2011). The effect of chewing gum's flavor on salivary flow
rate and pH. *Dental Research Journal, 8*(Suppl. 1), S71–S75.

Keller, H. H., Carrier, N., Slaughter, S., et al. (2017). Making
the Most of Mealtimes (M3): protocol of a multi-centre
cross-sectional study of food intake and its determinants in
older adults living in long term care homes. *BMC Geriatrics,
17*(15). doi:10.1186/s12877-016-0401-4.

Kobayashi, K., Ryu, M., Izumi, S., et al. (2017). Effect of oral cleaning using mouthwash and a mouth moisturizing gel on bacterial number and moisture level of the tongue surface of older
adults requiring nursing care. *Geriatrics & Gerontology International, 17,* 116–121. doi:10.1111/ggi.12684.

Li, C., Zhang, Q., Ng, L., et al. (2016). *Oral care measures for preventing nursing home-acquired pneumonia.* Cochrane Oral
Health Group. doi:10.1002/14651858.CD012416.

Lilley, L. L., Harrington, S., Snyder, J. S., et al. (2011). *Pharmacology
for Canadian health care practice* (2nd Canadian ed.). Toronto:
Elsevier Canada.

Liu, B., Dion, M. R., Jurasic, M. M., et al. (2012). Xerostomia and
salivary hypofunction in vulnerable elders: prevalence and etiology. *Oral Surgery, Oral Medicine, Oral Pathology and Oral
Radiology, 114*(1), 52–60. doi:10.1016/j.oooo.2011.11.014.

Madhavan, A., Lagorio, L. A., Crary, M. A., et al. (2016). Prevalence
of and risk factors for dysphagia in the community dwelling
elderly: A systematic review. *The Journal of Nutrition, Health &
Aging, 20*(8), 806–815. doi:10.1007/s12603-016-0712-3.

McElhaney, J., Murray, S., Donnelly, M. L., et al. (2011). Prevention in acute care for seniors. *British Columbia Medical Journal,
53*(2), 86–87.

National Institutes of Health. (2014). *Aging changes in the senses.* Retrieved from https://medlineplus.gov/ency/article/004013.htm.

Neyens, J., Halfens, R., Spreeuwenberg, M., et al. (2012). Malnutrition is associated with an increased risk for falls and impaired
activity in elderly patients in Dutch residential long-term care
(LTC): A cross-sectional study. *Gerontology and Geriatrics,
56*(1), 265–269. doi:10.1016/j.archger.2012.08.005.

Nogueiras, R., Romero-Picó, A., Vazquez, M. J., et al. (2012). The
opioid system and food intake: Homeostatic and hedonic mechanisms. *Obesity Facts, 5*(2), 196–207. doi:10.1159/000338163.

Ontario Long Term Care Association (OLTCA). (2016). *This is
long-term care 2016.* Retrieved from http://www.oltca.com/
OLTCA/Documents/Reports/TILTC2016.pdf.

Peterson, G. (2015). Aged care: Unintentional weight loss in the
elderly. *Australian Pharmacist, 34*(1), 31–33.

Registered Nurses' Association of Ontario (RNAO). (2011). *Prevention of constipation in the older adult population.* Toronto, ON:
Author.

Registered Nurses' Association of Ontario (RNAO). (2008). *Oral
health: Nursing assessment and interventions.* Toronto, ON:
Author.

Rugg-Gunn, A. J., & Do, L. (2012). Effectiveness of water fluorida-
tion in caries prevention. *Community Dentistry and Oral Epidemiology, 40*(s2), 55–64. doi:10.1111/j.1600-0528.2012.00721.x.

Sauer, A. C., Alish, C. J., Strausbaugh, K., et al. (2016). Nurses
needed: Identifying malnutrition in hospitalized older adults.
NursingPlus Open, 2, 21–25. doi:10.1016/j.npls.2016.05.001.

Statistics Canada. (2013). *Persons in low income before tax.* Retrieved
from http://www.statcan.gc.ca/tables-tableaux/sum-som/l01/
cst01/famil41a-eng.htm?sdi=low%20income.

Statistics Canada. (2015a). *Chapter 3. Low income across groups of
people.* Retrieved from http://www.statcan.gc.ca/pub/75f0002m/
2012001/chap3-eng.htm.

Statistics Canada. (2015b). *Oral health: Edentulous people in 2007 to
2009.* Retrieved from http://www.statcan.gc.ca/pub/82-625-x/
2010001/article/11087-eng.htm.

Statistics Canada. (2016). *Percentage overweight or obese (body
mass index 25 kg/m² or more), by age group and sex, household population aged 18 or older, Canada excluding territories,
2004, 2005 and 2008.* Retrieved from http://www.statcan.gc.ca/
pub/82-229-x/2009001/status/desc/abm-desc4.2-eng.htm.

Sura, L., Madhavan, A., Carnaby, G., et al. (2012). Dysphagia in
the elderly: management and nutritional considerations. *Clinical Interventions in Aging, 2012*(7), 287–298. doi:10.2147/CIA.
S23404.

Touhy, T. A., & Jett, K. F. (2013). *Ebersole & Hess' toward healthy
aging: human needs and nursing response* (p. 179). St. Louis:
Elsevier Health Sciences.

Vandewee, K., Clays, E., Bocquaert, I., et al. (2010). Malnutrition
and associated factors in elderly hospital patients: a Belgian
cross-sectional, multi-centre study. *Clinical Nutrition: Official
Journal of the European Society of Parenteral and Enteral Nutrition, 29*(4), 469–476. doi:10.1016/j.clnu.2009.12.013.

Watanabe, N., Omori, I. M., Nakagawa, A., et al. (2011). Mirtazapine versus other antidepressive agents for depression. *The
Cochrane Library,* doi:10.1002/14651858.CD006528.pub2.

Watkins, R., Goodwin, V. A., Abbott, R. A., et al. (2017). Attitudes, perceptions and experiences of mealtimes amongst residents and staff in care homes for older adults: A systematic review of the qualitative literature. *Geriatric Nursing*, 1–9. doi:10.1016/j.gerinurse.2016.12.002.

White, J. V., Guenter, P., Jensen, G., et al. (2012). Consensus statement of the Academy of Nutrition and Dietetics/American Society for Parenteral and Enteral Nutrition: characteristics recommended for the identification and documentation of adult malnutrition (undernutrition). *Journal of the Academy of Nutrition and Dietetics*, *112*(5), 730–738. doi:10.1016/j.jand.2012.03.012.

World Health Organization. (2017). *Diet, nutrition and the prevention of chronic diseases. Report of the joint WHO/FAO expert consultation.* Retrieved from http://www.who.int/dietphysicalactivity/publications/trs916/summary/en/.

Zou, Y. M., Lu, D., Liu, L. P., et al. (2016). Olfactory dysfunction in Alzheimer's disease. *Neuropsychiatric Disease and Treatment*, *12*, 869–875. doi:10.2147/NDT.S104886.

Hydration and Continence

Upon completion of this chapter, the reader will be able to:

- Identify risk factors for dehydration.
- Discuss interventions to prevent or treat dehydration.
- Define *urinary* and *fecal incontinence.*
- List factors contributing to urinary and fecal incontinence.
- Explain the types of urinary incontinence and their causes.
- Discuss nursing interventions for urinary and fecal incontinence.

GLOSSARY

Dehydration   A harmful reduction in the amount of water in the body.

Detrusor   A body part that pushes down, such as the bladder muscle.

Incontinence   The inability to control excretory function.

Micturition   Urination.

Transient   Temporary.

THE LIVED EXPERIENCE

"UI (urinary incontinence) is like being a bad kid or a big baby."

"There's nothing that can be done. Well, I don't think there is anything else but a diaper."

"Sometimes I have to wet my bed before they get here, you know, and they are all busy and I have to wait for somebody, then I can't control it."

"I do something that is very wrong. I try not to drink too much but that's so wrong. So how can you drink a lot, you would be soaked all the time."

Comments from participants in a study of living with urinary incontinence in long-term care (MacDonald & Butler, 2007).

HYDRATION

HYDRATION MANAGEMENT

Hydration management is the maintenance of an adequate fluid balance, which prevents complications resulting from abnormal or undesirable fluid levels (Mentes & Kang, 2013). Water, a commodity that is accessible and available to almost all people, is often overlooked as an essential part of nutrition. Water's functions in the body include thermoregulation, dilution of water-soluble medications, facilitation of renal and bowel function, and creation of requisite conditions for and maintenance of metabolic processes.

Daily needs for water can usually be met through the intake of fluids with meals and by social drinks. However, a significant number of older persons (up to 85% of those 85 years of age and older) drink less than 1 litre of fluid per day. Older persons, with the exception of those requiring fluid restrictions, should consume at least 1,500 to 2,000 mL of fluid per day (Registered Nurses' Association of Ontario [RNAO], 2011).

Maintenance of the balance between fluid intake and fluid output (fluid intake equals fluid output) is essential to health, regardless of a person's age (Bunn et al., 2015). Age-related changes, medication use, functional impairments, and comorbid medical illness place some older persons at risk for changes in fluid balance and especially for dehydration (Popkin et al., 2010). A comprehensive hydration management guideline as well as intervention strategies can be found on the ConsultGeri website (https://consultgeri.org). Detailed recommendations for care planning to reduce the risk of dehydration and to maintain hydration are available on the Registered Nurses' Association of Ontario (RNAO) *Long-Term Care Best Practices Toolkit* website (http://ltctoolkit.rnao.ca/).

DEHYDRATION

Dehydration results from insufficient fluid intake, is indicated by elevated directly measured serum osmolality, and undermines the health of older people (Hooper et al., 2016). Dehydration is a geriatric syndrome frequently associated with common diseases (e.g., diabetes, respiratory illness, and heart failure) and with frailty (Hooper et al., 2016).

Dehydration is a problem among older persons in all settings. Not only is dehydration a significant risk factor for delirium, thromboembolic complications, infections, and kidney stones, it also contributes to constipation and obstipation, falls, medication toxicity, renal failure, seizure, electrolyte imbalance, hyperthermia, and delayed wound healing (Gupta & Ashraf, 2012; Martins & Fernandes, 2012). Due to a lack of understanding of the pathogenesis and consequences of dehydration in older persons, dehydration in these persons is often attributed to poor care by long-term care (LTC) home staff, physicians, or both. However, for most older people, dehydration is a result of increased fluid loss combined with decreased fluid intake due to decreased thirst.

Risk Factors for Dehydration

Most healthy older persons maintain adequate hydration. However, physical or emotional illness, surgery, trauma, or conditions with higher physiological demands increase the risk of dehydration. At that time, the limited capacity of the homeostatic mechanisms to maintain fluid balance can put the older person's fluid balance at risk (Prowle et al., 2010).

Age-related changes in the thirst mechanism, a decrease in total body water, and decreased kidney function increase the risk for dehydration. Total body water (TBW) decreases with age. In young adults, TBW is about 60% of body weight in men and 52% in women. In older people, TBW decreases to about 52% of body weight in men and 46% of that in women. The loss of muscle mass with age increases the proportion of fat cells. This loss is greater in women because they have a higher percentage of body fat and less muscle mass than men have. Because fat cells contain less water than muscle cells contain, older people have a lower volume of intracellular fluid. Furthermore, thirst sensation diminishes, resulting in the loss of an important defence against dehydration. Creatinine clearance also declines with age, and the kidneys are less able to concentrate urine. These changes are more pronounced among persons with illnesses that affect kidney function (see Chapter 6).

Risk factors for dehydration include the use of medications that directly affect renal function and fluid balance (e.g., diuretics, laxatives, and angiotensin-converting enzyme inhibitors) and the use of psychoactive medications that have anticholinergic effects (dry mouth, urinary retention, and constipation). The concurrent use of four or more medications is also a risk factor (Rolland & Morley, 2016).

Functional deficits, communication and comprehension problems, oral problems, dysphagia, depression, dementia, hospitalization, low body weight, diagnostic procedures that necessitate fasting, inadequate assistance with fluid intake, diarrhea, fever, vomiting, infections, bleeding, draining wounds, artificial ventilation, fluid restrictions, high environmental temperature, and multiple comorbidities have all been

| BOX 9.1 | Simple Screen for Dehydration |

Drugs
End of life
High fever
Yellow urine turns dark
Dizziness (orthostasis)
Reduced oral intake
Axillae dry
Tachycardia
Incontinence (fear of)
Oral problems
Neurological impairment (confusion)
Sunken eyes

Source: Thomas, D., Cote, T., Lawhorne, L., et al. (2008). Understanding clinical dehydration and its treatment. *Journal of the American Medical Directors Association, 9*(5), 292–301.

noted as risk factors for dehydration in older people (Rolland & Morley, 2016; Burns, 2016). Nothing-by-mouth (NPO) periods for diagnostic tests and surgical procedures should be avoided or made as short as possible for older persons, and adequate fluids should be given once procedures are completed. Research has determined that consuming clear liquids (e.g., water, apple juice, black tea, black coffee) 2 to 3 hours before surgery does not increase gastric residual volume or the risk for aspiration (Brown & Heuberger, 2014). Box 9.1 presents a simple screen for dehydration.

Hyponatremia is a decrease in sodium plasma concentration (<135 mmol/L), caused by an excess of water relative to solute. Differential diagnosis includes the syndrome of inappropriate antidiuretic hormone (SIADH) (Thomas & Fraer, 2016). Selective serotonin reuptake inhibitors (SSRIs) increase the risk of hyponatremia, the risk being greatest in the first 2 weeks of treatment. Monitoring the sodium level and fluid intake of individuals taking recently prescribed SSRIs is important. Changes in mental status, including lethargy or acute confusion, should be investigated immediately (see Chapter 21). Other risk factors include certain medications, such as thiazide and loop diuretics, and comorbidities such as renal and hepatic insufficiencies, congestive heart failure, and respiratory infections. Hyponatremia is especially common in older persons (Soiza et al., 2014).

 IMPLICATIONS FOR GERONTOLOGICAL NURSING AND HEALTHY AGING

ASSESSMENT

Prevention of dehydration is essential, but the assessment of dehydration in older people is complex; clinical signs may not appear until dehydration is advanced. Attention to risk factors is very important for identifying possible dehydration and intervening early. In addition, the minimum data set has 12 triggers for dehydration-fluid maintenance and 7 additional risk factors. Older people and their caregivers should be taught about the need for fluids and about the signs and symptoms of dehydration. Acute episodes of vomiting, diarrhea, or fever should be quickly recognized and treated. Older persons over the age of 85 years who have experienced volume deficits, weight loss, malnutrition, or infections are at a high risk for dehydration, as are older persons with dementia, delirium, and functional impairments.

Older people may not always show the typical signs of dehydration (Shimizu et al., 2012). Skin turgor, assessed at the sternum and commonly included in the assessment of dehydration, is an unreliable marker in older persons because of the loss of subcutaneous tissue that occurs with aging. Dry mucous membranes in the mouth and nose, longitudinal furrows on the tongue, orthostasis, speech incoherence, weakness of extremities, dry axillae, and sunken eyes may indicate dehydration.

Laboratory tests for suspected dehydration include blood urea nitrogen (BUN) and tests for sodium, creatinine, glucose, and bicarbonate. Osmolarity should be either directly measured or calculated. While most cases of dehydration have elevated levels of BUN, there are many other causes of an elevated BUN (Thomas et al., 2008). Changes in body weight should also be assessed, as they indicate changes in hydration.

INTERVENTIONS

Interventions for dehydration are derived from a comprehensive assessment and consist of risk identification and hydration management (Wakefield et al., 2008). Hydration management involves both acute and ongoing management of oral intake. Oral hydration is the first treatment approach for dehydration.

Individuals with mild to moderate dehydration who can drink and do not have significant mental or physical compromise due to fluid loss may be able to replenish fluids orally. Water is considered the best fluid for this purpose, but other clear fluids may also be offered, depending on the person's preference.

Rehydration methods depend on the severity and type of dehydration and may include either intravenous administration or hypodermoclysis, an infusion of isotonic fluids into the subcutaneous space. A general rule is to replace 50% of the loss within the first 12 hours (1 litre per day in afebrile older persons) or a sufficient quantity to relieve tachycardia and hypotension. Further fluid replacement can be administered over a longer period.

Hypodermoclysis is safe, easy to administer, and a useful alternative to intravenous administration for persons with mild to moderate dehydration, particularly those with altered mental status. Normal saline (0.9%), half-normal saline (0.45%), a 5% dextrose in water infusion (D5W), or Ringer's solution can be used (Smithard & Leslie, 2016). Because hypodermoclysis can be administered in almost any setting, hospital admission may be avoided.

Ongoing management of oral intake includes the following five steps: (1) calculate a daily fluid goal; (2) compare the person's current intake to the amount calculated, to evaluate the person's hydration status; (3) provide fluids consistently throughout the day; (4) plan for at-risk individuals; and (5) perform fluid regulation and documentation (Mentes, 2012) (Box 9.2).

URINARY CONTINENCE

BLADDER FUNCTION

Normal bladder function requires an intact brain and spinal cord, competent lower urinary tract function, motivation to maintain continence, functional ability to recognize voiding signals and use a toilet, and an environment that facilitates the process. A full bladder increases pressure and alerts the spinal cord and the brainstem centre to the need to micturate. Social training then dictates whether **micturition** should be attended to or should be postponed (e.g., until there is an opportunity to seek out toilet facilities). However, when bladder contents reach 500 mL or more, the pressure is such that the urge to void becomes more difficult to control. As volume increases, emptying the bladder becomes an uncontrollable act.

Age-Related Changes in Bladder Function

Bladder changes that occur with aging include decreased capacity, increased irritability, contractions during filling, and incomplete emptying. These changes may lead to frequency, nocturia, urgency, and vulnerability to infection. The warning period between the desire to void and actual micturition is shortened. This shorter warning period—combined with illness, cognitive impairments, problems in manipulating clothing, or difficulty in walking to the toilet or handling a bedpan or urinal—can affect an older person's ability to maintain continence.

URINARY INCONTINENCE

Urinary **incontinence** is the involuntary loss of urine (Dowling-Castronovo & Bradway, 2012), and it is an important yet neglected geriatric syndrome. Because of its high prevalence and chronic but preventable nature, urinary incontinence (UI) is most appropriately considered a public health problem (Lawhorne et al., 2008)—a stigmatized, underreported, underdiagnosed, and undertreated condition that is erroneously thought to be part of normal aging (National Institute for Health and Clinical Excellence, 2006).

Individuals may not seek treatment for UI, because they are embarrassed by the problem or because they do not know that successful treatments are available. Women who are members of ethnocultural minorities may be less knowledgeable about UI than nonminority women are. For example, a study of women living in the general community found that Korean American women were less knowledgeable about UI and had more-negative attitudes toward it when compared to another study population consisting of Caucasian, African American, and Hispanic women (Kang, 2009). Men may be unlikely to report UI to their primary care providers because they feel that UI is a woman's condition. Nurses caring for older persons in all practice settings should be prepared to assess the person for urine control and implement nursing interventions that promote continence (Dowling-Castronovo & Bradway, 2012). *Incontinence: Breaking the Silence*, a fact sheet for public education, is available from the

---

BOX 9.2 Ongoing Management of Oral Intake

1. Calculate a daily fluid goal. All older persons should have an individualized fluid goal determined by a documented standard for daily fluid intake (minimum 1,500 mL of fluid per 24 hours).
2. Compare the person's current intake to the fluid goal to evaluate hydration status.
   a. Provide fluids consistently throughout the day and when the patient is awake at night (75–80% of fluids delivered at meals and 20–25% during nonmeal times such as medication administration or snack times).
   b. Offer a variety of fluids, and offer fluids that the person prefers.
   c. Standardize the amount of fluid offered with medication administration (at least 100 mL).
3. Plan for at-risk individuals.
   a. Provide fluid rounds midmorning and midafternoon.
   b. Provide a minimum of four 250-mL glasses of fluid throughout the day.
   c. Organize "happy hours" or tea times, when residents can gather to consume additional fluids and socialize.
   d. Modify fluid containers according to the person's abilities (e.g., lighter cups and glasses or plastic water bottles with straws, attach cupholders to wheelchairs or chairs to hold cups or bottles).
   e. Ensure that fluids are accessible to residents at all times (e.g., full water pitchers, fluid stations, beverage carts in congregate areas or at nursing stations).

   f. Allow adequate time and staff for feeding or assisting with eating; meals can provide two-thirds of daily fluids.
      (1) Offer the patient a sip of fluid every two to three mouthfuls of food.
      (2) Offer the patient fluids at the end of each meal to cleanse and refresh the mouth.
   g. Monitor hydration during hot weather.
   h. Encourage family members to participate in feeding and in offering fluids.
4. Perform fluid regulation and documentation. (Frequency of documentation of fluid intake depends on the setting and the individual's condition.)
   a. Teach patients to use a urine colour chart to monitor hydration if they are able to do so.
   b. Know the volumes of fluid containers to accurately calculate fluid consumption.
   c. Document complete intake, including hydration habits.
   d. Document accurate intake and output including the amount of fluid consumed, any difficulties with consumption, and the amount, gravity, and colour of urine.
   e. Observe continence products used by incontinent persons for amount and frequency of urine, for colour changes, and for odour, and report variations from the person's normal pattern.

Source: Adapted from Mentes, J. C. (2012). Managing oral hydration. In M. Boltz, E. Capezuti, T. Fulmer, et al. (Eds.), *Evidence-based geriatric nursing protocols for best practice* (4th ed.). New York: Springer; Registered Nurses' Association of Ontario (RNAO). (n.d.). *RNAO Best Practices Toolkit Implementing and Sustaining Change in Long-Term Care: Care Planning for Hydration Management.* Retrieved from http://ltctoolkit.rnao.ca/resources/continence-and-constipation-assessment-and-management.

RNAO (http://rnao.ca/bpg/fact-sheets/incontinence-breaking-silence).

Epidemiology of Urinary Incontinence

Millions of adults worldwide are affected by UI. In Canada, 50% of adults report symptoms of urge incontinence. Women are more likely than men to have UI (14% versus 9%). In addition, UI is more common among older persons; at age 85 years or older, 19% of men and 22% of women experience UI (Ramage-Morin & Gilmour, 2013). An estimated 60 to 90% of LTC home residents are incontinent (Wagg et al., 2016).

Urinary incontinence is more prevalent than diabetes, Alzheimer's disease, and many other chronic conditions that receive more attention and treatment. Incontinence is also costly; the Canadian Urinary Bladder Survey estimated that UI cost Canadians $2.3 billion in 2014 (The Canadian Continence Foundation, 2014). A recent study of UI in LTC homes reported that staff education and staff perceptions of UI treatment's effectiveness influenced care intervention in LTC homes. Enabling factors included teamwork and the experience of success (French et al., 2017).

Consequences of Urinary Incontinence

Urinary incontinence affects quality of life and has physical, psychosocial, and economic consequences; UI is associated with falls, skin irritations and infections, urinary tract infections (UTIs), and pressure ulcers. It also affects self-esteem and increases the risk for depression, anxiety, social isolation, and avoidance of sexual activity. Older persons with UI experience a loss of dignity, loss of independence, and loss of self-confidence, as well as feelings of shame and embarrassment (Dowling-Castronovo & Bradway, 2012). The psychosocial impact of UI affects both the person and family caregivers. Three instruments are available to assess the psychological effects of UI: the Incontinence Impact Questionnaire (Uebersax et al., 1995), the International Consultation on Incontinence Questionnaire–Lower Urinary Tract Symptoms Quality of Life (ICIQ-LUTSqol) (Avery et al., 2004), and the Male Urinary Symptom Impact Questionnaire (Robinson & Shea, 2002).

Risk Factors for Urinary Incontinence

Cognitive impairment, limitations in daily activities, and institutionalization are associated with higher risks of UI. Stroke, diabetes, obesity, poor general health, and comorbidities are also associated with UI (Wagg et al., 2016). Pregnancy, childbirth, menopause, and hysterectomy are other factors that contribute to UI. Urinary incontinence can also be exacerbated by medications that increase urinary output and by sedative-hypnotic medications, which produce drowsiness, confusion, or limited mobility, thus dulling the desire to urinate.

In a study of LTC home residents with dementia, 48% had UI upon admission, and 81% had UI 6 months after admission. Dementia does not cause UI but affects the ability of the person to recognize the urge to void and to find a washroom in which to do so. Mobility problems and dependency in transfers are better predictors of continence status than is dementia, which suggests that persons with dementia may be able to remain continent as long as they are mobile. Making toilets easily visible, helping persons go to the washroom at regular intervals, and implementing prompted voiding protocols can help promote continence for people with dementia.

Box 9.3 presents risk factors for UI.

Types of Urinary Incontinence

Incontinence is classified as either **transient** (acute) or established (chronic). Transient incontinence has

---

BOX 9.3	Risk Factors for Urinary Incontinence

- Age
- Immobility, functional limitations
- Diminished cognitive capacity (dementia, delirium)
- Medications (anticholinergics, sedatives, diuretics)
- Smoking
- High caffeine intake
- Obesity
- Constipation, fecal impaction
- Pregnancy, vaginal delivery, episiotomy
- Low fluid intake
- Environmental barriers
- High-impact physical exercise
- Diabetes
- Stroke
- Parkinson's disease
- Hysterectomy
- Pelvic muscle weakness
- Childhood nocturnal enuresis
- Prostate surgery
- Estrogen deficiency
- Arthritis
- Hearing and vision impairments

Sources: Adapted from Dowling-Castronovo, A., & Bradway, C. (2012). Urinary incontinence. In Boltz, E., et al. (Eds.), *Evidence-based geriatric nursing protocols for best practice* (4th ed.). New York: Springer.

---

a sudden onset, is present for 6 months or less, and is usually caused by treatable factors, such as UTIs, delirium, constipation and stool impaction, and increased urine production caused by metabolic conditions such as hyperglycemia and hypercalcemia. *Iatrogenic* (treatment-induced) incontinence is a type of transient UI that results from the use of restraints, limited fluid intake, bedrest, or intravenous fluid administration. The use of diuretics, anticholinergics, antidepressants, sedatives, hypnotics, calcium channel blockers, and alpha-adrenergic agonists and blockers can also lead to transient UI (Dowling-Castronovo & Bradway, 2012).

Established UI may have either a sudden or a gradual onset and is categorized into the following types:

- *Urge incontinence* (overactive bladder) is defined as involuntary urine loss that occurs soon after feeling an urgent need to void. The bladder muscles are overactive and cause a sudden urge to void—the "gotta go right now" syndrome (Das et al, 2016). The defining characteristics of urge incontinence include the loss of moderate to large amounts of urine before reaching a toilet and an inability to suppress the need to urinate. Urinary frequency and nocturia may also be present. Postvoid residual urine reveals a small amount of urine left in the bladder after voiding. Urge incontinence is the most common type of UI in older persons (Dowling-Castronovo & Bradway, 2012).

- *Stress incontinence* (outlet incompetence) is defined as an involuntary loss of less than 50 mL of urine during actions that increase intra-abdominal pressure (e.g., coughing, sneezing, exercising, lifting, and bending). Stress incontinence is more common in women because of their short urethras and poor pelvic-muscle tone (as a result of pregnancies); it occurs in men who have undergone prostatectomy and radiation treatment. Postvoid residual urine is low (Dowling-Castronovo & Bradway, 2012).

- *Urge* or *stress UI with high postvoid residual incontinence* (formerly called "overflow incontinence") is what occurs when the bladder does not empty normally and becomes overdistended (beyond regular distention when filled with a normal amount of urine). This condition is accompanied by frequent or nearly constant urine loss (dribbling). Its symptoms include hesitancy in starting urination, slow urine stream, infrequent urination or small volumes of urine, a feeling of incomplete bladder emptying, and large volumes of postvoid residual urine. Persons with diabetes and men with enlarged prostates are at risk for this type of UI. The use of calcium channel blockers, anticholinergics, and adrenergics also contributes to symptoms.

- *Functional incontinence* is defined as a situation in which the lower urinary tract is intact but the individual is unable to reach a toilet because of environmental barriers, physical limitations, or severe cognitive impairment. The person may be dependent on others for assistance in reaching a toilet but have no genitourinary problems other than incontinence. Older persons in institutions have higher rates of functional incontinence (Dowling-Castronovo & Bradway, 2012).

Functional incontinence may also occur in the presence of other types of UI.

- *Mixed incontinence* is defined as a combination of more than one type of UI, usually stress and urge. Mixed incontinence is the most prevalent type of incontinence in older women; with increasing age, older women with stress incontinence begin to experience urge incontinence.

 IMPLICATIONS FOR GERONTOLOGICAL NURSING AND HEALTHY AGING

Nurses in all practice settings with older persons should be prepared to assess continence and implement nursing interventions that promote continence.

ASSESSMENT

Continence must be routinely addressed in the initial assessment of every older person, yet many people do not bring up their concerns about incontinence, and many health care providers do not ask. Health care providers must begin to change their thinking about incontinence and acknowledge that it can be cured or treated to minimize its detrimental effects. Nurses are often the ones to identify UI, but neither nurses nor physicians have been particularly aggressive in its management.

Assessment is multidimensional; it includes a health history, targeted physical examination, urinalysis, and a determination of postvoid residual urine. More extensive examinations are considered after the initial findings are assessed. A thorough health history should focus on the medical, neurological, and genitourinary history; functional assessment; cognitive assessment; psychosocial effects; strategies currently used to control UI; medication review of both prescribed and over-the-counter medications; detailed exploration of the symptoms of the UI; and associated symptoms and other factors. In care facilities, an environmental assessment including the accessibility of bathrooms, room lighting, and the use of aids such as raised toilet seats or commodes is also important.

In an LTC home, the completed minimum data set may trigger the Resident Assessment Protocol for incontinence. Several tools can be used for comprehensive continence assessment, treatment, and evaluation for LTC home residents. The Continence, History, Assessment, Medications, Mobility, and Plan (CHAMMP) tool was developed by certified wound, ostomy, and continence nurses to guide comprehensive continence assessment and the implementation of individualized care plans in LTC homes (Bucci, 2007) (Fig. 9.1). The International Consultation on Incontinence Questionnaire-Urinary Incontinence-Short Form (ICIQ-UI-SF) is another instrument that can be used to evaluate UI (Timmermans et al., 2016).

One of the best ways to establish the presence of incontinence problems and to describe them is with a voiding diary, the "gold standard" for obtaining objective information about voiding patterns and the frequency and severity of UI episodes (Dowling-Castronovo & Bradway, 2012). Older persons living in the community can usually keep a voiding diary without much difficulty. In LTC homes, voiding diaries are usually maintained by the staff. The character of the urine (colour, odour, sediment, clearness) and any difficulty the person has starting or stopping the urinary stream should be recorded. The person's ability to accomplish activities of daily living (such as reaching and using a toilet) and his or her finger dexterity for manipulating clothing should be documented.

INTERVENTIONS

Behavioural

Continence can be improved when appropriate care is provided. A number of behavioural interventions have a good basis in research and can be implemented by nurses without extensive and expensive evaluation. These treatments are viewed as healthy bladder behaviour skills (Dowling-Castronovo & Bradway, 2012). These interventions will do no harm; if they bring no improvement, further evaluation can be sought. Behavioural techniques such as scheduled voiding, prompted voiding, bladder training, biofeedback, vaginal weight training, and pelvic floor muscle exercises (PFMEs) are recommended as first-line treatment for UI (Box 9.4.) The selection of a modality and interventions will depend on a comprehensive assessment, the type of incontinence and its underlying cause, and whether the goal is to cure or to minimize the extent of the incontinence. Interventions and treatment planning for UI should involve the

---

BOX 9.4   Research for Evidence-Informed Practice: Incontinence Improves in Older Women After Intensive Pelvic Floor Muscle Training: An Assessor-Blinded Randomized Controlled Trial

Problem: Urinary incontinence (UI) is a major problem in older persons and impacts quality of life. The prevalence of UI increases with age.

Methods: An assessor-blinded randomized controlled trial in two centres was completed. The study was 20 weeks in duration, one group receiving high-intensity pelvic floor muscle training (PFMT), the other group receiving bladder training.

Findings: Eighty-three women participated in the study. Both groups improved over the intervention period. The PFMT group reported significantly lower amounts of leakage on the stress test.

Application to nursing practice: Nurses have the opportunity to encourage exercises such as pelvic floor muscle strength and motor exercises with older persons who have UI. Nurses should have a knowledge of exercises that can have a significant effect in improving UI.

Source: Sherburn, M. et al. (2011). Incontinence improves in older women after intensive pelvic floor muscle training: An assessor-blinded randomized controlled trial. *Neurology and Urodynamics, 30,* 317–324. doi:10.1002/nau.

---

interprofessional team and everyone involved with the person's care. Physiotherapy and occupational therapy, restorative programs, or all should be part of the treatment plan for persons with impaired mobility. Box 9.5 lists nursing interventions in the treatment of UI that focus on supportive measures and restorative therapeutic modalities.

- *Scheduled (timed) voiding* is used to treat urge and functional UI in both cognitively intact and cognitively impaired older persons. The scheduling or timing of voiding is based on the voiding patterns shown in the person's bladder diary or on common voiding patterns (i.e., voiding upon arising, before and after meals, and at midmorning, midafternoon, and bedtime). Generally, regular toileting is scheduled at 2- to 4-hour intervals. People can be taught to do this routinely, or they can be helped to the bathroom at the scheduled intervals.
- *Prompted voiding* combines scheduled voiding with monitoring, prompting, and verbal reinforcement.

CHAMMP TOOL

(Continence, History, Assessment, Medications, Mobility, Plan)

C Resident is continent? Yes ___ No ___

H Medical / Surgical History:

    a. Diagnosis often associated with continence? Yes ___ No ___
        ___ BPH (prostate) ___ Diabetes ___ MS
        ___ CHF ___ Fracture ___ Osteoporosis
        ___ Constipation ___ Heart Disease ___ Pain
        ___ Contractures ___ HTN ___ Parkinson's
        ___ CVA ___ Immobility ___ Spinal Cord Injury
        ___ Dementia ___ Kidney Stones ___ UTI (last 90 days)
        ___ Depression
    b. Recent Acute Medical Condition (last 30 days)? Yes ___ No ___
        If yes, date and type:
    c. Recent Surgery (last 30 days)? Yes ___ No ___
        If yes, date and type:
    d. Surgical History: Hysterectomy ___ Bladder Repair ___ Prostate (TURP) ___ Other ___
    e. Lab Data ___ Urodynamic Studies ___ Imaging Studies ___
        Date and type:

A Assessment of Urinary Incontinence:

    Trigger Event (surgery, accident, other)? Yes ___ No ___
    Leak urine when cough, sneeze, laugh, stand up, change position? Yes ___ No ___
    Urge to go (Need to be there NOW)? Yes ___ No ___
    Wet without feeling the need to go? Yes ___ No ___
    Number of night time voids? ___
    Leak only at night? Yes ___ No ___
    Difficult to start or stop stream? Yes ___ No ___
    Weak stream? Yes ___ No ___
    Dribbling? Yes ___ No ___
    Products used? _____

M1 Medications:

    a. Current Medication:

___ Anticholinergic	___ Diuretic	___ Narcotic
___ Antidepressant	___ Hypnotic	___ OTC Cold Remedies
___ Antihypertensive	___ Laxative	___ Sedative
___ Other:		

    b. Medications to treat Incontinence:

___ Antibiotic	___ Estrogen	___ Proscar
___ Detrol	___ Flomax	___ Sanctura
___ Ditropan	___ Imipramine	___ VESIcare
___ Enablex	___ Other:	

M2 Mobility Status: I Independent, A Assist, D Dependent

___ Ambulation	___ Dressing	___ Toileting
___ Transfer		

    Can access bedpan, BSC, urinal, toilet independently ___ Yes ___ No

P Plan of care:

    a. Resident is motivated to toilet: ___ Yes ___ No ___ Not oriented
    b. Resident is candidate for treatment program? Yes ___ No ___
    If no, reason:
    c. Care Plan interventions: (Circle Suggestions)
        ° Incontinence, functional–Prompted voiding, behavioral modification (i.e., timed voiding), restorative toileting, physical and/or occupational therapy, environmental modifications
        ° Incontinence, overflow–clean intermittent catheterization
        ° Incontinence, stress–pelvic muscle exercises, behavior modification, medications
        ° Incontinence, urge–pelvic muscle exercises, behavior modification, medication
        ° Incontinence, mixed (stress and urge)–pelvic muscle exercises, behavior modification, medications
        ° Incontinence, total–check and change
    d. Bladder treatment initiated (date):
    Nurse Signature: _____ Date: _____

FIGURE 9.1 Continence, History, Assessment, Medications, Mobility, and Plan (CHAMMP) tool. *Source:* Bucci, A. (2007). Be a continence champion: Use the CHAMMP tool to individualize the plan of care. *Geriatric Nursing, 28*(2), 123.

BOX 9.5   Nursing Interventions and Support Measures in the Treatment of Urinary Incontinence

- Appropriate attitude
- Accessible toilets and toilet substitutes (bedpan, urinal, commode)
- Avoidance of iatrogenic conditions (urinary tract infections, constipation or impaction, excessive sedation, medications adversely affecting the bladder or urethral function)
- Protective undergarments
- Absorbent bed pads
- Behavioural techniques: bladder training, scheduled (timed) voiding, prompted voiding, biofeedback, pelvic floor muscle exercises, vaginal weight training
- Good skin care

With a cognitively intact person, the objective is to increase self-initiated voiding and decrease the episodes of UI. With a cognitively impaired person, caregivers should regularly ask whether he or she needs assistance in using the toilet. The person is assisted to the toilet if he or she requests. Positive feedback is provided after successful voiding.

- In a systematic review of randomized trials of interventions in LTC home residents with UI, Fink et al. (2008) concluded that prompted voiding is associated with modest short-term improvements in daytime UI among these residents.

Newly admitted LTC home residents should be thoroughly assessed for continence, and those who are incontinent yet able to use the toilet should undergo a 3- to 5-day trial of prompted voiding. The trial can help demonstrate a person's response to toileting and determine patterns of and symptoms associated with the incontinence. Residents who are unresponsive to toileting programs or are unable or unwilling to participate in toileting can be provided with supportive management, including the use of absorbent pads and briefs, and with attention to the prevention of skin breakdown (Zarowitz & Ouslander, 2007; Lawhorne et al., 2008).

Continence programs in LTC homes are required by regulations in some provinces. Monitoring and the documentation of continence status in relation to implemented continence care should be a quality-of-care indicator for LTC homes (Registered Nurses' Association of Ontario [RNAO], 2007).

- *Bladder training* aims to increase the interval between the urge to void and voiding. This method is appropriate for people with urge UI who are cognitively intact and independent in toileting. The person follows an established voiding schedule until UI episodes cease. The interval between voidings is then extended, and techniques (e.g., pelvic floor muscle exercises) for overcoming the urge to urinate and for postponing urination are taught.

- *Pelvic Floor Muscle Exercises* (PFMEs), also called *Kegel exercises*, involve repeated voluntary pelvic floor muscle contraction. The targeted muscle is the pubococcygeal muscle, which forms the support for the pelvis and surrounds the urethra, and rectum and the vagina for women. The goal of the repetitive contractions is to strengthen the muscle and decrease UI episodes. PFMEs are recommended for stress, urge, and mixed UI in older women and have also been shown to be helpful for men who have undergone prostatectomy. Contractions should be repeated 30 to 100 times a day; the contraction is held for 10 seconds and followed by 10 seconds of relaxation.

Correct identification of the pelvic floor muscles and compliance with the exercise regimen are key to success. Improvement may not be noted until 2 to 4 weeks of exercising have been successfully completed. To help the person identify the correct muscle groups, the caregiver can tell the person to try to tighten the anal sphincter, as if controlling the passage of flatus or feces, and then to tighten the urethral muscles, vaginal muscles, or both, as if stopping the flow of urine. The stomach, thigh, or buttock muscles should not be contracted, since this increases intra-abdominal pressure. This exercise may be taught during a vaginal or rectal examination, when the clinician helps the patient identify the pelvic muscles by having him or her "squeeze" the clinician's gloved examination finger (Healy et al., 2013).

- *Biofeedback* may be helpful in identifying the correct muscles and visualizing the strength and time of the contraction (Newman, 2014).

- *Vaginal weight training* is an alternative for women who have difficulty identifying the pelvic floor muscles. The woman wears graded-weight vaginal balls or cones for two 15-minute periods each day or uses them in addition to doing PFMEs. When the weighted ball or cone is placed in the vagina, the pelvic floor muscle contractions keep it from slipping out. Although this technique involves less time and is more easily taught than PFMEs, discomfort and difficulties inserting the objects have been noted as deterrents to its use.

Lifestyle Modifications

Several lifestyle factors are associated with either the development or exacerbation of UI. Lifestyle modifications that can diminish UI include modification of dietary factors (e.g., increased fluid intake, avoidance of caffeine), weight reduction, smoking cessation, bowel management, and physical activity. Recent research has found that coffee and tea consumption has limited or no effect on incontinence, but guidelines generally recommend limiting caffeine intake (Tettamanti et al., 2011). Box 9.6 presents other recommendations to community-dwelling older persons for controlling or eliminating UI.

Absorbent Products

A variety of protective undergarments and adult briefs are available for the older person who is incontinent. Disposable types come in several sizes determined by hip and waist measurements or as a one-size-fits-all garment. Many of these undergarments look like regular underwear and contribute more to dignity than does the standard "diaper." Referring to protective undergarments as "diapers" is demeaning and infantilizing to older people and should be avoided. Some individuals may prefer to use absorbent products in addition to toileting interventions to maintain "social continence."

Urinary Catheters

External catheters (condom catheters) are used in male patients who are incontinent and cannot be toileted. Long-term use of external catheters can lead to fungal skin infection, penile skin maceration, edema, fissures, contact burns from urea, phimosis, UTIs, and septicemia. The catheter should be removed and replaced daily, the meatal area washed with soap and water, and the penis washed, dried, and aired to

---

BOX 9.6 Helpful Recommendations to Community-Dwelling Older Persons for Controlling or Eliminating Urinary Incontinence

- Empty the bladder completely before and after meals and at bedtime.
- Urinate whenever the urge arises; never ignore it.
- Try a schedule of urinating every 2 hours during the day and every 4 hours at night, which is often helpful in retraining the bladder. The use of an alarm clock may be necessary.
- Drink 1.5–2.0 L of fluid before 20:00 hours each day to help the kidneys function properly. Limit fluids after supper to 125–250 mL, except in very hot weather.
- Eliminate or reduce the consumption of coffee, tea, brown cola, and alcohol, since they have a diuretic effect.
- Take prescription diuretics in the morning upon rising.
- Limit the use of sleeping pills, sedatives, and alcohol; they decrease the sensation of urinating and can increase incontinence, especially at night.
- Lose weight if overweight.
- Try doing pelvic floor muscle exercises, which are often helpful for women with stress, urge, and mixed UI. They may also be helpful for men after prostatectomy.
- Make sure the toilet is nearby, has a clear path to it, and has good lighting, especially at night. Grab bars or a raised toilet seat may be needed.
- Dress protectively with cotton underwear and protective pants or incontinent pads if necessary.

---

prevent irritation, maceration, pressure ulcers, and skin breakdown. If the catheter is not sized appropriately and is not applied and monitored correctly, strangulation of the penile shaft can occur.

Intermittent catheterization may be used in persons with urinary retention related to a weak **detrusor** muscle (e.g., diabetic neuropathy), a blockage of the urethra (e.g., benign prostatic hypertrophy), or reflex incontinence related to a spinal cord injury. The goal is to maintain a urine volume of 300 mL or less in the bladder. Most of the research on intermittent catheterization has been conducted with children or young adults with spinal cord injuries, but the procedure may be useful for older persons who are able to self-catheterize. Intermittent catheterization is an important alternative to indwelling catheterization.

Clinical guidelines indicate that indwelling catheters are not appropriate for long-term (i.e., more than 30 days) management. Continuous indwelling catheter use is indicated for urethral obstruction or urinary retention and in patients to whom the following apply:

- Surgical or pharmacological interventions are inappropriate or unsuccessful.
- Intermittent catheterization to treat retention is contraindicated.
- Changes of bedding, clothing, and absorbent products may be painful or disruptive for a patient with an irreversible medical condition (such as a terminal disease).
- Skin integrity is severely impaired.
- Patient lives alone either without a caregiver or with a caregiver who is unable to routinely change the patient's absorbent pads, protective undergarments, and bed or chair linens (Newman & Palmer, 2003; Johnson & Ouslander, 2006).

Regulatory standards for LTC homes follow these same guidelines, and the use of indwelling catheters must be justified on the basis of medical conditions and the failure of other efforts to maintain continence. The use of indwelling catheters in hospitals is often unjustified, and they are used inappropriately (for example, for the convenience of staff) or left in place too long. The misuse of catheterization should be considered a medical error. About one in four indwelling catheters in hospitalized patients aged 70 years or older and one in three patients aged 85 years or older turns out to be unnecessary (Inelmen et al., 2007). Urinary catheterization is a risk factor for delirium (see Chapter 21), and catheterization without a specific medical indication is associated with a greater risk of death and longer hospital stays (Fakih et al., 2010).

Long-term catheter use increases the risk of recurrent urinary tract infections, leading to urosepsis, urethral damage in men secondary to urethral erosion, urethritis or fistula formation, and bladder stones or cancer. Urinary tract infections (UTIs) are the most common infections among residents of LTC homes. Asymptomatic bacteria in the urine are considered benign in older people and should not be treated with antibiotics. Screening of urine cultures should not be performed for asymptomatic patients. Symptomatic UTIs necessitate antibiotic treatment, but it is important to pay attention to the range of symptoms older people may present (fever, dysuria, flank pain, abdominal pain, new-onset incontinence, decreased appetite, changes in mental status, or even respiratory distress).

Pharmacological

Medications are not considered first-line treatment; behavioural therapies are more effective and should be implemented first (Richter et al., 2010). Pharmacological treatment including anticholinergic-antimuscarinic (antispasmodic) agents—toterodine, trospium chloride, oxybutynin, darifenacin, flavoxate, and solifenacin succinate—may be indicated for urge UI and overactive bladder. Oxybutynin is the most commonly prescribed medication in Canada for urinary urgency (Wallis et al., 2016). There is no evidence of the superiority of any one medication (Hartmann et al., 2009). Most antispasmodic medications may not be effective at the doses tolerated by older persons; they are poorly tolerated by older persons because of anticholinergic adverse effects, sedation, and weakness (Wallis et al., 2016). Undesirable side effects of anticholinergic medications (such as dry mouth and eyes, constipation, confusion, and the precipitation of glaucoma) are problematic in older people. For older persons, dosages should be very low at the start of treatment and titrated slowly, with careful attention to side effects and medication interactions. Many patients discontinue medications prematurely (Wallis et al., 2016).

Medications for the treatment of benign prostatic hypertrophy include alpha-adrenergic blockers and 5-alpha-reductase inhibitors. Alpha-adrenergic blockers are usually the therapy of choice in early, mild disease. Saw palmetto, an herbal preparation reported to have 5-alpha-reductase inhibitor activity and often used to treat lower urinary symptoms attributed to benign prostatic hypertrophy, has been found to have limited effectiveness (Barry et al., 2011).

Nonsurgical Devices

Stress incontinence can be treated with intravaginal support devices, pessaries, and urethral plugs. Primarily used to prevent uterine prolapse, a pessary is a device that is fitted into the vagina and exerts pressure to elevate the urethro-vesical junction of the pelvic floor. The patient is taught to insert and remove the pessary, much as a diaphragm used for contraception is inserted and removed. The pessary is removed weekly or monthly for cleaning with soap and water and then reinserted. Adverse effects include vaginal infection, low back pain, and vaginal mucosal erosion. Another concern is the danger of forgetting to remove the pessary.

Surgical

Surgical intervention is appropriate for some conditions of incontinence. Surgical suspension of the bladder neck (sling procedure) is effective in 80 to 95% of women who elect to have this surgical corrective procedure. In men, outflow obstruction incontinence secondary to prostatic hypertrophy is generally corrected by prostatectomy. Sphincter dysfunction resulting from nerve damage following surgical trauma or radical perineal procedures is 70 to 90% repairable through sphincter implantation. Periurethral bulking—the injection of collagen or polytetrafluoroethylene into the periurethral area to increase pressure on the urethra—has been added to the number of surgical procedures that address UI. This procedure adds bulk to the internal sphincter and closes the gap that allowed leakage to occur.

FECAL AND BOWEL INCONTINENCE

Fecal incontinence (FI) is defined as the continuous or recurrent uncontrolled passage of fecal material for at least 1 month in a mature person. Its prevalence is difficult to determine with accuracy, since many people are reluctant to discuss this disorder and because many health care providers do not ask about it. Prevalence varies with the study population. The Canadian Study of Health and Aging indicated a prevalence of 4% among community-dwelling adults aged 65 years or older (AlAmeel et al., 2010). Other estimated prevalence rates are 2 to 17% in community-dwelling older people, 50 to 65% in older persons living in LTC homes, and 33% in older persons in hospital. Higher prevalence rates are found among patients with diabetes, irritable bowel syndrome, stroke, multiple sclerosis, and spinal cord injury (Roach & Christie, 2008).

Often, FI is associated with UI, and as many as 50 to 70% of patients with UI also have FI. It can be transient (in episodes of diarrhea, acute illness, or fecal impaction) or persistent. Like UI, FI has devastating social ramifications for the individuals who experience it and for their families. Both UI and FI have similar contributing factors, including damage to the pelvic floor as a result of surgery or trauma, neurological disorders, functional impairment, immobility, and dementia.

 ## IMPLICATIONS FOR GERONTOLOGICAL NURSING AND HEALTHY AGING

ASSESSMENT

For most patients, FI can be improved and in many cases resolved. In many cases, multiple factors interact to cause FI. Assessment should include a complete history (as is done in UI assessment, described earlier in this chapter) and investigation of the following: diet, stool consistency and frequency, use of laxatives or enemas, surgical and obstetrical history, use of medications that could exacerbate FI, and the effect of FI on the person's quality of life. A focused physical examination (with attention to the gastro-intestinal system) and a bowel record are also necessary. A digital rectal examination should be performed to identify the presence of any mass, impaction, or occult blood.

Because FI is often associated with fecal impaction, reports of diarrhea in older persons must be thoroughly assessed before using antidiarrheal medications, which further complicate the problem of fecal impaction. Digital rectal examination for impacted stool and an abdominal plain film will confirm the presence of impacted stool. Stool analysis for *Clostridium difficile* toxin should be ordered for patients who develop new-onset diarrhea with incontinence (Whitehead et al., 2014). Additional tests may be indicated by assessment findings. Comprehensive assessment seeks to identify underlying and potentially treatable causes of FI, such as fecal loading, infection, inflammatory bowel disease, lower gastro-intestinal cancer, and rectal prolapse. Maintenance of healthy bowel function and prevention of constipation are discussed in Chapter 8.

BOX 9.7   Bowel Training Program

Obtain a bowel history, complete a bowel record, and establish a schedule for the bowel training program that is comfortable and conforms to the patient's lifestyle.

Ensure adequate fibre intake (to normalize stool consistency).

1. Recommendations for adequate fibre intake:
   a. Add high-fibre foods (dried fruit and beans, vegetables, whole-grain products) to the person's diet.
   b. Add 15–45 mL of bran to the person's diet one or two times per day, or administer a bulk laxative (e.g., Metamucil, Benefibre, Prodiem). Titrate the dosage, based on the person's response.
   c. Use the following recipe for a natural laxative: 250 mL wheat bran, 250 mL applesauce, and 250 mL prune juice. Mix and store in refrigerator. Start with 15 mL per day and increase slowly until the desired effect is achieved (see Chapter 8).

Ensure adequate fluid intake (to normalize stool consistency).

1. Recommendations for adequate fluid intake:
   a. The person should drink 2–3 litres daily (unless contraindicated).
   b. The person should consume 4 ounces of prune, fig, or pear juice (or a warm fluid) daily as a stimulus (e.g., 30–60 minutes before established time for defecation).

Encourage exercise:

1. Pelvic tilt and modified sit-ups for abdominal strength.
2. Walking for general muscle tone and cardiovascular system.
3. A more vigorous program if appropriate.

Facilitate bowel movements.:

1. Establish a regular routine and time for bowel movements, depending on person's schedule. The best times are 20–40 minutes after regularly scheduled meals, when the gastrocolic reflex is active.
2. Attempts at evacuation should be made daily within 15 minutes of the established time and whenever the person senses rectal distension.
3. Promote normal posture for defecation (i.e., sitting on the toilet or commode; for persons who are unable to get out of bed, a left-side lying position).
4. Instruct the person to contract the abdominal muscles and "bear down."
5. Have the person lean forward to increase intra-abdominal pressure by using compression against the thighs.
6. Stimulate the anorectal reflex and rectal emptying if necessary, by one of the following actions:
   a. Administer an enema or insert a rectal suppository into the rectum 15–30 minutes before the planned bowel movement. (The suppository should be placed against the bowel wall.)
   b. Insert a gloved, lubricated finger into the anal canal, and gently dilate the anal sphincter.

INTERVENTIONS

Interventions depend on the underlying cause of FI. Condition-specific interventions for treatable causes of FI should be implemented first. Nursing interventions are aimed at managing bowel continence, restoring bowel continence, or both, and for persons with intractable FI, preserving health and dignity. Therapies similar to those used to treat UI, such as environmental manipulation (for access to toilet), diet alterations, habit-training schedules, improvement in transfer and ambulation ability, sphincter-training exercises, biofeedback, medications, or surgery to correct underlying defects, are effective in the treatment of FI.

Keeping accurate bowel records and identifying triggers that initiate incontinence are important. For example, eating a meal stimulates defecation 30 minutes following the completion of the meal, or defecation is stimulated after a morning cup of coffee. If its patterns are identified, FI can be controlled by preparation. Placing the person on the toilet or commode or having a bedpan available at a given time following the trigger event facilitates defecation. The judicious use of nonirritant laxatives can help to promote complete rectal emptying. Box 9.7 describes a bowel training program.

As in the treatment of UI, goals must be realistic. It cannot be stated too often or too strongly that the nurse must always provide immaculate skin care to incontinent persons, because the person's self-esteem and skin integrity depend on it. When FI is intractable, interventions are aimed at preserving the person's dignity and independence and providing psychological and emotional support. Patients may require advice about skin care, talking to friends and family, and obtaining and using continence products. Problems with toilet access can be addressed through the clear indication of location and by environmental modifications. Patients can be referred to support groups. The National Collaborating Centre for Acute Care recommends a review of symptoms every 6 months (National Collaborating Centre for Acute Care [NCCAC], 2007).

SUMMARY

Gerontological nurses play a pivotal role in continence care. It is important that nurses and other health care providers understand the risk factors for incontinence, the causes of incontinence, and evidence-informed protocols for interventions. Health promotion, public education, comprehensive assessments of incontinence, education of informal and formal caregivers, and evidence-informed interventions should be part of individualized care for all older people experiencing symptoms of incontinence.

KEY CONCEPTS

- Age-related changes in the thirst mechanism, a decrease in total body weight, and decreased kidney function increase the risk for dehydration in older persons.
- Most healthy older persons maintain adequate hydration, but physical or emotional illness, surgery, trauma, or conditions of physiological demands increase the risk for dehydration.
- Urinary incontinence is not a part of normal aging; it is a symptom of an underlying problem and calls for thorough assessment.
- Urinary incontinence can be minimized or cured, and many therapeutic modalities for its treatment are available for nurses to implement.
- Health promotion teaching, identification of risk factors, comprehensive assessments, education of informal and formal caregivers, and use of evidence-informed interventions are basic continence competencies for nurses.
- A number of interventions for urinary incontinence are applicable to the management of fecal incontinence.

ACTIVITIES AND DISCUSSION QUESTIONS

1. Explain the problems associated with dehydration in the older person.
2. Identify the signs and symptoms of dehydration.
3. Discuss interventions to prevent and treat dehydration.
4. Discuss risk factors for urinary incontinence in older persons.
5. Conduct a urinary incontinence history with a partner or with an older person.
6. Explain what measures can be taken to cure or decrease the incidence or impact of urinary or fecal incontinence in the community and in long-term care settings.
7. Devise a nursing care plan for an older person with urinary or fecal incontinence.

RESOURCES

Agency for Healthcare Research and Quality (AHRQ). Nursing Standard of Practice Protocol: Urinary incontinence (UI) in older adults admitted to acute care.
https://www.guideline.gov/summaries/summary/43941/urinary-incontinence-in-older-adults-admitted-to-acute-care-in-evidencebased-geriatric-nursing-protocols-for-best-practice

Agency for Healthcare Research and Quality (AHRQ). Prevention of urinary and fecal incontinence in adults.
https://archive.ahrq.gov/downloads/pub/evidence/pdf/fuiad/fuiad.pdf

Canadian Society of Intestinal Research. Research summaries and patient information.
http://www.badgut.com

Hydration Management
https://consultgeri.org/geriatric-topics/hydration-management

Regional Geriatric Program Central. Professional and patient education resources for hydration and continence.
http://www.rgpc.ca/resources/

Registered Nurses' Association of Ontario (RNAO). Continence Care and Bowel Management.
http://ltctoolkit.rnao.ca/resources/continence-and-constipation-assessment-and-management

Registered Nurses' Association of Ontario (RNAO). Promoting Continence Using Prompted Voiding.
http://rnao.ca/bpg/guidelines/promoting-continence-using -prompted-voiding

The Canadian Continence Foundation
http://www.canadiancontinence.ca/EN/?index.html

The Canadian Nurse Continence Advisors. Standards of practice, continuing education, and pamphlets and video clips for patient education.
http://www.cnca.ca

For additional resources, please visit *http://evolve .elsevier.com/Canada/Ebersole/gerontological/*

REFERENCES

AlAmeel, T., Andrew, M. K., & MacKnight, C. (2010). The association of fecal incontinence with institutionalization and mortality in older adults. *American Journal of Gastroenterology*, 105(8), 1830–1834. doi:10.1038/ajg.2010.77.

Avery, K., Donovan, J., Peters, T. J., et al. (2004). ICIQ: a brief and robust measure for evaluating the symptoms and impact of urinary incontinence. *Neurourology and Urodynamics*, 23(4), 322–330. doi:10.1002/nau.20041.

Barry, M. J., Meleth, S., Lee, J. Y., et al. (2011). Effect of increasing doses of saw palmetto extract on lower urinary tract symptoms: A randomized trial. *The Journal of the American Medical Association*, 306(12), 1344–1351. doi:10.1001/jama.2011.1364.

Brown, L., & Heuberger, R. (2014). Nothing by mouth at midnight: Saving or starving? A literature review. *Gastroenterology Nursing*, 37(1), 14–23. doi:10.1097/SGA.0000000000000018.

Bucci, A. (2007). Be a continence champion: Use the CHAMMP tool to individualize the plan of care. *Geriatric Nursing*, 28(2), 120–124. doi:10.1016/j.gerinurse.2006.12.002.

Bunn, D., Jimoh, F., Wilsher, S. H., et al. (2015). Increasing fluid intake and reducing dehydration risk in older people living in long-term care: a systematic review. *Journal of the American Medical Directors Association*, 16(2), 101–113. doi:10.1016/j.jamda.2014.10.016.

Burns, J. (2016). Patient safety and hydration in the care of older people. *Nursing Older People*, 28(4), 21–24. doi:10.7748/nop .28.4.21.s21.

The Canadian Continence Foundation. (2014). *Incontinence: A Canadian perspective*. Peterborough, ON: Author.

Das, R., Buckley, J., & Williams, M. (2016). Assessing multiple dimensions of urgency sensation: The University of South Australia Urinary Sensation Assessment (USA2). *Neurourology and Urodynamics*, doi:10.1002/nau.22992.

Dowling-Castronovo, A., & Bradway, C. (2012). Urinary incontinence. In M. Boltz, E. Capezuti, T. Fulmer, et al. (Eds.), *Evidence-based geriatric nursing protocols for best practice* (5th ed.). New York, NY: Springer.

Fakih, M. G., Shemes, S. P., Pena, M. E., et al. (2010). Urinary catheters in the emergency department: Very elderly women are at high risk for unnecessary utilization. *American Journal of Infection Control*, 38(9), 683–688. doi:10.1016/j.ajic.2010.04.219.

Fink, H. A., Taylor, B. C., Tacklind, J. W., et al. (2008). Treatment interventions in nursing home residents with urinary incontinence: a systematic review of randomized trials. *Mayo Clinic Proceedings. Mayo Clinic*, 83(12), 1332–1343. doi:10.1016/S0025 -6196(11)60781-7.

French, B., Thomas, L. H., McAdam, J., et al. (2017). Client and clinical staff perceptions of barriers to and enablers of the uptake and delivery of behavioural interventions for urinary incontinence: qualitative evidence synthesis. *Journal of Advanced Nursing*, 73(1), 21–38. doi:10.1111/jan.13083.

Gupta, N., & Ashraf, M. Z. (2012). Exposure to high altitude: a risk factor for venous thromboembolism? *Seminars in Thrombosis and Hemostasis*, 38(2), 156–163. doi:10.1055/s-0032-1301413.

Hartmann, K. E., McPheeters, M. L., Biller, D. H., et al. (2009). *Treatment of overactive bladder in women. Evidence Report/ Technology Assessment No. 187. AHRQ Publication No. 09–E017*. Rockville, MD: Agency for Healthcare Research and Quality.

Healy, F., Barry, E., & O'Sullivan, S. (2013). Physiotherapy service provision and its effectiveness after obstetric anal sphincter injuries. *Journal of the Association of Chartered Physiotherapists in Women's Health*, 113, 30–41.

Hooper, L., Bunn, D. K., Downing, A., et al. (2016). Which frail older people are dehydrated? The UK DRIE Study. *The Journal of Gerontology Series A, Biological Sciences*, 71(10), 1341–1347. doi:10.1093/gerona/glv205.

Inelmen, E., Giuseppe, S., & Giuliano, E. (2007). When are indwelling catheters appropriate in elderly patients? *Geriatrics*, 62(10), 18–22.

Johnson, T., & Ouslander, J. (2006). The newly revised F-Tag 315 and surveyor guidance for urinary incontinence in long-term care. *Journal of the American Medical Directors Association*, 7(9), 594–600. doi:10.1016/j.jamda.2006.08.007.

Kang, Y. (2009). Knowledge and attitudes about urinary incontinence among community-dwelling Korean American women. *Journal of Wound Ostomy Continence Nursing*, 36(2), 194–199. doi:10.1097/01.WON.0000347662.33088.c9.

Lawhorne, L., Ouslander, J., Parmelee, P., et al. (2008). Urinary incontinence: A neglected geriatric syndrome in nursing facilities. *Journal of the American Medical Directors Association*, 9(1), 9–35. doi:10.1016/j.jamda.2007.08.003.

MacDonald, C., & Butler, L. (2007). Silent no more: elderly women's stories of living with urinary incontinence in long-term care. *Journal of Gerontological Nursing*, 33(1), 14–20.

Martins, S., & Fernandes, L. (2012). Delirium in elderly people: A review. *Frontiers in Neurology*, 3, 101. doi:10.3389/fneur .2012.00101.

Mentes, J. C. (2012). Managing oral hydration. In E. Capezuti, M. Mezey, T. Fulmer, et al. (Eds.), *Evidence-based geriatric nursing protocols for best practice* (4th ed.). New York: Springer.

Mentes, J. C., & Kang, S. (2013). Hydration management. *Journal of Gerontological Nursing*, 39(2), 11–19. doi:10.3928/0098913 4-20130110-01.

National Collaborating Centre for Acute Care (NCCAC) (2007). *Faecal incontinence: The management of faecal incontinence in adults. National Clinical Guideline.* London, UK: Author. Retrieved from http://www.nice.org.uk/nicemedia/live/11012/36582/36582.pdf.

National Institute for Health and Clinical Excellence (2006). *Urinary incontinence: The management of urinary incontinence in women.* London, UK: RCOG Press. Retrieved from http://www.nice.org.uk/nicemedia/live/10996/30281/30281.pdf.

Newman, D. K. (2014). Pelvic floor muscle rehabilitation using biofeedback. *Urologic Nursing, 34*(4), 193.

Newman, D. K., & Palmer, M. H. (2003). The state of the science on urinary incontinence. *American Journal of Nursing, 3*(Suppl.), 1–58.

Popkin, B. M., D'Anci, K. E., & Rosenberg, I. H. (2010). Water, hydration and health. *Nutrition Reviews, 68*(8), 439–458. doi:10.1111/j.1753-4887.2010.00304.x.

Prowle, J. R., Echeverri, J. E., Ligabo, E. V., et al. (2010). Fluid balance and acute kidney injury. *Nature Reviews. Nephrology, 6*(2), 107–115. doi:10.1038/nrneph.2009.213.

Ramage-Morin, P. L., & Gilmour, H. (2013). *Urinary incontinence and loneliness in Canadian seniors. Health Reports, 24(10)* (pp. 3–10). Ottawa: Statistics Canada.

Registered Nurses' Association of Ontario (RNAO) (2007). *Continence/constipation workshop for RNs in long-term care: A facilitator's guide.* Toronto, ON: Author.

Registered Nurses' Association of Ontario (RNAO) (2011). *Prevention of constipation in the older adult population.* Toronto, ON: Author.

Richter, H. E., Burgio, K. L., Brubaker, L., et al. (2010). Continence pessary compared with behavioral therapy or combined therapy for stress incontinence: a randomized controlled trial. *Obstetrics and Gynecology, 115*(3), 609–617. doi:10.1097/AOG.0b013e3181d055d4.

Roach, M., & Christie, J. (2008). Fecal incontinence in the elderly. *Geriatrics, 63*(2), 13–22. doi:10.1016/0016-5085(95)27031-0.

Robinson, J. P., & Shea, J. A. (2002). Development and testing of a measure of health-related quality of life for men with urinary incontinence. *Journal of the American Geriatric Society, 50*(5), 935–945. doi:10.1046/j.1532-5415.2002.50223.x.

Rolland, Y., & Morley, J. E. (2016). Frailty and polypharmacy. *The journal of Nutrition, Health & Aging, 20*(6), 645–646. doi:10.1007/s12603-015-0510-3.

Shimizu, M., Kinoshita, K., Hattori, K., et al. (2012). Physical signs of dehydration in the elderly. *Internal Medicine, 51*, 1207–1210. doi:10.2169/internalmedicine.51.7056.

Smithard, D., & Leslie, P. (2016). Role of hypodermoclysis in clinical care. *Perspectives of the ASHA Special Interest Groups, 1*(13), 81–88. doi:10.1044/persp1.SIG13.81.

Soiza, R. L., Cumming, K., Clarke, J. M., et al. (2014). Hyponatremia: special considerations in older patients. *Journal of Clinical Medicine, 3*(3), 944–958. doi:10.3390/jcm3030944.

Tettamanti, G., Altman, D., Pedersen, N. L., et al. (2011). Effects of coffee and tea consumption on urinary incontinence in female twins. *An International Journal of Obstetrics and Gynaecology, 118*(7), 806–813. doi:10.1111/j.1471-0528.2011.02930.x.

Thomas, D. R., Cote, T. R., Lawhorne, L., et al. (2008). Understanding clinical dehydration and its treatment. *Journal of the American Medical Directors Association, 9*(5), 292–301. doi:10.1016/j.jamda.2008.03.006.

Thomas, C. P., & Fraer, M. (2016). *Syndrome of inappropriate antidiuretic hormone secretion.* Retrieved from http://emedicine.medscape.com/article/246650-overview.

Timmermans, L., Falez, F., Melot, C., et al. (2016). Use of the International Consultation on Incontinence Questionnaire-Urinary Incontinence-Short Form (ICIQ-UI-SF) for an objective assessment of disability determination according to the Modified Katz Scale: a prospective longitudinal study. *The Italian Journal of Urology and Nephrology, 68*(4), 317–323.

Uebersax, J. S., Wyman, J. F., Shumaker, S. A., et al. (1995). Short forms to assess life quality and symptom distress for urinary incontinence in women: The Incontinence Impact Questionnaire and the Urogenital Distress Inventory. Continence Program for Women Research Group. *Neurology & Urodynamics, 14*(2), 131–139.

Wagg, A. S., Hunter, K. F., Poss, J. W., et al. (2016). From continence to incontinence in nursing home care: the influence of a dementia diagnosis. *Alzheimer's & Dementia: The Journal of the Alzheimer's Association, 12*(7), 265–266. doi:10.1016/j.jalz.2016.06.476.

Wakefield, B. J., Mentes, J., Holman, J. E., et al. (2008). Risk factors and outcomes associated with hospital admission for dehydration. *Rehabilitation Nursing Journal, 33*(6), 233–241.

Wallis, C. J., Lundeen, C., Golda, N., et al. (2016). Anticholinergics for overactive bladder: temporal trends in prescription and treatment persistence. *Canadian Urological Association Journal, 10*(7–8), 277. doi:10.5489/cuaj.3526.

Whitehead, W. E., Rao, S. S. C., Lowry, A., et al. (2014). Treatment of fecal incontinence: State of the science summary for the National Institute of Diabetes and Digestive and Kidney Diseases workshop. *American Journal of Gastroenterology, 110*(1), 138–146. doi:10.1038/ajg.2014.303.

Zarowitz, B. J., & Ouslander, J. G. (2007). The application of evidence-based principles of care in older persons (issue 6): Urinary incontinence. *Journal of the American Medical Directors Association, 8*(1), 35–45. doi:10.1016/j.jamda.2006.09.011.

Upon completion of this chapter, the reader will be able to:

- Identify age-related changes that affect rest, sleep, and activity.
- Discuss the importance of sleep and activity to the health and well-being of older persons.
- Describe nursing assessment relevant to rest, sleep, and activity.
- Explain nursing interventions useful in the promotion of rest, sleep, and activity.

🔆 **GLOSSARY**

Circadian rhythm   The regular recurrence of certain phenomena in cycles of approximately 24 hours.

Insomnia   Disturbed sleep pattern (difficulty falling asleep, staying asleep, or feeling restored following sleep) in the presence of adequate opportunity and circumstances for sleep.

Nocturia   Excessive urination at night.

Non–rapid eye movement sleep   The first four stages of sleep.

Obstructive sleep apnea   Repetitive cessation (>10 seconds) of respiration during sleep.

Rapid eye movement sleep   Wakeful and active form of sleep, during which dreaming occurs or tension is discharged.

🔆 **THE LIVED EXPERIENCE**

You know, I never get a decent night's sleep. I wake up at least four times every night, and I just know I won't get back to sleep. I really don't want to keep taking pills for sleep, but when I lie there awake, I just think of all the difficult times and situations I can't manage. After a while, I'm really in a stew about everything.

   Richard, a 67-year-old recent retiree

This is really beginning to tire me out. Richard keeps waking me at night because he can't sleep. I try to tell him to get up and read or something. I really need my sleep if I'm going to get to work on time. I wonder if Richard needs to see a doctor. Maybe he is depressed about being retired and alone while I'm at work. I'll talk to him about it.

   Clara, Richard's wife

Rest, sleep, and activity depend on one another. Inadequacy of rest and sleep affects any activity, be it an activity requiring strenuous exertion or an activity of daily living. Activity, in turn, is necessary to maintain physical and physiological integrity (such as that of cardiopulmonary endurance and function and that of musculo-skeletal strength, agility, and structure), and it helps people obtain adequate sleep. Rest, sleep, and activity contribute greatly to overall physical and mental well-being.

REST AND SLEEP

The human organism needs rest and sleep to conserve energy, prevent fatigue, provide organ respite, and relieve tension. Rest occurs with sleep in sustained unbroken periods, whereas sleep is an extension of rest. Both are physiological and mental necessities for the preservation of life. Our lives proceed in a series of rhythms that influence and regulate physiological function, chemical concentrations, performance, behavioural responses, moods, and the ability to adapt.

Gerontologists are now studying the relevance of age-related changes in **circadian rhythm** to health, illness, and the process of aging. It is clear that body temperature, pulse, blood pressure, neurotransmitter excretion, and hormonal levels change significantly and predictably in a circadian rhythm. With aging, there is a reduction in the amplitude of all these circadian endogenous responses. The most important and obvious biorhythm is the circadian sleep–wake rhythm. Abnormalities of this endogenous cycle may be responsible for some of the sleep difficulties of old age. Complaints of sleep difficulty are common, since aging is associated with changes in the amount of sleep, sleep quality, and specific sleep disorders, such as **insomnia,** sleep apnea, restless legs syndrome, and circadian rhythm disturbances (Merilahti et al, 2016; Fernandes-Barbosa et al., 2016).

The predictable pattern of normal sleep is called *sleep architecture* (Garcia-Molina et al., 2016). The body progresses through five stages of the normal sleep pattern, which consists of **rapid eye movement (REM) sleep** and **non–rapid eye movement (NREM) sleep** (Box 10.1). The amount of deep sleep (stages 3 and 4) contributes to how rested and refreshed a person feels the next day. Sleep architecture changes in aging; less time is spent in stages 3 and 4, and more time is spent in stage 1. These declines start between 20 and 30 years of age, going against the stereotype that sleep disturbances occur only in older persons. Time spent in REM sleep also declines with age, and transitions between stages 1 and 2 are more common.

As a result, older persons' sleep is lighter, more fragmented, and characterized by frequent awakenings (Merilahti et al., 2016). Older people report more time in bed, reduced total sleep time, prolonged sleep latency (i.e., the amount of time it takes to fall asleep), more frequent awakenings, increased wakefulness after the onset of sleep, and increased frequency of daytime naps (Cefalu, 2004) (Box 10.2). Sleep deprivation and fragmentation of sleep in older persons may promote the experience of pain and adversely affect cognitive functioning, respiratory function, and general health status (Nowakowski & Ancoli-Israel, 2011). These concerns are greater when older persons are in hospital or reside in long-term care (LTC) homes (FitzGerald et al., 2017; Merilahti et al., 2016).

BOX 10.1   Sleep Structure

Four Stages of Non–Rapid Eye Movement Sleep

Stage 1
Lightest level
Between being awake and falling asleep
Light sleep

Stage 2
Onset of sleep
Disengagement from surroundings
Regular breathing and heart rate
Lowering of body temperature

Stages 3 and 4
Sleep is at deepest and most restorative level.
Blood pressure drops.
Breathing becomes slower.
Muscles are relaxed.
Blood supply to muscles increases.
Tissue growth and repair occurs.
Energy is restored.
Hormones (such as growth hormone, essential for growth and development [including muscle development]) are released.

Rapid Eye Movement Sleep
Takes up 25% of sleep
First occurs about 90 minutes after falling asleep.
Recurs about every 90 minutes, getting longer throughout the night.
Provides energy to brain and body.
Supports daytime performance.
Brain is active and dreams occur.
Eyes dart back and forth.
Muscles relax and body becomes immobile

Source: Adapted from National Sleep Foundation. (2017). *What happens when you sleep?* Retrieved from https://sleepfoundation.org/how-sleep-works/what-happens-when-you-sleep.

BOX 10.2   Age-Related Sleep Changes

- More time is spent in bed awake before falling asleep.
- Total sleep time and sleep efficiency are reduced.
- Awakenings are frequent, increasing after age 50 years (>30 minutes of wakefulness after sleep onset)
- Person naps in the daytime.
- Circadian rhythm changes
- Sleep is subjectively and objectively lighter (i.e., more stage 1, less stage 4, more disruption).
- Rapid eye movement sleep is shorter and less intense.
- Frequency of abnormal breathing events increases.
- Frequency of leg movements during sleep increases.

Source: Adapted from Subramanian, S., & Surani, S. (2007). Sleep disorders in the elderly. *Geriatrics, 62*(12), 10–32.

BOX 10.3   Factors Contributing to Sleep Problems in Older Adults

- Age-related changes in sleep architecture
- Comorbidities (cardiovascular disease, diabetes, pulmonary disease, musculo-skeletal disorders), CNS disorders (Parkinson's disease, seizure disorder, dementia), GI disorders (hiatal hernia, GERD, PUD), urinary disorders (incontinence, BPH)
- Depression, anxiety, delirium, psychosis
- Medications
- Life stressors
- Limited exposure to sunlight
- Environmental noises, health care organizational routines
- Poor sleep hygiene
- Lack of exercise
- Excessive napping
- Caregiving for a dependent person
- Sleep apnea
- Restless legs syndrome
- Periodic leg movement
- REM sleep behaviour disorder
- Alcohol consumption
- Smoking

BPH, benign prostatic hyperplasia; CNS, central nervous system; GERD, gastro-esophageal reflux disease; GI, gastro-intestinal; PUD, peptic ulcer disease; REM, rapid eye movement.
Source: Adapted from Subramanian, S., & Surani, S. (2007). Sleep disorders in the elderly. *Geriatrics, 62*(12), 10–32.

Older people may not be exposed to adequate amounts of bright outdoor light, particularly in certain climates or in LTC homes. Bright-light therapy (exposure to bright outdoor light or to an indoor light box later in the afternoon) may assist in resetting the circadian rhythm (van Maanen et al., 2016).

Older persons who are in good general health, have positive moods, and engage in active lifestyles and meaningful activities report better sleep and express fewer sleep complaints. Poor sleep is not an inevitable consequence of aging; poor sleep is an indicator of health status and calls for further investigation.

SLEEP DISORDERS

Sleep disorders include insomnia, sleep apnea, restless legs syndrome, and rapid eye movement sleep behaviour disorder.

Insomnia

Insomnia is a subjective perception of insufficient or nonrestorative sleep (Subramanian & Surani, 2007; Araújo et al., 2017). Insomnia can be classified as sleep-onset insomnia, sleep-maintenance insomnia, or nonrestorative sleep (awakening without feeling refreshed or rested). Insomnia has a high prevalence in older persons and results from numerous factors (Box 10.3).

Comorbid medical and psychiatric conditions contribute to insomnia in older persons. The most common reason for interrupted sleep is **nocturia** (Vaughan et al., 2016). Gastro-esophageal reflux disease (GERD) is also a common cause of sleeplessness. During REM sleep, more acid is produced. Because the esophageal sphincter at the gastric inlet is more relaxed in older persons, acid refluxes into the esophagus, which does not have the same protective lining as the stomach has. Over time, the lining of the esophagus becomes scarred, and protective secretions emerge into the back of the throat, resulting in frequent coughing during sleep. Treatment includes elevating the head of the bed (not just the mattress) 18–20 cm (7–8 inches) so that gravity keeps the secretions in the lower part of the esophagus. Other treatments for GERD include the use of proton pump inhibitor (PPI) medications and education on the avoidance of caffeine and alcohol. Although PPI therapy is highly effective for the treatment of GERD, its long-term use has been associated with an increased risk of hip fractures (Yang et al., 2006).

Sleep problems among older persons with dementia can include sleeping too much or too little, wandering during the night, or rising earlier than usual (Lo et al., 2016). Subramanian and Surani reported that "Disturbances in rest–activity rhythm where nighttime sleep is severely fragmented and daytime activity is disrupted by multiple napping episodes are prominent and disabling symptoms in Alzheimer's disease" (Subramanian & Surani, 2007, p. 16). Anxiety and depression also contribute to insomnia (see Chapter 24). There is some evidence that nonpharmacological complementary therapies (such as light therapy) and daytime activities help people with dementia sleep better, and bedtime music and reduced ambient noise at night may also be helpful for those with dementia (Brown et al., 2013).

The side effects of many common medications used by older people could also include sleep disturbances and insomnia (Box 10.4). A medication review is always indicated when sleep complaints are investigated.

Sleep Apnea

Sleep apnea is a condition in which people stop breathing while asleep. Apnea (complete cessation of respiration) and hypopnea (partial decrease in respiration) result in hypoxemia and changes in autonomic nervous system activity. The result is increased systemic and pulmonary arterial pressure and changes in cerebral blood flow. The episodes are generally terminated by an arousal (a brief awakening), which results in fragmented sleep and excessive daytime sleepiness. Other symptoms of sleep apnea include loud periodic snoring, gasping and choking on awakening, unusual nighttime activity (such as sitting upright or falling out of bed), morning headache, poor memory and intellectual functioning, and irritability and personality change. If the person has a sleeping partner, it is often the partner who reports the nighttime symptoms.

The two types of sleep apnea are **obstructive sleep apnea** and *central sleep apnea*. Obstructive sleep apnea (OSA), caused by obstruction of the upper airway, is the most common; central sleep apnea (CSA) is due to central nervous system or cardiac dysfunction. Sleep apnea affects an estimated 5% of older men and women in Canada (Statistics Canada, 2010).

BOX 10.4 Medications That Can Cause Insomnia

Antidepressants
- Selective serotonin reuptake inhibitors
- Monoamine oxidase inhibitors
- Bupropion
- Venlafaxine

Antihypertensives
- Clonidine beta-blockers (propranolol, atenolol)
- Methyldopa
- Reserpine

Anticholinergics
- Ipratropium (Atrovent)

Antineoplastics
- Medroxyprogesterone
- Interferon
- Leuprolide

Sympathomimetic Amines
- Bronchodilators
- Xanthine derivatives (theophylline)
- Decongestants (pseudoephedrine, phenylpropanolamine)

Hormones
- Thyroid preparations
- Cortisone
- Progesterone

Psychotropics
- Phenytoin
- Topiramate
- Levodopa

Miscellaneous
- Alcohol
- Nicotine
- Opiates
- Quinidine
- Cough and cold medications
- Anacin
- Diuretics (If used late in the day, they cause nocturia, waking the person.)

Source: Adapted from Zee, P., & Bloom, H. (2006). Understanding and resolving insomnia in the elderly. *Geriatrics* (Suppl May), 1–12.

In LTC homes, the prevalence of OSA has been estimated to be as high as 70 to 80% (Rose et al., 2010). The age-related decline in the activity of the upper-airway muscles, which results in compromised pharyngeal patency, predisposes older persons to

BOX 10.6   Sleep Diary

Instructions: Record the following for 2 to 4 weeks:
1. The number of times a call for assistance is made (e.g., concerning the bathroom, pain medication, and subjective symptoms of inability to sleep)
2. Whether the person appears to be asleep or awake when checked during the night
3. Time and dosage of sleep medication
4. Time the person awakens in the morning
5. Where the person falls asleep in the evening
6. Duration of daytime naps

BOX 10.7   Sleep Hygiene Rules

1. Limit daytime naps to 30 minutes.
2. Avoid stimulants (caffeine and nicotine) before sleeping.
3. Daily exercise.
4. Avoid consuming spicy foods, fried meals, and carbonated drinks before bedtime.
5. Ensure adequate exposure to natural light during the day and darkness at night, as this will help maintain a healthy sleep-wake cycle.
6. Establish a regular bedtime routine, including relaxation techniques such as having a warm bath, reading a book, or doing light stretches.
7. Ensure the sleep environment is pleasant; for optimal sleep, have the bedroom at a cool temperature (between 15.5° to 19.4° Celsius); turn off TVs, and avoid light from computer and cell phone screens.

Source: Adapted from National Sleep Foundation. (2017). How can I improve my sleep hygiene? Retrieved from https://sleepfoundation.org/sleep-topics/sleep-hygiene.

BOX 10.8   Nonpharmacological Therapies for Sleep Disorders

Behavioural Therapy
Behavioural therapy is stimulus control therapy. The bedroom should be used only for sleep and for sexual activity. The goal is to strengthen the person's emotional perception of the bedroom as a place for sleeping instead of a place for experiencing insomnia.

Relaxation Techniques
Relaxation techniques include progressive relaxation exercises, guided imagery, meditation, and electromyographic biofeedback. The goal is to minimize the physical and emotional stressors that affect sleep.

Temporal Control Therapy
The goal is to promote the consistency of the sleep-wake cycle by maintaining a set time to go to bed and get up, regardless of the quality and quantity of sleep. Daytime napping is to be avoided.

Sleep Restriction Therapy
Time spent in bed should be limited to actual sleeping. Mild sleep deprivation is allowed to develop, which is expected to enhance the ability to sleep.

Exercise
Regular exercise during the day enhances the ability to sleep. Exercise is to be avoided in the 4 hours before bedtime.

Light Therapy
Light therapy consists of exposure to natural light, the use of a light box, and the elimination of nighttime light (especially in health care settings).

Source: Chaperon, C., Farr, L., & LoChiano, E. (2007). Sleep disturbance of residents in a continuing care retirement community. Journal of Gerontological Nursing, 33(10), 21–28; Zee, P., & Bloom, H. (2006). Understanding and resolving insomnia in the elderly. Geriatrics (Suppl May), 1–12.

therapy, and relaxation therapy are all effective and produce sustained positive effects. These behavioural treatments have been reported to be effective and practical treatments for chronic insomnia in older persons (Buysse et al., 2011). Tai chi also improves an older person's sleep quality (Nguyen & Kruse, 2012). Box 10.8 presents other nonpharmacological therapies for sleep disorders.

In all health care settings, the promotion of a good sleep environment is important. A sleep improvement protocol (including do-not-disturb periods; provision of usual bedtime routines; and soft music, relaxation techniques, massage, and aromatherapy) may improve sleep. An interprofessional approach to identifying sources of noise and light, such as equipment and staff interactions, can result in modification without compromising the patient's safety and quality of care (Missildine, 2008). Because a full sleep cycle of 90 minutes can have a positive influence on sleep effectiveness, any effort to allow sufficient time for a full sleep cycle is important (Missildine et al., 2010). Box 10.9 provides suggestions for promoting sleep for older persons who live in LTC homes.

Aromatherapy, such as the use of essential oils, has been mentioned as beneficial in sleep promotion

BOX 10.9 Suggestions for Promoting Sleep in Long-Term Care Homes

- Limit the resident's intake of caffeine before bedtime.
- Provide a light snack or warm beverage before bedtime.
- Maintain a quiet environment: soft lights, quiet music, and limited noise and staff intrusions.
- Reduce interruptions for medication administration by modifying the dosing schedule.
- Discontinue invasive treatments (e.g., use of Foley catheters, percutaneous gastrostomy tubes, or intravenous lines) when possible.
- Encourage the resident to go the bathroom before bedtime, and assist the resident when help is needed.
- Give pain medication before bedtime for residents with pain.
- Provide regular exercise or walking programs during the day.
- Encourage the resident to stay out of bed and out of the bedroom for as long as possible before bedtime.
- Maintain a sleep schedule based on the resident's needs and wishes.
- Encourage the resident to rise and get out of bed every morning at a regular time.
- Maintain a comfortable temperature in room; provide blankets as needed.
- Provide meaningful activities during the daytime.

Source: Adapted from Cefalu, C. (2004). Evaluation and management of insomnia in the institutionalized elderly. *Annals of Long-Term Care, 12*(6), 25.

(Forrester et al., 2014). Outdoor physical activities for LTC residents can promote well-being, activity, and sleep. An example of such an activity program for older persons is that offered at Oliver Woods Wellness Park in British Columbia.

Pharmacological Interventions

Medications may be used in combination with behavioural interventions, but they must be chosen carefully, started at the lowest possible dosage, and monitored closely to avoid untoward effects in older persons. Older persons should be educated on the proper use of medications and on their side effects. Sedatives and hypnotics, including benzodiazepines and barbiturates, should be avoided. Over-the-counter medications such as diphenhydramine (Benadryl) and Tylenol PM (containing diphenhydramine), often thought to be relatively harmless, should be avoided

because of their antihistaminic and anticholinergic side effects.

Benzodiazepine receptor agonists (such as zolpidem, eszopiclone, and zaleplon) have shorter half-lives for older persons than other insomnia prescription medications (Subramanian & Surani, 2007). However, they also have undesirable effects and a narrow safety margin and should be used in the short term only. Because of the rapid action of these medications, they should be taken immediately before bedtime. Recent research reported that hospitalized patients who took zolpidem had a fall rate that was more than four times higher than those of patients who did not take that medication. Precautions against falls should be taken for people who take sleeping medications (Kolla et al., 2012). Ramelteon, a melatonin receptor agonist that promotes sleep via action on the circadian system, can be used for individuals who have difficulty falling asleep.

ACTIVITY

Activity is a direct use of energy—in voluntary, involuntary, physical, and mental ways—that alters a person's micro- and macroenvironment. Few factors contribute as much to health in aging as physical activity. One of the goals of promoting healthy aging is having more people participate in regular physical activity to improve functional fitness and overall physical and mental health (Canadian Society for Exercise Physiology [CSEP], 2011). Regular physical activity throughout life is likely to enhance health and functional status as a person ages. It also decreases the number of persistent or chronic illnesses and the mobility and functional limitations that are often assumed to be part of aging.

Physical activity is important for all older people, not just those who are active and healthy. Studies have found that increasing physical activity improves health outcomes for persons with persistent illnesses (regardless of severity) and for those with functional impairment (Bauman et al., 2016). The benefit of exercise for frail LTC residents diagnosed with illnesses ranging from arthritis to lung disease and dementia has also been shown (Gallaway et al., 2017).

Despite a large body of evidence about the importance of physical activity for maintaining and improving function, it was found that only 13% of older persons were accumulating at least 150 minutes per week of moderate to vigorous physical activity, as per public health guidelines (Schmidt et al., 2016). The levels of physical activity among older persons in Canada have not improved significantly over the past 5 years (Statistics Canada, 2016). Inactivity poses serious health hazards to young and old alike. It can lead to hypertension, coronary artery disease, osteoporosis, obesity, tension, chronic fatigue, premature aging, depression, poor musculature, inadequate flexibility, and decreased cognitive function (Pederson & Saltin, 2016). Many older people mistakenly believe that they are too old to begin an active fitness program. Even a small amount of time (e.g., 30 minutes of moderate activity several days a week) can improve health.

 IMPLICATIONS FOR GERONTOLOGICAL NURSING AND HEALTHY AGING

ASSESSMENT

Exercise counselling and an assessment of functional abilities should be part of the health assessment of all older persons. The purpose of screening is to (1) identify medical problems while allowing the individual to achieve the maximal benefit from physical activity; (2) identify functional limitations that will be addressed in the exercise program; and (3) minimize injury and other serious harmful effects. Two tools, the Exercise Assessment and Screening for You (EASY) tool (Resnick et al., 2008b) and the Physical Activity Readiness Questionnaire (PAR-Q) (http://uwfitness.uwaterloo.ca/PDF/par-q.pdf), can be used to screen older persons before the older person is started on a moderate program of physical activity. Depending on the results of the initial screening, older persons may need to be evaluated by their primary care provider. Frail or vulnerable older adults will also need close monitoring to ensure benefit without compromising safety.

INTERVENTIONS

Suggestions for exercise programs are based on the person's preference and medical history. Exercise programs should include the following components (Resnick et al., 2008a; Cadore et al., 2013):

- *Endurance exercises* are composed of continuous movement involving large muscle groups for a minimum of 10 minutes. These exercises increase breathing and heart rates and improve the health of the heart, lungs and circulatory system. Examples of endurance exercises are swimming, bicycling, brisk walking, tennis, dancing, and gardening. Endurance exercises should initially be of short duration and gradually increased.
- *Strength (resistance) exercises* build muscles and increase muscle strength by moving or lifting something that poses resistance, such as hand or ankle weights or resistance bands. The exercises should be performed at least twice a week.
- *Balance exercises* improve standing and gait and help prevent falls. Tai chi has been shown to be of benefit for older people (Box 10.10).
- *Flexibility exercises* keep the body limber and increase range of motion. These exercises should be performed at least 3 days a week. Yoga is a form of exercise that can be practised regardless of one's condition.

Nonambulatory older people can also engage in physical activity and may benefit the most from an exercise program in terms of function and quality of life. Both muscle weakness and atrophy are functionally relevant and are reversible through exercise in nonambulatory older persons (Resnick et al., 2008a). Upper-extremity cycling, marching in place, stretching, range-of-motion exercise, water-based activities, and chair yoga are examples of exercises for nonambulatory older persons. For older persons who reside in LTC homes, participation in self-care activities improves functioning and also contributes to greater staff, family, and resident satisfaction (Resnick et al., 2008b). The restorative care (Res-Care) intervention, a self-efficacy–based approach to restoring or maintaining residents' physical function, can be used as a model for restorative care in LTC homes (Resnick et al., 2008b).

The older person may be able to integrate activity into daily life rather than doing specific exercises. An example is walking to the store instead of driving there. Older persons limited to residential homes

BOX 10.10   Research for Evidence-Informed Practice: Randomized Controlled Trial of Tai Chi for Balance, Sleep Quality, and Cognitive Performance in Older Individuals

Problem: Older persons often avoid or minimize physical activity because of balance problems, muscle weakness, and impaired gait. These factors are also the most significant risk factors for falling, which leads to poor health consequences and limited mobility for older persons. This study evaluated the effects of tai chi on balance, sleep quality, and cognitive performance in community-dwelling older persons. The study included 102 participants from 60 to 79 years of age and living in a large city.

Method: Participants were divided into two groups. The intervention group performed tai chi; the non–tai chi group served as a control group. Participants in the tai chi group were assigned a 6-month tai chi training program, which included 60-minute practice sessions twice a week for 6 months. Participants in the control group were instructed to maintain their daily activities and not to start a new exercise program. Three instruments were used to collect data: The Falls Efficacy Scale, to measure fear of falling; the Pittsburgh Sleep Quality Index (PSQI), to measure the quality and pattern of sleep; and the Trail Making Test, to measure motor speed and visual attention.

Findings: The 6-month tai chi program had a positive effect on the intervention group. Sleep quality, balance, and cognitive performance all improved as measured by the PSQI. Tests of balance and cognitive performance showed that tai chi could improve the balance and cognitive function of older persons. Tai chi may be a beneficial exercise for improving sleep, cognitive performance, and balance in older persons living in the community.

Source: Nguyen, M. H., & Kruse, A. (2012). A randomized controlled trial of tai chi for balance, sleep quality and cognitive performance in elderly Vietnamese. *Clinical Interventions in Aging, 7*, 185–290. doi:10.2147/CIA.S32600.

should also be encouraged to increase their amount of walking. First they might walk only from the bed to the bathroom; with time, down the hall; and eventually around the total facility or even outside. Restorative walking programs and other exercise programs should be integral activity in all LTC homes.

When especially low-intensity exercise is needed, the person can exercise for 2 to 3 minutes, rest for 2 to 3 minutes, and continue this pattern for 15 to 20 minutes. The Public Health Agency of Canada (2003) provides an excellent resource and also offers educational materials on exercise at https://www.canada.ca/en/public-health/services/health-promotion/healthy-living/physical-activity.html.

Exercise Prescription

As noted earlier, most older persons do not exercise regularly. Motivational interventions are important when encouraging older persons to begin an exercise program, and such interventions should be continued to ensure that the person stays with the program. Emphasis on the immediate benefits of regular exercise (i.e., improvement of current health and quality of life) can be an important motivator for the patient. A list of safety tips for exercise should also be provided. Suggestions for exercise programs for older persons are presented in Box 10.11.

SUMMARY

This chapter has discussed separately the older person's need for rest and sleep and need for activity. It is apparent that each area influences the function of the other. The quality and the overall perception of life can be augmented when nurses monitor these specific functions and provide support or assistance according to the identified problems. Gerontological nurses must be knowledgeable about age-related changes in sleep and activity and about the effect of lifestyle on these changes. Many older people may have misconceptions about sleep and exercise, and the nurse can assess persons' beliefs and understanding and can provide education to enhance their optimal well-being.

The assessment of sleep, the chosen level of activity, and the design of interventions must be grounded in evidence-informed knowledge and applied to meet the needs of each person. Common practices (such as the use of hypnotics for sleep) without thorough assessment, or a person's confinement to a wheelchair because there is no one to help maintain his or her walking skills, lead to disabling and preventable problems for older people. Improvement of function is possible for even the frailest older person, and gerontological nurses must incorporate the health promotion activities discussed here into any plan of care for an older person.

BOX 10.11　Suggestions for Exercise Programs for Older Persons

- Provide appropriate screening before beginning an exercise program.
- Provide information on the benefits of exercise, emphasizing short-term benefits such as better sleep.
- Clarify the misconceptions associated with exercise (e.g., fatigue, injury).
- Assess the person for declines in function, and discuss how exercise can minimize these declines.
- Assess the person's barriers to exercise and how to overcome them.
- Provide an "exercise prescription" that specifies which exercises the person should perform and how often.
- Pursue both daily and long-term goals.
- Goals should be specific and achievable and should match the older person's perceived needs and health and cognitive abilities, as well as the person's interests.
- Allow the person to choose the types of exercise to do, and design the program so that the person can follow it at home or elsewhere when formal training ends.
- Provide self-monitoring methods to assist in visualizing progress.
- Group-based programs and exercise with a "buddy" may be more successful than exercising alone.
- Try to make the program fun and entertaining for the person (e.g., walking while listening to favourite music, socializing with friends).
- Discuss the potential side effects of exercise and any symptoms that should be reported.
- Follow up frequently on progress, and provide reinforcement.
- Begin with low-intensity physical activity for sedentary older persons.
- Initiate low-intensity activities in short sessions (less than 10 minutes), and include warm-up and cool-down periods with active stretching.
- Progress from low to moderate intensity to obtain maximum benefits, but change the level of activity gradually.
- Lifestyle activities (e.g., raking, gardening) can build endurance when performed for at least 10 minutes.

Source: Data from Cress, M., Buchner, D., Prohaska, T., et al. (2005). Best practices for physical activity programs and behavior counseling in older adult populations. *Journal of Aging & Physical Activity, 13*(1), 61–74; Schneider, J. K., Eveker, A., Bronder, D., et al. (2006). Exercise training program for older adults: Incentives and disincentives for participation. *Journal of Gerontological Nursing, 29*(9), 21–31; Struck, B., & Ross, K. (2006). Health promotion in older adults: Prescribing exercise for the frail and home bound. *Geriatrics, 61*(5), 22–27.

KEY CONCEPTS

- Rest and sleep are restorative, recuperative, and necessary for the preservation of life. Many persistent and chronic conditions can interfere with the quality and quantity of sleep.
- Complaints of sleep difficulties should be thoroughly investigated and not attributed to age. Nonpharmacological interventions should always be considered in any plan of care to improve sleep.
- Activity is an indication of an individual's health and wellness; the inability to exercise, do physical work, or perform activities of daily living is one of the first indicators of decline.
- Lack of physical activity increases the risk for many medical conditions experienced by older persons. Exercise can be done by individuals who are ambulatory, chairbound, or bedridden and should include endurance exercises, strength training, balance exercises, and flexibility exercises.
- The benefits of exercise include maintenance of functional ability, enhanced self-confidence and self-sufficiency, decreased depression, improvement in general lifestyle, maintenance of mental functional capacity, and decreased risk for medical problems.
- Exercise counselling and an exercise prescription should be taken into consideration for all older persons.

ACTIVITIES AND DISCUSSION QUESTIONS

1. Discuss the age-related changes that affect rest, sleep, and activity in older persons.
2. Describe the assessment of an older person for adequacy or inadequacy of rest, sleep, and activity.
3. Develop an exercise prescription for an older person residing in the outside community.

4. Discuss nursing interventions for promoting rest, sleep, and activity.
5. Devise a nursing care plan for an older person who has insomnia.

RESOURCES

Canadian Society for Exercise Physiology. Canada's Physical Activity Guide to Healthy Active Living
http://www.csep.ca/cmfiles/guidelines/csep_guidelines _handbook.pdf

Canadian Physical Activity Guidelines For Older Adults – 65 Years & Older
https://www.participaction.com/sites/default/files/ downloads/Participaction-Canadian-physical-activity -guidelines-older-adult.pdf

Physical Activity Readiness Questionnaire (PAR-Q)
http://www.uwfitness.uwaterloo.ca/PDF/par-q.pdf

Public Health Agency of Canada. Educational materials on exercise
https://www.canada.ca/en/public-health/services/health -promotion/healthy-living/physical-activity.html

University of Western Ontario. *BioPsychoSocial assessment tools for the elderly – Assessment summary sheet*
https://instruct.uwo.ca/kinesiology/9641/Assessments/ Biological/EASY.html

For additional resources, please visit *http:// evolve.elsevier.com/Canada/Ebersole/gerontological/*

REFERENCES

Araújo, T., Jarrin, D. C., Leanza, Y., et al. (2017). Qualitative studies of insomnia: Current state of knowledge in the field. *Sleep Medicine Reviews, 31*, 58–69. doi:10.1016/j.smrv.2016.01.003.

Aurora, N., Zak, R. S., Maganti, R. K., et al. (2010). Best practice guide for the treatment of REM sleep behavior disorder (RBD). *Journal of Clinical Sleep Medicine: JCSM: Official Publication of the American Academy of Sleep Medicine, 6*(1), 85–95.

Bauman, A., Merom, D., Bull, F. C., et al. (2016). Updating the evidence for physical activity: Summative reviews of the epidemiological evidence, prevalence, and interventions to promote "Active Aging." *The Gerontologist, 56*(Suppl. 2), S268–S280. doi:10.1093/geront/gnw031.

Bloom, H. G., Ahmed, I., Alessi, C. A., et al. (2009). Evidence-based recommendations for the assessment and management of sleep disorders in older persons. *Journal of the American Geriatric Society, 57*(7), 761–789. doi:10.1111/j.1532-5415.2009.02220.x.

Brooks, P., & Peever, J. (2008). Glycinergic and GABAA–mediated inhibition of somatic motor neurons does not mediate rapid eye movement sleep motor atonia. *The Journal of Neuroscience: The Official Journal of the Society for Neuroscience, 28*(14), 3535–3545. doi:10.1523/JNEUROSCI.5023-07.2008.

Brown, C., Berry, R., Tan, M., et al. (2013). A critique of the evidence base for non-pharmacological sleep interventions for persons with dementia. *Dementia (Basel, Switzerland), 12*(2), 210–237. doi:10.1177/1471301211426909.

Buysse, D., Germain, A., Moul, D. E., et al. (2011). Efficacy of brief behavioral treatment for chronic insomnia in older adults. *Archives of Internal Medicine, 171*(10), 887–895. doi:10.1001/archinternmed.2010.535.

Cadore, E. L., Rodríguez-Mañas, L., Sinclair, A., et al. (2013). Effects of different exercise interventions on risk of falls, gait ability, and balance in physically frail older adults: a systematic review. *Rejuvenation Research, 16*(2), 105–114. doi:10.1089/rej.2012.1397.

Canadian Society for Exercise Physiology (CSEP). (2011). *Canadian physical activity guidelines for older adults (65 years and older)*. Retrieved from http://www.csep.ca/home.

Cefalu, C. (2004). Evaluation and management of insomnia in the institutionalized elderly. *Annals of Long-Term Care, 12*(6), 25–32.

Chaperon, C., Farr, L., & LoChiano, E. (2007). Sleep disturbance of residents in a continuing care retirement community. *Journal of Gerontological Nursing, 33*(10), 21–28.

Dugger, B. N., Boeve, B. F., Murray, M. E., et al. (2012). Rapid eye movement sleep behavior disorder and subtypes in autopsy-confirmed dementia with Lewy bodies. *Movement Disorders: Official Journal of the Movement Disorder Society, 27*(1), 72–78. doi:10.1002/mds.24003.

Fernandes Barbosa, K. T., de Oliveira, R. L., Maria, F., et al. (2016). Sleep quality in elderly patients in outpatient care. *Journal of Nursing UFPE/Revista de Enfermagem UFPE, Feb*(Suppl. 2), 756–761. doi:10.5205/reuol.6884-59404-2-SM-1.1002sup201609.

FitzGerald, J. M., O'Regan, N., Adamis, D., et al. (2017). Sleep-wake cycle disturbances in elderly acute general medical inpatients: Longitudinal relationship to delirium and dementia. *Alzheimer's & Dementia: Diagnosis, Assessment & Disease Monitoring, 7*, 61–68. doi:10.1016/j.dadm.2016.12.013.

Forrester, L. T., Maayan, N., Orrell, M., et al. (2014). Aromatherapy for dementia. *The Cochrane Database of Systematic Reviews, (2)*, CD003150. doi:10.1002/14651858.CD003150.pub2.

Gallaway, P. J., Miyake, H., Buchowski, M. S., et al. (2017). Physical activity: A viable way to reduce the risks of mild cognitive impairment, Alzheimer's Disease, and vascular dementia in older adults. *Brain Sciences, 7*(2), 22. doi:10.3390/brainsci7020022.

Garcia-Molina, G., Vissapragada, S., Mahadevan, A., et al. (2016). Probabilistic characterization of sleep architecture: Home Based study on healthy volunteers. *Engineering in Medicine and Biology Society (EMBC), 2016 IEEE 38th Annual International Conference of the IEEE, 2834–2838.* doi:10.1109/EMBC.2016.7591320.

Kerr, D., & Wilkinson, H. (2010). *Providing good care at night for older people: practical approaches for use in nursing and care homes.* London, UK: Jessica Kingsley Publishers.

Kolla, B. P., Lovely, J. K., Mansukhani, M. P., et al. (2012). Zolpidem is independently associated with increased risk of inpatient falls. *Journal of Hospital Medicine, 8*(1), 1–6. doi:10.1002/jhm.1985.

Lo, J. C., Groeger, J. A., Cheng, G. H., et al. (2016). Self-reported sleep duration and cognitive performance in older adults: A systematic review and meta-analysis. *Sleep Medicine, 17,* 87–98. doi:10.1016/j.sleep.2015.08.021.

Merilahti, J., Viramo, P., & Korhonen, I. (2016). Wearable monitoring of physical functioning and disability changes, circadian rhythms and sleep patterns in nursing home residents. *IEEE Journal of Biomedical and Health Informatics, 20*(3), 856–864. doi:10.1109/JBHI.2015.2420680.

Missildine, K. (2008). Sleep and the sleep environment of older adults in acute care settings. *Journal of Gerontological Nursing, 34*(6), 15–21. doi:10.3928/00989134-20080601-06.

Missildine, K., Bergstrom, N., Meininger, J., et al. (2010). Sleep in hospitalized elders: a pilot study. *Geriatric Nursing, 31*(4), 263–271. doi:10.1016/j.gerinurse.2010.02.013.

Nguyen, M. H., & Kruse, A. (2012). A randomized controlled trial of Tai chi for balance, sleep quality and cognitive performance in elderly Vietnamese. *Clinical Interventions in Aging, 7,* 185–190. doi:10.2147/CIA.S32600.

Nowakowski, S., & Ancoli-Israel, S. (2011). Acute and emergent events in the sleep of older adults. *Acute and emergent events in sleep disorders,* 247-263.

Ohayon, M. M., O'Hara, R., & Vitiello, M. V. (2012). Epidemiology of restless legs syndrome: A synthesis of the literature. *Sleep Medicine Review, 16*(4), 283–295. doi:10.1016/j.smrv.2011.05.002.

Pederson, B. K., & Saltin, B. (2016). Exercise as medicine – evidence for prescribing exercise as therapy in 26 different chronic diseases. *Scandinavian Journal of Medicine and Science in Sports, 25*(S3), 1–72. doi:10.1111/sms.12581.

Public Health Agency of Canada. (2003). *Physical activity guide for older adults.* Retrieved from https://www.canada.ca/en/public-health/services/health-promotion/healthy-living/physical-activity.html.

Rajki, M. (2012). *Sleep problems in older adults.* Retrieved from http://occupational-therapy.advanceweb.com/Features/Articles/Sleep-Problems-in-Older-Adults.aspx.

Resnick, B., Petzer-Aboff, I., Galik, G., et al. (2008a). Barriers and benefits to implementing a restorative care intervention in nursing homes. *Journal of the American Medical Directors Association, 9*(2), 102–108. doi:10.1016/j.jamda.2007.08.011.

Resnick, B., Ory, M., Hora, K., et al. (2008b). The Exercise Assessment and Screening for You (EASY) tool: Application in the oldest old population. *American Journal of Lifestyle Medicine, 2*(5).

Rose, K. M., Fagin, C. M., & Lorenz, R. (2010). Sleep disturbances in dementia: what they are and what to do. *Journal of Gerontological Nursing, 36*(5), 9–14. doi:10.3928/00989134-20100330-05.

Schmidt, L., Rempel, G., Murray, T. C., et al. (2016). Exploring beliefs around physical activity among older adults in rural Canada. *International Journal of Qualitative Studies in Health & Well-Being, 11,* doi:10.3402/qhw.v11.32914.

Statistics Canada. (2010). *What is the impact of sleep apnea on Canadians?* Retrieved from https://www.canada.ca/en/public-health/services/chronic-diseases/sleep-apnea/what-impact-sleep-apnea-on-canadians.html.

Statistics Canada. (2016). *Physical activity during leisure time, by age group and sex (Number of persons).* Retrieved from http://www.statcan.gc.ca/tables-tableaux/sum-som/l01/cst01/health77a-eng.htm.

Subramanian, S., & Surani, S. (2007). Sleep disorders in the elderly. *Geriatrics, 62*(12), 10–32. Retrieved from https://www.ncbi.nlm.nih.gov/pubmed/18069880.

van Maanen, A., Meijer, A. M., van der Heijden, K. B., et al. (2016). The effects of light therapy on sleep problems: A systematic review and meta-analysis. *Sleep Medicine Reviews, 29,* 52–62. doi:10.1016/j.smrv.2015.08.009.

Vaughan, C. P., Fung, C. H., Huang, A. J., et al. (2016). Differences in the association of nocturia and functional outcomes of sleep by age and gender: A cross-sectional, population-based study. *Clinical Therapeutics, 38*(11), 2386–2393. doi:10.1016/j.clinthera.2016.09.009.

Winkelman, J., Allen, R., Tenzer, P., et al. (2007). Restless legs syndrome: Nonpharmacologic and pharmacologic treatments. *Geriatrics, 62*(10), 13–16. doi:10.1001/archneur.56.12.1526.

Yang, Y. X., Lewis, J. D., Epstein, S., et al. (2006). Long-term proton pump inhibitor therapy and risk of hip fracture. *JAMA: The Journal of the American Medical Association, 296*(24), 2947–2953. Retrieved from http://jamanetwork.com/journals/jama/fullarticle/204783.

Zee, P. C., & Bloom, H. G. (2006). Understanding and resolving insomnia in the elderly. *Geriatrics* (May 2006). Retrieved from https://www.researchgate.net/publication/265198932_Understanding_and_Resolving_Insomnia_in_the_Elderly.

LEARNING OBJECTIVES

Upon completion of this chapter, the reader will be able to:

- Identify normal age-related changes of the integument and feet.
- Identify skin and foot problems commonly found in later life.
- Use standardized tools to assess the skin and feet of older persons.
- Identify preventive, maintenance, and restorative measures for skin and foot health.

GLOSSARY

Debride   To remove dead or infected tissue, usually from a wound.

Emollient   A medication that softens and smoothes the skin.

Eschar   Black, dry, dead tissue.

Hyperemia   Redness caused by increased blood flow, such as in an area of infection.

Maceration   Tissue that is overhydrated and subject to breakdown.

Slough   Dead tissue that has become wet, appearing as yellow to white and fibrous.

Tissue tolerance   The amount of pressure a tissue (i.e., skin) can endure before it breaks down, as in a pressure injury.

Xerosis   Very dry skin.

THE LIVED EXPERIENCE

I can't thank you enough for helping me with my feet. I have been to the podiatrist, but no one has made them, and me, feel so good. I feel like I can walk forever now.

   Tom, age 86 years

Gerontological nurses have an instrumental role in promoting the health of the skin and the feet of the persons who seek their care. These areas of function may often be overlooked when the focus is on management of disease or acute problems. However, preservation of the integrity of the skin and the functioning of the feet is essential to well-being. To promote healthy aging, the nurse needs information about common problems encountered by the older person and skill in developing effective interventions for both acute and chronic conditions.

INTEGUMENT

Integument is defined as the natural covering of an organism or organ. The skin, an example of integument, is the largest organ of the body and has several physiological functions, including maintaining a

BOX 11.1   Physiological Functions of the Skin

- Protects underlying structures
- Regulates body temperature
- Serves as a vehicle for sensation
- Stores fat
- Is a component of the metabolism of salt and water
- Is a site for two-way gas exchange
- Is the site for the production of vitamin D, when exposed to sunlight

homeostatic environment and protecting the body from exposure to heat, cold, water, trauma, friction, and pressure (Box 11.1). Healthy skin is durable, pliable, and strong enough to protect the body by absorbing, reflecting, cushioning, and restricting various substances and forces that might enter and alter its function, yet it is sensitive enough to relay subtle messages to the brain. When the integument malfunctions or is overwhelmed, discomfort, disfigurement, or death may ensue. Nurses can recognize and prevent many of the sources of danger to an older person's skin in the promotion of the best possible health.

Many skin problems are seen as people age, both when people are in health and when they are compromised by illness or limited mobility. Skin problems seen in older persons are influenced by the environment and by age-related changes (see Chapter 6). The most common skin problems for older persons are xerosis, pruritus, seborrheic keratosis, herpes zoster, and cancer. People who are immobilized or medically fragile, such as residents in long-term care (LTC) or residential homes, are at a higher risk for fungal infections and pressure injuries, both major threats to wellness.

COMMON SKIN PROBLEMS

Xerosis

Xerosis is extremely dry, cracked, and itchy skin. Xerosis is the most common skin problem experienced by older people. The thinner epidermis of older skin makes it less efficient, thus allowing more moisture to escape. Inadequate fluid intake worsens xerosis, as the body will pull moisture from the skin in an attempt to combat systemic dehydration. Xerosis

occurs primarily in the extremities, especially the legs, but can affect the face and trunk as well.

Exposure to environmental elements such as artificial heat, decreased humidity, harsh soaps, and frequent hot baths or hot tub use, contributes to skin dryness. Nutritional deficiencies and smoking can also lead to dehydration of the outer layer of the epidermis.

Hospitals and LTC homes accelerate the development of xerosis in older persons through routine baths, the use of drying soap, prolonged bed rest, and the action of bed linen on the person's skin (LeBlanc et al., 2016). For persons with incontinence, the skin must be protected from both the burning of urine or feces and from the excess dryness that arises from the frequent washing and drying.

Pruritus

One of the consequences of xerosis is *pruritus*, that is, itchy skin. It is a symptom, not a diagnosis or disease, and is a threat to skin integrity because of the person's attempts to relieve it by scratching. Pruritus is aggravated by perfumed detergents, fabric softeners, heat, sudden temperature changes, pressure, vibration, electrical stimuli, sweating, restrictive clothing, fatigue, exercise, and anxiety. If rehydration of the stratum corneum is not sufficient to control itching, cool compresses or oatmeal or Epsom salt baths may be helpful. Failure to control the itching increases the risk for eczema, excoriations, cracks in the skin, inflammation, and infection. Pruritus also may accompany systemic disorders such as chronic renal failure, biliary or hepatic disease, and iron deficiency anemia. The nurse should be alert for signs of infection.

Herpes Zoster

Herpes zoster (HZ), or shingles, is a viral infection frequently seen in older persons. Immunosuppressed older people and those with a history of chicken pox are at greatest risk for the reactivation of dormant varicella-zoster virus within the sensory ganglia. However, HZ can occur in healthy people as well. It always occurs along a nerve pathway, or *dermatome*. The more dermatomes involved, the more serious the infection, especially if it involves the head. Involvement with the eye is always a medical emergency, owing to the possibility of scarring and blindness (Public Health Agency of Canada [PHAC], 2013). In most cases, the severity of the infection increases with age.

The onset of HZ may be preceded by chills, fever, gastro-intestinal disturbance, malaise, and pain or paresthesias. Before diagnosis, the person may complain of pain, tingling, and a painful rash (PHAC, 2013). The area where the eruption *will* occur is burning, painful, or tender, and this is often a predictive sign.

During the healing process, clusters of papulovesicles develop along a nerve pathway. The lesions themselves eventually rupture, crust over, and resolve. Scarring may result, especially if scratching or poor hygiene leads to a secondary bacterial infection. Shingles is infectious until it becomes crusty. The condition may be very painful and pruritic, and as many as 20% of older persons may have postherpetic neuralgia (PHN) lasting weeks or months after the acute infection resolves. The pain of PHN is difficult to control and can significantly affect the person's quality of life (see Chapter 16). As of January 2017, shingles vaccinations in Ontario are free for adults aged 65 to 70 years (Government of Ontario, 2016).

IMPLICATIONS FOR GERONTOLOGICAL NURSING AND HEALTHY AGING

Gerontological nurses are in a perfect position to promote healthy skin in older persons. In embracing this position, they can significantly improve older persons' quality of life and comfort.

XEROSIS

Because age-related changes are one of the major causes of xerosis, nurses need to pay attention to the environment and provide preventative treatment to maintain healthy skin. Maintaining the environment's humidity at about 60% is a start. The challenge is to find ways to rehydrate the epidermis (Box 11.2).

Skin can be hydrated only with water. Topical skin products can help retain natural moisture in the skin. Most lubricants such as creams, lotions, and **emollients** work by trapping moisture and are most effective when applied to towel-patted, damp skin

---

> **BOX 11.2 Tips to Older Persons for Maintaining Healthy Skin**
>
> - Watch for any break in the skin, and initiate treatment as soon as possible.
> - Use a humidifier to keep the room humid.
> - Use only tepid water for bathing, and limit time in the water.
> - Use only mild skin cleansers without perfume or lanolin.
> - Pat dry; do not rub.
> - Do not add bath oil to water, to minimize risk of slipping.
> - Apply moisturizers as often as necessary to maintain continuous coverage.
> - Choose clothing made of soft cotton or other nonabrasive materials.
> - Maintain systemic hydration (a balance between fluid intake and hydration status).
> - Protect skin from exposure to cold temperatures.

---

immediately after a bath. Bath oils and other hydrophobic preparations may also be used to hold in moisture. Oils can be directly applied to moist skin; water-laden emulsions without perfumes or alcohol are best.

To prevent excessive loss of moisture and natural oil during bathing, only tepid water temperatures and superfatted soaps or skin cleansers without hexachlorophene or alcohol should be used. Soap products such as Cetaphil, Dove, Tone, and Caress soaps, or bath washes such as Jergens, Neutrogena, or Oil of Olay, help prevent the loss of the protective lipid film from the skin surface. The use of deodorant soaps and detergents containing alcohol as a drying agent should be avoided, except in the axilla and groin.

In cases of extreme dryness, petroleum jelly can be applied to the affected areas before bed, and the skin will be smoother and have more moisture in the morning. Oils and ointments with zinc oxide are designed to coat the skin and replace the skin's natural oil barrier. These products are often used to prevent excoriations from feces or urine; however, they can be applied only to skin that is clean and intact.

Pruritus

When xerosis leads to pruritus, the goal of treatment is to reduce and alleviate the itching. If rehydration of the epidermis is not sufficient to control itching, then cool compresses or baths with oatmeal or Epsom salts may be helpful. Nurses should educate patients on the importance of hydration and skin protection to prevent scratching. Failure to control the itching increases the risk for eczema, excoriations, cracks in the skin, inflammation, and infection. Nurses should be alert to signs of infection and rough, scaly, or flaky skin. Pharmacological treatment can be used if necessary.

Herpes Zoster

Most care and treatment for herpes zoster is medical, involving the prompt initiation of antiviral medications and optimal pain management. Nursing care includes providing both emotional support during the outbreak and education in regard to reducing secondary infections and cross-contamination. Weeping and ruptured vesicles should be covered with an absorbent yet nonadherent product, such as gauze. If the gauze adheres to the skin, warm normal saline applied to it will help release it. Hands, bedding, towels, and clothing should be washed before and after contact.

Postherpetic neuralgia (PHN) requires optimal pain management. The pain may persist for many months or even years; it may be severe and interfere with sleep and activities of daily living, resulting in weight loss, fatigue, and depression. Tricyclic antidepressants, tramadol (Ultram), long-acting opioids, or anticonvulsants (i.e., gabapentin [Neurontin] or pregabalin [Lyrica]) can decrease the pain of PHN. If topical therapy is indicated, capsaicin cream (Zostrix) or a lidocaine patch (Lidoderm) may lessen the pain (Fashner & Bell, 2011).

Given the frequent occurrence of herpes zoster in older persons and its associated morbidity, prevention should be considered. The zoster vaccine significantly boosts immunity to the varicella-zoster virus in older persons (Tseng et al., 2011). Additionally, the zoster vaccine can significantly reduce the burden of illness and the incidence of PHN (Tseng et. al., 2011).

PREMALIGNANT CONDITIONS OF THE SKIN

Older people can have premalignant conditions of the skin, some of which lead to skin cancer. The most common of these conditions are keratoses and photodamage to the skin.

KERATOSES

A *keratosis* is a thick, scaly, or crusty patch of skin and is associated with frequent exposure to the sun. There are two types of keratoses: seborrheic and actinic.

Seborrheic keratosis is a benign growth that appears mainly on the trunk, face, neck, and scalp as single or multiple lesions. One or more lesions are present on nearly all adults older than 65 years of age, and the lesions are more common in men. A person may have dozens of these benign lesions. A seborrheic keratosis is a waxy, raised, verrucous lesion that is flesh-coloured or pigmented in various sizes (Fig. 11.1). The lesions have a "stuck on" appearance, as if they could be scraped off. If there are cosmetic concerns, seborrheic keratoses may be removed by a dermatologist. A variant seen in darkly pigmented persons occurs mostly on the face and appears as numerous small, dark, and possibly taglike lesions (see http://www.dermatlas.com).

An *actinic keratosis* is a precancerous lesion that may become a squamous cell carcinoma. It is characterized by rough, scaly, sandpaper-like patches that are pink to reddish-brown on an erythematous base (Shoimer et al., 2010). Lesions may be single or

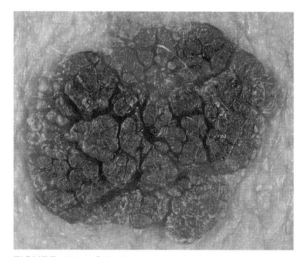

FIGURE 11.1 Seborrheic keratosis in an older person. *Source:* Habif, T. P. (2004). *Clinical dermatology: A color guide to diagnosis and therapy* (4th ed.). St. Louis: Mosby.

multiple and may be painless or mildly tender. Actinic keratosis is found on the face, lips, hands, and forearms, areas of sun exposure in everyday life. Risk factors are age and fair complexion. A person with actinic keratoses should be monitored by a dermatologist every 6 to 12 months for any change in the appearance of the lesions. Early recognition, treatment, and removal of the lesion are easy yet very important.

PHOTODAMAGE TO THE SKIN

Although exposure to sunlight is necessary for the production of vitamin D, the sun is also the most common cause of skin damage and skin cancer. With accumulating years of sun exposure, the risk of damage to the skin is significantly increased for older persons. The damage results from prolonged exposure to ultraviolet light (photo or solar) from the environment or from tanning booths. Although the amount of sun-induced damage varies with skin type and genetics, much of the associated damage is preventable. Ideally, preventive measures begin in childhood, but clinical evidence has shown that by limiting a person's sun exposure and having the person regularly use sunscreen, some measures can be effective at any time.

SKIN CANCERS

Worldwide, one of every three diagnosed cancers are skin cancers (*neoplasms*), growths on the skin (World Health Organization, 2017). The three most common skin cancers are basal cell cancer, squamous cell cancer, and melanoma; each is named for the type of skin cell from which it arises.

Skin cancer generally develops in the epidermis (the outermost layer of skin), so a tumour is usually clearly visible, making most skin cancers detectable in the early stages. Nonmelanoma skin cancer represents approximately 30% of all new cancer cases in Canada (Canadian Cancer Society, 2017a); in 2014, about 76,100 Canadians were diagnosed with nonmelanoma skin cancer (PHAC, 2014).

Most of these skin cancers are curable; the type with the greatest potential to cause death is melanoma (Canadian Cancer Society, 2017a). Persons with a history of sunburn, tanning bed use, skin cancer, exposure to carcinogenic materials, sun sensitivity, or a depressed immune system are at particular risk. Treatment depends on the type of cancer, the stage of the cancer, and the thickness and location of the lesion (Canadian Cancer Society, 2017b).

BASAL CELL CARCINOMA

Basal cell carcinoma and squamous cell carcinoma are the most common types of skin cancer in Canada, making up 80% of all cases of nonmelanoma skin cancers in the country (Canadian Cancer Society, 2017a). A basal cell lesion can be triggered by extensive sun exposure (especially that leading to sunburn), chronic irritation, and chronic ulceration of the skin. Basal cell carcinoma usually begins as a pearly papule with prominent telangiectasis (pattern or widened tiny blood vessels) or as a scarlike area with no history of trauma. It may be indistinguishable from squamous cell carcinoma and is diagnosed by biopsy. Basal cell carcinoma grows slowly, and metastasis is rare. Early detection and treatment are necessary to minimize disfigurement.

SQUAMOUS CELL CARCINOMA

Squamous cell carcinoma is the second most common skin cancer; however, it is aggressive and has a high incidence of metastasis if not identified and treated promptly. Squamous cell cancer is more prevalent in fair-skinned, older men who live in sunny climates and is usually found on the head, neck, or hands. Individuals in their midsixties who have been or are chronically exposed to the sun (e.g., persons who work outdoors, athletes) are at high risk for this type of cancer. Less common causes include persistent stasis ulcers, scars from injury, and exposure to chemical carcinogens. The lesion begins as a firm, irregular, fleshy, pink nodule that becomes reddened and scaly, much like actinic keratosis, but may increase rapidly in size. The lesions may also be hard and wart-like, with a grey top and a horny texture, or they may be ulcerated and indurated, with raised, defined borders. Because the lesions can appear so differently, they are often overlooked or thought to be insignificant. The best advice to give older persons, especially those who live in sunny climates, is to be regularly screened by a nurse practitioner, family physician, or dermatologist.

MELANOMA

Melanoma, a neoplasm of melanocytes, is the least common skin cancer, but it has a high mortality rate because of its ability to metastasize quickly. Blistering sunburns before the age of 18 years are thought to damage Langerhans cells, which affects the skin's immune response and increases the risk for a later melanoma. The legs and backs of women and the backs of men are the most common sites. Two-thirds of melanomas develop from pre-existing moles; only one-third arise alone. A melanoma lesion has a multicoloured, raised appearance with an asymmetrical, irregular border. It may appear to be of any size, but, much like an iceberg, its surface diameter does not necessarily reflect its size beneath the surface. It is treatable if caught very early, before it has a chance to invade surrounding tissue. If a nurse finds any questionable lesions upon assessment, the person should be referred to a dermatologist immediately. A common approach to assessing potential lesions is the ABCDE method (Box 11.3).

 IMPLICATIONS FOR GERONTOLOGICAL NURSING AND HEALTHY AGING

Gerontological nurses have an active role in the prevention and early recognition of skin cancers. This role may include working within community awareness and education programs, working in screening clinics, and providing direct care. In promoting skin health, nurses should be vigilant in observing the skin for any changes that require further evaluation. Several applications for electronic devices—Spot Check, Skin of Mine, Skin Prevention, Mole Detective 2, and Skin Scan—can be helpful in the detection of skin cancer (Ferrero et al., 2013).

By far the most important preventive nursing intervention is educating the older person about the risks caused by photodamage and smoke damage. Preventive strategies include using sunscreen, wearing protective clothing, and limiting sun exposure (Box 11.4).

Secondary prevention of skin cancer is early diagnosis. Following a thorough clinical screening, the older person, the family, the care aides, or all parties can be taught to perform regular checks of the skin, watching for signs of change and the need to contact a primary care provider or dermatologist promptly. For the person with keratosis and multiple freckles (*nevi*), photographs of the body parts may be useful references. The adage "When in doubt, get it checked" is an important one, and regular screenings should be a part of the health care of all older persons.

SKIN PROBLEMS ASSOCIATED WITH CARDIOVASCULAR PROBLEMS

Diabetes and hypertension are common problems for aging persons (see Chapters 17 and 20). A complication of both of these conditions is *vascular insufficiency*, which includes arterial insufficiency and is also called peripheral or lower-extremity artery disease; another is *venous insufficiency*. Vascular insufficiency may lead to serious skin infections and lesions, from mild stasis dermatitis to ulceration and gangrene. In promoting healthy aging, nurses need to be aware of the signs of vascular insufficiency and protect the person's limb and skin from further injury.

ARTERIAL INSUFFICIENCY

Peripheral artery disease (PAD) affects about 202 million people worldwide (Hussain et al., 2016). The disease is often caused by increased atherosclerotic plaques, which lead to ischemia of the limb and can lead to severe infections and limb loss. Many persons with PAD, whether diagnosed or not, complain of pain or muscle fatigue when they exercise. In more severe cases, the lower extremity can be extremely painful when the person is walking or when the legs are elevated (a condition called *intermittent claudication*). The person's pain is relieved only when the legs are returned to a dependent position (because of increased arterial flow downward) or when the person stops walking and rests, thus eliminating the extra circulatory demands made by exercise. Risk factors for PAD include obesity, coronary artery disease, smoking, dyslipidemia, hypertension, and diabetes.

As a result of PAD, the slightest trauma to a lower extremity, such as that caused by bumping the side of a wheelchair, can result in an arterial ulcer, which is very difficult and sometimes impossible to heal without surgical intervention. Pain is a significant problem, because the ulcer increases the pain already experienced from the arterial insufficiency.

VENOUS INSUFFICIENCY

Venous insufficiency (VI) is usually a consequence of a deep venous thrombosis that occurred in the past. The most important risk factors of VI are uncontrolled diabetes and venous hypertension with impaired

functioning of the valves within the veins. Skin tissue becomes vulnerable to insignificant trauma, such as an insect bite or the pressure from snug elastic-topped ankle socks. These insignificant traumatic events may also precipitate venous ulcer formation, or ulceration can develop spontaneously.

The first sign of VI may be edema of the lower extremities, which can become particularly troublesome and can affect functioning. Later in the process, the skin on the lower half of the extremity develops a brownish discoloration caused by the leakage of iron from red blood cells. In people with dark-pigmented skin, the discoloured skin is darker than the surrounding skin.

Venous ulcerations are painful and difficult to heal (Maddox, 2012). Although they are most often found over the outer malleolus, they can become quite extensive. The characteristics of venous ulcers are summarized in Table 11.1.

IMPLICATIONS FOR GERONTOLOGICAL NURSING AND HEALTHY AGING

The most important aspect of caring for the person with VI and PAD is to ensure that a proper and timely diagnosis is made and that treatment is consistent. To promote the health of the person's lower extremities, nurses must stay alert for signs of potential problems and take prompt action to minimize tissue damage. If ulcers develop, treatment must be consistent with evidence-informed practice. Nurses can also help older persons reduce risk factors whenever possible, for example, by encouraging smoking cessation and careful control of hypertension. Nurses can help reduce the incidence of ulcerations by protecting an affected limb from accidental injury.

A complaint of lower-extremity pain at rest necessitates a prompt referral to a vascular surgeon. Since the symptoms and problems associated with PAD are the result of ischemia of the extremity, interventions that promote circulation, such as finding ways for the older person to dangle his or her feet, are helpful. In the LTC setting, caregivers must recognize that a resident may be refusing to elevate the lower extremities because doing so causes sudden and severe pain.

TABLE 11.1 Comparison of Arterial and Venous Insufficiency of the Lower Extremities

CHARACTERISTICS	ARTERIAL INSUFFICIENCY	VENOUS INSUFFICIENCY
Location	Between toes or on tips of toes Over phalangeal heads and on heels Lateral malleolus or pretibial area (in diabetic patients), over metatarsal heads, on sides or soles of feet	Lower calf and ankle (especially medial malleolus)
Appearance	Well-defined edges Black or necrotic tissue Deep, pale base Nonbleeding	Uneven edges Ruddy granulation tissue Superficial Bleeding
Pain	Extreme pain with elevation of leg (relieved by dependent position) Persistent pain Constant severe pain with complete occlusion of blood supply	Deep muscle pain if DVT develops Relieved by elevation
Pulses	Absent or weak	Normal
Associated changes in leg and foot	Thin, shiny, dry skin Thickened toenails Absence of hair growth Temperature variations (cooler if there is no cellulitis) Elevational pallor Dependent rubor	Firm edema Reddish-brown discoloration of skin Evidence of healed ulcers Dilated and tortuous superficial veins

DVT, Deep vein thrombosis.

A person may be more comfortable sleeping in a recliner, where the feet can dangle. If an ulcer develops, the emphasis should be on preventing it from worsening. The wound should be kept warm and covered, but compression is contraindicated. The goals of care are to maximize function, relieve edema and pain, and treat the ulcer as needed. Treatment usually consists of a combination of therapies, such as leg elevation whenever the person is sitting and support stockings worn during waking hours. Although the stockings are usually considered uncomfortable, wearing them should nonetheless be encouraged. Support stockings are now available in an assortment of colours, including skin tones that are more acceptable than the traditional white. For maximal effect, support stockings should be put on before the person gets out of bed. They should extend to the top of the leg and be prevented from "rolling," since constriction is increased at the roll. Treatment of the venous ulcer includes managing the exudate and preventing worsening.

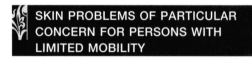

SKIN PROBLEMS OF PARTICULAR CONCERN FOR PERSONS WITH LIMITED MOBILITY

Persons with limited mobility, compromised immunity, or both are at particular risk for fungal skin infections and pressure injuries.

CANDIDIASIS

The fungus *Candida albicans* (referred to as yeast) is present on the skin of any healthy person. However, under certain circumstances and in the right environment, a fungal infection can develop. Persons who are obese, are malnourished, are receiving antibiotic or steroid therapy, or have diabetes are at increased risk. *Candida* grows especially well in areas that are moist, warm, and dark, such as in skinfolds, in the axilla and groin, under pendulous breasts, at the corners of the mouth, and in the vagina.

When it occurs inside the mouth, a *Candida* infection is referred to as *thrush* and is associated with poor hygiene and immunocompromise, such as that seen in persons engaged with long-term steroid use (e.g., because of chronic obstructive pulmonary disease), people who are receiving chemotherapy, or people who are infected with human immunodeficiency virus or have developed acquired immunodeficiency syndrome. In the mouth, candidiasis appears as irregular, white, flat to slightly raised patches on an erythematous base that cannot be scraped off. The infection can extend down into the throat and cause painful swallowing. In severely immunocompromised persons, the infection can extend down the entire gastro-intestinal tract.

On the skin, a *Candida* infection usually manifests as maculo-papular and glazed; it is dark pink on persons with less pigmentation and is greyish on persons with more pigmentation. If the infection is advanced, the central area may be completely red or dark (or both) and weeping, with characteristic bright red, dark, or bright red and dark satellite lesions (distinct lesions a short distance from the centre). At that point, the skin may be edematous, itching, and burning.

The best approach to managing fungal infections is to prevent them. The key to prevention is limiting the conditions that encourage fungal growth. People who are at risk are those who are bedridden, incontinent, obese, or diaphoretic. It is important to pay attention to the adequate drying of target areas of the body after bathing, prompt management of incontinent episodes (see Chapter 9), the use of loose-fitting cotton clothing and underwear, and the avoidance of incontinence products that are tight or have plastic that touches the skin.

One of the best ways to dry hard-to-reach, vulnerable areas is with a hair dryer set on low. A folded dry washcloth or a cotton sanitary pad can be placed under the breasts or between skinfolds to allow exposure to air and light. Cornstarch should never be used because it promotes the growth of *Candida* organisms. Optimizing nutrition and glycemic control are also important.

The goal of treatment is to eradicate the infection. Eradication requires not only the use of prescribed antifungal medication but also the active involvement of nurses or caregivers in reducing or eliminating the conditions that create the problem.

The affected area of the skin must be cleansed carefully with a mild soap or cleansing agent (such as Cetaphil) and dried thoroughly before antifungal preparations are applied. Antifungal preparations are available as powders, creams, and lotions. Because creams and lotions trap moisture, powder is recommended. These preparations are usually needed for 7 to 14 days or until the infection has completely cleared. Antifungal medications include miconazole (Micatin), clotrimazole (Canesten, Clotrimaderm, Lotriderm), nystatin (Mycostatin), and econazole (Ecostatin).

PRESSURE INJURIES

According to the Registered Nurses' Association of Ontario, a pressure injury is "any lesion caused by unrelieved pressure that results in damage to underlying tissue. Pressure injuries usually occur over a bony prominence and are staged to classify the degree of tissue damage observed" (Registered Nurses' Association of Ontario [RNAO], 2011, p. 19). As tissue is compressed, blood is diverted, and blood vessels are forcibly constricted by the persistent pressure on the skin and underlying structures; thus, cellular respiration is impaired, and cells die from ischemia and anoxia. Intervention at any point in this development can stop the advancement of the pressure injury. Just how much pressure can be endured by tissue (**tissue tolerance**) is highly variable between body locations and persons. Tissue tolerance is inversely affected by moisture, friction, shearing, amount of pressure, and age, and is directly related to malnutrition, anemia, and low arterial pressure.

The prevalence of pressure injuries is quite high in later life. The Canadian Institute of Health Information reported that between 2011 and 2012, 2.4%, 14.1%, and 6.7% of patients experienced a pressure injury in home care, complex continuing care, and LTC settings, respectively (Canadian Institute of Health Information [CIHI], 2013). Pressure injuries are highly preventable; however, they remain commonly prevalent, particularly in LTC settings (Pham et al., 2011). According to some researchers, pressure injuries are associated with adverse effects on health, social well-being, quality of life, and high treatment costs—approximately US$3.3 billion per year in 2008 (Pham et al., 2011).

Risk Factors

Persons who are frail, nonambulatory, and/or neurologically impaired are at the greatest risk for the development of a pressure injury. The most important predictors of pressure injuries are severity of illness and involuntary weight loss owing to problems of poor nutrition, especially dehydration, hypoproteinemia, and vitamin deficiencies. Other important indicators of increased risk are impaired sensory feedback systems (which prevent discomfort from being noticed) and impaired mobility or immobilization by sedation. Nevertheless, most pressure injuries are considered preventable.

Pressure injuries can develop anywhere on the body but are most frequently seen on posterior aspects, especially the sacrum, coccyx, knees, heels, and toes (RNAO, 2011). Secondary areas of breakdown include the lateral condyles of the knees and ankles. The pinna of the ears is also subject to breakdown, as are the elbows and the scapulae. If a person is lying prone, the knees, shins, and pelvis sustain undue pressure.

Heels are particularly apt to develop pressure injuries, since heels are small surfaces that receive a high degree of pressure. People who have peripheral vascular insufficiency and are immobile are at high risk for heel ulcers. In the acute care setting, patients who are supine for prolonged periods during surgical procedures may leave the operating room with newly acquired pressure injuries.

For many older persons, an ulcer will prolong recovery and lengthen rehabilitation. Complications include sepsis, the need for grafting, and the need for amputation; even death can occur (Box 11.5).

The development of pressure injuries is a dynamic process that makes constant vigilance and reassessment necessary, and nurses have an extremely important role in preventing them and in assessing the skin. The Braden Scale (Fig. 11.2) and the Norton Scale are risk assessment tools frequently used in the clinical setting to identify persons who are at high risk for pressure injuries (Bergstrom et al., 1994; Norton, 1996).

BOX 11.5	**Examples of Complications of Pressure Injuries**

- Local infection of wound or surrounding tissue
- Loss of function
- Tetanus
- Extension of the infection to the bone: osteomyelitis
- Systemic infection: septicemia
- Extended period of acute and continuous medical and nursing care

---

 IMPLICATIONS FOR GERONTOLOGICAL NURSING AND HEALTHY AGING

Of all health care providers, nurses are the most responsible for the prevention and treatment of pressure injuries and other interruptions in skin integrity. Nurses are in an ideal position to implement preventive measures, identify early signs, and implement appropriate interventions to prevent skin breakdown and promote healing. Failure to take these actions jeopardizes the health and life of the person receiving care. The nurse can inform other health care providers of the need for prevention, recommended treatments, evaluation of the status of the wound or wounds, and the adequacy of interventions. A detailed Best Practice Guideline can be found at http://rnao.ca/events/skin-and-wound-care-resourcestools-ltc-toolkit.

ASSESSMENT

Assessment begins with a detailed head-to-toe skin examination and an analysis of laboratory test findings (Box 11.6). Laboratory values that have been correlated with risk for the development and poor healing of pressure injuries include those that indicate anemia and poor nutritional status. Visual and tactile inspection of the entire skin surface, with special attention to bony prominences, is essential. Special attention must be paid to affected areas when an individual uses orthotic devices such as corsets, braces, prostheses, postural supports, splints, slings, or casts.

The nurse will look for any interruption in skin integrity or other changes, including **hyperemia** (redness). Any pressure should be relieved and the area reassessed in 1 hour. Redness may be less noticeable on darkly pigmented persons than on lightly pigmented persons; it may be necessary to look for induration, darkening, or a shadowed appearance. Pressure areas should be palpated for changes

Braden Scale for Predicting Pressure Sore Risk

Resident's Name _____   Evaluator's Name _____

		Date of assessment					
SENSORY PERCEPTION Ability to respond meaningfully to pressure-related discomfort	**1. Completely Limited** Unresponsive (does not moan, flinch or grasp) to painful stimuli, due to diminished level of consciousness or sedation. OR limited ability to feel pain over most of body.	**2. Very Limited** Responds only to painful stimuli. Cannot communicate discomfort except by moaning or restlessness. OR has a sensory impairment that limits the ability to feel pain or discomfort over ½ of body.	**3. Slightly Limited** Responds to verbal commands, but cannot always communicate discomfort or the need to be turned. OR has some sensory impairment which limits ability to feel pain or discomfort in 1 or 2 extremities.	**4. No Impairment** Responds to verbal commands. Has no sensory deficit which would limit ability to feel or voice pain or discomfort.			
MOISTURE Degree to which skin is exposed to moisture	**1. Constantly Moist** Skin is kept moist almost constantly by perspiration, urine, etc. Dampness is detected every time patient is moved or turned.	**2. Very Moist** Skin is often, but not always, moist. Linen must be changed at least once a shift.	**3. Occasionally Moist** Skin is occasionally moist, requiring an extra linen change approximately once a day.	**4. Rarely Moist** Skin is usually dry. Linen only requires changing at routine intervals.			
ACTIVITY Degree of physical activity	**1. Bedfast** Confined to bed.	**2. Chairfast** Ability to walk severely limited or non-existent. Cannot bear own weight and/or must be assisted into chair or wheelchair.	**3. Walks Occasionally** Walks occasionally during day, but for very short distances with or without assistance. Spends majority of each shift in bed or chair.	**4. Walks Frequently** Walks outside the room at least twice a day and inside room at least every 2 hours during waking hours.			
MOBILITY Ability to change and control body position	**1. Completely Immobile** Does not make even slight changes in body or extremity position without assistance.	**2. Very Limited** Makes occasional slight changes in body or extremity position, but unable to make frequent or significant changes independently.	**3. Slightly Limited** Makes frequent though slight changes in body or extremity position independently.	**4. No Limitation** Makes major and frequent changes in position without assistance.			

FIGURE 11.2 Braden Scale for Predicting Pressure Sore Risk. *Source:* Regional Geriatric Program of Toronto. (n.d.). *Braden scale for predicting pressure sore risk.* Copyright, Braden and Bergstrom, 1988. Reprinted with permission. All rights reserved. Retrieved from http://rgp.toronto.on.ca/torontobestpractice/Bradenscaleforpredictingpressuresorerisk.pdf.

Continued

	1. Very Poor	2. Probably Inadequate	3. Adequate	4. Excellent			
NUTRITION Usual food intake pattern	Never eats a complete meal. Rarely eats more than 1/3 of any food offered. Eats 2 servings or less of protein (meat or dairy products) per day. Takes fluids poorly. Does not take a liquid dietary supplement. OR is NPO and/or maintained on clear liquids or IVs for more than 5 days.	Rarely eats a complete meal and generally eats only about 1/2 of any food offered. Protein intake includes only 3 servings of meat or dairy products per day. Occasionally will take a dietary supplement. OR receives less than optimum amount of liquid diet or tube feeding.	Eats over half of most meals. Eats a total of 4 servings of protein (meat or dairy products) each day. Occasionally will refuse a meal, but will usually take a supplement if offered. OR is on tube feeding or TPN regimen, which meets most of nutritional needs.	Eats most of every meal. Never refuses a meal. Usually eats a total of 4 or more servings of meat and dairy products. Occasionally eats between meals. Does not require supplementation.			
FRICTION AND SHEAR	1. Problem Requires moderate to maximum assistance in moving. Complete lifting without sliding against sheets is impossible. Frequently slides down in bed or chair, requiring frequent repositioning with maximum assistance. Spasticity, contractures or agitation lead to almost constant friction.	2. Potential Problems Moves feebly or requires minimum assistance. During a move skin probably slides to some extent against sheets, chair restraints, or other devices. Maintains relatively good position in chair or bed most of the time but occasionally slides down.	3. No Apparent Problem Moves in bed and chair independently and has sufficient muscle strength to lift up completely during move. Maintains good position in bed or chair.				
				Total Score			

© Copyright Barbara Braden and Nancy Bergstrom, 1988.

Note: (Braden, 2001)
15 to 18 = At Risk
13 to 14 = Moderate Risk
10 to 12 = High Risk
≤ 9 = Very High Risk

Assessment Schedule:
Very High to High Risk = minimum monthly
Moderate Risk = q3months
Low/No Risk = q6months

Consider other resident factors that will also increase risks, e.g., advanced age, uncontrolled pain, underlying disease conditions, low albumin and HGB.

FIGURE 11.2, cont'd

BOX 11.6 Risk Assessment and Prevention of Pressure Injuries

- Carry out a daily head-to-toe assessment of persons who are at risk for skin breakdown; pay particular attention to bony prominences.
- Assess risk for pressure injury development with a valid and reliable tool, such as the Braden Scale for Predicting Pressure Sore Risk (Fig. 11.2).
- Assess persons who have restricted mobility for pressure, friction, and shearing forces, in all positions and during lifting, turning, and repositioning.
- Develop a collaborative, individualized plan of care based on assessment data, identified risk factors, and the patient's goals.
- Use proper positioning, transferring, and turning techniques.
- Avoid massaging over bony prominences.
- Protect and promote skin integrity through hydrating the skin, minimizing force and shear during cleansing, using protective barriers to reduce friction, and so on.

Source: Adapted from the Registered Nurses' Association of Ontario (RNAO). (2011). *Risk assessment and prevention of pressure injuries* (Rev. ed.). Toronto, ON: RNAO.

BOX 11.7 Key Aspects of Assessment of a Pressure Injury

1. Stage and size (width, depth, length)
2. Location
3. Surface area (length × width) (mm^2, cm^2)
4. Odour
5. Sinus tracts, undermining, tunnelling
6. Exudate
7. Condition of surrounding tissue
8. Condition of wound edges (e.g., smooth and white, or irregular and pink)
9. Wound bed (warmth, moisture, odour, amount, and colour of exudates)

in temperature and tissue resilience. Blisters or pimples (with or without hyperemia) and scabs over weight-bearing areas in the absence of trauma should be considered suspect.

Existing pressure injuries are assessed with each dressing change, and detailed assessment is repeated as needed (Box 11.7). The purpose of the assessment is to carefully evaluate the effectiveness of treatment. If there are no signs of healing from week to week or if worsening is seen, then either the treatment is insufficient or the wound has become infected; in either case, treatment must be changed.

Pressure Injury Classification

Pressure injuries are classified according to the scale developed and updated by the National Pressure Ulcer Advisory Panel (2014). The scale encompasses suspected injury, pressure injury stages 1 through 4, and "unstageable" pressure injury (Fig. 11.3). An ulcer is always classified by the highest stage; this means that the wound is documented at the stage that represents the maximum damage that has occurred. As the wound heals, it fills with granulation tissue composed of endothelial cells, fibroblasts, collagen, and an extracellular matrix. Muscle, subcutaneous fat, and dermis are not replaced. The staging of a pressure injury cannot be reversed; that is, a stage IV pressure injury that is healing is not reclassified as stage III and then stage II; it remains defined as a (healing) stage IV pressure injury. Wounds that are covered in black (**eschar**) or yellow fibrous (**slough**) necrosis cannot be staged, because it is not possible to determine the condition of the underlying wound bed. These wounds are documented as unstageable. Once the dead tissue has been removed (**debrided**), the wound can be staged.

Careful and detailed documentation of the condition of the skin is required at the onset of the problem and at intervals during its treatment.

INTERVENTIONS

The goal of nurses is to help maintain skin integrity against the various environmental, mechanical, and chemical assaults that are potential causes of breakdown. In promoting the healthy aging of all persons, nurses focus on prevention by taking action to eliminate friction and irritation to the skin (such as that caused by shearing); to reduce moisture so that tissues do not **macerate;** and to displace body weight from prominent areas in order to facilitate circulation to the skin. Nurses should assess the frequency of position changes, add pillows so that skin surfaces do not touch, and establish a turning schedule if needed. They should also be familiar with the various types of supportive surfaces and dressings so that the most effective products are used.

Stage I

Erythema not resolving within thirty
(30) minutes of pressure relief.
Epidermis remains intact.
REVERSIBLE WITH INTERVENTION.

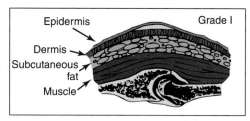

Stage II

Partial-thickness loss of skin layers
involving epidermis and possibly
penetrating into but not through
dermis. May present as blistering
with erythema and/or induration;
wound base moist and pink;
painful; free of necrotic tissue.

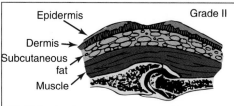

Stage III

Full-thickness tissue loss extending
through dermis to involve
subcutaneous tissue. Presents as
shallow crater unless covered by
eschar. May include necrotic tissue,
undermining, sinus tract formation,
exudate, and/or infection. Wound
base is usually not painful.

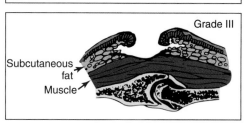

Stage IV

Deep tissue destruction extending
through subcutaneous tissue to fascia,
possibly involving muscle layers, joint,
and/or bone. Presents as a deep
crater. May include necrotic tissue,
undermining, sinus tract formation,
exudate, and/or infection. Wound
base is usually not painful.

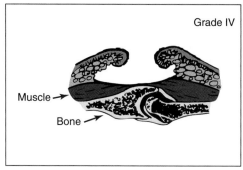

Unstageable

A wound that is covered by eschar or
slough, preventing the visualization
of the wound bed.

FIGURE 11.3 Pressure sore development.

Nutritional intake should be monitored, as well as serum albumin, hematocrit, and hemoglobin levels. Diets high in protein, carbohydrates, and vitamins are necessary to maintain and promote tissue growth. If the patient lacks appetite, appetite stimulants may be prescribed. Nurses can promote nutritional health by ensuring that dining is a pleasant experience for the person (see Chapter 8).

It is not always possible to prevent interruptions in skin integrity that are caused by overwhelming conditions. Fortunately, the state of the science of wound care is well developed, and evidence-informed guidelines are available. Sources of information include the websites of the Registered Nurses' Association of Ontario (http://www.rnao.ca) and Wounds Canada (Canadian Association of Wound Care) (https://www.woundscanada.ca).

Consultation with a wound care nurse-specialist is advisable for wounds that are extensive or non-healing. Specialized nurses such as enterostomal therapists or nurse practitioners, who may work at wound centres or with surgeons, provide consultation in hospitals, LTC homes, offices, and clinics (see Chapter 2).

HEALTHY FEET

Feet influence the older person's physical, psychological, and social well-being. Feet carry the body's weight, hold the body erect, coordinate and maintain balance in walking, and must be adaptable enough to conform to changing walking surfaces. Little attention is given to a person's feet until they interfere with moving and ultimately the ability to remain independent. Promoting healthy feet and good care of the feet can alleviate disability and pain and lessen the risk of falling.

COMMON FOOT PROBLEMS

The human foot is a complex structure with many bones, joints, tendons, muscles, and ligaments. Some foot irregularities and problems are inherited; however, many problems occur because of wear and tear, the shoes the person wears, or misuse of the feet.

Older feet, subjected to a lifetime of stress, may not be able to continue to adapt, and inflammatory changes in bone and soft tissue can occur. Foot health and function may reflect systemic disease or give early clues to physical illness. Changes in the nails or skin of the feet or the recurrence of infections may be precursors of more serious health problems.

Major abnormalities occur gradually. Rheumatological disorders (such as the various forms of arthritis) usually affect other joints but can also affect the feet. Gout is a systemic disease that occurs most often in the joint of the great toe (see Chapter 18). Both diabetes and venous insufficiency (VI) commonly cause lower-extremity problems that can quickly become life-threatening.

Without proper care and treatment, these conditions become disabling and threaten the person's mobility and independence. Care of the feet requires a team approach that includes the older person, the nurse, the podiatrist, and the person's primary health care provider. Nurses have the opportunity to promote healthy aging by applying their knowledge of the common problems of the feet and their skills in foot care.

Corns and Calluses

Corns and *calluses* are both growths of compacted skin that occur as a result of prolonged pressure, usually from ill-fitting, tight shoes. Corns are cone shaped and develop on the top of the toe joints as the result of the rubbing of the shoe on the joint. Calluses are thickened and hardened parts of the skin as a result of repeated friction or pressure. Soft corns form between opposing surfaces of the toes from prolonged squeezing. Corns and calluses can interfere with the ability to walk and to wear shoes comfortably. Once a corn forms, continued pressure on it will cause pain. Unless the friction and pressure are relieved, the corn will continue to enlarge and cause increasing pain.

Many older persons self-treat corns and calluses with over-the-counter preparations to remove the corn temporarily. However, chemical burns and ulcerations from these products can result in the loss of toes or a leg for a person with diabetes, neurological impairment, or poor circulation in the lower extremities. Some people use razor blades and scissors to remove the affected tissue; this is very dangerous and is never recommended. Oval corn pads, moleskin, or lambswool, with a hole cut in the centre for the corn, can be used for more proper treatment. Irritation from soft corns between the toes can be eased by loosely wrapping a small amount of lambswool around the involved toe, or cotton balls can be placed between the toes. Gel pads are also useful in protecting the toes from friction and pressure. For persons who are prone to developing calluses, daily lubrication of the feet is important. For persons with VI and diabetes, foot care should be performed only by a trained nurse, a physician, or a podiatrist.

Mild corns may resolve themselves when pressure is removed and tight shoes are replaced by larger shoes with a better fit. Bigger or resistant corns may need to be surgically removed by a podiatrist. For persons at high risk, such as those with diabetes or VI, corns are not usually removed because of the risk of poor wound healing at the surgical site.

Bunions

Bunions are bony deformities that develop from the longstanding squeezing together of the first (great or big) and second toes. Bony prominences develop over the medial aspect of the joint of the great toe and, at times, at the lateral aspect of the fifth metatarsal head (*tailor's bunion* or *bunionette*). Heredity may be a factor in their development. Walking can be markedly compromised by any of these defor-mities. Bunions may be treated with corticosteroid injections, anti-inflammatory pain medications, or surgery if necessary. Shoes that provide forefoot space (e.g., running shoes) and sandals work well, or a custom-made shoe could be considered. Nurses can promote comfort by helping the person find shoes that properly support and protect the foot.

Hammer Toes

A *hammer toe* is a toe that is permanently flexed, giving it a clawlike appearance. The condition is a result of muscle imbalance and pressure from the great toe slanting toward the second toe. The toe then contracts, leaving a bulge on top of the joint. It is aggravated by poor-fitting shoes and is often seen in conjunction with bunions. This condition limits the ability to walk and restricts balance and comfort. As with bunions, treatment includes professional orthot-ics or specially designed protective devices; properly fitting, nonconstricting shoes; or surgical intervention.

Fungal Infections

Fungal infections are very common on the aging foot, and the incidence increases with age. These infections may affect the skin of the foot as well as the nails. Nail fungus, or *onychomycosis*, is characterized by degen-eration of the nail plate, change in the colour of the nail (to yellow or an opaque brown), and brittleness and thickening of the nail (Fig. 11.4). A fine, powdery

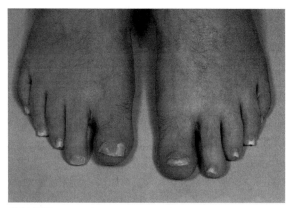

FIGURE 11.4 Onychomycosis: Yellowing, crumbling, and thickening of the toenails. *Source:* Bolognia, J., Jorizzo, J. L., & Rapini, R. (2003). *Dermatology.* St Louis: Mosby (Fig. 77.15B).

collection of fungus forms under the centre of the nail, separating the layers and pushing the nail up, causing the sides of the nail to dig into the skin like an ingrown toenail. Culturing is the only definitive way to diagnose onychomycosis. Several oral medications are available but are expensive and of limited effec-tiveness, need to be taken for 3 to 12 months, and are potentially toxic to the liver and heart. When nails are involved, a cure is difficult to impossible because of limited circulation.

Another common fungal infection is *tinea pedis* (athlete's foot). Many of the causes of candidia-sis are also causes of this infection. Tinea pedis is treated as any other fungal infection is treated. Feet, especially the area between the toes, should be kept dry and clean and regularly exposed to sun and air. Topical application of antifungal powders, in addition to the hygiene measures already noted, is the usual treatment.

 IMPLICATIONS FOR GERONTOLOGICAL NURSING AND HEALTHY AGING

Gerontological nurses should advocate the best foot health possible. Foot care is a prime factor in the maintenance of mobility and independence. Nursing care of the older person with foot problems should be directed toward maintaining optimal comfort and function, removing possible mechanical irritants, and decreasing the likelihood of infection. The nurse has to assess the feet for clues of functional ability and their owner's well-being (Box 11.8). Nurses can iden-tify potential and actual problems and make referrals or seek assistance from the primary care provider or podiatrist as needed.

Gerontological nursing care includes the observa-tion of gait, postural deformities, physical limitations, the position of the foot with the heel strike, and the type of shoe worn and its condition, including sole wear. Assessment also includes an inspection of the feet for irritation, abrasions, and other lesions; hazards to the maintenance of adequate circulation to the lower extremities and the existing circulatory status; and the individual's general mobility. Peri-odic assessment of the feet is especially important for persons with diabetes, heart disease, VI, thyroid or

BOX 11.8 Essential Aspects of Foot Assessment

Observation of Mobility
- Gait
- Use of assistive devices
- Footwear type and pattern of wear

Past Medical History
- Neuropathies
- Musculo-skeletal limitations
- Vascular insufficiency
- Vision problems
- Falls
- Pain affecting movement

Bilateral Assessment
- Colour
- Circulation and warmth
- Pulses
- Structural deformities
- Skin lesions
- Lower-extremity edema
- Evidence of scratching
- Rash or excessive dryness
- Condition and colour of toenails

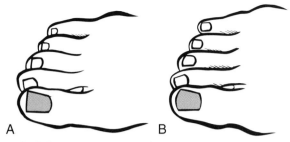

FIGURE 11.5 Cutting toenails. A, Correct angle and shape. B, Incorrect angle and shape.

renal conditions, and any neurological impairment, such as reduced or absent sensations resulting from a stroke.

CARE OF TOENAILS

Poor close vision, difficulty bending, obesity, or increased thickness of the nails makes self-care of the toenails difficult. Care of the feet and nails of persons in the LTC setting is the nurse's responsibility. Nails that become too long will begin to interfere with stockings, hose, or shoes. Ideally, toenails should be trimmed after the bath or shower when they are soft, but if this is not possible, soaking the feet for 20 to 30 minutes before care is sufficient. Nails should be clipped straight across and even with the top of the toe, with the edges filed slightly (to remove sharpness) but not to the point of rounding (Fig. 11.5). The foot care of persons with diabetes should be done only by a podiatrist or a trained registered nurse, and special care must be taken to prevent accidental damage or trauma to the skin (Registered Nurses' Association of Ontario (RNAO), 2007). Persons with diabetes or

peripheral neuropathy should never have pedicures from commercial establishments.

Nails that are neglected become long and curved. Hard, thickened nails indicate inadequate nutrition to the nail matrix because of trauma or poor circulation. Once the nail becomes thickened, it will remain so. Thick, hard nails split easily, causing trauma, pain, and possibly infection. Any attempt by the nurse or other caregiver to cut these nails may result in further damage to the matrix or precipitate an infection. These conditions should be brought to the attention of a podiatrist.

An ingrown toenail is a fragment of nail that pierces the skin at the edge of the nail. This problem is often a consequence of the hypertrophy of the nail with onychomycosis, improper cutting of the nail, or pressure exerted on the toes by tight hosiery or shoes. Ingrown toenails should be referred to a podiatrist because of the risk of infection. Temporary relief can be provided by inserting a small piece of cotton under the affected nail corner.

Nursing interventions include helping the older person understand the necessity of appropriate foot-wear and helping the person obtain such footwear. For persons with diabetes or other neurological impairments, the shoes should cover and protect the foot entirely without pressure areas. For persons with arthritis, firm soles are more comfortable than soft soles and may decrease pain associated with walking (Dahmen et al., 2014).

Shoes should be functional; that is, they should cover, protect, and stabilize the foot and provide maximum toe space to prevent bunions, corns, and calluses. One foot is usually larger than the other. Feet lengthen slightly with age; one foot is usually larger than the other, and the feet are largest in the afternoon. Thus, shoes should be fitted to the largest foot, and afternoon purchases are advised. Fabric shoes are not recommended for persons with diabetes or VI as they do not provide enough support. Low-heeled shoes place less stress on the legs and back than completely flat shoes do.

Slip-on shoes are helpful for those who are unable to bend or lace shoes, but care must be taken that the person's feet will not accidentally slip out of the shoes, which can lead to a fall. Velcro closures are useful for those who have limited finger dexterity. Custom-made shoes, although expensive, may be necessary for persons with bunions or any other deformity.

SUMMARY

Gerontological nurses have an instrumental role in promoting the health of the skin and feet of the older person, but this is sometimes overlooked when dealing with other, more immediately life-threatening problems. However, preservation of the integrity of the skin and the functioning of the feet is essential to mobility, well-being, and quality of life. To promote healthy aging, the nurse needs to be able to assess common skin and foot problems encountered by older people and to develop effective interventions both for acute and for persistent conditions.

KEY CONCEPTS

- The skin is the largest and most visible organ of the body and has multiple roles in maintaining health.
- Maintaining adequate moisture and skin lubrication will reduce the incidence of xerosis and other skin problems.
- The best way to minimize the risk for skin cancer is to avoid prolonged sun and smoke exposure.
- Prompt treatment of persons with herpes zoster infection is needed to lessen the risk of postherpetic neuralgia.
- Problems of the skin and feet may reflect systemic disease.
- Mobility is fundamental to independence; therefore, care of the feet and toenails is an important concern for the gerontological nurse.

- A pressure injury is documented by stage, which indicates the degree of tissue damage; a healing ulcer retains its original staging.
- A pressure injury that is covered in dead tissue (eschar or slough) cannot be staged until it has been debrided.
- Darkly pigmented persons will not display the "typical" erythema of a stage I pressure injury or early VI; therefore, closer vigilance is necessary for these persons.
- Persons with VI, diabetes, or peripheral neuropathy are at special risk for serious skin problems.
- Foot care for older people with diabetes should always be performed by a podiatrist or a trained registered nurse.

ACTIVITIES AND DISCUSSION QUESTIONS

1. Describe the common skin and foot problems an older person is likely to experience.
2. Describe the nurse's responsibility in maintaining the patient's skin integrity.
3. List several interventions that apply to skin and foot care.
4. Develop a nursing care plan for an older person experiencing xerosis and pruritus.

RESOURCES

Hartford Institute for Geriatric Nursing
https://consultgeri.org/

National Pressure Ulcer Advisory Panel
http://www.npuap.org

Registered Nurses' Association of Ontario (RNAO). *Reducing foot complications for people with diabetes* *http://rnao.ca/sites/rnao-ca/files/Foot_Compl_Diabetes _Updated.pdf*

Registered Nurses' Association of Ontario (RNAO). *Risk assessment & prevention of pressure ulcers* *http://rnao.ca/sites/rnao-ca/files/Risk_Assessment_and _Prevention_of_Pressure_Ulcers.pdf*

Wounds Canada (Canadian Association of Wound Care)
http://www.woundscanada.ca

For additional resources, please visit *http:// evolve.elsevier.com/Canada/Ebersole/gerontological/*

REFERENCES

Bergstrom, N., Allman, R., Alvarez, O. M., et al. (1994). *Treatment of pressure ulcers.* Clinical practice guideline no. 15, AHCPR pub no. 95-0652. Rockville, MD: U.S. Department of Health and Human Services, Public Health Service, Agency for Health Care Policy and Research.

Canadian Cancer Society. (2017a). *Melanoma: deadliest type of skin cancer is on the rise.* Retrieved from https://www.cancer .ca/en/about-us/for-media/media-releases/national/2014/201 4-canadian-cancer-statistics/?region=on.

Canadian Cancer Society. (2017b). *Treatment of melanoma.* Retrieved from http://www.cancer.ca/en/cancer-information/ cancer-type/skin-melanoma/treatment/?region=on.

Canadian Institute for Health Information (CIHI). (2013). *Compromised wounds in Canada.* Retrieved from https://secure.cihi.ca/ free_products/AiB_Compromised_Wounds_EN.pdf.

Dahmen, R., Buijsmann, S., Siemonsma, P. C., et al. (2014). Use and effects of custom-made therapeutic footwear on lower-extremity-related pain and activity limitations in patients with rheumatoid arthritis: A prospective observational study of a cohort. *Journal of Rehabilitation Medicine, 46*(6), 561–567. doi:10.2340/16501977-1807.

Fashner, J., & Bell, A. (2011). Herpes Zoster and postherpetic neuralgia: Prevention and management. *American Family Physician, 83*(12), 1432–1437. Retrieved from www.aafp.org/afp/ 2011/0615/p1432.html.

Ferrero, N. A., Morrell, D. S., & Burkhart, C. N. (2013). Skin scan: a demonstration of the need for FDA regulation of medical apps on iPhone. *Journal of the American Academy of Dermatology, 68*(3), 515–516. doi:10.1016/j.jaad.2012.10.045.

Government of Ontario. (2016). *Shingles vaccine free for Ontario seniors.* Retrieved from https://news.ontario.ca/mohltc/en/ 2016/12/shingles-vaccine-free-for-ontario-seniors.html.

Hussain, M. A., Lindsay, T. F., Mamdani, M., et al. (2016). Sex differences in the outcomes of peripheral arterial disease: A population-based cohort study. *Canadian Medical Association Journal, 4*(1), E124–E131. doi:10.9778/cmajo.20150107.

LeBlanc, K., Kozell, K., Martins, L., et al. (2016). Is twice-daily skin moisturizing more effective than routine care in the prevention of skin tears in the elderly population? *J Wound Ostomy Continence Nurs, 43*(1), 17–22. doi:10.1097/WON.0000000000000195.

Maddox, D. (2012). Effects of venous leg ulceration on patients' quality of life. *Nursing Standard, 26*(38), 42–49. doi:10.7748/ ns2012.05.26.38.42.c9111.

National Pressure Ulcer Advisory Panel. (2014). *Pressure ulcer stages revised, February 2014.* Retrieved from http://www.npuap.org.

Norton, D. (1996). Calculating the risk: Reflections on the Norton Scale. *Advances in Wound Care, 9*(6), 38–43. https:// www.ncbi.nlm.nih.gov/pubmed/9069755.

Pham, B., Stern, A., Chen, W., et al. (2011). Preventing pressure ulcers in long-term care: A cost-effectiveness analysis. *Archives of Internal Medicine, 171*(20), 1839–1847. doi:10.1001/ archinternmed.2011.473.

Public Health Agency of Canada (PHAC). (2013). *Fact sheet – shingles (Herpes zoster).* Retrieved from https://www.canada.ca/en/ public-health/services/infectious-diseases/fact-sheet-shingles -herpes-zoster.html.

Public Health Agency of Canada (PHAC). (2014). *Non melanoma skin cancer.* Retrieved from https://www.canada.ca/en/public -health/services/chronic-diseases/cancer/non-melanoma-skin -cancer.html.

Registered Nurses' Association of Ontario (RNAO) (2007). *Reducing foot complications for people with diabetes.* Toronto, ON: RNAO.

Registered Nurses' Association of Ontario (RNAO) (2011). *Risk assessment & prevention of pressure ulcers.* Toronto, ON: RNAO.

Shoimer, I., Rosen, N., & Muhn, C. (2010). Current management of actinic keratoses. *Skin Therapy Letter, 15*(5), 5–7. Retrieved from http://www.skintherapyletter.com/2010/15.5/2.html.

Tseng, H. F., Smith, N., Harpaz, R., et al. (2011). Herpes zoster vaccine in older adults and the risk of subsequent herpes zoster disease. *JAMA: The Journal of the American Medical Association, 305*(2), 160–166. doi:10.1001/jama.2010.1983.

World Health Organization (WHO). (2017). *Skin Cancers.* Retrieved from http://www.who.int/uv/faq/skincancer/en/index1.html.

CHAPTER 12

Maintaining Mobility and Environmental Safety

CHAPTER

LEARNING OBJECTIVES

Upon completion of this chapter, the reader will be able to:

- Discuss the effects of impaired mobility on general function and quality of life.
- Specify risk factors for impaired mobility.
- Identify older persons at risk for falls, and list several interventions to reduce fall risk.
- Understand the negative effects of restraints, and discuss appropriate alternatives for safety promotion and fall risk reduction.
- Identify factors in the environment that contribute to the safety and security of the older person.
- Relate strategies for protecting the older person from injury and accidents.
- Develop a nursing care plan appropriate for an older person at risk of falling.

GLOSSARY

Agility The ability to change the body's position efficiently.

Orthostatic (postural) hypotension A drop in blood pressure occurring when a person assumes an upright position after being in a lying-down position.

Proprioception The sense, independent of vision, of movements and position of the body in space.

Sarcopenia The loss of skeletal muscle mass, strength, and function.

Syncope A brief lapse in consciousness, caused by transient cerebral hypoxia.

THE LIVED EXPERIENCE

After that fall last year when I slipped in the bathroom, I feel so insecure. I find myself taking small, shuffling steps to avoid falling again, but it makes me feel awkward and clumsy. When I was younger, I never worried about falling, but now I'm so afraid I will break a bone or something.

Betty, age 75 years

MOBILITY

Mobility is the capacity for movement within the immediate and larger-scale environment. Older persons move more slowly and purposefully, sometimes with more forethought and caution. This chapter focuses on the maintenance of maximal mobility, both in health and in the presence of various disorders; the assessment of gait and mobility status; the negative consequences of restraints; measures to achieve safety without using restraints; causes and consequences of falls in older persons; reduction of the risk of falling; and aids and interventions that are useful when mobility is impaired. Specific information will be provided to promote a safe environment for older persons in all health care settings and in the community. Challenges related to transportation and driving as essential aspects of environmental mobility are also included. Chapter 10 provides a further discussion about activity and exercise, and bone and joint problems affecting mobility are addressed in Chapter 18.

AGE-RELATED CHANGES IN MOBILITY AND AGILITY

Mobility and **agility** are affected by the strength of the muscles, flexibility, postural stability, vibratory sensation, cognition, and perceived stability. With aging, changes occur in muscles and joints, particularly those of the back and the legs. Strength and flexibility of muscles and endurance decrease, especially if there is a decrease in activity. Movements and range of motion become more limited and are less fluid, and joints change as the regeneration of tissue slows and muscle wasting occurs. Normal wear and tear reduces the smooth cartilage of joints. Proper management of persistent illnesses and maintenance of healthy lifestyles can forestall the onset of mobility limitations for older persons.

Sarcopenia, a loss of skeletal muscle mass, strength, and function, is thought to be related to aging and contributes to mobility impairments and disability. Sarcopenia is therefore a marker of frailty (Weber et al., 2010). Some gait changes that are thought to be associated with aging include a narrower standing base, wider side-to-side swaying when walking, slower responses, a greater reliance on **proprioception,** diminished arm swing, and increased care in gait. Steps are slower, and there is a decrease in step height (lifting of the foot when taking a step). These changes are less pronounced in people who remain active and at a desirable weight. A sedentary lifestyle, excess weight, and smoking are all associated with mobility problems (Agahi et al., 2016). Health promotion programs to address these factors contribute to improving the mobility and functional status of older persons. Even for frail older persons, exercise and strength training will improve mobility and function (see Chapter 10).

Because of aging and a variety of comorbidities, older persons are vulnerable to becoming immobilized. Various degrees of immobility are often

---

BOX 12.1	Consequences of Immobility

- Dehydration
- Bronchial pneumonia
- Contractures
- Deep venous thrombosis
- Constipation
- Pressure ulcers
- Incontinence
- Hypothermia
- Iatrogenic complications
- Disability
- Institutionalization
- Loss of independence
- Isolation and depression

---

temporary or the permanent consequences of illnesses, falls, and fractures. Immobility, a common problem for older persons in hospital or residing in institutions, can have severe consequences (Box 12.1).

Older people frequently have limited environmental mobility because of a lack of transportation or the loss of their driver's licence. Impairment of mobility is highly associated with poor outcomes and quality of life for older people (Davis et al., 2015). Therefore, the maintenance of mobility and safety for older persons is one of the most important components of gerontological nursing.

DISORDERS AFFECTING MOBILITY

To prevent problems associated with immobility, nurses need to pay special attention to common conditions that accompany the normal changes of aging, as well as to disorders that occur more frequently in older persons. Osteoporosis, gait disorders, Parkinson's disease, stroke, and arthritic conditions markedly affect movement and functional capacities (see Chapter 18). Mobility may also be limited by paresthesias, amputations, neuromotor disturbances, fractures, joint problems, and illnesses that deplete the person's energy.

FALLS

A fall is "an unplanned descent to the floor (or extension of the floor, e.g., trash can or other equipment) with or without injury to the patient" (Lake et al.,

2010). Zecevic et al., (2006) compared the definition of a fall and reasons for falls and concluded that the terms *slips*, *trips*, and *falls* are used interchangeably. It is therefore important to define a fall in words that older persons understand. Unfortunately, falls are a common and often devastating problem for older people and cause a tremendous amount of morbidity and mortality (Ambrose et al. 2013). This section discusses the significance of falls for the older person, the risk factors of falling, and different nursing assessments.

FALLS: A SIGNIFICANT GERIATRIC SYNDROME

Among older persons, falls are the leading cause of death by injury and the most common cause of non-fatal injuries and hospital admissions for trauma (Canadian Institute for Health Information [CIHI], 2017). Approximately 20 to 30% of seniors fall each year (Public Health Agency of Canada [PHAC], 2014). The number of falls of older persons that result in serious injury are increasing dramatically, and falls are a serious public health problem (PHAC, 2014). In Canada, self-reported injuries due to falls have increased by 43% between 2003 and 2010, and the number of deaths due to falls increased by 65% between 2003 and 2008 (PHAC, 2014). In addition, 95% of all hip fractures are directly caused by falls (PHAC, 2014).

In response to rising fall-related sentinel events in health care organizations, several national and international professional organizations and governments have established fall-prevention guidelines based on systematic reviews of research evidence on best practices for working with older persons. The Canadian Public Health Association has engaged community organizations in fall prevention for older persons (Markle-Reid et al., 2015). The Registered Nurses' Association of Ontario (RNAO) developed a Best Practice Guideline, *Prevention of Falls and Fall Injuries in the Older Adult* (RNAO, 2011), that includes practices for addressing education and post-fall prevention. Internationally, one of the most widely adopted guidelines is the American Geriatrics Society's *Guideline for the Prevention of Falls in Older Persons*, prepared in collaboration with the British Geriatrics Society and the American Academy of Orthopaedic Surgeons (American Geriatrics Society

et al., 2001). In addition, most provinces and territories have implemented mandatory reporting of falls that occur in long-term care (LTC) settings.

FACTORS CONTRIBUTING TO FALLS

Falls are a geriatric syndrome and a symptom of a problem or underlying issue, but they become the core of the problem when they occur. The etiology of falls is multifactorial; falls may indicate neurological, sensory, cognitive, medication-related, osteoporotic, or musculo-skeletal problems, or may indicate impending physical illness. The cause of a fall is usually an interaction between an environmental factor, such as a wet floor, and an intrinsic factor, such as limited vision, cognitive impairment, or a gait problem. In health care settings, iatrogenic factors (such as limited staffing), a lack of toileting programs, and the use of restraints and side rails can also interact to increase the risk of falls.

Risk factors for falls can be categorized as intrinsic (person specific) or extrinsic (environmental specific). Some of these risk factors are presented in Table 12.1.

Older persons often have gait patterns that are stiffer and less coordinated (Ambrose et al., 2013). Women with functional impairment and those who take medications are at higher risk for falling than those who are not impaired or who do not take medications. Chronic diseases and periods of symptoms such as vertigo contribute to a high fall risk (Ambrose et al., 2013). In inpatient settings, the most common causes of patient falls are inadequacies in patient assessment and communication, in footwear, and in environmental safety and security (Wolf, 2016). A relationship may exist between urinary tract infections and falls, particularly in LTC residents with dementia (Nicolle, 2016). In addition, insomnia is a fall risk factor for older people in LTC homes who may get out of bed during the night while drowsy (Verdelho & Bentes, 2017).

Even if a fall does not result in injury, it contributes to a loss of confidence that leads to reduced physical activity, increased dependency, and social withdrawal. Fear of falling may restrict an person's life space (the area in which an individual carries on activities) and is an important predictor of general functional decline and a risk factor for future falls. Frequent falls contribute significantly to the downward spiral in frail

TABLE 12.1   Fall Risk Factors for Older Persons

INTRINSIC FACTORS	EXTRINSIC FACTORS
Age	Home environment
Gender	• Cluttered home
Gait	• Loose rugs
Balance	• Poor lighting
Strength	• Lack of
Vision	bathroom safety
Cognition	equipment
Dizziness or vertigo	Footwear
Cardiovascular diseases and	• Slippers that
conditions (orthostatic hypotension,	provide no
hypertension, atrial fibrillation)	support
Medications (polypharmacy,	
psychotropics, diabetic medications,	
NSAIDs, cardiovascular medications)	
Depression	
Dementia	

NSAIDs, Nonsteroidal anti-inflammatory drugs.
Sources: Adapted from Public Health Agency of Canada (PHAC). (2015); Griffith, L., Sohel, N., Walker, K., et al. (2012). Consumer products and fall-related injuries in seniors. *Canadian Journal of Public Health, 103*(5), e332–e337; Ambrose, A. F., Paul, G., Hausdorff, J. M. (2013). Risk factors for falls among older persons: A review of the literature. *Maturitas, 75*(1), 51–61. doi:10.1016/j.maturitas.2013.02.009; Slattum, P. W. & Ansello, E. F. (2013). Case study: Medications as a risk factor in falls by older persons with and without intellectual disabilities. *Activities in Geriatrics and Gerontology Education and Research, 28*(1).

older people (Ambrose et al., 2013). Nursing staff may also contribute to their older patients' fear of falling by telling them not to get up by themselves or by using restrictive devices to keep them from independently moving about (Lane & Harrington, 2011). A more appropriate nursing response would be to assess fall risk and design individual prevention interventions and safety plans that enhance mobility and independence and reduce the risk of falls (RNAO, 2011).

 IMPLICATIONS FOR GERONTOLOGICAL NURSING AND HEALTHY AGING

ASSESSMENT

Comprehensive assessments (with attention to the conditions and situations noted above) and nursing observations of function are essential in assessing fall risk and premobilization safety. Nurses are most likely to have greater opportunities to observe the older persons' functioning, whether in the community or in a health care facility. Older people may be reluctant to share information about falls for fear of losing independence, so gerontological nurses must use judgement and empathy in eliciting information about falls, assuring the person that there are many ways to increase safety and maintain independence.

Assessment is an ongoing and comprehensive process that includes assessments of the older person who is at risk for falls or who has had a fall, the environment and situational circumstances, and the person's knowledge about falls and their prevention (RNAO, 2011).

Assessment of Fall Risk

A variety of instruments for assessing the risk of fall are available. Assessments of fall risk provide general information about a person's risk factors but must be combined with an individual assessment, so that appropriate fall risk-reduction interventions can be developed and modifiable risk factors identified and managed. In addition, any "almost fall" or "near miss" situation needs to be assessed as well, as such an event could have led to a fall.

The Hendrich II Fall Risk Model (Fig. 12.1), an instrument that has been validated with skilled nursing and rehabilitation populations, provides a determination of the risk of falling (Miller, 2008). This determination is based on gender, mental and emotional status, symptoms of dizziness, and known categories of medications that increase risk (Hendrich, 2016). The tool screens for the risk of falls and has been integral to postfall assessments for the prevention of falls (Hendrich, 2016).

The Morse Fall Scale (MFS) (Morse et al., 1989) is widely used in hospitals and other inpatient settings (http://ltctoolkit.rnao.ca/resources/assessment-tools/morse-falls-scale). A rapid and simple method of assessing a patient's likelihood of falling, the MFS consists of six variables that are easy to score and has predictive validity and interrater reliability (Network of Care, n.d.).

The Berg Balance Scale measures balance ability in older people whose balance function is impaired

Hendrich II Fall Risk Model ™

RISK FACTOR	RISK POINTS	SCORE
Confusion/Disorientation/Impulsivity	4	
Symptomatic Depression	2	
Altered Elimination	1	
Dizziness/Vertigo	1	
Gender (Male)	1	
Any Administered Antiepileptics (anticonvulsants): (Carbamazepine, Divalproex Sodium, Ethotoin, Ethosuximide, Felbamate, Fosphenytoin, Gabapentin, Lamotrigine, Mephenytoin, Methsuximide, Phenobarbital, Phenytoin, Primidone, Topiramate, Trimethadione, Valproic Acid)[1]	2	
Any Administered Benzodiazepines:[2] (Alprazolam, Chloridiazepoxide, Clonazepam, Clorazepate Dipotassium, Diazepam, Flurazepam, Halazepam[3], Lorazepam, Midazolam, Oxazepam, Temazepam, Triazolam)	1	
Get-Up-and-Go Test: "Rising from a Chair" If unable to assess, monitor for change in activity level, assess other risk factors, document both on patient chart with date and time.		
Ability to rise in single movement - No loss of balance with steps	0	
Pushes up, successful in one attempt	1	
Multiple attempts but successful	3	
Unable to rise without assistance during test If unable to assess, document this on the patient chart with the date and time.	4	
(A score of 5 or greater = High Risk)	TOTAL SCORE	

© 2013 AHI of Indiana, Inc. All rights reserved. United States Patent No. 7,282,031 and U.S. Patent No. 7,682,308.

Reproduction of copyright and patented materials without authorization is a violation of federal law.

On-going Medication Review Updates:

Levetiracetam (Keppra) was not assessed during the original research conducted to create the Hendrich Fall Risk Model. As an antiepileptic, levetiracetam does have a side effect of somnolence and dizziness which contributes to its fall risk and should be scored (effective June 2010).

The study did not include the effect of benzodiazepine-like drugs since they were not on the market at the time. However, due to their similarity in drug structure, mechanism of action and drug effects, they should also be scored (effective January 2010).

Halazepam was included in the study but is no longer available in the United States (effective June 2010).

FIGURE 12.1 The Hendrich II Fall Risk Model, a fall-risk assessment tool recommended by the Hartford Institute for Geriatric Nursing. © 2012 AHI of Indiana Inc. All Rights Reserved. US Patent Nos. 7, 282, 031 and 7, 682, 308. Federal laws prohibit the replication, distribution or clinical use expressed or implied without written permission from AHI of Indiana, Incorporated.

by assessing the performance of "functional tasks" (American Academy of Health and Fitness, n.d.). It is an effective tool for assessing balance in older persons who have had a stroke (Saso et al., 2016) and is recommended by the RNAO (http://ltctoolkit.rnao.ca/resources/assessment-tools/berg-balance-scale). In the LTC setting, the Minimum Data Set (MDS) calls for information about a history of falls and hip fractures in the previous 180 days, and the fall-related Resident Assessment Protocol provides an excellent overview of fall risk and fall assessment (see Chapter 5).

It is recommended that all persons over 65 years of age be asked at least once a year about falls (Harris & Garcia, 2016) (Table 12.2). A history of falls is an important predictor of future falls, and any older person who reports a fall should be observed with the brief, performance-based Fall Risk Assessment Tool (Tiedemann et al., 2010). The Tinetti balance scale has also been tested and validated to predict fall risk and was found to have 70% sensitivity and 52% specificity, indicating that it is a useful tool for preventative interventions (Raîche et al., 2000; Tinetti, 2003).

An older person who is seen after a fall, who shows abnormalities of gait or balance and impaired performance on any fall risk assessment test, or who has had recurrent falls should have a comprehensive fall evaluation (Box 12.2).

Environmental Assessment

Assessment of home safety and environmental factors should always be included in a comprehensive fall assessment of community-dwelling older persons.

A home safety assessment should include a fall, injury, fire, and crime risk assessment. Older persons with Alzheimer's disease may present with additional risk factors for injuries. Hurley and colleagues (2004) describe a home safety/injury model for persons with Alzheimer's disease and their caregivers. Table 12.3 provides suggestions for assessment of safety in the home environment.

Environmental barriers often discourage ambulation in various settings. In the outside environment, steps and curbs may be too high. Buses, subway trains, elevators, revolving doors, and escalators may move too rapidly for a slower-moving older person to enter and exit comfortably. Thus, the older person may find the interactional world gradually shrinking as a result

of factors that are beyond his or her control. Fortunately, the Canadian government has made a concerted effort to encourage the elimination of environmental barriers for disabled people (e.g., by modifying public transit entrances and exits, sidewalk amenities), and this has had a beneficial effect on older and disabled persons as they negotiate the environment (http://www.mah.gov.on.ca). Accessibility standards can be found on the Canadian Standards Association Group website, (http://www.csagroup.org/).

Assessment After a Fall Has Occurred

Postfall assessments (PFAs) are essential to the prevention of future falls and the implementation of risk-reduction programs, particularly in health care settings. If the older person cannot tell you about the circumstances of the fall, information should be obtained from witnesses. The purposes of the PFA are to identify the underlying cause of the fall and to assist in implementing appropriate individualized risk-reduction interventions (Gillespie et al., 2012). Box 12.3 provides information for a PFA that can be used in health care facilities.

RESTRAINTS

Restraints are "physical, chemical or environmental measures used to control the physical or behavioural activity of a person or a portion of his/her body" (College of Nurses of Ontario, 2017). *Physical restraints* limit a person's movement (for example, bed rails that cannot be opened by the patient) (College of Nurses of Ontario, 2017). *Chemical restraints* use medication, particularly psychotropics, that are given without specific indications, given in excessive doses that affect functioning, used as sole treatment without behavioural interventions, or administered for the convenience of staff. *Environmental restraints* control a person's mobility (e.g., seclusion, a secure unit or garden, or a time-out room.)

Restraints have been used historically for the "protection" of the patient and for the security of the patient and staff. Restraints were used to control the behaviour of individuals with mental illness considered to be dangerous to themselves or others (Evans et al., 2003). Some common reasons for restraining patients were to prevent falls, altered mental status, the patient's harming of self or others, wandering,

TABLE 12.2   Clinical Assessment and Management of Fall Risk for Older Persons

ASSESSMENTS	MANAGEMENT
Circumstances of previous falls*	Changes in environment and activity, to reduce the likelihood of recurrent falls
Medication use • High-risk medications (e.g., benzodiazepines, other sleep medications, antipsychotics, antidepressants, anticonvulsants, or class IA antidysrhythmics)*†‡ • Four or more medications‡	Review and reduction of medications
Vision • Acuity <20/60 • Decreased depth perception • Decreased contrast sensitivity • Cataracts	Ample lighting without glare; avoidance of multifocal glasses while walking; referral to ophthalmologist
Postural blood pressure (after ≥5 minutes supine, immediately after standing, and 2 minutes after standing)‡ ≥20 mm Hg (or ≥20%) drop in systolic pressure, with or without symptoms, either immediately upon standing or after 2 minutes of standing	Diagnosis and treatment of underlying cause if possible; review and reduction of medications; modification of salt restriction; adequate hydration; compensatory strategies (e.g., elevation of head of bed, rising slowly, or dorsiflexion exercises); pressure stockings; pharmacological therapy if previously listed strategies fail
Balance and gait†‡ • Person's report or observation of unsteadiness • Impairment on brief assessment	Diagnosis and treatment of underlying cause if possible; reduction of medications that impair balance; environmental interventions; referral to physiotherapist for assistive devices and for gait and progressive balance training
Targeted neurological examination • Impaired proprioception* • Impaired cognition* • Decreased muscle strength†‡	Diagnosis and treatment of underlying cause if possible; increase in proprioceptive input (with assistive device or appropriate footwear); reduction of medications that adversely affect cognition; caregivers' awareness of cognitive deficits; reduction of environmental risk factors; referral to physiotherapist for gait, balance, and strength training
Targeted musculo-skeletal examination • Legs (joints and range of motion) • Feet*	Diagnosis and treatment of underlying cause if possible; referral to physiotherapist for strength, range of motion, and gait and balance training (and assistive devices); appropriate footwear; referral to podiatrist
Targeted cardiovascular examination† • **Syncope** • Arrhythmia (if known cardiac disease, abnormal electrocardiogram, and/or syncope)	Referral to cardiologist; carotid-sinus massage • Syncope (in the case of syncope)
Evaluation of home hazards (after hospital discharge)†‡	Removal of loose rugs Use of night lights, nonskid bathmats, and stair rails Other interventions as necessary

*Recommendation is based on observational data indicating an association with an increased risk of falls.
†Recommendation is based on one or more randomized controlled trials of a single intervention.
‡Recommendation is based on one or more randomized controlled trials of a multifactorial intervention strategy that included this component.
Source: Tinetti, M. (2003). Clinical practice: Preventing falls in elderly persons. *New England Journal of Medicine, 348*(1), 42–49.

BOX 12.2   Research for Evidence-Informed Practice: Reducing Inpatient Falls in Long-Term Care: Evaluation of the Impact of a Nurse Training Program

Objective: Researchers aimed to reduce long-term care residents' incidence of falls by 25% within 1 year and hoped to reduce any associated adverse outcomes.

Methods: A Plan-Do-Study-Act methodology was used. A nurse training program led by the team and geriatricians supported nurses in using multifactorial fall risk assessment. Each biweekly training session lasted 45 minutes. The program itself lasted for 12 months and included discussions about the definition of a fall and on the assessment, complications, and risk factors of falls. At baseline, residents' incidence of falls was measured before the program started,

and the same data were collected after 12 months.

Findings: Pretraining data showed inadequate fall assessments and high fall incidences of 18.19 +/- 3.46 per 1,000 resident-bed days. After the intervention, the incidence of falls was reduced significantly, to 13.36 +/- 2.89 ($p < 0.001$) per 1,000 resident-bed days.

Conclusion: The training program improved nurses' knowledge of fall risk, risk assessments, and risk implications. The number of falls was significantly reduced during the 1-year period by 34%.

Source: Singh, I., & Okeke, J. (2016). Reducing inpatient falls in a 100% single room elderly care environment: Evaluation of the impact of a systematic nurse training programme on falls risk assessment (FRA). *British Medical Journal Quality Improvement Reports, 5*(1). doi:10.1136/bmjquality.u210921 .w4741.

TABLE 12.3   Assessment and Interventions of the Home Environment for Older Persons

ASSESSMENT	INTERVENTION
Bathroom	
Necessary safety equipment	Use elevated toilet seat, grab bars, nonslip mats.
Difficulty getting in and out of tub	Use bath bench, transfer bench, hand-held shower nozzle, rubber bath mat, hydraulic-lift bath seat.
Water temperature too high	Check water temperature before bath; set hot-water thermostat to 48.8°C or lower. Use a bath thermometer.
Doorway too narrow	Remove door and use curtain; leave wheelchair at door and use walker.
Bedroom	
Rolling bed	Remove wheels; block against wall.
Bed too low	Use leg extensions, blocks, second mattress, adjustable-height hospital bed.
Insufficient lighting	Use bedside light, night light, flashlight attached to walker or cane.
Sliding rugs	Remove; tack down; use rubber–back rugs; use two-sided tape.
Slippery floor	Use nonskid wax, no wax, rubber-soled footwear, indoor-outdoor carpet.
Thick rug edge or doorsill	Install metal strip at edge; remove doorsill; tape down edge.
Need for nighttime calls	Use a bedside phone, cordless phone, intercom, buzzer; Lifeline alert service.
Kitchen	
Open flames and burners	Substitute microwave oven or electrical toaster oven.
Difficult access to items	Place commonly used items in easy-to-reach areas; use adjustable-height counters, cupboards, and drawers.
Hard-to-open refrigerator	Install foot lever.
Difficulty seeing	Use adequate lighting, utensils with brightly coloured handles.

Continued

TABLE 12.3 Assessment and Interventions of the Home Environment for Older Persons—cont'd

ASSESSMENT	INTERVENTION
Living Room	
Chairs are too low or soft or both	Place board under cushion; use pillow or folded blanket to raise seat, blocks or platform under legs, good armrests to push up on, back and seat cushions.
Swivel and rocking chairs	Block motion.
Obstructing furniture	Relocate or remove to clear paths.
Extension cords	Run cords along walls; eliminate unnecessary cords; place cords under sturdy furniture; use power strips with circuit breakers.
Telephone	
Difficult to reach	Use cordless phone; inform friends to let phone ring 10 times; clear path; use answering machine and return call.
Difficult to hear ringing	Use headset, speaker phone.
Difficult to dial numbers	Use preset numbers, large buttons with large numbers on phone, voice-activated dialing.
Steps	
Difficulty managing stairs and steps	Use stair guide or lift, elevator, ramp (permanent, portable, or removable).
No handrails	Install on at least one side.
Loose rugs	Remove or nail down to wooden steps.
Difficult to see	Ensure adequate lighting; mark edge of steps with brightly coloured tape.
Unable to use walker on stairs	Keep a second walker or wheelchair at top or bottom of stairs.
Home Management	
Difficulty managing laundry	Sit on stool to access washer and dryer; have good lighting; fold laundry sitting at table; on stairs, carry laundry in bag; use cart; use a laundry service.
Difficulty managing the mail	Have an easy-to-access mailbox; keep a mail basket on door.
Difficulty managing housekeeping	Assess safety and manageability; use no-bend dust pan, lightweight all-surface sweeper; provide with resources for assistance if needed.
Difficulty controlling thermostat	Mount in accessible location; choose large-print numbers; use remote-controlled thermostat.
Safety	
Difficulty locking doors	Use remote-controlled door lock, door wedge, hook and chain locks.
Difficulty opening door and knowing who is there	Use automatic door openers, lever door handles, intercom at door.
Difficulty opening and closing windows	Install and use lever and crank handles.
Difficulty hearing alarms	Use blinking lights, vibrating surfaces.
Difficulty seeing owing to insufficient lighting	Place lighting 30–60 cm from object being viewed; change bulbs when dim; ensure adequate lighting in stairways and hallways; use night lights.

Source: Modified from Lane, J. P. (1995). Rehabilitation engineering research center on technology evaluation and transfer center for assistive technology, University at Buffalo. *Technology and Disability, 4*(2), 137–148.

BOX 12.3 Post-Fall Assessment

History

Ask the patient for or about the following:

- Description of the fall by the individual or witness
- Individual's opinion of the cause of the fall
- Circumstances of the fall (trip or slip)
- Individual's activity at the time of the fall
- Presence of comorbid conditions, such as a previous stroke, Parkinson's disease, osteoporosis, seizure disorder, sensory deficit, joint abnormalities, depression, or cardiac disease

Medication Review

Ask the patient for the following information:

- Associated symptoms (e.g., chest pain, palpitations, lightheadedness, vertigo, fainting, weakness, confusion, incontinence, or dyspnea)
- Time of day and location of the fall
- Presence of acute illness

Physical Examination

Observe or examine the following:

- Vital signs (postural blood pressure changes, fever, or hypothermia)
- Head and neck (visual impairment, hearing impairment, nystagmus, bruit)
- Heart (arrhythmia or valvular dysfunction)
- Neurological signs (altered mental status, focal deficits, peripheral neuropathy, muscle weakness, rigidity or tremor, and impaired balance)
- Musculo-skeletal signs (arthritic changes; reduced range of motion; podiatric deformities or problems; swelling, redness, or bruises; abrasions; pain on movement; and shortening and external rotation of lower extremities)

Functional Assessment

Observe and inquire about the following:

- Functional gait and balance (rising from a chair, walking, turning, and sitting down)
- Balance test findings, mobility, use of assistive devices or personal assistance, extent of ambulation, use of restraints, and prosthetic equipment used
- Activities of daily living (bathing, dressing, transferring, and toileting)

Environmental Assessment

Look for the following:

- Existing staffing patterns, unsafe practice in transferring, delay in response to call light
- Faulty equipment
- Incorrect use of bed and chair alarms
- Call light not within reach
- Wheelchair and bed unlocked
- Inadequate supervision
- Clutter (walking paths not clear)
- Dim lighting
- Glare
- Uneven flooring
- Wet, slippery floors
- Poorly fitting seating devices
- Inappropriate footwear or eyewear

---

agitation, and interference with treatment. However, in recent years, the use of physical and chemical restraints has come under careful scrutiny, both legal and ethical, and they are now prohibited in some provinces and territories (Ontario Regulation 79/10 [2010]). There is no evidence in the literature of the efficacy of physical restraints in maintaining safety, preventing the disruption of treatment, preventing falls, or controlling behaviour. In fact, research over the past 20 years, primarily in LTC settings, has shown that the practice of physical restraint is ineffective and hazardous (Bleijlevens et al., 2016). Physical restraints, intended to prevent injury, do not protect patients from falling, wandering, or removing tubes and other medical devices. Physical restraints may actually exacerbate many of the problems for which they are used and can cause serious injury as well as emotional and physical problems. Furthermore, research also indicates that physical restraints are associated with higher mortality rates, injurious falls, health care–associated infections, incontinence, contractures, pressure ulcers, agitation, and depression.

Although the prevention of falls is most frequently cited as the primary reason for using restraints, restraints do not prevent serious injury and may even increase the risk of injury and death. Injuries occur as a result of the patient's attempting to remove the restraint or attempting to get out of bed. The most common mechanism of restraint-related death is asphyxiation; that is, the person is suspended by a restraint from a bed or chair, and the ability to inhale is inhibited by gravitational chest compression (Boltz et al., 2016). Restraints are a source of great physical and psychological distress to older persons, and they may intensify agitation and contribute to depression. A significant reduction in restraint use has largely been a result of the combination of research-based clinical evidence, increased knowledge about restraint alternatives, advocacy groups' efforts, and changed standards and regulations in regard to restraints. Restraint-free care is now the standard of practice and an indicator of quality care in all health care settings.

Because of the movement toward freedom from restraints and the promotion of the least restrictive environment, safety plans are essential. Many of the suggestions on safety and fall risk reduction in this chapter can be used to promote a safe and restraint-free environment. Implementing best-practice nursing care in a restraint-free environment calls for the recognition and assessment of physical and psychosocial concerns and for interventions to address those concerns. Consultation with advanced-practice nurses when implementing alternatives to restraints has been most effective (Boltz et al., 2016). Alternative to restraints are presented in Boxes 12.4 and 12.5.

SIDE RAILS

The use of side rails is also coming under scrutiny through nursing research. Historically, side rails have been used to prevent falling from the bed, but careful evaluation has led to discontinuing their use. Side rails are no longer viewed as simply attachments to a patient's bed but are considered restraints accompanied with the concerns discussed above. When side rails impede the person's desired movement or activity, they meet the definition of a restraint. Evaluation of the proper use of side rails before applying them is necessary.

FALL PREVENTION AND REDUCTION

The prevention and reduction of falls consists of eliminating or reducing the risk of physical and psychological harm associated with falls in older people. The most effective programs are often a combination of several interventions.

FALL REDUCTION INTERVENTIONS

Successful approaches to fall risk reduction include education of health care providers about fall risk reduction, multifactorial assessment, and interventions directed at the identified risk factors (Ayton et al., 2017). Fall risk reduction is the shared responsibility of all health care providers caring for older persons. It also calls for the patient (as well as informal and formal caregivers) to be educated in all aspects of environmental hazards and to become aware that falling may be an indication of underlying problems.

The choice of the most appropriate interventions to reduce the risk of falls depends on appropriate assessment at various intervals according to the person's changing condition. Best Practice Guidelines in falls prevention and management can be found at http://ltctoolkit.rnao.ca/clinical-topics/falls-prevention and https://consultgeri.org/geriatric-topics/falls.

The RNAO provides excellent resources on preventing falls in older persons, including the nursing Best Practice Guideline entitled *Prevention of Falls*

BOX 12.4   Alternatives to Using Restraints

- Work with the interprofessional team.
- Lower the bed to the lowest level, or use a bed that is specially designed to be low to the floor.
- Use a concave mattress.
- Use bed boundary markers to mark the edges of the bed (such as mattress bumpers, a rolled blanket, or "swimming noodles" under sheets).

- Place a soft floor mat or mattress by the bed to cushion any falls.
- Use a water mattress to reduce movement to edge of bed.
- Have the person at risk sleep on a mattress on the floor.
- Remove the wheels from the bed.

BOX 12.4   Alternatives to Using Restraints—cont'd

- Clear the floor of debris and excessive furniture, and make sure it is not wet or slippery.
- Place nonskid strips on the floor next to the bed, and ensure nonskid flooring.
- Place the call bell within the person's reach, and make sure the person can use it.
- Provide visual reminders to encourage the person to use the call bell.
- Use night lights in the room and bathroom.
- Use identification bracelets or door signs to identify persons at risk for falling.
- Inform all staff of fall risk, and put fall risk and fall risk–reduction interventions on the person's care plan.
- Involve family and all staff in fall risk–reduction education and activities.
- Assess ambulation ability; refer to physiotherapy for walking, strengthening, or both.
- Have ambulation devices within reach, and make sure the person knows how to use them properly.
- Use bed, chair, or wrist alarms, or use a patient-worn sensor alarm (a position-sensitive, lightweight alarm worn above the knee).
- Keep the person in a supervised area or room within view of the nursing station.
- Check for orthostasis (a systolic drop greater than 20 mm Hg, greater than 10 mm Hg after 2 minutes of standing, or both).

- If the person is able, he or she should walk at every opportunity possible.
- Establish a toileting plan, and take the person to the bathroom frequently.
- Make sure the person knows the location of the bathroom (leave the door open so he or she can see the toilet, or put a picture of a toilet on the door); clear a path to the bathroom.
- Know the person's sleeping patterns—if the person is usually up during the night, get the person up into a chair, and keep him or her at the nursing station.
- Be especially alert at change-of-shift times.
- Understand that very few people spend all day in bed; activity is necessary.
- Provide diversional activities (catalogues, puzzles, busy box).
- Wedge cushions—or materials that promote sitting in an upright position without restraints—into the wheelchair; occupational therapy can be helpful.
- Arrange for a family member or a sitter to be with the person, especially at high-risk times.
- See that the person wears his or her eyeglasses, hearing aids, or dentures.
- Have the person sleep wearing shoes, rubber-soled slippers, or socks with nonskid treads.
- Ensure that pain is well managed.
- Provide a trapeze to enhance mobility in bed.

BOX 12.5   Restraint Alternatives: Tubes, Lines, and Other Medical Devices

- Determine whether the device is really necessary.
- Show and explain the tubes to the patient preoperatively, which may be effective in decreasing anxiety about devices.
- Remove tubes and lines as soon as possible; Foley catheters should be used only if the person needs intensive output monitoring or has an obstruction.
- Use guided exploration and a mirror to help the person understand what is in place and why.
- Provide comfort care to the site (oral and nasal care, anchoring of tubing, topical anaesthetic).
- Consider alternatives (replace intravenous [IV] tubing with heparin lock, deliver medications intramuscularly, subcutaneously); consider intermittent IV administration, hypodermoclysis, or analgesic pumps.

- Use camouflage: clothing or elastic sleeves, a temporary air splint (occupational therapy can be helpful), or skin sleeves to prevent IV tube dislodgement.
- Use diversional activity aprons (zipping and unzipping, threading exercises, dials and knobs), a busy box, or a therapeutic activity kit.
- Hang IV bags behind the person's field of vision.
- Replace a nasogastric (NG) tube with a percutaneous endoscopic gastrostomy (PEG) tube if necessary, but obtain a comprehensive speech therapy swallowing evaluation. If an NG tube is used, use as small a lumen as possible to minimize irritation; consider taping with occlusive dressings.
- Cover the PEG tube or abdominal incisions and other tubes with abdominal binder and sweat pants.
- Use a modified soft collar for tracheotomy protection.

and Fall Injuries in the Older Adult (http://www.rnao
.org). The RNAO (2011) recommends the following
interventions:

- Gait training and correct use of assistive devices
- Medication review (particularly psychotropics)
- Exercise programs that include balance training
- Assessment and treatment of postural hypoten-
sion and cardiovascular disorders
- Environmental hazard modification
- Staff education

EXERCISE

Exercise programs have shown effectiveness in reducing falls and fall-related injuries in older persons
who live in the community (Shier et al., 2016). For
older people, the relationship between exercise and
fall risk reduction is strong, particularly when combined with balance training. Although the best type,
duration, and intensity of exercise have not been
determined, exercise programs must be at least 10
weeks in duration, must be individualized, and must
include balance training for benefit. Group exercises
may also be effective. Further research is needed to
evaluate the effect of exercise in LTC settings, as well
as the effect of other programs, such as tai chi (see
Chapter 10).

ENVIRONMENTAL MODIFICATIONS

Environmental modifications alone have not been
shown to reduce falls, but they may be of benefit in
risk reduction when included as part of a multifactorial program. However, research indicates that a home
safety assessment and modifications to prevent injurious falls could produce considerable health gain and
are highly cost-effective for older people (Pega et al.,
2016).

MEDICATION REVIEW

The reduction of medications is an important component of effective fall-reducing programs in both
community and LTC homes. Medications, including
over-the-counter medications and herbals, should
be reviewed, and only those that are essential should
be used (see Chapter 21). The risk of falls increases
with the use of four or more medications, particularly
antipsychotics and benzodiazepines (both long- and
short-acting).

BEHAVIOUR AND EDUCATION PROGRAMS

Used alone, behaviour and education programs do
not reduce falls, but they are recommended as part of
multifactorial intervention programs. Information on
fall risk factors and risk-reduction strategies should
be provided to older persons, health care providers,
and caregivers. Many excellent sources of information
on interventions to reduce fall risks are available for
both consumers and professionals (see the end of this
chapter).

ASSISTIVE DEVICES

Research on multifactorial interventions, including
the use of assistive devices, has indicated that they
are of benefit in fall risk reduction. It is important
to provide instruction in the correct use of assistive
devices and to supervise their use. Many devices are
designed for specific benefits. When the correct device
is obtained, the older person will need assistance in
learning how to use it correctly; this assistance should
be provided by specialists in occupational therapy or
physiotherapy. Nurses can supervise older persons'
use of assistive devices. Some of these devices can also
be used to facilitate safe transfers from one location
to another; for example, a correctly used walker or a
sit-to-stand device can reduce the risk of falls when
an older person is being transferred from a bed to a
chair or vice versa.

The following principles and recommendations
should be followed when caring for persons who are
using assistive devices:

- Advise the person who is using a cane to do the
following: Place the cane firmly on the ground
before taking a step, and do not place the cane
too far ahead. Put all the weight on the unaffected
leg, and then move the cane and the affected leg
a comfortable distance forward. With the weight
supported by the cane and the affected leg, step
through with the unaffected leg.
- Older persons should always wear low-heeled,
nonskid shoes. It is best to have people wear the
kind of shoes they are accustomed to wearing, and
consideration should be given to properly fitted
orthotic shoes, as appropriate.
- Advise the person to do the following when using a
cane on stairs: Step up with the unaffected leg and
down with the affected leg. Use the cane as support

when lifting the affected leg. Bring the cane up to the step just reached before climbing another step. When descending, place the cane on the next step down, move the affected leg down, and then move the unaffected leg down.

- Advise patient who is using a walker to do the following: Stand upright and lift or roll the walker with both hands a step's length ahead. Lean slightly forward and hold the arms of the walker for support. Step toward it with the weaker leg, and then bring the stronger leg forward. Do not climb stairs with a walker.
- Every assistive device must be adjusted to the individual's height; the top of a cane should align with the crease of the wrist.
- Choose a size and shape of cane handle that fits comfortably in the person's palm; like a tight shoe, it will be a constant irritant if it is not properly fitted.
- Cane tips are most secure when they are flat across the bottom and have a series of concentric rings. Replace tips frequently because they wear out, and a worn tip is insecure.
- Wheelchairs are a necessary adjunct at some level of immobility. General safety tips for preventing fall-related injuries can be applied to both power and manual wheelchairs. Caregivers and wheelchair users need to remember to always lock the brakes of the chair when transferring to or from another location. Inform the user never to reach for an object if he or she has to move to the edge of the seat to reach it. Also, instruct the user not to reach for an object that is on the floor. These actions may cause a fall. It is important that a professional evaluate the wheelchair for proper fit and provide training in its proper and safe use. Often, physiotherapists and occupational therapists can assist in wheelchair mobility programs.
- Discuss safety in regard to the use of motorized scooters or wheelchairs and the use of helmets.

OTHER INTERVENTIONS

Other interventions include assessment and treatment of osteoporosis to reduce fracture rates (see Chapter 18). Older people with osteoporosis are more likely to sustain serious injury from a fall. The use of hip protectors for the prevention of hip fractures in high-risk persons may be considered, but further research is needed to determine their effectiveness (Ferrari et al., 2016). Formal vision assessment is also an important intervention to identify remediable visual problems. Poor visual acuity, reduced contrast sensitivity, decreased visual field, cataracts, and use of nonmiotic glaucoma medications have all been associated with falls. Although there is a significant relationship between visual problems and falls, little research has been done on intervention for visual problems as a part of fall risk-reduction programs.

ENVIRONMENTAL SAFETY

A safe environment is one in which a person is capable (with reasonable caution) of carrying out activities of daily living and instrumental activities of daily living, as well as life-enriching activities, without fear of attack, accident, or imposed interference. It is the responsibility of nurses, other health care team members, and all community members to ensure a safe environment for older individuals. Table 12.3 describes home environment assessments and interventions.

Vulnerability to environmental risks increases as people become less physically or cognitively able to recognize or cope with real or potential hazards. Older persons and their caregivers need to be knowledgeable about risks and interventions to avoid unsafe behaviours and situations.

VULNERABILITY TO ENVIRONMENTAL TEMPERATURES

Given a growing problem with the supply and costs of energy, many older persons are exposed to temperature extremes in their own dwellings. Environmental temperature extremes pose a serious risk to older persons in declining physical health. Preventive measures entail paying attention to impending changes of season, as well as strategies to protect the person from extremes of temperature. Early intervention in extreme temperature exposure is crucial, because excessively high or low body temperatures further impair thermoregulatory function and can be lethal.

Sensorineural changes in thermoregulation diminish the older person's awareness of temperature changes and may impair behavioural and thermoregulatory responses to dangerously high or low environmental temperatures (see Chapter 6). Furthermore, many of the medications taken by older people affect thermoregulation by affecting the ability of blood vessels to vasoconstrict or vasodilate, both of which are thermoregulatory mechanisms. Other medications inhibit neuromuscular activity, suppress metabolic heat generation, or dull awareness (e.g., tranquilizers and pain medications). Alcohol is notorious for inhibiting thermoregulatory function by affecting vasomotor responses in either hot or cold weather.

Combined economic, behavioural, and environmental factors may create a dangerous thermal environment in which older persons are subjected to temperature extremes from which they cannot escape or that they cannot change. Caregivers and family members should be aware that people are vulnerable to temperature extremes if they are unable to shiver, sweat, take in sufficient liquids, move about, put on or take off clothing, adjust bedcovers, or adjust the room temperature. They may also be a lack of control of blood supply to the skin. A temperature that may be comfortable for a young and active person may be too cold or too warm for a frail older person.

Economic conditions often determine whether an older person living in the community can afford air conditioning or adequate heating. Older people are the most vulnerable to adverse health effects due to prolonged heat exposure (Kenney et al., 2014). Global warming will increase the risks of extreme heat–related events in the future; local governments and communities must coordinate their response strategies to protect older persons.

Hyperthermia

When body temperature rises above normal ranges because of environmental or metabolic heat loads, a clinical condition called heat illness, or *hyperthermia,* occurs. Hyperthermia is a temperature-related illness and is classified as a medical emergency. The numerous deaths of older people from high temperature extremes could be almost entirely prevented with education and caution. Most of these problems occur in the homes of people who do not have air conditioning, but older persons who are residing in LTC homes and have multiple physical problems

may be especially vulnerable to high temperatures. Older people with cardiovascular disease, diabetes, or peripheral vascular disease, and those taking certain medications (anticholinergics, antihistamines, diuretics, beta-blockers, antidepressants, or antiparkinsonian medications) are at risk. Instructions on how one can prevent hyperthermia when the ambient temperature exceeds 32°C are presented in Box 12.6.

Hypothermia

Hypothermia is a medical emergency necessitating comprehensive assessment of neurological activity, oxygenation, renal function, and fluid and electrolyte balance. The term "hypothermia" literally means "low heat," but it is used clinically to describe core temperatures below 35°C. A healthy individual exposed to a severely cold environmental condition for a prolonged period will tend to become hypothermic. A person with impaired thermoregulatory ability is left without protection at room temperatures that may be comfortable for a younger person. The more prolonged the exposure or severe the impairment, the less thermoregulatory responses can defend against heat loss.

Older people are particularly predisposed to hypothermia, because the opportunity for heat loss frequently coexists with the decline in heat generation and conservation responses. Such coexistence occurs frequently among persons who are homeless or cognitively impaired, persons injured in falls, and persons with cardiovascular, adrenal, or thyroid dysfunction. Other risk factors include excessive alcohol use, exhaustion, poor nutrition, inadequate housing, and the use of sedatives, anxiolytics, phenothiazines, and tricyclic antidepressants.

Unfortunately, a dulling of awareness accompanies hypothermia, and the person experiencing it rarely recognizes the problem or seeks assistance. For very old and frail persons, environmental temperatures below 18°C may cause a serious drop in core body temperature to 35°C or less. The numerous factors that increase the risk of hypothermia in older persons are listed in Box 12.7.

In normal temperatures, heat in a person is produced in sufficient quantities by the cellular metabolism of food, the friction produced by contracting muscles, and blood flow. Paralyzed or immobile

BOX 12.6 Preventing Hyperthermia

- Keep out of the sun. If your house is cooler than outdoors, stay inside.
- If you must go out into the sun, shade yourself with an umbrella or a wide-brimmed hat that is well ventilated (to allow the sweat on your head to evaporate).
- Drink lots of water. How much water you should drink depends on how much you are sweating.
- If it is sunny, keep the house cooler by pulling down awnings or closing outdoor shutters over your windows, or keep the curtains or blinds closed.
- If the house has two stories, keep the upper-storey windows slightly open, to draw excess heat up and out.
- If the house is hot, try to spend a few hours in an air-conditioned space such as a shopping mall or a cooling centre. Rest in cool shade periodically.
- Take a cool bath or shower.
- At night, if the outdoor temperature is cooler, open all the windows. If you have fans that fit into the windows, use them to bring down the temperature faster.

- Use fans to evaporate sweat and cool the body, but doing so may not be effective or may have the opposite effect if the temperature and humidity are both very high.
- Limit physical activity (especially if you are in an at-risk group), particularly during the middle of the day, when the heat is greatest.
- Avoid liquids that are high in sugar or alcohol, as they can increase the amount of water lost by the body.
- Consider taking in extra salt if you experience heat cramps, if so advised by your doctor, or if you have to work in the heat and are sweating a lot (even though most people's diets contain enough salt to make up for losses in sweat).
- Ask your doctor or pharmacist about the possible side effects of any medications you take during periods of extreme heat.
- Offer to help and check up on your neighbours, especially those who may be on their own and who may not be in a position to take these precautions.

Source: Adapted from Health Canada. (2011). *Extreme heat events guidelines: Technical guide for health care workers.* Ottawa, ON: Water, Air and Climate Change Bureau, Healthy Environments and Consumer Safety Branch, Health Canada. Retrieved from http://www.psno.ca/uploads/1/0/1/9/10197937/extremeheateventguidelines-technicalguide_000.pdf.

BOX 12.7 Factors That Increase the Risk of Hypothermia in Older Persons

Thermoregulatory Impairment
- Failure to vasoconstrict promptly on exposure to cold
- Failure to sense cold
- Failure to respond behaviourally to protect oneself against cold
- Diminished or absent shivering to generate heat
- Reduced cold-induced metabolic heat production

Conditions That Decrease Heat Production
- Hypothyroidism, hypopituitarism, hypoglycemia, malnutrition
- Immobility or decreased activity (e.g., stroke, paralysis, parkinsonism, dementia, arthritis, fractured hip, coma)
- Diabetic ketoacidosis

Conditions That Increase Heat Loss
- Open wounds, generalized inflammatory skin conditions, burns

Conditions That Impair Central or Peripheral Control of Thermoregulation
- Stroke, brain tumour, Wernicke's encephalopathy, subarachnoid hemorrhage
- Uremia, neuropathy (e.g., diabetes, alcoholism)
- Acute illness (e.g., pneumonia, sepsis, myocardial infarction, congestive heart failure, pulmonary embolism, pancreatitis)

Medications That Interfere With Thermoregulation
- Tranquilizers (e.g., phenothiazines)
- Sedative-hypnotics (e.g., barbiturates, benzodiazepines)
- Antidepressants (e.g., tricyclics)
- Vasoactive medications (e.g., vasodilators)
- Alcohol (causes superficial vasodilation; may interfere with carbohydrate metabolism and judgement)
- Others medications (e.g., methyldopa, lithium, morphine)

Source: Adapted from Mallet, M. L. (2002). Pathophysiology of accidental hypothermia. *Oxford Journals of Medicine, 95*(12), 775–785; National Collaborating Centre for Environmental Health. (2010). *Drugs.* Retrieved from http://www.ncceh.ca/en/major_projects/heat_advice/drugs.

persons are unable to generate significant heat by muscle activity and become cold even at normal room temperatures. It is important to closely monitor body temperature in older people. When exposed to cold temperatures, older people with some degree of thermoregulatory impairment are at high risk for hypothermia if they undergo surgery, are injured in a fall or accident, or are lost or left unattended in a cool place. Persons who are emaciated and have poor nutritional status lack insulation and fuel for metabolic heat-generating processes, so they may be chronically hypothermic. Box 12.8 lists factors and

---

BOX 12.8   Factors Associated With Low Body Temperature in Older Persons

Aging
- Increased risk of thermoregulatory dysfunction
- Increased risk of acute and persistent conditions that predispose to hypothermia

Low Environmental Temperature
- Increased risk of hypothermia if lower than 18°C

Thinness and Malnutrition
- Less thermal insulation and higher ratios of surface area to volume in very thin people
- Decreased metabolic rate (by 20–30%) if malnutrition is prolonged

Poverty
- Inadequate clothing, low environmental temperature
- Increased risk of thinness and malnutrition
- Secondary to poor housing conditions and inadequate heat

Living Alone
- Associated with poverty, delayed detection of hypothermia, and delayed rescue if person falls

Nocturia and Night Rising
- Associated with falls; if rescue is delayed, hypothermia may develop as heat is conducted away from the body to the cold floor

Orthostatic Hypotension
- Indicates autonomic nervous system impairment; dizziness and postural instability are associated with falls

Source: Worfolk, J. B. (1997). Keep frail elders warm. *Geriatric Nursing, 18*(1), 7–11.

---

situations that may induce low basal body temperatures in older people.

 IMPLICATIONS FOR GERONTOLOGICAL NURSING AND HEALTHY AGING

Recognition of the clinical signs and severity of hyperthermia and hypothermia is an important nursing responsibility; nurses are responsible for keeping frail older people comfortable and for preventing these problems. It is important to closely monitor body temperature in older people and to pay particular attention to both lower and higher readings as compared with a person's baseline. The potential risk of hypothermia makes prevention important and early recognition vital.

Detecting hyperthermia and hypothermia among home-dwelling older people is sometimes difficult (unlike detection in the clinical setting) because no one measures body temperature. For persons exposed to low temperatures in the home or outdoors, confusion and disorientation may be the first overt signs of hypothermia. As his or her judgement becomes clouded, the person may remove clothing or fail to seek shelter, and hypothermia can progress to profound levels. For this reason, regular contact with home-dwelling older people during cold or hot weather with extreme temperatures is crucial. Persons with pre-existing alterations in thermoregulatory ability should be monitored even in mildly cool weather. Specific interventions to prevent hypothermia are shown in Box 12.9.

TRANSPORTATION

Even though an older person might be physically able to move about, there may be many hindrances to that person's full use of public space. Available transportation is critical to the ability of older people to remain independent and functional. The lack of accessible transportation may contribute to other problems, such as social withdrawal, poor nutrition, or the neglect of health care. A "crisis in mobility" exists for many older people because of the lack of an automobile, an inability to drive, limited access to public transportation, health factors, geographical location,

BOX 12.9 Nursing Interventions to Prevent Hypothermia in Frail Older People

Desired Outcomes
- Hands and limbs warm
- Body relaxed, not curled
- Body temperature >36°C
- No shivering
- No complaints of cold

Interventions
- Maintain a comfortably warm ambient temperature no lower than 18°C. Many frail older people will require much higher temperatures.
- Provide generous quantities of clothing and bed covers. Layer the clothing and bed covers for best insulation. Be careful not to judge the person's needs by how you feel working in a warm environment.
- Limit the time the person sits by cold windows.
- Provide a head covering whenever possible—in bed, out of bed, and particularly outdoors.
- Cover the person well during bathing. The standard covering—a light bath blanket over the naked body—is not enough protection for a frail older person.
- Cover a naked person with heavy blankets for transfer to and from showers; dry the person quickly and thoroughly before leaving shower room; cover the person's head with a dry towel or hood while wet.
- Dry wet hair quickly with warm air from an electric dryer; never allow the hair of a frail older person to air-dry.
- Use absorbent pads for incontinence rather than allowing urine to wet large areas of clothing, sheets, and bed covers.
- Provide the person with as much exercise as possible to generate heat from muscle activity.
- Provide hot high-protein meals and bedtime snacks to add heat and sustain heat production throughout the day and as far into the night as possible.

Source: Worfolk, J. B. (1997). Keep frail elders warm. *Geriatric Nursing, 18*(1), 7–11.

or economic considerations. Culturally and ethnically diverse older people and rural residents may experience more difficulty getting around.

Older persons may desire increased contact with friends and relatives. Even more crucial is the need to reach medical services, shopping areas, and service agencies. If mobility is hampered, both security and the sense of belonging to the mainstream of society

may be blocked. The emphasis on a "barrier-free" (structurally revised) transportation system and reduced fares has been helpful to many older people, but some cannot avail themselves of public transportation because of physical disability or residence in a high-crime area.

Many provinces and territories provide subsidized transportation to help older people reach social services, nutrition sites, health services, emergency or medical care facilities, recreational centres, mental health services, adult day programs, physical and vocational rehabilitation centres, continuing education classes, and library services. Although transportation can often be found for special needs (e.g., to attend health care appointments), transportation for pleasure or recreation may be virtually impossible to find. Senior centres offer a wide range of activities for older people, as well as transportation services. Nurses can refer older people to local services and aging-related organizations for information on resources and financial assistance.

DRIVING

Driving is one of the instrumental activities of daily living for most older people, because it is often essential for obtaining necessities. Yet, driving is a highly complex activity that requires a variety of visual, motor, and cognitive skills (Mathias & Lucas, 2009). Assessments of functional capacities often neglect this important activity. Giving up driving is a major loss for an older person in regard to independence, pleasure, and feelings of competence and self-worth. Giving up driving has been associated with decreased social integration, fewer out-of-home activities, increased depressive and anxiety symptoms, decreased quality of life, and a greater risk of being placed in an LTC facility (Carr & Ott, 2010; Siren & Hakamies-Blomqvist, 2009). Many older people depend on driving to obtain basic needs, and the inability to drive can cause depression and isolation. For many, alternate transportation is not readily available; consequently, they may continue driving beyond the time at which it becomes unsafe.

Age-related changes in driving skills—vision changes, cognitive impairment, and various medical illnesses and functional impairments—are all factors related to driving safety for older persons.

The procedures and regulations for driver's licence renewal vary across the country and may include repeated renewal, renewal in person rather than electronically or by mail, and vision and road tests.

The issue of older people driving is the subject of a great deal of public discussion (Ackerman et al., 2011). Many older drivers and their families struggle with issues and conversations related to continued safety in driving.

Older drivers typically drive fewer miles than younger drivers do, and they tend to drive less at night, less in adverse weather conditions, and less in congested areas. Generally, they choose familiar routes, and fewer older drivers speed or drive after drinking alcohol than do drivers of other ages. However, when compared with younger age groups, older people have more accidents per mile driven, and older drivers and passengers are three times more likely than younger people to die after a motor vehicle crash. The leading cause of injury-related death among drivers 65 to 74 years of age is motor vehicle accidents; for those older than 75 years of age, motor vehicle accidents are the second leading cause of death, after falls (Hooyman & Kiyak, 2011). Age-related changes—including vision changes, cognitive impairment, and various medical illnesses and functional impairments—are safety factors for older persons.

IMPLICATIONS FOR GERONTOLOGICAL NURSING AND HEALTHY AGING

Gerontological nurses should encourage open discussions about driving with the older person and his or her family, should identify impairments that affect driving, correct these when possible, and offer alternatives for transportation. Vehicle modifications, sensory aids, driving training for older persons, and driving assessment programs are helpful in promoting safe driving.

Driving evaluations can help determine if an older person's driving ability is affected (Canadian Association of Occupational Therapists [CAOT], n.d.). Evaluations of older persons include a screening evaluation and an on-road evaluation. The clinical evaluation consists of the following:

- Visual screening, to check if a person's eyes meet the standards for driving, the person's ability to move the eyes, the person's ability to judge distance, and the person's peripheral vision.
- Movement and strength assessment, to ascertain whether the person's arms and legs have enough movement and strength to control all features of the car. The need for adaptive equipment is also assessed.
- Perceptual and cognitive screening, to measure the person's reaction time. Screening includes other tests to assess the person's memory, problem-solving ability, and interpretation of what is seen.

The on-road evaluation involves assessing the following:

- Physical skill and endurance to drive and navigate the vehicle
- Awareness of and ability to identify potential hazards
- Efficiency with which the eyes move to take in necessary information
- Responses to traffic environments

KEY CONCEPTS

- Mobility provides opportunities for exercise, exploration, and pleasure, and is crucial to maintaining independence.
- Ease of mobility is thought to be the most visible measure of overall health and capacity for survival.
- Changes with aging in bones, muscles, and ligaments affect balance and gait and increase instability.
- Gait disorders are often an obvious index of systemic problems and should be investigated thoroughly.
- A thorough nursing assessment must include assessment of fall risk, balance, and gait, as well as intrinsic, extrinsic, and iatrogenic factors.
- Fall risk–reduction interventions are among the most important proactive measures for preserving the health and functioning of the older person.
- Physical restraints have numerous negative consequences for the health and well-being of the older person. Restraint-free care, fall risk–reduction interventions, and a safe environment are essential to the best care.

- Transportation for the older person is critical to physical, psychological, and social health.

ACTIVITIES AND DISCUSSION QUESTIONS

1. Put your shoes on the wrong feet, then ask another student to analyze your gait.
2. Wear eyeglasses (or borrow a pair from someone), then walk up and down a flight of stairs.
3. Evaluate the safety of your living quarters, using Table 12.3 as a guide.
4. Discuss your activities that increase your vulnerability to falls.
5. Discuss falls you have had and their consequences. Consider how it might have been different if you were 80 years old.
6. Obtain a wheelchair and sit in it for 20 minutes with a restraining belt around your waist. Discuss your feelings with a partner. Reverse the process with your partner.
7. Discuss the risks for hypothermia and strategies for its prevention.
8. Discuss why the nurse might need to ensure safety for an older person in hospital, and identify several alternative measures that might be appropriate for ensuring the person's safety.
9. Explore the transportation options in the person's community, and discuss how these may help or interfere with the older person's independence and opportunities for social engagement.

RESOURCES

Canadian Automobile Association (CAA). *Seniors driving* *https://www.caa.ca/seniors/*

CSA Group (Canadian safety standards) *http://www.csagroup.org/*

Health Canada (2011). *Extreme heat events guidelines: Technical guide for health care workers* *http://www.psno.ca/uploads/1/0/1/9/10197937/ extremeheateventguidelines-technicalguide_000.pdf*

National Institute for Health and Care Excellence. *Falls in older people: Assessing risk and prevention* *https://www.nice.org.uk/guidance/cg161*

Older Driver Safety *http://www.olderdriversafety.ca/*

Public Health Agency of Canada (PHAC). *Seniors falls in Canada: Second report* *https://www.canada.ca/en/public-health/services/health -promotion/aging-seniors/publications/publications -general-public/seniors-falls-canada-second-report.html*

Public Health Agency of Canada (PHAC). *The safe living guide—A guide to home safety for seniors* *https://www.canada.ca/en/public-health/services/health -promotion/aging-seniors/publications/publications -general-public/safe-living-guide-a-guide-home-safety -seniors.html*

Registered Nurses' Association of Ontario (RNAO). *Prevention of falls and fall injuries in the older adult* *http://rnao.ca/sites/rnao-ca/files/Prevention_of_Falls _and_Fall_Injuries_in_the_Older_Adult.pdf*

Scott, V. (2007). *World Health Organization Report: Prevention of falls in older age. Falls prevention: Policy, research and practice* *http://www.who.int/ageing/projects/5.Intervention, %20policies%20and%20sustainability%20of%20falls %20prevention.pdf*

Scott, V., Peck, S., & Kendall, P. (2004). *Prevention of falls and injuries among the elderly: A special report from the Office of the Provincial Health Officer* *http://www.health.gov.bc.ca/library/publications/year/ 2004/falls.pdf*

Veterans Affairs Canada. *Falls prevention* *http://www.veterans.gc.ca/eng/services/health/promotion/ fallsp*

For additional resources, please visit *http:// evolve.elsevier.com/Canada/Ebersole/gerontological/*

REFERENCES

Ackerman, M. L., Crowe, M., Vance, D. E., et al. (2011). The impact of feedback on self-rated driving ability and driving self-regulation among older adults. *The Gerontologist*, *51*(3), 367–378. doi:10.1093/geront/gnq082.

Agahi, N., Fors, S., Fritzell, J., et al. (2016). Smoking and physical inactivity as predictors of mobility impairment during late life: Exploring differential vulnerability across education level in Sweden. *The Journals of Gerontology. Series B, Psychological Sciences and Social Sciences*, gbw090. doi:10.1093/geronb/gbw090.

American Academy of Health and Fitness. (n.d.). *Berg Balance Scale.* Retrieved from http://www.aahf.info/pdf/Berg_Balance _Scale.pdf.

American Geriatrics Society, British Geriatrics Society, & American Academy of Orthopaedic Surgeons. (2001). Guideline for the prevention of falls in older persons. *Journal of the American Geriatrics Society, 49*(5), 664–672. doi:10.1046/j.1532-5415 .2001.49115.x.

Ambrose, A. F., Paul, G., & Hausdorff, J. M. (2013). Risk factors for falls among older adults: A review of the literature. *Maturitas, 75*(1), 51–61. doi:10.1016/j.maturitas.2013.02.09.

Ayton, D. R., Barker, A. L., Morello, R. T., et al. (2017). Barriers and enablers to the implementation of the 6-PACK falls prevention program: A pre-implementation study in hospitals participating in a cluster randomised controlled trial. *PLoS ONE, 12*(2), e0171932. doi:10.1371/journal.pone.0171932.

Bleijlevens, M. H., Wagner, L. M., Capezuti, E., et al. (2016). Physical restraints: Consensus of a research definition using a modified delphi technique. *Journal of the American Geriatrics Society, 64*(11), 2307–2310. doi:10.1111/jgs.14435.

Boltz, M., Capezuti, E., Fulmer, T. T., et al. (Eds.), (2016). *Evidence-based geriatric nursing protocols for best practice.* New York: Springer Publishing Company.

Canadian Association of Occupational Therapists (CAOT). (n.d.). *What is included in a driving evaluation?* Retrieved from http:// www.olderdriversafety.ca/consumer/safe_driving_strategies/ index.html.

Canadian Institute for Health Information (CIHI). (2017). *Preventing falls: Improving the health and quality of life of Canadians.* Retrieved from https://www.cihi.ca/en/health-system -performance/quality-of-care-and-outcomes/patient-safety/ preventing-falls-improving-the.

Carr, D. B., & Ott, B. R. (2010). The older adult driver with cognitive impairment: "It's a very frustrating life." *JAMA: The Journal of the American Medical Association, 203*(16), 1632–1641. doi:10.1001/jama.2010.481.

College of Nurses of Ontario. (2017). *Practice Standard: Restraints.* Retrieved from: https://www.cno.org/globalassets/docs/prac/ 41043_restraints.pdf.

Davis, J. C., Bryan, S., Best, J. R., et al. (2015). Mobility predicts change in older adults' health-related quality of life: Evidence from a Vancouver falls prevention prospective cohort study. *Health and Quality of Life Outcomes, 13*, 101. doi:10.1186/ s12955-015-0299-0.

Evans, D., Wood, J., & Lambert, L. (2003). Patient injury and physical restraint devices: a systematic review. *Journal of Advanced Nursing, 41*(3), 274–282. doi:10.1046/j.1365-2648.2003.02501.x.

Ferrari, S., Reginster, J. Y., Brandi, M. L., et al. (2016). Unmet needs and current and future approaches for osteoporotic patients at high risk of hip fracture. *Archives of Osteoporosis, 11*(1), 37. doi:10.1007/s11657-016-0292-1.

Gillespie, L. D., Robertson, M. C., Gillespie, W. J., et al. (2012). Interventions for preventing falls in older people living in the community. *The Cochrane Database of Systematic Reviews*, (11), CD007146, doi:10.1002/14651858.CD007146.pub3.

Griffith, L., Sohel, N., Walker, K., et al. (2012). Consumer products and fall-related injuries in seniors. *Canadian Journal of Public Health, 103*(5), e332–e337. Retrieved from http://www.jstor.org/ stable/canajpublheal.103.5.e332.

Harris, P., & Garcia, M. B. (2016). To fall is human: Falls, gait, and balance in older adults. In *New directions in geriatric medicine* (pp. 71–90). New York: Springer International Publishing.

Hendrich. (2016). *Fall risk assessment for older adults: The Hendrich II Risk Model.* Retrieved from https://consultgeri.org/try-this/ general-assessment/issue-8.pdf.

Hooyman, N., & Kiyak, H. (2011). *Social gerontology: A multidisciplinary perspective.* Boston, MA: Pearson Education.

Hurley, A., Gauthier, A., Horvath, K., et al. (2004). Promoting safer home environments for persons with Alzheimer's disease: The home safety/injury model. *Journal of Gerontological Nursing, 30*(6), 43–51.

Kenney, W. L., Craighead, D. H., & Alexander, L. M. (2014). Heat waves, aging, and human cardiovascular health. *Medicine & Science in Sports & Exercise, 46*(10), 1891–1899. doi:10.1249/ MSS.0000000000000325.

Lake, E. T., Shang, J., Klaus, S., et al. (2010). Patient falls: Association with hospital magnet status and nursing unit staffing. *Research in Nursing & Health, 33*(5), 413–425. doi:10.1002/ nur.20399.

Lane, J. P. (1995). Rehabilitation engineering research center on technology evaluation and transfer center for assistive technology, University at Buffalo. *Technology and Disability, 4*(2), 137–148.

Lane, J., & Harrington, A. (2011). The factors that influence nurses' use of physical restraint: A thematic literature review. *International Journal of Nursing Practice, 17*(2), 195–204.

Markle-Reid, M. F., Dykeman, C. S., Reimer, H. D., et al. (2015). Engaging community organizations in falls prevention for older adults: Moving from research to action. *Canadian Journal of Public Health, 106*(4), 189–196. doi:10.17269/cjph.106.4776.

Mathias, J. L., & Lucas, L. K. (2009). Cognitive predictors of unsafe driving in older drivers: A meta-analysis. *International Psychogeriatrics, 21*(4), 637–653. doi:10.1017/S1041610209009119.

Miller, C. (2008). *Nursing for wellness in older adults.* Philadelphia: Lippincott Williams & Wilkins.

Morse, J., Morse, R., & Tylko, S. (1989). Development of a scale to identify the fall-prone patient. *Canadian Journal of Aging, 8*(4), 336–377. Retrieved from https://www.researchgate.net/profile/ Janice_Morse/publication/7105715_The_modified_Morse_ Fall_Scale/links/548494430cf283750c370838.pdf.

Network of Care. (n.d.). *Morse Fall Scale.* Retrieved from http:// www.networkofcare.org/library/Morse%20Fall%20Scale.pdf.

Nicolle, L. E. (2016). Urinary tract infections in the older adult. *Clinics in Geriatric Medicine, 32*(3), 523–538. doi:10.1016/ j.cerg.2016.03.002.

Ontario Regulation 79/10. (2010). *Long-term care homes act, 2007.* Retrieved from http://www.e-laws.gov.on.ca/html/source/regs/ english/2010/elaws_src_regs_r10079_e.htm#BK132.

Pega, F., Kvizhinadze, G., Blakely, T., et al. (2016). Home safety assessment and modification to reduce injurious falls in community-dwelling older adults: Cost-utility and equity analysis. *Injury prevention*, *22*(6), 420–426. doi:10.1136/injuryprev-2016-041999.

Public Health Agency of Canada (PHAC). (2014). *Seniors' falls in Canada: Second report*. Retrieved from https://www.canada.ca/en/public-health/services/health-promotion/aging-seniors/publications/publications-general-public/seniors-falls-canada-second-report.html.

Raîche, M., Hébert, R., Prince, F., et al. (2000). Screening older adults at risk of falling with the Tinetti balance scale. *The Lancet*, *356*(9234), 1001–1002. doi:10.1016/S0140-6736(00)02695-7.

Registered Nurses Association of Ontario (RNAO). (2011). *Prevention of falls and fall injuries in the older adult*. Retrieved from http://rnao.ca/sites/rnao-ca/files/Prevention_of_Falls_and_Fall_Injuries_in_the_Older_Adult.pdf.

Saso, A., Moe-Nilssen, R., Gunnes, M., et al. (2016). Responsiveness of the Berg balance scale in patients early after stroke. *Physiotherapy Theory and Practice*, *32*(4), 251–261. doi:10.3109/09593985.2016.1138347.

Shier, V., Trieu, E., & Ganz, D. A. (2016). Implementing exercise programs to prevent falls: Systematic descriptive review. *Injury Epidemiology*, *3*(1), 16. doi:10.1186/s4021-016-0081-8.

Siren, A., & Hakamies-Blomqvist, L. (2009). Mobility and wellbeing in old age. *Topics in Geriatric Rehabilitation*, *25*(1), 3–11. doi:10.1097/TGR.0b013e31819147bf.

Tiedemann, A., Lord, S. R., & Sherrington, C. (2010). The development and validation of a brief performance-based fall risk tool for use in primary care. *Journals of Gerontology*, *65A*(8), 896–903. doi:10.1093/gerona/glq067.

Tinetti, M. E. (2003). Clinical practice. Preventing falls in elderly persons. *New England Journal of Medicine*, *348*(1), 42–49. Retrieved from http://www.medicine.emory.edu/ger/bibliographies/geriatrics/bibliography45_files/Preventing_Falls_in_the_Elderly_Persons.pdf.

Verdelho, A., & Bentes, C. (2017). Insomnia in dementia: A practical approach. In *Neuropsychiatric symptoms of cognitive impairment and dementia* (pp. 263–277). Gewerbestrasse, Switzerland: Springer International Publishing.

Weber, J., Gillain, S., & Petermans, J. (2010). Sacropenia: A physical marker of frailty. *Revue Medicale de Laige*, *65*(9), 514–520.

Wolf, L. (2016). *Balancing the complexity of patient falls: Implementing quality improvement and human factors/ergonomics and systems engineering strategies in healthcare* (Doctoral dissertation, Loughborough University).

Zecevic, A., Salmoni, A., Speechley, N., et al. (2006). Defining a fall and reasons for falling: Comparisons among the views of seniors, health care providers, and the research literature. *The Gerontologist*, *46*(3), 367–376. Retrieved from https://academic.oup.com/gerontologist/article/46/3/367/565294.

LEARNING OBJECTIVES

Upon completion of this chapter, the reader will be able to:

- Discuss the advantages of using standardized assessment tools in gerontological nursing.
- Contrast different formats used to collect assessment data.
- Describe the range of tools used in a comprehensive gerontological assessment.
- Begin to develop the skills needed to select an evidence-informed and appropriate tool for a specific assessment situation and use it correctly.
- Identify key components of assessing older persons.

GLOSSARY

Activities of daily living (ADLs) Those tasks necessary to maintain one's health and basic personal needs.

Instrumental activities of daily living (IADLs) Those tasks necessary to maintain one's home and independent living, such as shopping, cooking, managing medications, using the phone, doing housework,

driving or using public transportation, and managing finances.

Report by proxy One person (the proxy) answering questions or providing information for another person, based on the first person's knowledge of the second person.

THE LIVED EXPERIENCE

"After 2 months in [large rehab facility] I could not stay any longer, so they ship you home. But before they ship you home, they want to have somebody out here that's going to take over and look after you. They couldn't find anyone. So, I came home with nothing. I called several agencies. But I could not get anyone; they did not service this area. They couldn't help me. After 6 weeks, I found someone from Red Cross who came and gave me a shower. And they did that for once a week for 10 weeks. But after 10 weeks, I was on my own again. Then I went to my Dr. and he asked me what I did for therapy. I said 'Nothing". He said "that is ridiculous," so he got on the phone with someone and then they called me from a community hospital that I should go there on Wednesday. But I have no way of getting all the way there. It's difficult being on your own.

A 70-year-old woman who had a stroke

ASSESSING OLDER PERSONS

One of the most important functions of gerontological nurses is to conduct skilled and detailed assessments of the older person. Assessment of older

persons is different from assessment of younger adults in that it is more complex and detailed and takes longer to complete. Comprehensive assessments are usually performed by a nurse-led interprofessional health care team. A gerontological assessment has a number of components, including the collection of physical data as well as the integration of biological, psychosocial, cognitive, and functional information.

GERONTOLOGICAL ASSESSMENT

Assessing the older person requires the nurse to listen patiently, allow for pauses, ask questions that are not often asked, obtain data from all available sources, and recognize the normal changes of aging (see Chapter 6). Furthermore, the assessment of older persons takes more time because of the increased medical and social complexity and must be paced according to the stamina of the person. Both the quality of the assessment and the time required to complete the assessment depend on the nurse's experience. Novice nurses should neither expect nor be expected to perform assessments proficiently, but the skills and information they acquire will increase over time. According to Benner (1984), assessment is a task for the expert. However, by following some basic guidelines and learning how to use select assessment tools, nurses at all skill levels can obtain reasonably reliable data.

Over the years, nurses and others have developed tools to facilitate and standardize the collection of assessment data. (A number of the tools used in the gerontological setting are presented in this chapter.) The use of these tools increases the likelihood of obtaining more reliable data. Data collection is followed by data analysis and identifying priority nursing diagnoses. The nursing diagnoses provide the basis for selecting nursing interventions to address the person's needs.

Assessments are conducted in every nursing setting. In most settings, a standardized electronic format is routinely used. For example, the Minimum Data Set is a standardized comprehensive geriatric assessment and is mandatory in most Canadian long-term care homes, rehabilitation settings, and home care settings (see Chapter 5). Which assessments are completed depends on both the setting and the purpose of the assessment. Some tools are derived directly from the gerontological literature; other tools are modified to meet the particular needs of the older person in a particular setting.

DATA COLLECTION

Three approaches are used for collecting assessment data: self-report, **report by proxy**, and observation.

In the self-report approach, the person verbally answers direct questions (or responds to written questions) about his or her health status. Often, the person's ability to self-report is overestimated.

In the report-by-proxy approach, information is obtained indirectly by the nurse's asking another person (such as a spouse, child, or caregiver) to report his or her observations. This approach is used when a person who is cognitively impaired requires an assessment, but it tends to underestimate the older person's abilities and health.

In the observational approach, the nurse collects and records the data as observed. Physical examination and performance-based functional assessment are examples of observational measures. Observation is probably the most accurate data collection method, but it is limited in that it presents only a snapshot in time.

Regardless of the type or format of the tool used, the following guidelines should be observed:

- Collect the data at a time when the older person is at his or her best whenever possible.
- Use standardized tools correctly; training may be required.
- Do not direct the way the question is answered, to avoid biasing the response; novice nurses need to ask questions in a way that avoids bias.
- Obtain more information only if necessary to complete the assessment.
- Ask more-personal questions—such as questions about sexual functioning—in a sensitive manner.
- Record responses accurately, using the person's own words where possible; do not analyze data while they are being collected. (For example, if the person says, "I have a runny nose," do not record "Patient has a cold" until the analysis of the data is completed.)

Ideally, assessment tools should be used to gather baseline data before the older person has a health crisis. Periodically, the person can be reassessed with the same tools. For example, a person with an altered mental status as a result of illness or medication should be reassessed when the underlying problem has been resolved.

HEALTH ASSESSMENT

HEALTH HISTORY

The initiation of the health history marks the beginning of the nurse-patient relationship and the assessment process. This assessment begins with a review of what the person reports as the problem, known as the "chief complaint"; this is considered to be objective information recorded in the person's own words. With an older person, the complaint is likely to be vague or less straightforward (for example, "I don't feel well").

The health history is best collected verbally during a face-to-face interview or by using the interview to review a written history completed by the person or the person's proxy beforehand; the latter method is usually faster. If the older person has limited proficiency in the language in which the interview is conducted, a trained interpreter is needed, and the interview will generally take about twice as long.

Any health history form or interview plan should include a profile, past medical history, review of symptoms and systems, medication history (prescribed and over-the-counter products such as herbals and dietary supplements), family history, and social history. The social history includes information about the person's living arrangements, economic resources to meet current health-related or food expenses, amount of support, community resources, and other social determinants of health. The health history also includes information on the person's functional status as measured by observation, self-report, or report by proxy.

When a more comprehensive assessment is indicated, additional information is collected on the person's cognitive and functional abilities, psychological well-being, caregiver support or burden, and patterns of health and health care. Areas frequently not addressed by the nurse or mentioned by the older person include sexual dysfunction, depression, incontinence, alcoholism, hearing loss, memory loss, and confusion. See Chapter 24 for a discussion of the assessment of alcohol use and misuse. Although not usually conducted by a nurse, a driving assessment may be recommended (see Chapter 12).

PHYSICAL ASSESSMENT

The next step in the health assessment is the physical assessment, which includes the evaluation of vital signs, mobility, and laboratory results. The techniques used in the physical examination apply to any age group. However, because of the complexity of older persons, head-to-toe examination is more difficult with older persons and can be burdensome for them. When performing a physical assessment, gerontological nurses must be able to quickly determine what information is most necessary (based on the chief complaint) and then work from there. When the chief complaint is unknown because of communication challenges (e.g., dementia or aphasia), a more thorough assessment is necessary.

A number of excellent tools have been developed specifically for assessing older persons who are frail, who exhibit signs or symptoms of common conditions, or who manifest both. Several tools are discussed or referred to in this chapter; however, these are some of the tools that are available. A list of additional evidence-informed tools is available at https://hign.org/ and the Try This Series.

COMPREHENSIVE ASSESSMENT FOR THE FRAIL AND MEDICALLY COMPLEX OLDER PERSON

A model for a comprehensive prioritized assessment that is especially useful for assessing frail older persons is FANCAPES (*F*luids, *A*eration, *N*utrition, *C*ommunication, *A*ctivity, *P*ain, *E*limination, and *S*ocialization) (Ellison et al., 2015). This model emphasizes the determination of basic needs and the individual's functional ability to meet these needs independently. It can be used in all settings and may be used in part or in whole, depending on the need. The nurse obtains comprehensive information in each section, guided by the questions provided in Table 13.1.

FUNCTIONAL ASSESSMENT

Whereas the emphasis of FANCAPES is on physical needs, a full functional assessment is more broad. A thorough functional assessment will help gerontological nurses promote healthy aging by the following:

- Identifying specific areas in which help is needed
- Identifying changes in abilities from one period to another
- Helping to determine the need for specific services
- Providing information that may help determine the safety of a particular living situation

TABLE 13.1 FANCAPES Assessment

ACRONYM	ASSESSMENT
F (Fluids)	• What is the person's current state of hydration? • Does the person have the functional capacity to consume adequate fluids to maintain optimal health, including the ability to sense thirst, obtain the needed fluids mechanically, and swallow and excrete fluids?
A (Aeration)	• Is the person's oxygen exchange adequate for full respiratory functioning, including the ability to maintain an oxygen saturation >96%? • Is supplemental oxygen required, and if so, is it possible for the person to obtain it? • What is the respiratory rate and depth at rest and during activity (talking, walking, exercising, and performing ADLs)? • What sounds are auscultated, palpated, and percussed, and what do they suggest?
N (Nutrition)	• What mechanical and psychological factors are affecting the person's ability to obtain and benefit from adequate nutrition? • What type and amount of food is consumed? • Does the person have the ability to bite, chew, and swallow? • What effect does oral health status or periodontal disease have on the person? • Do the dentures of an edentulous person fit properly, and does the person wear them? • Does the person understand the need for special diets? • Is the special diet designed to be consistent with the person's eating and cultural patterns? • Can the person afford the special foods needed? • Have preventive strategies been taught to persons who are at risk for aspiration, including those who are tube fed?
C (Communication)	• Is the person able to communicate his or her needs adequately? • Do the care providers understand the person's form of communication? • What is the person's ability to hear in various environments? • Are there any environmental situations in which the patient's understanding of the spoken word is inadequate? • Is the vision of the person who depends on lip-reading adequate? • Does the person have either expressive or receptive aphasia? If so, has a speech pathologist been made available? • What are the levels of the person's reading comprehension and auditory comprehension?
A (Activity)	• Is the person able to participate in the activities necessary to meet basic needs such as toileting, grooming, and meal preparation? • How much assistance does the person need, if any, and is someone available to provide such assistance? • Is the person able to participate in activities that address higher needs, such as the need for belonging or finding meaning in life? • Is the person able to voluntarily move about, either with or without assistive devices? • Does the person have the coordination, balance, ambulatory skills, finger dexterity, grip strength, and other capacities necessary to function fully in day-to-day life?
P (Pain)	• Is the person experiencing physical, psychological, or spiritual pain? • Is the person able to express pain and the desire for relief? • Do any cultural barriers make the assessment or the expression of pain difficult for the patient? • How does the person customarily attain pain relief?

Continued

TABLE 13.1	FANCAPES Assessment—cont'd
ACRONYM	**ASSESSMENT**
E (Elimination)	• Is the person having difficulty with bladder or bowel elimination? • Does the person lack control of elimination? • Does the environment interfere with the person's elimination and related personal hygiene? • Does the person need any assistive devices, and if so, are they available and functioning? • How are problems, if any, affecting the person's social functioning?
S (Socialization and social skills)	• Is the person able to negotiate relationships in society, give and receive love and friendship, and feel self-worth?

ADLs, Activities of daily living; *FANCAPES,* fluids, aeration, nutrition, communication, activity, pain, elimination, and socialization.
Sources: Adapted from Jett, K. F. (2013). Health assessment. In T. A. Touhy & K. F. Jett (Eds.), *Ebersole & Hess' toward healthy aging: Human needs and nursing response* (8th ed., pp. 104–117). St. Louis, MO: Mosby; Montgomery, J. & Mitty, E. (2008). Resident condition change: Should I call 911? *Geriatric Nursing, 29*(1), 15–26. doi:10.1016/j.gerinurse.2007.11.009.

Most functional assessment tools assess the individual's ability to perform the tasks needed for self-care and independent living. Self-care activities are known as **activities of daily living (ADLs)** and are most often identified as eating, toileting, ambulation, bathing, dressing, and grooming. Three of these activities (grooming, dressing, and bathing) entail higher cognitive function than the others.

Instrumental activities of daily living (IADLs) are tasks needed for independent living (e.g., cleaning, doing yard work, shopping, and managing money); they call for a higher level of cognitive and physical functioning than the ADLs do. Nurses must keep in mind that the interest and skills needed to perform specific ADLs and IADLs are influenced by social and cultural factors.

Numerous tools describe, screen, assess, monitor, and predict functional ability. Most of the tools result in a score of some kind—a rating of the person's ability (or inability) to complete the task alone or with assistance. However, ratings are not always sensitive enough to show small changes in function. The Katz Index, of which there are several versions, serves as a basic framework for most ADL measures (Katz et al., 1963). One version of the Katz Index is based on a three-point scale and scores persons as independent, assistive, dependent, or unable to perform. Another version of the Katz Index assigns one point to each ADL that the person can complete independently and records a zero if the person is unable to perform these activities. Scores range from 0 (totally dependent) to 6 (totally independent) (Wallace & Shelkey, 2007). A score of 4 indicates moderate impairment, whereas a score of 2 or less indicates severe impairment (Table 13.2). This tool is useful because it creates a common language about patient function for all caregivers involved in care planning.

The IADLs are considered to be activities that are more complex and that necessitate higher functioning than the ADLs. The original scoring tool for IADLs was developed by Lawton and Brody (1969). Both the original tool and its subsequent variations use self-reporting, reporting by proxy, and observation, with three levels of functioning (independent, assisted, and unable to perform). Box 13.1 gives an example of an instrument for rating IADLs.

In rehabilitation settings, the Barthel Index is commonly used to measure the amount of physical assistance required when a person can no longer carry out ADLs (Mahoney & Barthel, 1965). This index is especially useful for documenting the improvement of a person's ability. It classes functional status as either "independent" or "dependent," then further classifies the former as either "intact" or "limited" and the latter as either "needing a helper" or "unable" to do the activity at all. Training in the correct use and scoring of this tool is required.

The widely used Functional Independence Measure (FIM) is the most comprehensive functional assessment tool used in rehabilitation settings (Wallace et al., 2002). It includes measures of mobility, cognition, social functioning, and the ability to carry

TABLE 13.2	Katz Index of Independence in Activities of Daily Living	

ACTIVITIES	INDEPENDENCE (1 POINT)	DEPENDENCE (0 POINTS)
	No supervision, direction, or personal assistance	With supervision, direction, personal assistance, or total care
Bathing Points: ___	(1 point) Bathes self completely or needs help in bathing only one part of the body (i.e., back, genital area, or disabled extremity).	(0 points) Needs help with bathing more than one part of the body or with getting in or out of the tub or shower. Requires total bathing.
Dressing Points: ___	(1 point) Gets clothes from closets and drawers and puts on clothes and outer garments, complete with fasteners. May need help tying shoes.	(0 points) Needs help with dressing, or needs to be completely dressed by caregiver.
Toileting Points: ___	(1 point) Goes to toilet, gets on and off toilet, arranges clothes, and cleans genital area without help.	(0 points) Needs help going to the toilet or cleaning self, or uses a bedpan or commode.
Transferring Points: ___	(1 point) Moves in and out of bed or on and off chair unassisted. Mechanical transferring aids are acceptable.	(0 points) Needs help in moving from bed to chair, or requires a complete transfer.
Continence Points: ___	(1 point) Exercises complete self-control over urination and defecation.	(0 points) Is partially or totally incontinent of bowel, bladder, or both.
Feeding Points: ___	(1 point) Transfers food from plate to mouth without help. Preparation of food may be done by another person.	(0 points) Needs partial or total help with feeding, or requires parenteral feeding.
Total points Points: ___	6 = High (independent)	0 = Low (totally dependent)

Source: Katz, S., Down, T. D., Cash, H. R. et al. (1970). Progress in the development of the index of ADL. *Gerontologist, 10*(1), 20–30.

BOX 13.1	Instrumental Activities of Daily Living

1. Using the telephone
   I: Able to look up numbers, dial, and receive and make calls without help
   A: Able to answer phone or call operator in an emergency, but needs a special phone or help in a getting number or dialing
   D: Unable to use telephone
2. Travelling
   I: Able to drive own car or travel alone by bus or taxi
   A: Able to travel but not alone
   D: Unable to travel
3. Shopping
   I: Able to take care of all shopping with transportation provided
   A: Able to shop but not alone
   D: Unable to shop
4. Preparing meals
   I: Able to plan and cook full meals
   A: Able to prepare light foods, but unable to cook full meals alone
   D: Unable to prepare any meals
5. Housework
   I: Able to do heavy housework
   A: Able to do light housework, but needs help with heavy tasks
   D: Unable to do any housework
6. Taking medications
   I: Able to take medications in the right dose at the right time
   A: Able to take medications, but needs reminding or someone to prepare them
   D: Unable to take medications
7. Managing money
   I: Able to manage buying needs, write cheques, and pay bills
   A: Able to manage daily buying needs, but needs help managing chequing account and paying bills
   D: Unable to manage money

I, independent; A, assistance needed; D, dependent

Source: Duke University Center for the Study of Aging and Human Development. (1978). *Multidimensional Functional Assessment Questionnaire* (2nd ed.). With permission of Duke University.

out ADLs. It was developed through the work of a number of experts and has been thoroughly tested. The FIM is completed through the joint efforts of the interprofessional team and is used both for planning and for evaluating progress. Although considerable training is required to accurately use the FIM, its use is encouraged.

Performance Tests

The ADLs and IADLS can also be measured with performance tools. These tools overcome the problems associated with self-report and proxy report and yield a more objective measurement of performance. Performance tools take longer to use; again, the cut-offs are subjective and arbitrary. The three performance tests related to mobility are simple and quick: the ability to stand with feet together in a side-by-side manner and in tandem and semi-tandem positions; a timed walk of 2.5 metres (8 feet); and a timed rise from a chair and return to a seated position, repeated five times (Box 13.2).

Another performance test, the Timed Up & Go test, is a basic evaluation of functional mobility. It measures the time needed to rise from a chair, walk 3 metres, turn around, and then return to a seated position. This test has been used extensively in the field of clinical geriatrics to assess gait and balance (Beauchet et al., 2010).

MENTAL STATUS ASSESSMENT

Increasing age is accompanied by an increased rate of illnesses that affect the person's cognition (for example, Alzheimer's disease). Cognitive ability is also easily threatened by any disturbance in health. Altered or impaired mental status may be the first sign of physical illness, from a heart attack to a urinary tract infection. Gerontological nurses must be aware of the tools that are used in the assessment of mental status, especially in regard to cognitive ability and mood (see Chapter 21). The interprofessional team plays an important role in collecting data for a cognitive assessment.

Cognitive Measures

The commonly used cognitive measures are the Mini-Mental State Examination, the clock drawing test, the Mini-Cog, the Montreal Cognitive Assess-

ment, and the Cognitive Performance Scale and Cognitive Performance Scale 2.

Mini-Mental State Examination. The Mini-Mental State Examination (MMSE) was the first tool developed to screen for cognitive deficiencies such as those that occur in dementia or delirium (Folstein et al., 1975). It tests selected aspects of mental status, including orientation, short-term memory and attention, calculation ability, language, and construction. A score of 30 suggests no cognitive impairment, and a score of 24 or less suggests potential dementia; however, adjustments are needed for educational level. A plethora of psychometric studies have indicated that the MMSE does not confirm dementia, mild cognitive impairment, or delirium but can be used to rule out (screen) these conditions. The MMSE is neither the most accurate nor the more efficient tool with which to evaluate cognitive disorders, but it has provided a benchmark against which all newer tools can be measured (Mitchell, 2013).

Clock Drawing Test. The clock drawing test, which has been in use since 1992 (Tuokko et al., 1992), is a tool to identify the severity of cognitive impairment. This test requires the tested person to have some manual dexterity and thus would not be appropriate to use with persons who are limited in the use of their dominant hand or whose vision is impaired. The person is presented with a blank piece of paper or with a paper with a circle drawn on it. The individual is then asked to draw the face of a clock and then indicate 0345 hours (3:45 am) or some other selected time on the face of the clock. Scoring is based on both the position of the numbers and the position of the hands (Box 13.3). This tool does not establish criteria for dementia, but a poor performance indicates the need for further investigation.

Mini-Cog. The Mini-Cog is a tool used to determine a person's cognitive status. The Mini-Cog combines one of the functions tested by the MMSE (short-term memory recall) with the executive function tested by the clock drawing test. Recent studies have found that the usefulness of the Mini-Cog for detecting cognitive impairment in primary care is limited (Carnero-Pardo et al., 2013).

Montreal Cognitive Assessment. The Montreal Cognitive Assessment (MoCA) is designed to detect mild cognitive impairment. The MoCA consists of a brief

BOX 13.2   Functional Performance Tests

Standing Balance

Instructions for Semi-Tandem Stand:

1. Demonstrate the task. (The heel of one foot is placed to the side of the first toe of the other foot.)
2. Support one arm of the older person while he or she positions the feet as demonstrated above. The older person can choose which foot to place forward.
3. Ask if the person is ready, then release the support and begin timing.
4. Stop timing when the older person moves the feet or grasps the nurse for support, or when 10 seconds has elapsed.
   Start with the semi-tandem stand. If it cannot be done for 10 seconds, then the side-by-side test should be done. If the semi-tandem stand can be done for the requisite 10 seconds, carry out the full-tandem stand, following the same instructions as above, except that the full-tandem stand calls for placing the heel of one foot directly in front of the toes of the other foot.

Score	Full-tandem stand	Semi-tandem stand	Side-by-side stand
0	_____	<10 seconds or unable	<10 seconds or unable
1	_____	<10 seconds or unable	10 seconds
2	<3 seconds or unable	10 seconds	_____
3	3–9 seconds	10 seconds	_____
4	10 seconds	10 seconds	_____

Standing Balance score: _____

Walking Speed

1. Set up a 2.5 m (8 ft.) walking course with an additional 60 cm (2 ft.) at both ends free of any obstacles.
2. Place a 2.5 m (8 ft.) rigid carpenter's ruler to the side of the course.
3. Instruct the older person to "walk to the other end of the course at your normal speed, just like walking down the street to go to the store." Assistive devices should be used if needed.
4. Time two walks. The faster of the two is used as the score.

Score	Walking speed
0	Unable to complete course
1	>5.6 seconds
2	4.1–5.6 seconds
3	3.2–4.0 seconds
4	<3.2 seconds

Walking Speed score: _____

Chair Sit to Stands

1. Place a straight-backed chair next to a wall and ask the person to sit down.
2. Ask the person to fold the arms across the chest and stand up from the chair one time and sit down again. If successful, go to Step 3.
3. Ask the person to stand and sit five times as quickly as possible.
4. Note and record the time taken for the person to go from the initial sitting position to the final standing position at the end of the fifth stand.
   Scores are for the five rise-and-sits only. If the person performs fewer than five chair stands, the score is 0.

Score	Time to complete five chair sit to stands
0	Unable to complete five chair sit to stands
1	>16.6 seconds
2	13.7–16.5 seconds
3	11.2–13.6 seconds
4	<11.2 seconds

Chair Stands score: _____ **Total of all performance test scores (0–12):** _____

Source: Adapted from Bennett, J. A. (1999). Activities of daily living: Old-fashioned or still useful? *Journal of Gerontological Nursing, 25*(5), 22–29.

BOX 13.3   Clock Drawing Test

1. Ask the person to draw a circle on a blank piece of paper.
2. Ask the person to place the numbers 1 to 12 inside the circle, as they would appear on a clock.
3. Ask the person to place the clock hands to indicate 1545 hours (3:45 pm).

Performance	Score
Draws closed circle	1 point
Places numbers in correct positions	1 point
Includes all 12 correct numbers	1 point
Places hands in correct positions	1 point

Cognitively intact persons will rarely produce errors such as distorted contour or extraneous markings. Clinical judgement must be applied, but a low score indicates the need for further evaluation.

Source: Tuokko, H., Hadjistavropoulos, T., Miller, J. et al. (1992). The clock test: A sensitive measure to differentiate normal elderly from those with Alzheimer disease. Journal of the American Geriatric Society, 40(6), 579–584.

30-point test that takes about 10 minutes to complete (Nasreddine et al., 2005). The cognitive abilities it assesses include orientation, short-term memory, executive function, language ability, and visuospatial ability (Nasreddine et al., 2005). Scores on the MoCA range from 0 to 30; a score of 26 or higher is considered normal. The MoCA's advantages include its brevity, simplicity, and reliability as a screening test for Alzheimer's disease. In addition, it measures executive function, an important aspect of mental status that is affected in dementia. The MoCA also seems to work well in measuring executive functioning for those with Parkinson's disease and/or dementia and is free for nonprofit use (Smith et al., 2007; Kim et al., 2016). The MoCA is available at http://www.mocatest.org.

Cognitive Performance Scale

The Cognitive Performance Scale (CPS) and the Cognitive Performance Scale 2 (CPS2) are assessment tools created by interRAI, an international collaborative group that focuses on creative comprehensive assessment systems (interRAI, 2017). The CPS was initially used in residential care (Wellens et al., 2013); its scores range from 0 (no memory impairment) to 6 (severe memory impairment). The CPS has been shown to be highly correlated with the MMSE (interRAI, 2017). The CPS2 is a more up-to-date version of the CPS and is typically used in conjunction with other assessment tools in acute care. The CPS2 is a reliable screening tool for assessing cognitive impairment in older patients who are in hospital (Travers et al., 2013).

Delirium Index

The Delirium Index (DI), developed by McCusker and Cole, measures the severity of delirium, based on the observation of a patient. This index does not require any additional information from family members or other staff (McCusker & Cole, 2011). It was designed to be used in conjunction with the MMSE. The DI includes different categories measuring inattention, disorganized thinking, altered level of consciousness, disorientation in time and place, memory impairment, perceptual disturbances, psychomotor agitation, and psychomotor retardation (McCusker & Cole, 2011). The scoring is based on the sum of seven item scores.

Mood Measures

The above-mentioned tools are measures of cognitive ability. Other tools are needed to assess mood and especially to screen for depression, a common yet often unrecognized problem in older persons. Persons with untreated depression are more functionally impaired and will have prolonged periods in hospital, a lower quality of life, and earlier death (see Chapter 24). Persons with depression may appear as if they have dementia, and many persons with dementia are also depressed. The interconnection between the two syndromes calls for nurses' skill and sensitivity to ensure that older people receive the most appropriate and effective care possible (Goodarzi et al., 2017). Commonly used mood measures include the Geriatric Depression Scale and the Cornell Scale for Depression in Dementia. (See Chapters 21 and 24 for further discussion of cognitive assessment.)

Geriatric Depression Scale. The Geriatric Depression Scale (GDS), developed by Yesavage et al. (1982–1983), measures mood. It is a 30-item tool designed for older persons and is based almost entirely on psychological factors. The GDS has been extremely successful in determining the presence of depression, because it de-emphasizes physical complaints, sex drive, and

Geriatric Depression Scale: Short Form

Choose the best answer for how you have felt over the past week:

1. Are you basically satisfied with your life? YES / **NO**
2. Have you dropped many of your activities and interests? **YES** / NO
3. Do you feel that your life is empty? **YES** / NO
4. Do you often get bored? **YES** / NO
5. Are you in good spirits most of the time? YES / **NO**
6. Are you afraid that something bad is going to happen to you? **YES** / NO
7. Do you feel happy most of the time? YES / **NO**
8. Do you often feel helpless? **YES** / NO
9. Do you prefer to stay at home, rather than going out and doing new things? **YES** / NO
10. Do you feel you have more problems with memory than most? **YES** / NO
11. Do you think it is wonderful to be alive now? YES / **NO**
12. Do you feel pretty worthless the way you are now? **YES** / NO
13. Do you feel full of energy? YES / **NO**
14. Do you feel that your situation is hopeless? **YES** / NO
15. Do you think that most people are better off than you are? **YES** / NO

Answers in **bold** indicate depression. Score 1 point for each bolded answer.

A score > 5 points is suggestive of depression.
A score ≥ 10 points is almost always indicative of depression.

A score > 5 points should warrant a follow-up comprehensive assessment.

FIGURE 13.1 Geriatric Depression Scale (short form). *Source:* Greenberg, S.A. (2012). The Geriatric Depression Scale (GDS). *The Hartford Institute for Geriatric Nursing, Try This Series, 4.* Retrieved from https://consultgeri.org/try-this/general-assessment/issue-4.pdf.

appetite—the factors that are most affected by medications. The GDS is thought to measure depression in older persons more accurately than any other tools do. It cannot be used for assessing persons who have dementia or cognitive impairment. An updated, shorter (15-item) version is also available (Kurlowicz & Greenberg, 2007) (Fig. 13.1).

Cornell Scale for Depression in Dementia. The Cornell Scale for Depression in Dementia (CSDD) was developed specifically to assess the signs and symptoms of major depression in persons with dementia (Alexopoulos et al., 1988). The CSDD evaluates a broad spectrum of depressive signs and symptoms and includes items from other depression scales. Information is obtained by interviewing a caregiver as well as by directly observing and interviewing the person with dementia. A total score of 8 or more suggests significant depressive symptoms.

ASSESSMENT OF SOCIAL SUPPORTS

A comprehensive assessment includes an evaluation of the older person's social networks and supports. Assessment of social supports considers an individual's network of significant others, friends, and family and their ability to provide companionship and assistance in times of need. Tools to adequately measure social networks have been in development for a number of years. However, the many nuances and configurations of social support networks make standardized measurements difficult. One tool that has shown some usefulness is the Social Network and Support Scale in the International Mobility in Aging

Study (Bélanger et al., 2016; Phillips et al., 2016). This scale focuses on the emotional support and feelings of usefulness provided by the four cited types of social ties: friends, family members, children, and partners. Five Likert scale questions about social support are asked for each type of social tie. The maximum total score for social support is 20 for each type of social tie (Bélanger et al., 2016).

Caregiver Burden

A number of tools are specifically designed to measure the burden of the caregiver role (see Chapter 21). Caregiver burden assessment is vital to prevent potential family burnout and elder abuse. One of the most frequently used measures is the Caregiver Strain Index (CSI) (Fig. 13.2) (Gerritsen & Van Der Ende, 1994). The CSI identifies families that have potential

I am going to read a list of things that other people have found to be difficult. Would you tell me if any of these apply to you? (Give examples.)

	Yes = 1	No = 0
Sleep is disturbed (e.g., because is in and out of bed; wanders around at night)		
It is inconvenient (e.g., because helping takes so much time; it's a long drive over to help)		
It is a physical strain (e.g., because of lifting in and out of a chair; effort or concentration is required)		
It is confining (e.g., helping restricts free time; cannot go visiting)		
There have been family adjustments (e.g., because helping has disrupted routine; there has been no privacy)		
There have been changes in personal plans (e.g., had to turn down a job; could not go on vacation)		
There have been other demands on my time (e.g., from other family members)		
There have been emotional adjustments (e.g., because of severe arguments)		
Some behavior is upsetting (e.g., because of incontinence; has trouble remembering things; accuses people of taking things)		
It is upsetting to find has changed so much from his/her former self (e.g., he/she is a different person than he/she used to be)		
There have been work adjustments (e.g., because of having to take time off)		
It is a financial strain		
Feeling completely overwhelmed (e.g., because of worry about _____; concerns about how to manage)		
TOTAL SCORE (Count yes responses. Any positive answer may indicate a need for intervention in that area. A score of 7 or higher indicates a high level of stress.)		

FIGURE 13.2 Caregiver Strain Index. *Source:* Robinson, B. C. (1983). Validation of a caregiver strain index. *Journal of Gerontology, 38*(3), 344–348.

caregiving concerns. The tool comprises 13 questions that measure strain related to care provision within employment, financial, physical, social, and time domains. Positive responses to seven or more items on the index indicate a greater level of strain. The CSI can be used to assess individuals of any age who have assumed the role of caregiver for an older person.

ENVIRONMENTAL AND SAFETY ASSESSMENT

Environmental safety is an issue at all ages. Safety is especially important for persons who have limitations in cognition, mobility, vision, or hearing or who are at risk for a fall-related injury (see Chapters 12 and 19). Nurses in every setting are responsible for promoting the safety of the persons in their care. The most commonly used tools related to safety are (1) the listing of potential dangers and the status (present or absent) of the dangers and (2) the provision of suggestions or opportunities for reducing the potential dangers. Often, nurses think of safety as related to the risk for falling, but safety hazards include fires, poisoning, and problems with temperature (hypothermia or hyperthermia) as well. Unfortunately, many older persons who have lived in their homes for many years also face potential dangers from increased crime and victimization. See Chapter 12 for a detailed discussion of mobility and environmental safety, including premobilization assessment. See Chapter 19 for a description of several strategies and assessments to promote safety related to vision or hearing impairments.

INTEGRATED ASSESSMENTS

In some cases, an integrated approach is used rather than a collection of separate tools and assessments. The most well-known of these integrated tools is the Older American's Resources and Service tool (Fillenbaum & Smyer, 1981), which was taken into consideration in the development of the Minimum Data Set currently used in most facilities (see Chapter 5).

Older American's Resources and Service

The classic Older American's Resources and Service (OARS) instrument was designed to evaluate ability, disability, and the capacity level at which the person is able to function (Fillenbaum & Smyer, 1981). Each of its subscales—social resources, economic resources, physical health, mental health, and the ability to perform ADLs—can be used separately. The person's functional capacity in each area is rated on a scale of 1 (excellent) to 6 (completely impaired). At the conclusion of the assessment, a cumulative impairment score ranging from 6 (most capable) to 30 (total disability) is established. The information considered in each domain is listed below.

Social Resources. The social resources domain addresses the person's social skills and ability to negotiate and make friends. Is the person able to seek help from friends, family, and strangers? Is a caregiver available if needed? Who is the caregiver, and how long are they available? Does the person belong to any social network or group? How is the person's need for belonging met?

Economic Resources. Data about monthly income and sources are needed to determine the adequacy of income compared to the cost of living, including costs of food, shelter, clothing, medications, and small luxury items. This information can provide insight into the person's relative standard of living and can point to needs that might be alleviated by the use of additional resources.

Mental Health. Consideration is given to intellectual function, the presence or absence of psychiatric symptoms, and the amount of enjoyment and social interaction the person gets from life.

Physical Health. Diagnoses of major diseases, the type of prescribed and over-the-counter medications the person is taking, and the person's perception of his or her health status are evaluated. Physical health includes participation in regular vigorous activity (such as walking, dancing, or biking) daily or at least twice a week. Seriously impaired physical health is the result of the presence of one or more illnesses or disabilities that are severely painful or life-threatening or that require extensive care.

Activities of Daily Living. The ADLs included in the OARS are walking, getting into and out of bed, bathing, combing hair, shaving, dressing, eating, and getting to the bathroom on time by oneself. The IADLs include using the telephone, driving a car, hanging up clothes, obtaining groceries, taking medications, and having a correct knowledge of the required medication dosages.

Fulmer SPICES

The Fulmer SPICES is a tool for the overall assessment of older persons (Wallace & Fulmer, 2007). This tool has proved reliable and valid for persons in later life, whether in health or illness, living in acute or residential care homes, or living at home. The acronym "SPICES" refers to six common syndromes of the older person that require nursing interventions: *Sleep* disorders, *Problems* with eating or feeding, *Incontinence*, *Confusion*, *Evidence* of falls, and *Skin* breakdown. Several of these domains can be assessed in more depth with specific tools that assess sleep (see Chapter 10), nutrition (see Chapter 8), continence (see Chapter 9), cognition (see Chapter 21), mobility (see Chapter 12), and skin (see Chapter 11). Nurses are encouraged to make a 3 × 5-inch card with the SPICES acronym and use it as a reference when caring for older persons (https://hign.org/).

SUMMARY

This chapter is a brief overview of the standardized assessment tools that are commonly used in gerontological nursing. Whether a standardized tool or a new measure is being used, the goal is always to collect the most accurate data in the most efficient yet caring manner possible. Meeting this goal requires strong collaboration within the interprofessional team. The tools organize the collected data necessary for assessment and make it possible to compare the data over time. Some of the factors that complicate the assessment of the older person are the difficulty of differentiating the effects of aging from those of disease, the coexistence of multiple diseases, the underreporting of symptoms by older persons, atypical or nonspecific presentation of illness, and the increase in iatrogenic illnesses.

Over- and underdiagnoses occur when normal age changes, both physical and psychosocial, are not considered. Underdiagnosis is far more common in gerontological nursing. Many symptoms or complaints are ascribed to normal aging rather than to a health problem that may be developing. Assessing the older person who has multiple chronic conditions is also a challenge; the symptoms of one condition can exacerbate or mask the symptoms of another. The goal of gerontological nurses is to achieve the highest level of excellence in the care of older people; the use of validated assessment tools facilitates the attainment of this goal.

KEY CONCEPTS

- Assessment of the person's physical, cognitive, psychosocial, and environmental status is essential to meet the specific needs of the older person and to implement appropriate interventions.
- Collecting the data by self-report, by report by proxy, or through observation will affect the quality and quantity of the data.
- Knowledge of how to use a particular gerontological assessment tool is needed for its accurate use.
- Most comorbidities complicate the obtaining and interpreting of assessment data.

ACTIVITIES AND DISCUSSION QUESTIONS

1. Discuss the importance of the measurement of ADLs and IADLs for older persons.
2. Develop for each ADL a plan of interventions that could be used to compensate for ADL deficits and that would still foster an older person's independence.
3. Describe what makes an assessment tool effective.
4. Consider the limitations and challenges of using assessment tools for older persons.
5. Determine which tools would be most appropriate for assessing cognition in older persons who live in the community, in hospitals, or in LTC homes, and state the rationale for the choices.

RESOURCES

Geriatric Depression Scale
http://www.stanford.edu/~yesavage/GDS.html

Hartford Institute for Geriatric Nursing.
Evidence-informed geriatric assessment tools in the Try This assessment series (cost-free, web-based resources, including demonstration videos and a corresponding print series)
https://consultgeri.org/tools/try-this-series

Registered Nurses' Association of Ontario (RNAO). *Best Practice Guidelines and fact sheets on the assessment*

of pain, pressure ulcers, fall risk, delirium, dementia, depression, incontinence, and constipation
http://rnao.ca/bpg

For additional resources, please visit *http://evolve.elsevier.com/Canada/Ebersole/gerontological/*

REFERENCES

Alexopoulos, G. S., Abrams, R. C., Young, R. C., et al. (1988). The Cornell Scale for Depression in Dementia. *Biological Psychiatry*, 23(3), 271–284. Retrieved from http://www.scalesandmeasures.net/files/files/The%20Cornell%20Scale%20for%20Depression%20in%20Dementia.pdf.

Bélanger, E., Ahmed, T., Vafaei, A., et al. (2016). Sources of social support associated with health and quality of life: A cross-sectional study among Canadian and Latin American older adults. *British Medical Journal Open*, 6(6), e011503. doi:10.1136/bmjopen-2016-011503.

Benner, P. (1984). *From novice to expert*. Menlo Park, CA: Addison-Wesley.

Beauchet, O., Annweiler, C., Assal, F., et al. (2010). Imagined Timed Up & Go test: a new tool to assess higher-level gait and balance disorders in older adults? *Journal of the Neurological Sciences*, 294(1), 102–106. doi:10.1016/j.jns.2010.03.021.

Carnero-Pardo, C., Cruz-Orduña, I., Espejo-Martínez, B., et al. (2013). Utility of the Mini-Cog for detection of cognitive impairment in primary care: Data from two Spanish studies. *International Journal of Alzheimer's Disease*, 1-7. doi:10.1155/2013/285462.

Ellison, D., White, D., & Farrar, F. C. (2015). Aging population. *Nursing Clinics in North America*, 50(1), 185–213. doi:10.1016/j.cnur.2014.10.014.

Fillenbaum, G. G., & Smyer, M. A. (1981). The development, validity, and reliability of the OARS multidimensional functional assessment questionnaire. *Journal of Gerontology*, 36(4), 428–434. Retrieved from https://www.ncbi.nlm.nih.gov/pubmed/7252074.

Folstein, M. F., Folstein, S. E., & McHugh, P. R. (1975). Mini-mental state: A practical method for grading the cognitive state of patients for the clinician. *Journal of Psychiatric Research*, 12(3), 189–198. Retrieved from http://home.uchicago.edu/~tmurray1/research/articles/printed%20and%20read/mini%20mental%20state_a%20practical%20method%20for%20grading%20the%20cognitive%20state%20of%20patients%20for%20the%20clinician.pdf.

Gerritsen, J., & Van Der Ende, P. (1994). The development of a care-giving burden scale. *Age and Ageing*, 23, 483–491. Retrieved from https://www.ncbi.nlm.nih.gov/pubmed/9231943.

Goodarzi, Z. S., Mele, B. S., Roberts, D. J., et al. (2017). Depression case finding in individuals with dementia: A systematic review and meta-analysis. *Journal of the American Geriatrics Society*, 65(5), 937–948. doi:10.1111/jgs.14713.

interRAI. (2017). *Scales: Status and outcome measures*. Retrieved from http://www.interrai.org/scales.html.

Jett, K. F. (2013). Health assessment. In T. A. Touhy & K. F. Jett (Eds.), *Ebersole & Hess' toward healthy aging: Human needs and nursing response* (8th ed., pp. 104–117). St Louis, MO: Mosby.

Katz, S., Ford, A. B., Moskowitz, R. N., et al. (1963). Studies of illness in the aged: The index of ADL: A standardized measure of biological and psychosocial function. *Journal of the American Medical Association*, 185, 914–919. Retrieved from https://www.ncbi.nlm.nih.gov/pubmed/14044222.

Kim, J. I., Sunwoo, M. K., Sohn, Y. H., et al. (2016). The MMSE and MoCA for screening cognitive impairment in less educated patients with Parkinson's disease. *Journal of Movement Disorders*, 9(3), 152–159. doi:10.14802/jmd.16020.

Kurlowicz, L., & Greenberg, S. (2007). The Geriatric Depression Scale (GDS). The Hartford Institute for Geriatric Nursing, *Try This Series #4*. Retrieved from http://consultgerirn.org/uploads/File/trythis/try_this_4.pdf.

Lawton, M. P., & Brody, E. M. (1969). Assessment of older people: Self-maintaining and instrumental activities of daily living. *The Gerontologist*, 9(3), 179–186. Retrieved from https://academic.oup.com/gerontologist/article-abstract/9/3_Part_1/179/552574.

Mahoney, F. I., & Barthel, D. W. (1965). Functional evaluation: The Barthel Index. *Maryland State Medical Journal*, 14, 61–65. Retrieved from https://www.ncbi.nlm.nih.gov/pubmed/14258950.

McCusker, J., & Cole, M. (2011). *The delirium index: An instrument for measuring the severity of delirium*. Retrieved from http://www.smhc.qc.ca/ignitionweb/data/media_centre_files/510/Delirium%20Index%20July%2027_%202011.pdf.

Mitchell, A. J. (2013). The Mini-Mental State Examination (MMSE): an update on its diagnostic validity for cognitive disorders. In *Cognitive screening instruments* (pp. 15–46). London: Springer.

Montgomery, J., & Mitty, E. (2008). Resident condition change: Should I call 911? *Geriatric Nursing*, 29(1), 15–26. doi:10.1016/j.gerinurse.2007.11.009.

Nasreddine, Z. S., Phillips, N. A., Bédirian, V., et al. (2005). The Montreal Cognitive Assessment, MoCA: A brief screening tool for mild cognitive impairment. *Journal of American Geriatric Society*, 53, 695–699. doi:10.1111/j.1532-5415.2005.53221.

Phillips, S. P., Auais, M., Belanger, E., et al. (2016). Life-course social and economic circumstances, gender, and resilience in older adults: The longitudinal International Mobility in Aging Study (IMIAS). *SSM-Population Health*, 2, 708–717. doi:10.1016/j.ssmph.2016.09.007.

Smith, T., Gildeh, N., & Holmes, C. (2007). The Montreal Cognitive Assessment: Validity and utility in a memory clinic setting. *Canadian Journal of Psychiatry*, 52, 329–332. Retrieved from https://pdfs.semanticscholar.org/12a9/71d19e68520899034040d5942e7d7157cc83.pdf.

Travers, C., Byrne, G. J., Pachana, N. A., et al. (2013). Validation of the interRAI Cognitive Performance Scale against independent clinical diagnosis and the Mini-Mental State Examination in older hospitalized patients. *The Journal of Nutrition, Health and Aging*, 17(5), 435–439. doi:10.1007/s12603-012-0439-8.

Tuokko, H., Hadjistavropoulos, T., Miller, J., et al. (1992). The clock test: A sensitive measure to differentiate normal elderly from those with Alzheimer disease. *Journal of the American Geriatric Society, 40*(6), 579–584. Retrieved from https://www.ncbi.nlm.nih.gov/pubmed/1587974.

Wallace, D., Duncan, P. W., & Lai, S. M. (2002). Comparison of the responsiveness of the Barthel Index and the motor component of the Functional Independence Measure in stroke: The impact of using different methods for measuring responsiveness. *Journal of Clinical Epidemiology, 55*, 922–928. Retrieved from https://www.ncbi.nlm.nih.gov/pubmed/12393081.

Wallace, M., & Fulmer, T. (2007). Fulmer SPICES: An overall assessment tool for older adults. The Hartford Institute for Geriatric Nursing, *Try This Series #1*. Retrieved from http://consultgerirn.org/uploads/File/trythis/try_this_1.pdf.

Wallace, M., & Shelkey, M. (2007). Katz Index of Independence in activities of daily living (ADL). The Hartford Institute for Geriatric Nursing, *Try This Series #2*. Retrieved from http://consultgerirn.org/uploads/File/trythis/try_this_2.pdf.

Wellens, N. I. H., Flamaing, J., Tournoy, J., et al. (2013). Convergent validity of cognitive performance scale of the interRAI AcuteCare and Mini-Mental State Examination. *The American Journal of Geriatric Psychiatry, 21*(7), 636–645. doi:10.1016/j.jagp.2012.12.017.

Yesavage, J. A., Brink, T. L., Rose, T., et al. (1982–1983). Development and validation of a geriatric depression screening scale: A preliminary report. *Journal of Psychiatric Research, 17*(1), 37–49. Retrieved from http://home.uchicago.edu/~tmurray1/research/articles/at%20least%20read/development%20and%20validation%20of%20a%20geriatric%20depression%20screening%20scale_a%20preliminary%20report.pdf.

Safe Medication Use for Older Persons

LEARNING OBJECTIVES

Upon completion of this chapter, the reader will be able to:

- Explain age-related pharmacokinetic changes.
- Discuss potential use of chronotherapy for the older person.
- Describe medication use patterns and their implications for the older person.
- Explain the roles of the older person, caregiver, and social network in promoting medication compliance.
- List interventions that can help promote medication compliance.
- Identify diagnoses or symptoms for which psychotropic medications are prescribed.
- Discuss issues concerning psychotropic medication management in the older population.
- Develop a nursing care plan for older people who have been prescribed psychotropic medications.

GLOSSARY

Adverse effect or adverse event A harmful and undesired consequence of a medication or procedure, or a consequence of a drug or procedure other than that for which it is used (e.g., dry mouth); formerly called a "side effect."

Bioavailability The amount of medication available for effecting changes in target tissues.

Biotransformation A series of chemical alterations of a medication that occur in the body.

Complementary and alternative medicine Health practices that are not traditionally part of the biomedical health care model, such as acupuncture, chiropractic, hypnosis, massage therapy, and natural health products, such as herbal remedies, vitamins, homeopathic medicines, and nutrition therapies.

Delusion A false fixed belief that is not shared by others and guides the person's interpretation of events.

Half-life The time it takes after medication administration to inactivate half of the medication.

Hallucination A false sensory perception in the absence of a real stimulus (e.g., hearing voices that no one else can hear).

Iatrogenic Pertaining to the result of something that is done or given to a person in the context of health care.

Pharmacokinetics The movement of a medication in the body from its administration to its absorption, distribution, metabolism, and excretion.

Potentiation The strengthening of the effect of one or more substances (e.g., food or another medication) when they are used in combination.

Regimen A scheduled plan for taking medications (e.g., twice a day, with food).

Target tissue or target organ Tissue or organ intended to receive the greatest concentration of a medication or to be most affected by the medication.

Therapeutic window The range of the plasma concentration of a medication within which it is safe and effective.

Thought disorder Disturbance in a person's thought processes or way of thinking.

THE LIVED EXPERIENCE

It is so hard to keep track of my medications. I try arranging them in little cups to take with each meal, but then there are the ones that I take at odd times. Those are the easiest to forget. I get really confused and think sometimes I have taken them twice. I really wish I didn't have to take so many pills, but I'm not sure what would happen if I stopped any of them. I don't even know why I'm taking most of them.

Geraldo, 62 years old, hypertensive, and diabetic

MEDICATION USE FOR OLDER PERSONS

In Canada, persons 65 years of age and older are the largest users of prescription and over-the-counter (OTC) medications (Bernier, 2017). In 2011, 83% of community-dwelling Canadians aged 65 years or more were taking prescription medications; 33% of this group were taking five or more medications (Pannu et al, 2017). One study found that 26.5% of older persons used **complementary or alternative medicine** (CAM) therapy (Wood et al., 2010). In this chapter, the term "medication" refers to prescription and OTC medications and to herbal remedies. As people age, they are more likely to develop more complex health challenges, which is one reason the use of prescription medications tends to increase (Canadian Institute for Health Information [CIHI], 2011).

Unfortunately, the number of adverse drug reactions (ADRs) increases with the number of medications used. Also called adverse drug events, ADRs are a notable cause of hospital admission as well as a cause of **iatrogenic** mortality and morbidity for older persons (Perri, Menon, Deshpande, et al., 2005). How people use their prescribed medicines and other CAM or bioactive products depends on the person's unique characteristics, situations, beliefs, understanding about illness, function and cognition, perception of the necessity of the medications, severity of symptoms, reactions to the medications, finances, and access to medications, and the compatibility of such products with their lifestyle. Gerontological nurses have a responsibility to help minimize the risks of medication use for people in their care. Several resources on medication safety can be found at the Institute for Safe Medication Practices (ISMP), a non-profit organization devoted to the prevention of medication errors and to safe medication use (http://www.ismp.org/).

This chapter presents a review of changes in pharmacokinetics, pharmacodynamics, and medication use issues. The final section of this chapter discusses the use of psychotropic agents.

PHARMACOKINETICS

Pharmacokinetics refers to the movement of a medication in the body from the point of administration as it is absorbed, distributed, metabolized, and finally excreted. It is important for gerontological nurses to understand how pharmacokinetics may differ in older persons (Fig. 14.1). There is no conclusive evidence of an appreciable change in overall pharmacokinetics with aging; however, several changes with aging may have an effect on the process of pharmacokinetics (see Chapter 6). The four processes of pharmacokinetics (absorption, distribution, metabolism, and excretion) will be described in more detail.

ABSORPTION

In order for a medication to be effective, it must be absorbed into the bloodstream, the tissue, or both. The amount of time between the administration of the medication and its absorption depends on a number of factors, including the route of introduction (i.e., intravenous, oral, parenteral, transdermal, or rectal), **bioavailability**, and the amount of medication that passes into the body. An intravenous route will deliver the medication immediately to the bloodstream. Other quick routes for medication absorption include parenteral and transdermal routes and through mucous membranes such as the rectum and the oral mucosa. Orally administered medications are absorbed through the gastro-intestinal tract.

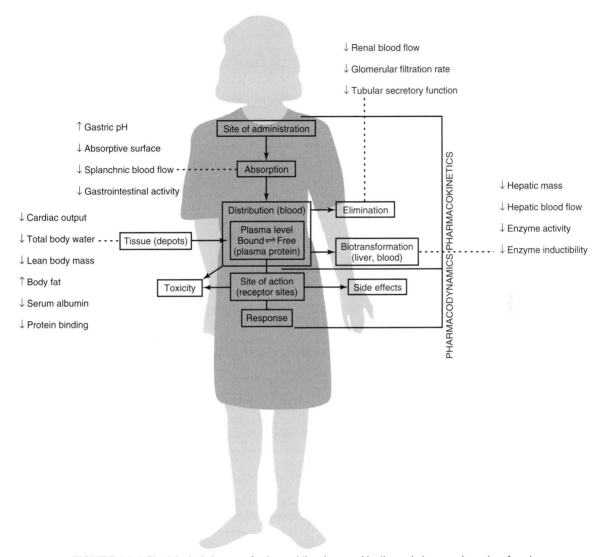

FIGURE 14.1 Physiological changes of aging and the pharmacokinetics and pharmacodynamics of medication use. *Sources:* Kane, R. L., Ouslander, J. G., & Abrass, I. B. (1984). *Essentials of clinical geriatrics.* New York: McGraw-Hill; Lamy, P. P. (1984). Hazards of drug use in the elderly: Commonsense measures to reduce them. *Postgraduate Medicine, 76*(1), 50–53; Vestal, R. E., & Dawson, G. W. (1985). Pharmacology and aging. In C. E. Finch & E. L. Schneider (Eds.), *Handbook of biology and aging.* New York: Van Nostrand Reinhold; Roberts, J., & Turner, N. (1988). Pharmacodynamic basis for altered drug action in the elderly. *Clinics in Geriatric Medicine, 4*(1), 127–149; Montamat, S. C., Cusack, B. J., & Vestal, R. E. (1980). Management of drug therapy in the elderly. *New England Journal of Medicine, 321*(5), 303–309.

A number of normal age-related physiological changes have implications for differences in both the prescription and the administration of medications for older persons (Shi & Klotz, 2011). The commonly diminished gastric pH will retard the action of acid-dependent medications. Delayed stomach emptying may diminish or negate the effectiveness of short-lived medications that could become inactivated before reaching the small intestine. The absorption of enteric-coated medications, which are specifically meant to bypass stomach absorption, may be delayed so that their action begins in the stomach, and this may produce gastric irritation or nausea.

Absorption is also influenced by changes in gastro-intestinal motility. If there is increased motility in the small intestine, the medication effect is diminished because of shortened contact time and therefore decreased absorption and effectiveness. Conversely, slowed intestinal motility can increase the contact time and thus the amount absorbed and, as a result, change the medication's effect. This increases the risk for adverse reactions or unpredictable effects.

Many prescription and OTC medications commonly taken by older persons can also affect the absorption of other medications. Antispasmodic medications slow gastric and intestinal motility. In some instances, the ingested medication's action may be useful, but when other medications are involved, it is necessary to consider the problem of medication absorption alterations due to medication–medication interaction. By binding the medication with elements and forming chemical compounds, antacids or iron preparations affect the availability of some medications for absorption. Medication–food interactions may either decrease or increase the amount absorbed. (Medication–herb interactions are presented in Table 14.1.) For example, when a bisphosphonate such as Fosamax is taken with food of any kind, absorption is reduced to only a few milligrams; therefore, the medication has no effect on the **target organ**, the bones.

Similarly, taking grapefruit juice with levothyroxine may delay the absorption of the medication (Bushra et al., 2011).

DISTRIBUTION

Once a medication is absorbed, it must be transported to the target organ to have any effect. Distribution depends on the availability of plasma protein in the form of lipoproteins, globulins, and especially albumin. As medications are absorbed, they bind with the protein and are distributed throughout the body. Normally, a predictable percentage of the absorbed medication is inactivated as it is bound to the protein. The remaining free medication is available in the bloodstream and has a therapeutic effect when an effective concentration is reached in the plasma.

Many older persons have an insignificant reduction in the serum albumin level. In others, especially those with prolonged illness or malnutrition (such as residents in long-term care homes), the serum albumin may be diminished. When this occurs, toxic levels of available free drug may accumulate unpredictably, especially for highly protein-bound medications with narrow **therapeutic windows**, such as phenytoin and warfarin (Ruscin, 2009).

Potential alterations of medication distribution in late life are related to changes in body composition, particularly decreased lean body mass, increased body fat, and decreased total body water. Decreased body water leads to higher serum levels of water-soluble medications such as digoxin, ethanol, and aminoglycosides. Adipose tissue nearly doubles in older men and increases by one half in older women; therefore, medications that are highly lipid soluble are stored in the fatty tissue, extending and possibly elevating the medication effect. This includes medications such as lorazepam, diazepam, chlorpromazine, phenobarbital, and haloperidol (Haldol).

METABOLISM

Biotransformation is the process by which the body modifies the chemical structure of medication. This process converts the compound to a metabolite that is more easily excreted later on. A medication will continue to exert a therapeutic effect as long as it remains in its original state or as an active metabolite. Active metabolites retain the ability to have a therapeutic effect, as well as the same or a greater chance of causing **adverse effects**. For example, the metabolites of acetaminophen (Tylenol) can cause liver damage with higher dosages (>4 g per 24 hours, or more than four extra-strength products) (National Library of Medicine, 2016). The duration of a medication's action is determined by the metabolic rate and is measured in terms of **half-life**, or how long the drug remains active in the body. The liver is the primary site of medication metabolism. With aging, the liver's activity, mass, volume, and blood flow are reduced (see Chapter 6). These changes result in a potential decrease in the liver's ability to metabolize medications such as benzodiazepines (e.g., lorazepam [Ativan] and diazepam [Valium]). These changes in the liver also result in a significant increase in the half-life of these

TABLE 14.1   Significant Medication–Food Interactions

MEDICATIONS	FOOD	MEDICATION–FOOD INTERACTION EFFECTS
Warfarin	High-protein diet	Raises serum albumin levels; decreases in INR
	Vegetables containing vitamin K	Interferes with effectiveness and safety of warfarin therapy
	Charbroiled vegetables and meat	Decreases warfarin activity
	Cooked onions	Increases warfarin activity
	Cranberry juice	Elevates INR without bleeding in older patient
	Leafy green vegetables	Potentiates development of thromboembolic complications
Monoamine oxidases	Tyramine-containing food[1]	Causes hypertensive crisis
Propranolol	Protein-rich food	Possibly increases serum level
Celiprolol	Orange juice	Inhibits intestinal absorption of drug
ACE inhibitors	(Empty stomach)	Increases absorption of drug
Ca2 channel drugs	Grapefruit juice	Increases drug bioavailability
Antibiotics	Milk products[2]	Prevents the absorption of some antibiotics; reduces drug bioavailability
Acetaminophen	Pectin	Delays absorption and onset of acetaminophen
NSAIDs	Alcohol	Increases potential risk of liver damage or stomach bleeding
	Beverages	Increases C_{max} and $AUC_{0-alpha}$ significantly[3]
Theophylline	High-fat meal	Increases drug bioavailability
	Caffeine	Increases risk of drug toxicity
Esomeprazole	High-fat meal	Reduces drug bioavailability
Cimetidine, rupatadine	With food (any type)	Increases drug bioavailability
Isoniazide	Plants, medicinal herbs, oleanolic acid	Exerts synergistic effect
Cycloserine	High-fat meals	Decreases the serum concentration
Esomeprazole	High-fat meal	Reduces drug bioavailability
Glimepiride	With breakfast	Allows for absolute drug bioavailability
Acarbose	At start of each meal	Allows for maximum drug effectiveness
Mercaptopurine	Cow's milk[4]	Reduces drug bioavailability
Tamoxifen	Sesame seeds	Negatively interferes with tamoxifen in inducing regression of established mcf-7 tumour size, but beneficially interacts with tamoxifen on bone in ovariectomized athymic mice
Levothyroxine	Grapefruit juice	Delays drug absorption[5]

ACE, Angiotensin-converting enzyme; *AUC,* area under the curve; *Ca2,* ionized calcium; C_{max}, maximum concentration; *INR,* international normalized ratio; *NSAIDs,* nonsteroidal anti-inflammatory drugs.

[1]Frankel, E.H. (2003). Basic concepts. In B. J. McCabe, E. H., Frankel, & J. J. Wolfe (Eds.), *Handbook of food-drug interactions* (p. 2). Boca Raton: CRC Press

[2]Ayo, J. A., Agu, H., & Madaki, I. (2005). Food and drug interactions: its side effects. *Nutrition & Food Science, 35*(4), 243–252. doi:10.1108/00346650510605630.

[3]Schmidt, L. E., & Dahloff, K. (2002). Food-drug interactions. *Drugs, 62*(10), 1481–1502. doi:10.2165/00003495-200262100-00005.

[4]Nekvindová, J., & Anzenbacher, P. (2007). Interactions of food and dietary supplements with drug metabolising cytochrome P450 enzymes. *Ceska a Slovenska Farmacie, 56*(4), 165–173.

[5]Hansten, P. D. (2004). Appendix II: Important interactions and their mechanisms. In B. G. Katzung, *Basic and clinical pharmacology* (9th ed., p. 1110). Boston: McGraw-Hill.

Source: Bushra, R., Aslam, N., & Khan, A. Y. (2011). Food-drug interactions. *Oman Medical Journal, 26*(2), 77–83. doi:10.5001/omj.2011.21. Retrieved from http://pubmedcentralcanada.ca/pmcc/articles/PMC3191675/.

medications. For example, the half-life of diazepam in a younger adult is about 37 hours but can be as long as 82 hours in an older person. If the dose and timing of these medications are not adjusted, the medication can accumulate, and the administration of a single dose can have significantly more effects (and longer effects) in an older person than in a younger person. Except in the rarest of circumstances, diazepam should not be used in an older population (American Geriatrics Society [AGS], 2015).

EXCRETION

Medications and their metabolites are excreted in sweat, saliva, and other secretions but are excreted primarily through the kidneys. However, many older persons may have comorbidities that affect the rate of excretion, and just as kidney function declines significantly in aging, so does the ability to excrete or eliminate medications in a timely manner. The considerably decreased glomerular filtration rate leads to a prolonged half-life of medication (that is, the amount of time required to eliminate the medication), which again presents opportunities for accumulation and increases the potential for toxicity or other adverse events (see Chapter 6). Although renal function cannot be estimated by the serum creatinine level, it can be approximated by the calculation of creatinine clearance. Reductions in dosages for renally excreted medications (e.g., allopurinol and vancomycin) are necessary when the creatinine clearance is reduced.

PHARMACODYNAMICS

Pharmacodynamics refers to the interaction between a medication and the body. The older a person becomes, the more likely is an altered or unreliable response of the body to medication. Although it is not always possible to explain the change in response, several mechanisms are known.

The aging process causes a decreased response to beta-adrenergic receptor stimulators and blockers; decreased baroreceptor sensitivity; and increased sensitivity to a number of medications, especially anticholinergics, benzodiazepines, narcotic analgesics, warfarin (Coumadin), and the cardiac medications diltiazem and verapamil (Briggs, 2005). If food–medication interactions occur, the problems become

worse. For example, drinking grapefruit juice while taking a statin such as Lipitor or taking any number of antibiotics may cause an unreliable response.

There is also a growing body of knowledge about the interaction of herbal preparations and currently prescribed medications. For example, the herbal extract of *Ginkgo biloba* is commonly thought to enhance cognitive function, but this herb will increase the potential for bleeding when an anticoagulant is used at the same time (Di Minno et al., 2017) (see Table 14.1). In addition to causing expected dry mouth, medications with anticholinergic properties can cause confusion, constipation, blurred vision, orthostatic hypotension, urinary retention, or heat stroke, even at low doses (Ruscin, 2009). The use of benzodiazepines is associated with an increased risk for accidental injury; thus, these medications are on the "do not use" list for older persons (AGS, 2015).

CHRONOPHARMACOLOGY

The normal biorhythms of the body and their differences in men and women can also affect pharmacokinetics and pharmacodynamics. The relationship of biological rhythms to variations in the body's response to medications is known as *chronopharmacology*. Although chronopharmacology has not yet been explored in relation to aging, it is a developing science that may lead to more effective medication therapy (Golombek et al., 2015). The best time to administer medications is now being considered to be influenced by the biorhythms of various physiological processes.

As discussed previously, absorption depends on gastric acid pH, the level of motility of the gastro-intestinal tract, and blood flow. All have been shown to have biorhythmical variations. The distribution of protein-bound medications depends on albumin and glycoproteins produced by the liver. During the day, albumin levels are high, but they are low in the early morning. Medication metabolism is also biorhythmical. Oxidation, hydrolysis, decarboxylation, and demethylation by liver enzymes demonstrate rhythmic variations. Renal elimination depends on kidney perfusion, glomerular filtration, and urine acidity and has shown rhythmic variation. The brain, heart, and blood cells also have varied rhythmicity,

TABLE 14.2 Rhythmical Influences on Disease and Physiological Processes

DISEASE OR PROCESS	RHYTHMICAL INFLUENCE
Allergic rhinitis	Symptoms worse in the morning
Arterial blood pressure	Circadian surge in the morning hours
Asthma	Greatest respiratory distress overnight (during sleep) Symptoms peak in early morning (0400–0500 hours)
Blood plasma	Plasma volume falls at night, thus hematocrit increases
Cancer	Tumour cells proliferate when normal cell miosis is low
Cardiac disease	Angina, myocardial infarction, and thrombolytic stroke occur in the first 4 hours after waking (peak at 0900 hours) (Prinzmetal's angina—during sleep).
Catecholamines	Increase in early morning
Fibrinolytic activity	Increase in early morning
Platelet activation	May result from abnormality in circadian rhythm, which affects cortisol levels, body temperature, and sleep–wake cycle
Gastric system	Gastric acid secretion peaks every morning (0200–0400 hours); circannual variability—incidence of gastric ulcers greater in winter
Osteoarthritis	Pain more severe in morning
Potassium excretion	Lowest in morning; highest in late afternoon
Rheumatoid arthritis	Pain more severe in late afternoon
Systemic insulin	Highest in afternoon

resulting in a cyclical response for beta-blockers, calcium channel blockers, angiotensin-converting enzyme (ACE) inhibitors, nitrates, and other similar medications. Medications such as Fosamax and Actonel must be taken on arising in the morning for maximum effectiveness (Brown, 2017). Table 14.2 shows some of the rhythmical influences on diseases and physiological processes.

The potential for decreasing individual doses of medications or the frequency of administration or both for older persons is the primary benefit of chronopharmacological therapy and may ultimately improve the therapeutic effect, decrease toxic effects, and improve compliance with a medication **regimen**. In addition, chronotherapeutics may be of financial benefit to the person (by reducing overall medication expense if lower or fewer doses are needed).

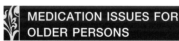

MEDICATION ISSUES FOR OLDER PERSONS

POLYPHARMACY

The number of administered medications that is "too many" is controversial. *Polypharmacy* is the use of a large number of medications, contraindicated or potentially inappropriate medications, or medications that are duplicated or unnecessary (Maggiore et al., 2010) (Fig. 14.2). The use of prescription medication increases with age (Reason et al., 2012). A Canadian study found that almost 27% of the older persons surveyed took more than five medications. Older persons who are subjected to polypharmacy are twice as likely as older persons taking one or two medications to report medication errors (Reason et al., 2012). Polypharmacy may be "accidental" when an existing medication regimen is not considered when new

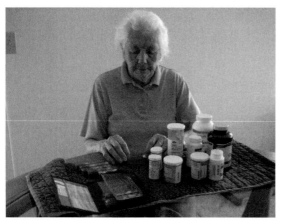

FIGURE 14.2 Polypharmacy. Courtesy Shannon Perry, Phoenix, AZ.

medications are prescribed or when any number of the thousands of OTC preparations and supplements are added to prescribed medications. The two major concerns with polypharmacy are the increased risks for medication interactions and for adverse events. Assessment and management of polypharmacy are competencies expected by the Canadian gerontological nursing *Standards of Practice* (Canadian Gerontological Nursing Association, 2010).

Medication Interactions

The more medications a person takes, the greater the possibility that one or more of the medications will interact with another medication, an herbal product or nutritional supplement, food, or alcohol. When two or more medications are given close together in time, the medications may **potentiate** one another, make one more effective, or make one or both less effective.

An interaction may result in altered pharmacokinetic activity or alterations in the absorption, distribution, metabolism, or excretion of one or more of the medications. Absorption can be delayed by medications that exert an anticholinergic effect. Tricyclic antidepressants act in this manner, decreasing gastrointestinal motility and interfering with the absorption of other medications. More than one medication may also compete to simultaneously occupy the necessary binding receptors, preventing one or the other from

reliably reaching the target organs and creating a varied bioavailability of one or both.

Interactions can also occur when two medications or foods are mixed together before administration. For example, medications are often crushed and delivered simultaneously through an enteral tube, yet the appropriate administration requires the nurse to know which medications are crushable and which medications can be administered together. For example, Fosamax and other bisphosphonates must be taken with a full glass of water 1 hour before any other medication, beverage, or food is ingested.

In pharmacodynamic interactions, one medication alters the body's response to another medication. This can be especially dangerous for older persons when two or more medications with the same effect are additive (that is, more potent taken together than when taken separately). Unless attention is paid to what the overall medication list includes, to when each medication is administered, and to what other products are taken, a harmful polypharmacy situation will occur. Nurses can lessen the likelihood of such a situation by monitoring the medications administered and by encouraging the older person to do the same.

Adverse Drug Reactions

Adverse drug reactions (ADRs) are unwanted pharmacological effects; they range from minor annoyances to death, and include allergic reactions. ADRs can sometimes be predicted from the pharmacological action of the medication (e.g., bone marrow depression from cancer chemotherapy; bleeding from Coumadin). Predictable ADRs can also occur when a person is started on a medication at a dosage that is inappropriately high or one that necessitates laboratory monitoring and adjustment (e.g., lithium or Coumadin).

All settings in which people take or are administered medications can have occurrences of ADRs. Up to 25% of all hospital admissions and emergency department visits are medication related, and older persons accounted for approximately 58% of all ADR-related hospital admissions between 2006 to 2007 and 2010 to 2011 (CIHI, 2013). Among the most common medications that lead to adverse reactions are anticoagulants, antibiotics, antineoplastic medications, nonsteroidal anti-inflammatory drugs,

TABLE 14.3	Examples of Drugs Considered Inappropriate for Older Persons
DRUG	**CONCERN**
Alprazolam (Xanax)	Rapid addiction, prolonged sedation effects, potential for confusion and falling
Amitriptyline (Elavil)	Strong anticholinergic and sedating properties, little effect on depression; with low dose, sometimes effective for neurogenic pain
Chlorpropamide (Diabinese)	Long lasting; danger of hypoglycemia is increased in older persons
Cimetidine (Tagamet)	Significant risk for ADRs with many substances and medications
Cyclobenzaprine (Flexeril)	Anticholinergic side effects, sedation, weakness
Diazepam (Valium)	Prolonged sedation, increasing fall risk and confusion risk
Diphenhydramine (Benadryl)	Excessive sedation, dry mouth, urinary retention, confusion
Dipyridamole (Persantine)	Orthostatic hypotension; no demonstrated effect on cognition
Disopyramide (Norpace)	May induce heart failure; strong anticholinergic effect
Doxepin (Sinequan)	Strong anticholinergic and sedating properties
Meperidine (Demerol)	Metabolite accumulation in older persons; can cause tremors and seizures
Oxybutynin (Ditropan)	Strong anticholinergic effect, confusion
Temazepam (Restoril)	Confusion, prolonged half-life

ADRs, Adverse drug reactions.
Source: Radcliff, S., Yue, J., Rocco, G., et al. (2015). American Geriatrics Society 2015 updated Beers Criteria for potentially inappropriate medication use in older adults. *Journal of the American Geriatrics Society, 63*(11), 2227–2246. doi:10.1111/jgs.13702.

and analgesics (CIHI, 2013). These medications are frequently prescribed to older persons. Because of the large number of medications taken by older persons in long-term care (LTC) settings and the high potential for residents to experience altered nutritional and fluid status, the risk for adverse reactions is of special concern to nurses working in these settings.

The use of medications that are considered inappropriate for older persons (Table 14.3) have also been found to increase the risk for ADRs and related hospitalizations. In a Canadian study by Morgan and colleagues, 37.2% of older persons were prescribed at least one inappropriate medication (Morgan et al., 2016). Older persons receiving medications from more than one prescriber are 1.3 times more likely to be hospitalized due to an ADR (CIHI, 2013).

Adverse drug reactions are not always predictable. An older person who is well controlled on a stable dose of a medication may undergo a change in physiology or environment that may alter the body's response to the medication. Changes in diet can also have a profound impact on medication effects. For example, decreased fluid intake can cause lithium toxicity (Oruch et al., 2014), and an increased intake of leafy green vegetables will counteract the anticoagulant effects of Coumadin and Aspirin (Masnoon et al., 2016). Some medications (e.g., antipsychotics, stimulants, anticholinergics) interfere with the body's ability to regulate temperature, such that exposure to hot weather can lead more easily to heat stroke (Ruscin, 2009). Other medications (e.g., sulfa medications, antidepressants, and many antipsychotics) are photosensitizing, and an increase in sun exposure can lead more quickly to sunburn than expected (Khandpur et al., 2016). Older persons whose fluid intake is decreased because of illness, because they cannot access fluids, or because their intake is inadequate in hot weather may quickly become volume depleted and develop increased sensitivity to the orthostatic hypotensive effects of alpha-blockers (e.g., phenothiazines and terazosin) or toxicity to antipsychotics (Jett, 2012).

BOX 14.1   Common Medications With the Potential to Cause Cognitive Impairment

Alcohol
Analgesics
Anticholinergics
Antidepressants
Antihistamines
Antiparkinsonian agents
Antipsychotics
Benzodiazepines
Beta-blockers
Digitalis, Lanoxin
Diuretics
Muscle relaxants
Sedatives, hypnotics

One of the most troublesome ADRs for the older person is medication-induced delirium and confusion. Polypharmacy with several psychotropic medications that have anticholinergic actions is perhaps the greatest precipitator of delirium as an adverse reaction (Morley, 2014). Too often, delirium goes unrecognized as an ADR and is instead perceived as a worsening of pre-existing dementia or even as new-onset dementia (see Chapter 21). Any time there is a change in an older person's function or cognitive abilities, the possibility of medication effect must be thoroughly evaluated. Box 14.1 contains a partial list of medications that have the potential to adversely affect cognitive functioning.

Another common adverse effect seen in older persons is lethargy, especially with the use of a number of the cardiovascular agents and antidepressants. Lethargy can be misinterpreted as a symptom of worsening cardiac, respiratory, or neurological conditions rather than as an ADR. Among other troublesome effects are those related to sexual functioning. Although they are not detailed in this chapter, many medications interfere with or contribute to sexual dysfunction in adults of any age. The medications that are most responsible are cardiovascular medications (antihypertensives and angiotensin-converting enzyme inhibitors) and psychotropic medications (antidepressants).

MISUSE OF MEDICATIONS

Medication misuse includes overuse, underuse, erratic use, and contraindicated use. Misuse of medications can occur for any number of reasons, from inadequate skills of the prescribers or the nurses who administer the medications, the misunderstanding of instructions, or inadequate funds to purchase prescribed medications. Although misuse of medications is often referred to as noncompliance, the term "misuse" is more descriptive of what is happening (see Chapter 24). It is important that gerontological nurses realize that the greater the number of medications taken, the greater is the potential for misuse. Wilcox et al. (1994) identified 20 medications that are considered inappropriate for older persons, including controversial cardiovascular agents (propranolol, methyldopa, and reserpine). The Beers Criteria identifies medications that carry a higher-than-usual risk when used with older persons (Beers, 1997). The Beers Criteria has been recommended as a "best practice" by several Canadian regulating and professional organizations and by the Hartford Institute of Geriatric Nursing. The list can be found at https://www.dcri.org/beers-criteria-medication-list/.

The misuse of a medication by the person taking it may be accidental (e.g., through misunderstanding or the inability to read labels or understand instructions), or it may be deliberate (e.g., through an attempt to make a prescription medication last longer, for financial reasons; because of cultural differences; or due to beliefs that the dose is too low or too high). When a person is labelled noncompliant, nurses may become frustrated with the individual for his or her inability to follow the plan of care and medication regime. Yet care providers tend to forget or ignore the reality that a person cannot and will not comply with a prescription or treatment plan under certain circumstances, such as when it is incompatible with the person's day-to-day life. For example, an individual cannot follow the instruction to "take medication three times per day with meals" if he or she eats only two meals each day (which is often the case with older persons).

Memory failures associated with noncompliance to medication regimens are generally of two types: (1) the person forgets to take the medications correctly (e.g., dose, route) and (2) the person experiences "prospective" recall failure, in which the person forgets to take the medication at the correct times, resulting in missed doses. The more frequently a medication must be taken, the less likely it will be taken as prescribed. With more and more medications available in once-a-day doses rather than doses to be taken three or four times each day, more people can take their medications as instructed.

Problems with regard to health literacy also limit a person's ability to correctly take medications (see Chapter 7). Many older persons, especially those from minority groups, have low levels of literacy; thus, written instructions should be at the Grade 3 level or lower. Limitations in vision will interfere with the reading of instructions, especially those on bottle labels; pharmacists can use large type or symbols to avoid this problem. The practice of nurses, physicians, and pharmacists giving rapid-fire directions is not effective when addressing most older persons, especially those with hearing impairments or normal age-related changes. It is also common for care providers to explain the treatment and give directions concerning medications when the person is physically uncomfortable or is about to be discharged from a care facility; to explain instructions in English even when the person has limited English proficiency; and to explain medication regimens while in a noisy or busy place. All of these practices can significantly reduce the clarity of the message and lead to consequent misuse of medications.

IMPLICATIONS FOR GERONTOLOGICAL NURSING AND HEALTHY AGING

ASSESSMENT

The initial step in ensuring that older persons use their medications safely and effectively is to conduct a comprehensive medication assessment. In some settings, a clinical pharmacist collects the medication history, but this assessment is more often completed through the combined efforts of the nurses and the prescribing health care provider (a nurse practitioner or physician).

Medication reconciliation is a formal process of comparing the prescribed medications to the medications the person is actually taking. This reconciliation is designed to prevent ADRs that occur as a result of miscommunication at times of transition in care (e.g., from one health care setting to another or from a health care setting to home) or when more than one physician is prescribing medication. Medication reconciliation on admission to, discharge from, or transfer between services is required by Canadian hospital accreditation standards. A medication reconciliation kit is available from the Institute for Safe Medication Practices website (http://www.ismp.org).

Ideally, it is best to use a "brown bag approach"—ask the person to bring in a bag containing all medications and other health products currently being taken or used. As each container of medication is taken out of the bag, the nurse asks the person how he or she actually takes the medication. By obtaining information in this manner rather than by following the written prescriptions, the nurse can determine if a misunderstanding or misuse is occuring. Another approach, associated with the review of systems or problems, is to ask questions such as, "What medication do you take for your heart? What medication do you take for your breathing?" Older people will often answer the above question with a description (e.g., "a little blue pill" or "a bad-tasting pill"). It is also important to ask about any prescribed medications the person is not currently using or is not refilling according to the prescription.

As the nurse learns what herbs, supplements, and OTC and prescribed medications the person takes, the assessment can continue. There is a great deal of information needed, but this assessment is vital to promote the health and well-being of the older person (Box 14.2). Through this assessment, nurses can learn of discrepancies between the prescribed dosage and the actual dosage, potential medication–medication and food–medication interactions, and potential or actual ADRs.

MONITORING AND EVALUATION

A significant part of a gerontological nurse's responsibilities consists of monitoring and evaluating the effectiveness of prescribed treatments and observing for signs of problems or iatrogenic complications. Monitoring and evaluating a situation involves observing and documenting observations, noting changes in physical and functional status (e.g., vital

BOX 14.2   Components of a Comprehensive Medication Assessment

Medications taken and prescribed, as described by patient, with names, doses, and frequency

Diagnosis associated with each medication

Beliefs regarding effectiveness and necessity of medications

Over-the-counter preparations, with doses, frequency, and reason taken

Herbals, with doses, frequency, and reason taken

Nutritional assessment (many food choices influence pharmacokinetics)

Nutritional supplements, with doses, frequency, and reason taken

Medication-related problems, such as side effects, difficulties with compliance

Ability to pay for and obtain prescription medications

Source of prescriptions

Persons involved in decision making regarding medications

Use of tobacco or nicotine in gum, patch, or forms of smoking

Use of alcohol, caffeine, and nonprescription medications

Medications borrowed from other persons

Recently discontinued medications

History of allergies, interactions, and adverse medication reactions

Strategies used to remember when to take medications as prescribed

Identification of malnutrition and hydration status

Recent medication blood levels, as appropriate

Recent measurements of liver and kidney functioning

Sources: Adapted from the Ontario College of Pharmacists. (2007). *Best possible medication history guidelines for medication reconciliation.* Toronto, Ontario, Canada: Ontario College of Pharmacists. Retrieved from http://www.ocpinfo.com/library/practice-related/download/Best%20 Possible%20Medication%20History.pdf; American Geriatrics Society. (2015). *Beers criteria for potentially inappropriate medication use in older adults.* Retrieved from http://www.americangeriatrics.org/press/ id:5907.

signs, performance of activities of daily living, sleeping, eating, hydrating, and eliminating) and changes in mental status (attention and alertness, memory, orientation, behaviour, mood, emotional display and affect, and content and characteristics of interactions). Monitoring also means ensuring that blood levels (such as fluids and electrolytes, albumin, and creatinine) are measured as needed. The following must be monitored on a schedule: thyroid-stimulating hormone levels for individuals taking thyroid replacement medication; international normalized ratios for those taking warfarin; periodic hemoglobin A1c levels for people with diabetes; serum digoxin level for individuals taking digoxin; and serum lithium levels for those prescribed lithium. Nurses need to promptly communicate their findings of potential problems to the person's nurse practitioner or physician.

PATIENT EDUCATION

Nurses are responsible for educating patients (individually or in small groups) about medication use, by way of setting goals and creating a treatment plan (Box 14.3). Older persons should be encouraged to ask questions and know what medication they are taking, how it will affect them, and what alternatives are available to them. Pamphlets and booklets written in lay terms, in appropriate language, and at an appropriate reading level should be available; if none are available, the nurse can develop a booklet or information sheet for the particular person. Information is best presented in bulleted lists rather than in paragraph form, and the type should be large and boldfaced. (See Chapter 7 for additional information about health education for older persons.)

Because of the complex needs of older persons, educating them about medications can be particularly challenging. The following tips may be helpful:

1. *Identify key persons:* Find out who, if anyone, manages the person's medications or assists with decision making. When applicable and with the person's permission, make sure that the support person is present during the education or teaching session..

2. *Ensure good environment:* Minimize distraction, and avoid competing with television or other sources for the person's attention. Make sure the person is comfortable and is not hungry, thirsty, tired, too warm or too cold, in pain, or in need of the bathroom.

3. *Determine best time:* Teach during the best time of the day for the person (i.e., when he or she is most alert, engaged, and energetic), and keep the sessions short and succinct.

4. *Communicate:* Ensure that you are understood. Make sure that the older person has his or her eyeglasses or hearing aids on if these are used. Use

---

BOX 14.3 Questions and Recommendations for Older Persons Taking Medications

- What is the name of each medication?
- What is the purpose of each medication?
- What is the dose per administration?
- What is the number of doses every day?
- What is the best time to take the medication?
- How should the medication be taken?
- Do food or fluid choices influence the absorption or metabolism of the medication?
- Can the medication be taken with other medications?
- Which medications can and cannot be taken together?
- Are any special techniques, devices, or procedures necessary to administer the medication?
- For how long should the medication be taken?
- What are the common side effects?
- If side effects occur, what should be done? What changes in administration are necessary? When should the medication be stopped? When should the physician or pharmacist (or both) be called?
- What can be done at home to watch for a therapeutic medication response?
- What should be done if a dose is missed?
- How many refills are allowed?
- How should the medication be stored?
- What nonprescription preparations should not be used with the present medication?
- Take all medications prescribed unless the physician states otherwise.
- If any new or unusual problems occur—such as shortness of breath, nausea, diarrhea, vomiting, sleepiness, dizziness, weakness, skin rash, or fever— stop taking the medication and report the problem.
- Never take medication prescribed for another person.
- Do not take medication that is more than 1 year old or past the expiration date on the container.
- Store medications in a safe place, preferably in the kitchen rather than in the bathroom, where moisture from bathing and (especially) showers may affect them.
- Do not keep medicines, especially sedatives and hypnotics, on the bedside stand; when you are sleepy, you may forget that you have already taken the medication.
- Do not place different medicines in the same container.
- Take a sufficient supply of all medicines in their individual containers when travelling away from home.
- Use a chart to keep track of medications.

---

simple and direct language, and avoid medical or nursing jargon (e.g., "intake"). Remain respectful at all times, and do not allow negative stereotypes to cloud communication. Encourage questions.

5. *Reinforce teaching:* Provide memory aids to reinforce teaching. Have actual medications or containers handy to visually illustrate directions. If appropriate, use written charts and lists with large letters and simple language, or charts with pictures of the medications and symbols for times of the day. After discharge, a follow-up phone call can help with assessing accurate medication usage or other problems with medications. A nurse's home visit to people at high risk for problems, such as those with cognitive deficits or those who have many medications for new conditions, reinforces education and provides assessment information.

6. *Evaluate teaching:* Have the person repeat back instructions and each medication's name, purposes, side effects, and times for administration. Have the patient describe his or her method for remembering to take the medicines and to mark off their ingestion.

7. *Avoid medication interactions:* Older people should be taught to obtain all their medications from the same pharmacy if possible, so that the pharmacist is able to watch for medication duplications and interactions. Additional information about recognizing and responding to early signs of ADRs may save lives.

MEDICATION ADMINISTRATION

Most older persons self-administer their medications; others receive them from family, friends, or health care providers. In LTC homes, the administration of medications is carried out by nurses. Regardless of the setting or the persons involved, several skills are needed for safe administration.

To ensure optimal safety, everyone who administers medication needs to take the "Ten Rights" into account. These ten rights are right medication, right patient, right dose, right time and frequency, right route, right reason, right documentation, right to refuse, right patient education, and right evaluation.

Several other factors need to be taken into consideration when administering medication or providing education to the older person.

Because of the high rate of arthritis and other debilitating conditions among older persons, it may be difficult or impossible for the older person to open a medication bottle, remove a medication bottle's cap, or break a tablet. Either the person or the nurse can ask the pharmacist to break the pills, dispense a smaller dose, or provide blister packages that are easy to open.

Many tablets and capsules are difficult to swallow because of their size or because they stick to the tongue, especially if the mouth is dry. A medication in liquid form is sometimes preferable and allows for flexible dosing; concentrations can be varied so that quantities of solution can be prepared and taken by the teaspoon or tablespoon, simple and commonly used household measurements. Crushing tablets or emptying the powder from capsules into fluid or food should not be done, unless specified by the pharmaceutical company or approved by a pharmacist; doing so may interfere with the effectiveness of the medication (causing either underdose or toxicity), create problems in administration, or injure the mouth or gastro-intestinal tract.

Some people have difficulty swallowing capsules. They can be advised to place the capsule onto the front of the tongue and swallow a fluid; this should wash the capsule to the back of the throat and down. Other persons do better taking pills or capsules with a semisolid food—such as applesauce, chocolate syrup, or peanut butter—as long as the substances do not interact.

Enteric-coated, extended-release, and sustained-release products allow absorption at different parts of the gastro-intestinal tract. Capsules containing these medications should never be broken, opened, or otherwise altered before administration, nor should pills be crushed before being taken. A transdermal patch, also called a transdermal delivery system, provides for a more constant rate of medication absorption and eliminates concern for gastro-intestinal absorption variation, gastro-intestinal tolerance, and medication interaction. Transdermal delivery systems are not recommended for persons who are noticeably underweight, because absorption is unpredictable owing to the reduced body fat.

Several supports are available for the older person who is self-administering medication. Pharmacists can prepare weekly doses of the required medication prepackaged in daily doses in easily opened containers, dossettes, or blister packs. Weekly calendars or tear-off-daily calendars will remind the older person to take daily medication. Clear envelopes or sandwich bags containing the medication can be affixed to the square on a calendar; each envelope or bag should state the medication's name, dose, and times it is to be taken that day. Commercial medication boxes are available for single or multiple doses by the day, week, or month, and some have medication administration alarms.

PSYCHOTROPIC MEDICATIONS

Psychotropic medications are those that alter brain chemistry, emotions, and behaviour. They include antipsychotics (formerly known as neuroleptics), antidepressants, mood stabilizers, anti-anxiety agents (anxiolytics), and sedative-hypnotic medications. This section provides an overview of psychotropic medications used to treat symptoms of disorders of behaviour, cognition, arousal, and mood in the gerontological population. This chapter also provides information on treating the movement disorders that may occur as a side effect of the use of antipsychotics.

PSYCHOTROPIC MEDICATION FOR OLDER PERSONS

Gerontological nurses, especially in LTC settings, are likely to care for older persons with mental health problems or cognitive impairment, especially depression, anxiety, and psychosis. The rate of depression for older persons 65 years old or older living in the community is about 10 to 15%; the rate is up to 44% in LTC settings (Government of Canada, 2016). Treatment for depression and other mental health problems has both pharmacological and nonpharmacological components.

Psychotropic medications can alter some behaviours and emotions; these medications can be prescribed only after thorough medical, psychological, and social assessments. These assessments should be done quickly to enable the individual to receive the appropriate treatment as soon as possible. Pharmacological interventions need to be supplemented by nonpharmacological measures such as counselling.

Nursing assessment before medication intervention contributes knowledge and baseline information that can optimize the patient's medical and psychological improvement. Issues to consider include the patient's medical status (and medications that might interact with psychotropics), mental status, ability to carry out ADLs and IADLs, and ability to participate in social activities and maintain satisfying relationships with others. The pharmacological treatment can include antidepressants, anti-anxiety medications or antipsychotics, or any combination of these medications.

ANTIDEPRESSANTS

Antidepressants are medications used to treat depression. In the past, the major antidepressants were monoamine oxidase inhibitors (MAOIs) and tricyclic antidepressants (TCAs), especially amitriptyline and doxepin (Sinequan). These medications had significant side effects, such as dry mouth, constipation, sedation, and urinary retention. The development of newer antidepression medications, such as selective serotonin reuptake inhibitors (SSRIs) and nonselective serotonin reuptake inhibitors (NSSRIs), has decreased the use of MAOIs and TCAs.

The SSRIs (e.g., Zoloft, Prozac) and NSSRIs are highly effective but have been implicated in serotonin syndrome, a potentially life-threatening ADR (Werneke et al., 2016). Serotonin syndrome manifests as changes in autonomic function and mental status as well as other neurological findings within 6 to 8 hours of starting or increasing serotonergic medications (Werneke et al., 2016). Taken in combination with St. John's wort (an herbal preparation taken for mild depression), SSRIs can also cause serotonin syndrome (Apaydin et al., 2016). Recognition and discontinuation of the causative medication is essential. Table 14.4 outlines the mild, moderate, and severe signs and symptoms of serotonin syndrome. Most SSRIs and NSSRIs cause initial problems with nausea or dry mouth. One side effect of the SSRIs that does not resolve with time is sexual dysfunction. The NSSRIs and other antidepressants, such as Effexor,

---

TABLE 14.4 Signs and Symptoms of Serotonin Syndrome

SEVERITY	AUTONOMIC SYMPTOMS	NEUROLOGICAL SYMPTOMS	MENTAL STATUS	OTHER
Mild	• Afebrile or low-grade fever • Tachycardia • Mydriasis • Diaphoresis or shivering	• Intermittent tremor • Akathisia • Myoclonus • Mild hyper-reflexia	• Restlessness • Anxiety	
Moderate	• Increased tachycardia • Fever (up to 41°C) • Diarrhea with hyperactive bowel sounds • Diaphoresis with normal skin colour	• Hyper-reflexia • Inducible clonus • Ocular clonus (slow continuous lateral eye movements) • Myoclonus	• Easily startled • Increased confusion • Agitation and hypervigilance	• Rhabdomyolysis • Metabolic acidosis • Renal failure • Disseminated intravascular coagulopathy (secondary to hyperthermia)
Severe	• Temperature often greater than 41°C (secondary to increased tone)	• Increased muscle tone (lower limbs greater than upper limbs) • Spontaneous clonus • Substantial myoclonus or hyper-reflexia	• Delirium • Coma	• As above

Source: Adapted from Botros, M., Wood, K., Negatu, Y., et al. (2016). Serotonin syndrome and critical care: A case report. *CHEST Journal, 150*(4S), 384A–384A. doi:10.1016/j.chest.2016.08.397; Werneke, U., Jamshidi, F., Taylor, D. M., et al. (2016). Conundrums in neurology: Diagnosing serotonin syndrome—a meta-analysis of cases. *BMC Neurology, 16*(1), 97. doi:10.1186/s12883-016-0616-1.

Wellbutrin, and Trazodone, are less likely to cause this problem and may be preferred by older persons who are sexually active.

Many older persons experience a therapeutic effect and significant relief from depression at lower doses of SSRIs because of age-related changes affecting the metabolism of medication. More than one trial of a medication, as well as some time, is often needed to find the optimal dose. Nurses can help older persons and their support persons monitor target symptoms and advocate for continued dose adjustments or changes until relief is obtained (see Chapter 24).

Gradually tapering doses is recommended when discontinuing SSRIs, because withdrawal effects that are self-limiting yet uncomfortable and distressing can occur, especially when medications are abruptly discontinued (Cosci, 2016). Discontinuation symptoms can include disequilibrium (e.g., dizziness, vertigo, ataxia), gastro-intestinal issues (e.g., nausea and vomiting), flulike symptoms (e.g., myalgia, fatigue), sensory disturbances (e.g., paresthesia), and sleep disturbances (e.g., insomnia, vivid dreams). Other psychological symptoms, such as anxiety and irritability, can occur (Cosci, 2016). When discussing the possibility of starting SSRIs, nurses can educate and inform the person about the side effects and possible withdrawal symptoms. This information is important in helping the person understand that these symptoms could be normal and that the medication is not an addictive substance.

ANTI-ANXIETY AGENTS

Medications designed for treatment of anxiety are referred to as anti-anxiety agents or *anxiolytics*. The decision to treat anxiety pharmacologically is based on the degree to which the anxiety interferes with the person's ability to function and on the person's feelings of discomfort.

Anxiolytics include benzodiazepines, buspirone, and beta-blockers. Antihistamines, especially diphenhydramine (Benadryl), are often used but are not recommended, owing to their anticholinergic effects. Antidepressants are usually the first-line pharmacological treatment for anxiety in older persons because of the risks associated with the use of benzodiazepines.

The most frequently used anxiolytic agents are the benzodiazepines. Older persons metabolize these medications slowly; thus, the medications remain in the bloodstream for long periods and can easily reach toxic levels. Adverse effects include drowsiness, dizziness, ataxia, mild cognitive deficits, and memory impairment. Signs of toxicity include excessive sedation, unsteady gait, confusion, disorientation, cognitive impairment, memory impairment, agitation, and wandering. Because these symptoms resemble those of dementia, people can easily be misdiagnosed once they start taking benzodiazepines. Benzodiazepines are highly addicting but are often prescribed because of their quick sedating effects for the highly anxious person. Because of the problems noted above, however, they should be avoided, except in extreme cases.

Lorazepam (Ativan), when prescribed in very low doses and for short periods, appears to be the least problematic benzodiazepine. It has the shortest half-life of the benzodiazepines and no active metabolites. Buspirone, which is not a benzodiazepine, is a safer alternative. Although dizziness is a side effect, it is often dose-related and resolves with time. Buspirone is best used for chronic anxiety and is not indicated for acute needs (see Chapter 24).

ANTIPSYCHOTICS

The term "psychosis" refers to a break with reality and may include **delusions**, **hallucinations**, and **thought disorders**. The person's behaviour is a response to this private reality—a reality that may be distressing and problematic for the person and those around him or her. Characteristically, psychosis occurs in schizophrenia as part of the typical presentation of the illness; however, some psychotic symptoms can also occur as part of mania, depression, some paranoid states, delirium, infection, and dementia.

A psychosis manifests as delusional beliefs, hallucinations, and thought disorders, which can cause extreme anxiety and bizarre behaviour. Antipsychotics, also known as neuroleptics, are medications used to treat psychotic symptoms. Older antipsychotics, referred to as *typical antipsychotics* or *first-generation antipsychotics*, include haloperidol, perphenazine, and chlorpromazine. The newer antipsychotics, referred to as *atypical antipsychotics* or *second-generation antipsychotics*, include risperidone, olanzepine, and Seroquel. When antipsychotics are prescribed to older persons, the atypical antipsychotics should be the first-line treatment because they cause fewer side effects. However, haloperidol is the first-line treatment when antipsychotics are used in the treatment of delirium if there is no previous evidence of Parkinson's disease or Lewy body dementia (Canadian Coalition for Seniors' Mental Health, 2014).

Unfortunately, antipsychotics are often misused by caregivers and health care providers in an attempt to control disruptive behaviours and are used without a careful assessment of the underlying cause of the behaviours.

When used appropriately and cautiously for psychotic illnesses, antipsychotics can provide a person with relief. Medications with the lowest side effects profile and at the lowest dose possible should be prescribed. Prescribing and using antipsychotics for persons with dementia is never recommended as a first-line treatment; nonpharmacological approaches should be considered as first-line treatments, even in conjunction with antipsychotics if necessary (Gitlin et al., 2012). In such a case, low doses, small increases in dose, and careful monitoring by an experienced nurse, nurse practitioner, or physician are necessary.

Although the atypical antipsychotics have a better side effect profile (e.g., fewer anticholinergic effects) than the typical antipsychotics have, older persons who take them may experience side effects (Amodeo et al., 2016). Some typical and atypical antipsychotics can cause orthostatic hypotension, thereby increasing the risk for falls. Anticholinergic effects are more likely with typical antipsychotics and are mild with atypical antipsychotics (except clozapine, which is strongly anticholinergic). Anticholinergic side effects include dry mouth, constipation, urinary retention, hypotension, and confusion. Careful nursing observation is essential for monitoring side effects and medication interactions whenever any of these medications is given.

Owing to antipsychotics' effects on the thermoregulatory centre of the brain, persons who take antipsychotics cannot tolerate excess environmental heat. Even mild elevations of core temperature can result in liver damage called *neuroleptic malignant syndrome*. This syndrome is a serious complication of taking antipsychotic medications. It is uncommon but has a mortality rate of 10 to 30% of people who experience it (Berman, 2011; Chandran et al., 2003). The most common clinical signs are abnormal blood pressure (typically hypertension), altered level of consciousness, diaphoresis, flushing, incontinence, muscle rigidity, tachycardia, and tachypnea (Berman, 2011). Common laboratory test findings include elevated creatine kinase levels due to rhabdomyolysis and leukocytosis (Berman, 2011). Other symptoms can include chorea (involuntary movements), generalized tonic-clonic seizures, mutism (inability to speak), opisthotonus (extreme hyperextension of the body, with the head and heels bent backward and the body bowed forward), positive Babinski's sign, trismus (motor disturbance of the trigeminal nerve), and increased transaminase levels (Chandran et al., 2003). The person taking antipsychotics must avoid or be protected from hyperthermia by staying in a cool environment, maintaining adequate hydration, being in a cool area when engaging in activity, and using a fan or taking a sponge bath should overheating occur. The person may or may not communicate his or her discomfort, so an assessment of body temperature is essential. Diuretics, coffee, alcohol, lithium, and uncontrolled diabetes decrease vascular volume, thereby decreasing the body's ability to sweat. Anticholinergics inhibit sweating and lead to further heat retention.

Movement Disorders

The most significant potential side effects of antipsychotics are movement disorders, also referred to as *extrapyramidal syndrome (EPS)* reactions—acute dystonia, akathisia, parkinsonian symptoms, and tardive dyskinesia. Although the risk for these side effects is lower with atypical antipsychotics, the effects do occur for some people.

Acute Dystonia. An acute dystonic reaction is an abnormal involuntary movement consisting of a slow and continuous muscular contraction or spasm. Involuntary muscular contractions of the mouth, jaw, face, and neck are common. The jaw may lock (trismus), the tongue may roll back and block the throat, the neck may arch backward (opisthotonos), or the eyes may close or be fixed in one position. These effects often create a feeling of needing to look up constantly without the ability to lower the eyes. Dystonias can be painful and frightening. An acute dystonic reaction may occur hours or days after antipsychotic medication administration or dosage increases and may last for minutes to hours.

Caregivers or others who are unfamiliar with EPS reactions often become alarmed. Although frightening, acute dystonia is usually not dangerous and is quickly relieved by anticholinergic medication such as benztropine, trihexyphenidyl, or diphenhydramine (Benadryl). These medications should be readily available to treat dystonic reactions in persons who are taking antipsychotics.

Akathisia. *Akathisia* refers to the compulsion to be in motion. Akathisia may occur at any time during therapy. People who are diagnosed with akathisia report feeling restless, being unable to be still, or having an unrelenting desire to move. Often this symptom is mistaken for worsening psychosis instead of the ADR that it is. Pacing, aimless walking, fidgeting, shifting weight from one leg to the other, and marked restlessness are characteristic behaviours for a person experiencing akathisia.

Parkinsonian Symptoms. The use of antipsychotics may cause symptoms that mimic Parkinson's disease. A bilateral tremor (as opposed to the unilateral tremor characteristic of true Parkinson's disease), bradykinesia, and rigidity that may progress to the inability to move may be observed. The person may have an inflexible facial expression and appear bored and apathetic and be mistakenly diagnosed as depressed. More common when higher-potency typical antipsychotics are given, parkinsonian symptoms may occur within weeks to months of the initiation of antipsychotic therapy.

Tardive Dyskinesia. People who have used antipsychotics continuously for at least 3 to 6 months are at risk for developing an irreversible movement disorder called *tardive dyskinesia (TD).* The risk of TD is considerably lower with the use of atypical antipsychotics. It usually appears first as wormlike movements of the tongue; grimacing, blinking, and frowning are other facial movements that occur. Slow, maintained, involuntary twisting movements of limbs, trunk, neck, face, and eyes (involuntary eye closure) have been observed. It is essential that nurses be attentive for early detection, so that changes to the psychotropic regimen can be made promptly.

Response to treatment is the most important consideration when psychotropics are taken. The person's subjective comments about feelings and symptoms and caregivers' observations of the person's behaviour are important data for evaluating the effectiveness of a medication.

MOOD STABILIZERS

Mood stabilizers are agents used for the treatment of bipolar disorders (formerly known as manic depression), which are characterized by periods of mania or hypomania and by periods of depression affecting the person's functioning. The symptoms of mania are euphoria (elation), disinhibition, impulsivity, distractibility, grandiosity, labile affect, pressured speech and flight of ideas, increased psychomotor activity, irritability that can result in anger, and decreased need for sleep. Hypomania, less extreme, is characterized by the same symptoms, but they last for a shorter time than in mania and do not markedly impair the person's functioning. For the older person, the symptoms of bipolar disorders are easily confused with the symptoms of moderate dementia (e.g., wandering, emotional lability) (see Chapter 24).

Lithium carbonate (Lithium), divalproex sodium (Epival) and carbamazepine (Tegretol) are mood-stabilizing medications. When a person with bipolar disorder or who is taking a mood stabilizer is being cared for, guidance from a psychiatrist is required. It is important to monitor patients who are taking lithium, as this medication interacts with other medications and certain foods. Lithium has a narrow therapeutic window, and toxicity can develop quickly. A low-salt diet will elevate the lithium level, and a high-salt diet will decrease it. Likewise, thiazide diuretics and nonsteroidal anti-inflammatory medications will elevate the serum lithium level. The side effects of lithium include fine resting tremor, fatigue, polyuria, and polydipsia. Nausea, vomiting, diarrhea, vertigo, muscle weakness, and sleepiness may occur when the medication is initiated, but these symptoms resolve. Symptoms of toxicity include gastro-intestinal symptoms, drowsiness, ataxia, tinnitus, blurred vision, confusion, muscle twitching, hyper-reflexia, and seizures; eventually, coma and death occur.

SUMMARY

This chapter reviewed age-related pharmacokinetic changes, medication compliance, and the use of psychotropic medications in the older population. All medications have indications, side effects, and interactions, as well as individual reactions. The nurse's advocacy role includes educating the older person and the family and determining whether the side effects are minimal and tolerable or whether they are serious. Asking the person about his or her experience and observing interactions, behaviour, mood, emotional responses, and daily habits provide data to delineate the problem, develop nursing diagnoses and interventions, and decide outcome criteria.

Medications occupy a central place in the lives of many older persons; cost, acceptability, interactions, unacceptable side effects, and the need to schedule medications appropriately all combine to create many difficulties. Nurses need to have a strong understanding of issues specific to the safe administration and consumption of medications in the older population in order to reduce the use of inappropriate medications and prevent or treat side effects and interactions. The nurse might also increase compliance through providing personally and culturally appropriate instructions.

Nurses in all health care settings are responsible for monitoring the overall health of older persons, being alert for the need for laboratory tests and other measures to ensure the correct dosage of several medications. Nurses are often the first care providers to assess medication use, evaluate outcomes, and teach older persons about safe medication use and self-administration.

KEY CONCEPTS

- The aging body responds to medication changes.
- Any medication has side effects. The therapeutic goal is to reduce the targeted symptoms without undesirable side effects.
- Medication–medication and medication–food incompatibilities are an increasing problem with aging.
- Polypharmacy is of serious concern for older persons.

- Medication misuse may be triggered by prescriber practices, individual self-medication and physiology, altered biodegradability, nutritional and fluid states, and inadequate assessment before prescribing.
- Nurses must consider the occurrence of a possible medication side effect immediately if they observe changes in the person's condition, including functional changes and changes in cognitive status.
- Chronotherapy uses the biorhythms of the body for the most effective medication therapy; it has the potential to decrease the dose, frequency, and cost of medication regimens and to improve compliance with medication therapy.
- The side effects of psychotropic medications vary significantly; thus, these medications must be selected and prescribed for the older person with care.
- The responses of the older person to treatment with psychotropic medications should be reduced distress, clearer thinking, and more appropriate behaviour.
- Older persons are particularly vulnerable to developing movement disorders with the use of antipsychotics.
- Any time a behavioural change in a person is noted, reversible causes must be sought and treated before medications are used.
- Dosages of medications must be carefully titrated for the individual, and the individual's responses must be accurately and consistently recorded.

ACTIVITIES AND DISCUSSION QUESTIONS

1. Describe the age-related changes that occur in the pharmacokinetics of the older person.
2. Explain the meaning of "chronotherapeutics." How applicable is chronotherapeutics to older persons?
3. Describe the medication use patterns of the older population. What can be done to correct or improve them?
4. Explain the role of the older person, the care provider, and the social network in medication compliance.

5. List a variety of measures that nurses can suggest to assist older persons with their medication use and compliance with their medication regimen.
6. List the most troublesome side effects of antipsychotic medications.
7. Describe what you would do to manage the following situation: Mrs. J. is calling out repeatedly for a nurse; although other patients are complaining, you simply cannot be available for long periods to quiet her.
8. Review the medications taken by an older person in the clinical setting. Use the Beers Criteria for Potentially Inappropriate Medication Use in Older Adults to determine if any of the medications are potentially contraindicated. Discuss your findings.

RESOURCES

The 2015 American Geriatrics Society Updated Beers Criteria for Potentially Inappropriate Medication Use in Older Adults
https://consultgeri.org/try-this/general-assessment/issue-16

Canadian Coalition for Seniors' Mental Health (CCSMH). *Guidelines on the assessment and treatment of depression, delirium, dementia, and suicide risk in older adults*
http://www.ccsmh.ca

Canadian Patient Safety Institute (CPSI). Medication safety
http://www.patientsafetyinstitute.ca/en/Topic/Pages/Medication-Safety.aspx

Government of Canada. *Medication matters: How you can help seniors use medication safely*
http://publications.gc.ca/site/eng/9.646877/publication.html

Government of Canada. *Sleeping pills and tranquilizers: Important information for seniors*
http://publications.gc.ca/site/eng/112429/publication.html

Information about medications used for Alzheimer's disease
http://www.alz.org

Institute for Safe Medication Practices (ISMP)
http://www.ismp.org/about/default.aspx

Institution for Safe Medication Practices Canada (ISMP Canada). Medication reconciliation in acute care: Getting started kit

https://www.ismp-canada.org/download/MedRec/Medrec_AC_English_GSK_V3.pdf

For additional resources, please visit *http://evolve.elsevier.com/Canada/Ebersole/gerontological/*

REFERENCES

American Geriatrics Society (AGS) 2015 Beers Criteria Update Expert Panel. (2015). American Geriatrics Society 2015 updated Beers Criteria for potentially inappropriate medication use in older adults. *Journal of the American Geriatrics Society, 63*(11), 2227–2246.

Amodeo, K., Schneider, R. B., & Richard, I. H. (2016). Call to caution with the use of atypical antipsychotics for treatment of depression in older adults. *Geriatrics, 1*(4), 33–41. doi:10.3390/geriatrics1040033.

Apaydin, E. A., Maher, A. R., Shanman, R., et al. (2016). A systematic review of St. John's Wort for major depressive disorder. *Systematic Reviews, 5*(1), 148. doi:10.1186/s13643-016-0325-2.

Beers, M. H. (1997). Explicit criteria for determining potentially inappropriate medication use by the elderly: An update. *Archives of Internal Medicine, 157*(14), 1531–1536.

Berman, B. D. (2011). Neuroleptic malignant syndrome. *The Neurohospitalist, 1*(1), 41–47. doi:10.1177/1941875210386491.

Bernier, N. F. (2017). *Improving prescription drug safety for Canadian seniors.* Retrieved from http://irpp.org/wp-content/uploads/2017/01/study-no61.pdf.

Briggs, G. C. (2005). Geriatric issues. In E. Youngkin, K. J. Sawin, J. Kissinger, et al. (Eds.), *Pharmacotherapeutics: A primary care guide.* Upper Saddle River, NJ: Prentice-Hall.

Brown, P. (2017). Osteoporosis and fracture prevention in primary care. In A. Connolly & A. Britton (Eds.), *Women's health in primary care* (pp. 230–241). Cambridge, UK: Cambridge University Press.

Bushra, R., Aslam, N., & Khan, A. Y. (2011). Food-drug interactions. *Oman Medical Journal, 26*(2), 77–83. doi:10.5001/omj.2011.21.

Canadian Coalition for Seniors' Mental Health (CCSMH). (2014). *The assessment and treatment of delirium: 2014 guideline update.* Toronto, ON: Author. Retrieved from: http://www.ccsmh.ca.

Canadian Gerontological Nursing Association. (2010). *Standards of Practice.* Toronto, ON: Author.

Canadian Institute for Health Information (CIHI). (2011). *Health care in Canada, 2011: A focus on seniors and aging.* Retrieved from https://secure.cihi.ca/free_products/HCIC_2011_seniors_report_en.pdf.

Canadian Institute for Health Information (CIHI). (2013). *Adverse drug reaction-related hospitalizations among seniors, 2006 to 2011.* Retrieved from https://secure.cihi.ca/free_products/Hospitalizations%20for%20ADR-ENweb.pdf.

Chandran, G. J., Mikler, J. R., & Keegan, D. L. (2003). Neuroleptic malignant syndrome: Case report and discussion. *Canadian Medical Association Journal, 169*(5), 439–442. Retrieved from https://www.researchgate.net/profile/David_Keegan2/publication/10584920_Neuroleptic_malignant_syndrome

_Case_report_and_discussion/links/54f25e9c0cf2b36214b1ab3e/Neuroleptic-malignant-syndrome-Case-report-and-discussion.pdf.

Cosci, F. (2016). Withdrawal symptoms after discontinuation of a noradrenergic and specific serotonergic antidepressant: A case report and review of the literature. *Personalized Medicine in Psychiatry*, *1*, 81–84. doi:10.1016/j.pmip.2016.11.001.

Di Minno, A., Frigerio, B., Spadarella, G., et al. (2017). Old and new oral anticoagulants: Food, herbal medicines and drug interactions. *Blood Reviews*, *31*(4), 193–203. doi:10.1016/j.blre.2017.02.001.

Gitlin, L. N., Kales, H. C., & Lyketsos, C. G. (2012). Managing behavioral symptoms in dementia using nonpharmacologic approaches: An overview. *Journal of the American Medical Association*, *308*(19), 2020–2029. doi:10.1001/jama.2012.36918.

Golombek, D. A., Pandi-Perumal, S. R., Brown, G. M., et al. (2015). Some implications of melatonin use in chronopharmacology of insomnia. *European Journal of Pharmacology*, *762*, 42–48. doi:10.1016/j.ejphar.2015.05.032.

Government of Canada. (2016). *Report on the social isolation of seniors*. Retrieved from https://www.canada.ca/en/national-seniors-council/programs/publications-reports/2014/social-isolation-seniors/page05.html.

Jett, K. (2012). Geropharmacology. In T. Touhy & K. Jett (Eds.), *Ebersole & Hess' Towards healthy aging: human needs and nursing response*. St. Louis: Mosby.

Khandpur, S., Porter, R. M., Boulton, S. J., et al. (2016). Drug-induced photosensitivity: New insights into pathomechanisms and clinical variation through basic and applied science. *The British Journal of Dermatology* (online), doi:10.1111/bjd.14935.

Maggiore, R. J., Gross, C. P., & Hurria, A. (2010). Polypharmacy in older adults with cancer. *The Oncologist*, *15*(5), 507–522. doi:10.1634/theoncologist.2009-0290.

Masnoon, N., Sorich, W., & Alderman, C. P. (2016). A study of consumer retention of key information provided by clinical pharmacists during anticoagulant counselling. *Journal of Pharmacy Practice and Research*, *46*(3), 227–244. doi:10.1002/jppr.1187.

Morgan, S. G., Hunt, J., Rioux, J., et al. (2016). Frequency and cost of potentially inappropriate prescribing for older adults: A cross-sectional study. *Canadian Medical Association Journal*, *4*(2), E346–E351. doi:10.9778/cmajo.20150131.

Morley, J. E. (2014). Inappropriate drug prescribing and polypharmacy are major causes of poor outcomes in long-term care. *Journal of the American Medical Directors Association*, *15*(11), 780–782. doi:10.1016/j.jamda.2014.09.003.

National Library of Medicine. (2016). *Drug record: Acetaminophen*. Retrieved from https://livertox.nih.gov/Acetaminophen.htm.

Oruch, R., Elderbi, M. A., Khattab, H. A., et al. (2014). Lithium: A review of pharmacology, clinical uses, and toxicity. *European Journal of Pharmacology*, *740*, 464–473. doi:10.1016/j.ejphar.2014.06.042.

Pannu, T., Sharkey, S., Burek, G., et al. (2017). Medication use by middle-aged and older participants of an exercise study: results from the Brain in Motion study. *BMC Complementary and Alternative Medicine*, *17*(1), 105. doi:10.1186/s12906-017-1595-5.

Perri, M., III, Menon, A. M., Deshpande, A. D., et al. (2005). Adverse outcomes associated with inappropriate drug use in nursing homes. *The Annals of Pharmacotherapy*, *39*(3), 405–411. doi:10.1345/aph.1E230.

Reason, B., Terner, M., McKeag, A. M., et al. (2012). The impact of polypharmacy on the health of Canadian seniors. *Family Practice*, *29*(4), 427–432. doi:10.1093/fampra/cmr124.

Ruscin, J. M. (2009). *Drug-related problems in the elderly*. Retrieved from http://www.merckmanuals.com/professional/geriatrics/drug_therapy_in_the_elderly/drug-related_problems_in_the_elderly.html#v1133742.

Shi, S., & Klotz, U. (2011). Age-related changes in pharmacokinetics. *Current Drug Metabolism*, *12*(7), 601–610. doi:10.2174/13890011796504527.

Werneke, U., Jamshidi, F., Taylor, D. M., et al. (2016). Conundrums in neurology: Diagnosing serotonin syndrome–a meta-analysis of cases. *BioMed Central Neurology*, *16*(1), 97. doi:10.1186/s12883-016-0616-1.

Wilcox, S. M., Himmelstein, D. U., & Woolhandler, S. (1994). Inappropriate drug prescribing for the community-dwelling elderly. *Journal of the American Medical Association*, *272*(4), 292–296. Retrieved from http://www.citizen.org/documents/1343.pdf.

Wood, A. K., Muntner, P., Joyce, C. J., et al. (2010). Adverse effects of complementary and alternative medicine use on antihypertensive medication adherence: Findings from CoSMO. *Journal of the American Geriatric Society*, *58*(1), 54–61. doi:10.1111/j.1532-5415.2009.02639.x.

LEARNING OBJECTIVES

Upon completion of this chapter, the reader will be able to:

- Define chronic illness and explain the differences between chronic illness and acute illness.
- Explain the concept of wellness in chronic illness.
- Discuss explanatory models of chronic illness.
- Discuss the factors that influence the experience of chronic illness.
- Explain strategies that have been used successfully to maintain maximal function and increase an individual's ability for self-care.
- Discuss nursing interventions to maximize wellness in the presence of chronic illness.

GLOSSARY

Care coordination An approach to health care in which all of a person's needs are coordinated with the assistance of a primary point of contact to make sure that the person gets the most appropriate treatment.

Case management The coordination of services on behalf of the patient or resident to ensure that the appropriate care is provided.

Exacerbation Worsening; in medicine, the term may refer to an increase in the severity of a disease or its signs and symptoms.

Exorbitant Exceeding that which is usual or proper.

Frailty "A state of vulnerability to poor resolution of homeostasis following a stress and is a consequence of cumulative decline in multiple physiological systems over a lifespan" (Clegg et al., 2013, p. 752).

Iatrogenesis A complication or side effect of the health care intervention, advice given, or the environment itself.

Trajectory The path followed by a body or an event moved along by the action of certain forces.

THE LIVED EXPERIENCE

"Because you understand my disease, you don't understand me. To understand that I am ill does not mean that you understand how I experience my illness. I am unique. I think and feel and behave in a combination that is unique to me. You do not understand me because you have a label for my disease or a plan for my treatment. It is not my disease or treatment that you need to understand. It is me."

(Jevne, 1993, p. 121)

CHRONIC ILLNESS

Chronic illnesses are "conditions that last a year or more and require ongoing medical attention and/or limit activities of daily living" (Hwang et al., 2001, p. 268). From a nursing perspective, "chronic illness is the irreversible presence, accumulation, or latency of disease states or impairments that involve the total human environment for supportive care and self-care, maintenance of function and prevention of further disability" (Curtin & Lubkin, 2006, pp. 6–7).

The rising prevalence and associated costs of chronic illness is a global health concern. Chronic illness accounts for over half of the global health burden (World Health Organization [WHO], 2012). By 2020, chronic illness will account for an estimated 80% of worldwide disease. It is estimated that up to 60% of Canadian older persons living in the community have two or more chronic conditions (CIHI, 2016; Mokraoui et al., 2016). A host of social determinants—especially education, income, gender, and ethnicity—influence levels of chronic illness (WHO, 2012). Chronic illnesses also exact significant personal costs and burdens due to a diminished quality of life for both the individual and his or her family and significant others. This chapter discusses chronic illness and the its implications for gerontological nursing and healthy aging. (For information on specific chronic illnesses, see Chapters 16 through Chapter 21.)

CHRONIC ILLNESS AND AGING

Many factors influence the rapid rise in the number of people with chronic illness, including the aging of the population; advances in medical sciences in extending the lifespan and in treating illness; and a rise in some chronic conditions, such as asthma and diabetes, in younger people (Public Health Agency of Canada [PHAC], 2009). The life expectancy of Canadians continues to rise and has now reached 80.7 years (Statistics Canada, 2015). Unfortunately, a longer life often means living longer with a chronic illness, especially for women, whose life expectancy is longer than that of men. Illnesses such as cancer, Alzheimer's disease, and diabetes; mental health challenges; and human immunodeficiency virus (HIV)

and acquired immunodeficiency syndrome (AIDS) are becoming chronic illnesses with which people will live for extended periods.

Chronic illnesses are common among older persons in Canada. Approximately one-quarter (24%) of Canadian older persons reported having received a diagnosis of three or more chronic conditions (multimorbidity) (CIHI, 2011). By the time a person has lived 50 years, he or she is likely to have at least one chronic condition. The most common chronic conditions for Canadians aged 65 years and older are high blood pressure (47%) and arthritis (27%) (CIHI, 2011). Those conditions also accounted for the three most common combinations of chronic conditions in older persons—14% had both high blood pressure and arthritis; 12% had both high blood pressure and heart disease; and 11% had both high blood pressure and diabetes (CIHI, 2011) (Fig. 15.1). Chronic illnesses in older people can be categorized as follows:

1. Nonfatal chronic illness—conditions such as osteoarthritis or hearing or vision impairments. These conditions contribute to disability and increased health care costs, but most individuals can live with them for many years.
2. Serious, potentially fatal chronic conditions—cancers, organ system failures, dementia, and stroke.
3. Frailty—a condition in which the body has few reserves left and in which any disturbance can cause multiple health conditions and costs (Xue, 2011; Clegg et al., 2013).

For the older person, having a chronic illness is not as important as its effect on functioning. The effect may be as little as an inconvenience or as great as an impairment of a person's ability to perform activities of daily living (ADLs) or instrumental activities of daily living (IADLs). Limitations in the ability to perform ADLs and IADLs occur more frequently among individuals over the age of 75 years, but recent trends show that the disability rate among older persons has declined and that the incidence of long-term disability has dropped dramatically (http://www.statcan.gc.ca). However, the health disparities that exist for many members of minority groups can reduce these gains (Koh et al., 2011) (see Chapter 4).

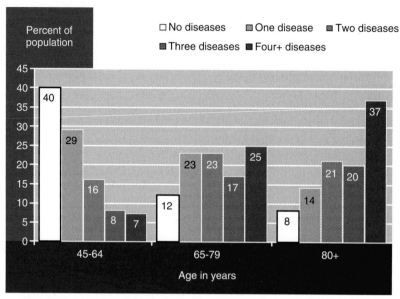

FIGURE 15.1 Percentage of persons in Canada aged 45 years and older who report selected chronic conditions. *Source:* Data from Gilmour, H., & Park, J. (2003). Dependency, chronic conditions and pain in seniors. *Health Reports, 16*(Suppl), 21–31. (Statistics Canada Catalogue no. 82-003.) Retrieved from http://www.statcan.gc.ca/pub/82-003-s/2005000/pdf/9087-eng.pdf.

ACUTE VERSUS CHRONIC ILLNESS

Chronic disorders and acute illnesses cannot really be separated, because so many conditions are intricately intertwined. Some acute disorders have chronic sequelae, and many commonly identified chronic disorders tend to intermittently flare up into acute problems and then move back into remission. Acute illnesses are those that occur suddenly, often without warning (e.g., stroke, myocardial infarction, hip fracture, or infection), and show signs and symptoms related to the disease process. These illnesses are usually treated aggressively and end in a relatively short time. Acute problems in later life can quickly cause death; at other times, the sequelae of the acute episode constitute a new or exacerbated chronic condition.

A chronic illness, on the other hand, continues indefinitely, is managed rather than cured, and requires the person to learn to live with the condition (Schulman-Green et al., 2012). If not triggered by an acute event, the onset of a chronic illness may be insidious and be identified only during a health screening. Symptoms of the effects of the illness or condition, including disabilities, may not appear for years. For example, a person with hypertension can develop enough heart damage to cause an acute episode of heart failure years later.

A person with a chronic illness may have episodic **exacerbation,** or the illness may remain in remission, with no symptoms for a long time (Touhy & Ebersole, 2014). People with chronic illness often continue to work and perform their usual activities early in their disease. Later, and with increasing age or frailty, the effects of the limitations increase. Many older people have several chronic disorders simultaneously (i.e., comorbidities) and have great difficulty managing the complexity of overlapping and often contradictory demands. Symptoms of chronic illness can interfere with many regular activities and routines, require medical regimens, disrupt patterns of living, and frequently make it necessary for the person to make significant lifestyle changes. Physical suffering, loss, worry, grief, depression, functional impairment, and increased dependence on family or friends for support are among the negative consequences of chronic illness (Nierenberg et al., 2016; Warner et al., 2017). One of the greatest fears of older people is the fear of being dependent on others as a result of chronic illness (Morse et al., 2016).

FRAILTY SYNDROME

Frailty is an independent geriatric syndrome that may be seen in older people with multiple comorbidities. It is "a state of vulnerability to poor resolution of homeostasis following a stress and is a consequence of cumulative decline in multiple physiological systems over a lifespan" (Clegg et al., 2013, p. 752). Frailty includes both physical and mental decline and leads to an increased risk for morbidity and mortality (Clegg et al., 2013). Frailty has also been linked to acute illness, falls, and hospitalization (Clegg et al., 2013; Lee et al., 2015).

Seven percent of older people are classified as frail; however, the prevalence of frailty increases up to 40% in persons aged 80 years and more. With the dramatic increase in the "oldest old" population, frailty is becoming common (Hao et al., 2016). Being female or African American and having less education and lower income are also associated with frailty (Salem et al., 2014).

Factors responsible for the pathogenesis of frailty include sarcopenia and related metabolic pathogenic factors, atherosclerosis, cognitive impairment, and malnutrition (Umegaki, 2016). Weight loss, fatigue, muscle weakness, slow or unsteady gait, and declines in activity are signs and symptoms of frailty (Clegg et al., 2013).

Frailty often goes unnoticed, as the symptoms are attributed to the aging process. Frailty can be assessed by using the Clinical Frailty Scale (accessed at the website listed at the end of this chapter). The identification of frailty during an early stage is important because specific interventions may prevent functional decline and other negative consequences. Interventions are aimed at maintaining homeostatic balance. They focus on resistance and balance exercises; nutritional support; treatment of depression, delirium, diabetes, osteoporosis, and hypertension; appropriate social support; aggressive treatment of pain; and treatment of early cognitive impairment (Muscedere et al., 2016).

PREVENTION OF CHRONIC ILLNESS

Research has shown that chronic illness and poor health are not inevitable consequences of aging. Many chronic illnesses are preventable through lifestyle choices or early detection and management of risk factors. Yet much remains to be learned about the distribution, risk factors, and effective measures to prevent or delay the onset of some chronic conditions. Some of these conditions can be managed with improved diet, exercise, medical treatment, or a combination of these. Health promotion activities and attention to healthy lifestyle habits can postpone and reduce morbidity for older people. Key strategies for improving the health of older people are presented in Box 15.1.

The common risk factors for most chronic illnesses are poor diet, inactivity, and smoking (Bauer et al., 2014). Eliminating these three risk factors would minimize a person's risks of having a stroke or developing heart disease, type 2 diabetes, and cancer (Health Canada, 2010). Public health efforts have traditionally focused on physical health, but health includes mental health as well. The promotion of cognitive health is an emerging public health priority and an essential feature of health-related quality of life (see Chapter 21). Public health efforts can help individuals avoid preventable illness and disability as they age. Health Canada's goals, as published in *Healthy Aging in Canada: A New Vision, a Vital Investment, From Evidence to Action*, are to increase the span of healthy life for all persons and to decrease disparities

BOX 15.1	Key Strategies for Improving the Health of Older People

Healthy lifestyle behaviours
Injury prevention
Delivery of culturally appropriate clinical preventive services
Immunization and preventive screenings
Self-management techniques for those with chronic illnesses

Source: Adapted from Public Health Agency of Canada [PHAC]. (2012). *The chief public health Officer's report on the state of public health in Canada 2010.* Retrieved from http://www.phac-aspc.gc.ca/cphorsphc-respcacsp/2010/fr-rc/cphorsphc-respcacsp-07-eng.php

in health outcomes among population subgroups (Health Canada, 2006). These goals can be achieved through the increased use of preventive health strategies and improved approaches to effectively treating health problems for all persons, regardless of age, ethnicity, or income. As a result of these efforts, older people have the potential to live longer and in better health. A focus on healthy aging requires nurses to implement health promotion and disease prevention activities.

CARE DELIVERY SYSTEM

The current health care system, with its focus on immediate medical needs to manage acute events (such as accidents, severe injury, and sudden bouts of illness) does not meet the needs of individuals with chronic illness, nor does it support health promotion and disease prevention. Each component of the health care system views the person from its own narrow window of care. No one entity, practice, facility, or agency is managing the entire disease, and certainly none is managing the illness experience of the person and family. Health insurance coverage for preventive health care services and rehabilitation, long-term care, and home care needed by persons with chronic illnesses is often limited. See Chapters 22 and 26 for a discussion of health care costs and funding for older people, as well as transitions in care across the continuum.

In addition to the problems mentioned above, health care providers sometimes lack the knowledge, awareness, and skills to care for the growing numbers of people with chronic illnesses. Most education programs for health care workers focus on episodic care in acute care settings (Fazio et al., 2016). The World Health Organization (2005) report, *Preparing a Health Care Workforce for the 21st Century: The Challenge of Chronic Conditions,* presents a training model and competencies for the care of people with chronic illness for all health care workers (Box 15.2).

THEORETICAL FRAMEWORKS FOR CHRONIC ILLNESS

Several theoretical frameworks—including the Chronic Illness Trajectory (Strauss & Glaser, 1975; Corbin & Strauss, 1988; Woog, 1992) and the

---

BOX 15.2   Competencies to Improve Care for Chronic Conditions

1. Patient-centred care
   - Interviewing and communicating effectively
   - Assisting changes in health-related behaviours
   - Supporting self-management
   - Using a proactive approach
2. Partnering
   - Partnering with patients
   - Partnering with other providers
   - Partnering with communities
3. Quality improvement
   - Measuring care delivery and outcomes
   - Adapting to change
   - Translating evidence into practice
4. Information and communication technology
   - Designing and using patient registries
   - Using electronic patient records
   - Using computer technologies
   - Communicating with partners
5. Public health perspective
   - Providing population-based care
   - Thinking in terms of systems
   - Working across the care continuum
   - Working in primary health care–led systems

Source: Data from World Health Organization (2005). *Preparing a health care workforce for the 21st century: The challenge of chronic conditions.* Geneva, Switzerland: Author. Retrieved from http://www.who.int/chp/knowledge/publications/workforce_report.pdf.

Shifting Perspectives Model of Chronic Illness (Paterson, 2001)—have been used to understand the effect of chronic illness and to organize nurses' responses in order to help persons with chronic illness. First, however, it is crucial that nurses caring for older people with chronic illness have a good understanding of wellness.

WELLNESS IN CHRONIC ILLNESS

A person's feeling of wellness is important when he or she is living with chronic illness. "Wellness in chronic illness" suggests that the person has an optimal level of functioning for achieving well-being and a good and satisfactory existence. Even for patients who have a chronic illness or are dying, an optimum level of wellness and well-being should be strived for.

Nurses working within a wellness model or approach focus on moving in a positive direction instead of a downward negative trajectory and the deterioration of the person's health. The older person may reach plateaus in his or her ascension to a higher level of wellness. The person may also regress because of an illness event, but the event can also be a stimulus for growth and a return to moving up the wellness continuum (see Chapter 1). Wellness is not a given; rather, it is a state of being and feeling that one strives to achieve through motivation and health practices.

The greatest factor in establishing wellness is adaptation. The maximization of life satisfaction requires an adaptation of lifestyle. The results of a qualitative study that explored the perceptions of nurses, older people, and families about living with a chronic illness in the community offered insight into the complexity and the adaptation (Ploeg et al., 2017). Participants spoke about the complexity of their experience of chronic illness and multicomorbidity, which included physical conditions and psychological conditions such as depression and anxiety; about the impacts of these conditions on the physical, psychological, and social domains of health; about managing many different medications for multiple conditions; about seeing numerous health and social care providers; and about health-related crises that led to transitions to and from the acute care sector. Participants described how they had to accept the realities of gradual health decline and set realistic goals. One older person explained, "I've adapted to it as it's happened…it's been a gradual thing. You know, you get this problem and then you get this problem and then you have another problem and …I've just dealt with it" (Ploeg et al., 2017). Building on the courage of older persons who are coping with chronic illnesses, disabilities, and other challenges is a good starting point for gerontological nurses.

CHRONIC ILLNESS TRAJECTORY

The **trajectory** model of chronic illness, conceptualized by Strauss and Glaser (1975), has long helped health care providers better understand the realities of chronic illness. Corbin and Strauss (1988) viewed the course of chronic illness as being on a trajectory that moved forward through eight phases: a preventive phase (pretrajectory), a definitive phase (trajectory onset), a crisis phase, an acute phase, a stable phase, an unstable phase, a downward phase, and a

dying phase (Table 15.1). The shape and stability of the trajectory is influenced by the combined efforts, attitudes, and beliefs held by the person, family members, significant others, and the involved health care providers. The key points of the model are based on the theoretical assumptions listed in Box 15.3. The person's perceptions of needs that are met and basic biological functional limitations are paramount to predicting movement along the illness trajectory (Corbin & Strauss, 1992).

THE SHIFTING PERSPECTIVES MODEL OF CHRONIC ILLNESS

The Chronic Illness Trajectory model described above views living with a chronic illness as a progression of phases that follow a predictable trajectory. The Shifting Perspectives Model of Chronic Illness (Paterson, 2001), derived from a synthesis of qualitative research findings, views living with chronic illness as an ongoing, continually shifting process in which the person moves between the perspectives of wellness in the foreground and illness in the foreground.

The Shifting Perspectives Model is more reflective of an "insider" perspective on chronic illness, as opposed to the more traditional "outsider" view. The model also changes the traditional view of the patient, from the traditional view of the patient as client to a view of the patient as a partner in care, and focuses on health within illness rather than on loss and burden (Larsen et al., 2006). People's perspectives on their chronic illnesses are neither right nor wrong but reflect their needs and situations. How people perceive the chronic illness at any given time influences how they interpret and respond to the disease, to themselves, to caregivers, and to situations affected by the illness (Paterson, 2001; Lindqvist et al., 2006).

Chronic illness contains elements of both illness and wellness, and people with chronic illness live in the "dual kingdoms of the well and the sick" (Donnelly, 1993, p. 6). The illness-in-the-foreground perspective is characterized by a focus on sickness, suffering, loss, and burden caused by the illness. This perspective occurs when a person is newly diagnosed, when new disease-related symptoms appear, when the illness is in an acute phase, or when there are perceived threats to the person's control (signs of disease

TABLE 15.1	The Chronic Illness Trajectory: Definitions of Phases and Goals
PHASE	**DEFINITION**
1. Pretrajectory	Before the illness course begins; the preventive phase; no signs or symptoms present
2. Trajectory onset	Signs and symptoms are present; includes diagnostic period
3. Crisis	Life-threatening situation
4. Acute	Active illness or complications that require hospitalization
5. Stable	Illness course—symptoms controlled by regimen
6. Unstable	Illness course—symptoms not controlled by regimen but not requiring hospitalization
7. Downward	Progressive deterioration of physical status, mental status, or both, characterized by increasing disability, symptoms, or both
8. Dying	Immediate weeks, days, and hours preceding death

Examples of Goals That Nurses Might Establish

1. To assist the person in overcoming a plateau during a comeback phase, by increasing the person's compliance with a regimen so that he or she might reach the highest level of functional ability possible within limits of the disability.
2. To assist a person in making the attitudinal and lifestyle changes needed to promote health and prevent disease.
3. To assist a person who is in a downward trajectory to make the adjustments and re-adjustments in everyday activities that are necessary to adapt to increasing physical deterioration.
4. To assist the person in an unstable phase to gain greater control over symptoms that are interfering with his or her ability to carry out everyday activities.
5. To assist a person in maintaining illness stability by finding a way to blend illness management activities with everyday life activities.

    Goals can be broken down into specific person-oriented objectives. Built into the objectives are the criteria that will be used to evaluate the effectiveness of each intervention.

Source: Woog, P. (1992). *Chronic illness trajectory framework: The Corbin and Strauss nursing model.* New York: Springer.

BOX 15.3	Key Points in the Chronic Illness Trajectory Framework

- The majority of health problems in late life are chronic.
- Chronic illnesses may be lifelong and entail lifetime adaptations.
- Chronic illness and its management often profoundly affect the lives and identities of both the person and the person's family or significant others.
- The management of the acute phase of illness is designed to stabilize physiological processes and promote a recovery (comeback) from the acute phase.

- The management of other phases of illness is designed primarily to maximize and extend the period of stability in the home, helped by family members and augmented by visits to and from health care providers.
- Maintaining stable phases is central to the work of managing chronic illness.
- The primary care nurse is often the coordinator of the numerous resources that may be needed to promote quality of life along the trajectory.

progression, lack of skills to manage the symptoms, disease-related stigma, or interactions with others that emphasize dependence and hopelessness). The illness-in-the-foreground perspective has a protective function, may assist in conserving energy, and helps

a person learn more about the illness and come to terms with it (Paterson, 2001).

Return to the wellness perspective calls for courage and resilience as well as the development of strategies and resources to adjust to the changes. Nurses can assist by understanding the person's perspective and providing education and support. The shift from illness to wellness is an active process triggered by the need to return to the wellness perspective.

In the wellness-in-the-foreground perspective, the focus is centred more on the self than on the disease and its consequences. The illness becomes part of who a person is but does not define the person. The illness is seen as an opportunity for growth and meaningful changes in relationships with the environment and others. This perspective is fostered by the patient's learning as much as possible about the illness, creating supportive environments, paying attention to his or her own patterns of response to the illness, and sharing knowledge of the disease with others.

With this perspective, the person is able to focus on the emotional, spiritual, and social aspects of life while still attending to disease management and the effects of the illness on his or her life. That the participants in a study of men with advanced prostate cancer were reluctant to describe themselves as ill suggests that having the wellness-in-the-foreground perspective is a desirable state (Lindqvist et al., 2006). Paterson (2001) suggested that the shifting perspectives model calls for an understanding of the person's perspective and why the person varies in his or her attention to symptoms. Health care providers who see the person with chronic illness as sick focus only on the disease and its symptoms and may not provide opportunities or support for wellness. Gerontological nurses must support persons with either perspective to optimize and sustain the wellness-in-the-foreground perspective.

Like the Shifting Perspectives Model of chronic illness, the person-centred care model focuses on partnership and on setting goals that are tailored to the individual person and his or her lifestyle. Person-centred care was conceptualized by Tom Kitwood (1997) to care for persons with dementia. Person-centred care considers each person's needs and preferences from a holistic perspective that includes associated relationships and the effect that other people or the physical environment (or a combination of these) may have on the person. Thus, this model of care emphasizes the person living with chronic illness, rather than the chronic illness itself.

 ## IMPLICATIONS FOR GERONTOLOGICAL NURSING AND HEALTHY AGING

Chronic illnesses are illnesses to live with, and nursing's response is one of long-term caring. The focus of treatment for chronic illness is seldom on cure but rather on care for the person. Nursing for chronic illness requires a different focus from that of acute care nursing, in which the emphasis is on attention to immediate and life-threatening needs and attempts to cure. "Chronic health problems are not fixable with shiny new technology, and do not promise the suspense, exhilarating hope, and dramatic ending that acute medical crises often do. They simply continue day after day, often invisible or misunderstood" (Hodges et al., 2001, p. 390).

ASSESSMENT

Assessment of the older person with a chronic illness involves the selection of appropriate tools, ongoing evaluation of responses and outcomes, careful observation, periodic monitoring, alert watchfulness, and most importantly, discussion and collaboration with the older person about his or her perceptions and the meaning of the illness. In the case of chronic illness and the great variability in its presentation and its impact on individual lifestyle, adequate assessment is critical. Assessment focuses on function and how the chronic illness affects function and well-being.

Functional assessments strive to identify the quantity and quality of disability in chronic illness. These assessments, although sometimes not specific to the medical treatment regimen, are often a good measure of the person's response and adaptation to persistent health problems. Disability assessment helps identify the gap between existing self-care abilities and needed self-care resources. The difference between abilities and needed resources identifies areas on which nursing care should focus. In this approach to assessment, nurses embrace the idea of illness as persistent; patients can achieve various degrees of adaptation, and nurses can help maximize people's function and therefore their quality of life. (See Chapter 13 for a discussion of comprehensive assessment and assessment instruments.)

Since many people with chronic illness manage their conditions in a community setting and may need assistance from different caregivers, assessment must also focus on the ability of family or significant others to assist and cope with caregiving. (See Chapter 23 for a discussion of the caregiving role.)

INTERVENTIONS

Interventions in the care of chronically ill persons must take into consideration the person's emotional responses, perspectives on the illness, individual needs, self-care ability, support from family and friends, and available resources, as well as the trajectory experience. Chronic illness affects all aspects of a person's life, and interventions must be holistic. Nursing recommendations for the care of persons with chronic illnesses are presented in Box 15.4.

BOX 15.4   Nursing Recommendations for the Care of Persons With Chronic Illness

- Come to know the person and what gives him or her meaning in life.
- Provide education about the illness and its management.
- Provide ongoing assessment, focusing on the prevention of complications.
- Relieve symptoms that interfere with function and quality of life.
- Help the person set realistic goals and expectations.
- Focus on potential rather than on limitations.
- Teach the skills required for effective self-care.
- Ensure the delivery of needed care and support for both the person and the person's family or significant others.
- Encourage the verbal expression of feelings.
- Provide support for losses, and facilitate the grieving process.
- Provide access to resources.
- Provide timely and appropriate referrals to suitable providers (or resources).
- Help the person balance the effects of treatment on quality of life.
- Maintain hope for the person through a supportive environment and by developing a caring, reciprocal relationship with the person.
- Help the person die with dignity and comfort.

CARING

Caring has historically been the foundation of nursing. The concept of caring has been studied by many nursing scholars. Roach's "five Cs" of caring offer a framework for understanding the meaning of caring. The five Cs are a way of understanding what the nurse is doing when he or she is caring, and they provide a comprehensive view of caring (Roach, 1992). The five Cs are as follows:

- Competence: having the ability and skills to provide required nursing care
- Compassion: sensitivity to the pain and brokenness of others
- Conscience: moral awareness, practising within the moral framework, doing what "ought" to be done, and advocating for conditions of justice
- Commitment: staying with the person on the journey; nursing as a lifelong commitment and way of life; doing the work of nursing because you want to, not because you have to
- Confidence: inspiring trust through caring

All five Cs must be actualized in caring. In other words, being competent in skills without compassion or being compassionate without adequate skills and knowledge does not demonstrate caring. Older persons with chronic illnesses are not seeking a cure; rather, they need care of the highest quality. Practising within this framework, nurses bring expertise in caring to meet the needs of older persons with chronic illnesses. Nursing's response of caring applies this expertise to helping people to adapt, continue to grow, and attain a level of wellness and wholeness despite chronic illnesses and functional limitations. Gerontological nurses know that understanding and caring for an older person who has a chronic illness and is facing long-term challenges require them to develop a close caring relationship and to accompany the person on his or her journey, day after day, with a focus on quality of life.

SPECIAL CONSIDERATIONS IN CHRONIC ILLNESS

Regardless of the nature of chronic conditions, special considerations need attention and must be actively addressed by nurses. The following is not a comprehensive discussion of these considerations but a touchstone for further examination and discussion.

This chapter will discuss fatigue and grieving in more depth. For a discussion of pain, which is common in most conditions, see Chapter 16; see Chapter 23 for a discussion of sexuality. See Chapter 16 for information about complementary and alternative resources, and see Chapter 25 for further descriptions of palliative care, loss, grief, dying, and death.

Fatigue

Fatigue is a common complaint of persons living with chronic illness, yet it is different from the normal feeling of being tired from activity. Fatigue from chronic illness affects every aspect of the person's life and may interfere with performing ADLs, as well as performing family and societal roles (Mueller-Schotte et al., 2016). Fatigue is often variable and unpredictable and is either ignored or assumed to be an inevitable part of the aging process. Instead, fatigue may be a symptom of the illness, a side effect of a medication, a symptom of depression, or all of these.

The goal of the nursing interventions is to find ways to decrease fatigue and help the person manage its effects on daily life (Mueller-Schotte et al., 2016; Zalai et al., 2016). The most important intervention is to acknowledge the person's experience of fatigue and any effects that this may cause in the person's daily life. The following instruments are available to assess fatigue: the Multidimensional Assessment of Fatigue scale, the Short Form 36 Vitality subscale, the Functional Assessment of Chronic Illness Therapy Fatigue scale, and the Profile of Mood States. It is also important to assess and treat depression that may be superimposed on the fatigue of chronic illness.

Discussing patterns of fatigue and identifying the precipitants is important. Gerontological nurses can encourage the person with a chronic illness to keep a health diary. The health diary may help the person develop self-awareness in regard to the perception and management of a chronic illness. It is also helpful to emphasize the signals of the body and to balance rest and activity (within limitations), to help conserve the person's energy for the most important or necessary activities. The diary may also assist the nurse in understanding the experience of the illness from the person's perspective, so that interventions can be tailored to the person's unique journey. Interventions for the person with fatigue include strategies

---

BOX 15.5 Interventions for Persons Experiencing Fatigue

- Set priorities, and make a list of daily activities identifying which activities are essential, optional, desirable, and transferable.
- Delegate activities and learn to accept help when needed.
- Anticipate needed resources, and determine the most efficient way to carry out important activities.
- Act during periods of peak energy.
- Pace activities by planning for rest and activity, breaking big tasks into smaller and more manageable ones, spreading activities out over the day and week, and resting for short periods before activity.
- Use relaxation strategies.
- Exercise appropriately to increase muscle strength and endurance. Consult a physiotherapist for specific therapeutic exercises that are appropriate for the type of illness.
- Consume a healthy, nutritious diet, and maintain normal body weight.

Source: Mueller-Schotte, S., Bleijenberg, N., van der Schouw, Y. T., et al. (2016). Fatigue as a long-term risk factor for limitations in instrumental activities of daily living and/or mobility performance in older persons after 10 years. *Clinical Interventions in Aging, 11,* 1579. doi:10.2147/CIA.S116741.

---

for energy conservation, an appropriate balance of exercise and rest, and adequate nutrition (Box 15.5). Nurses should listen carefully to what is most important to the older person, as well as to what responses are most useful. People with chronic illnesses are the experts on managing their illnesses and lifestyles.

Grieving

Grieving the loss of independence, control, status, activities, social roles, appearance, comfort, and one's identity as a healthy person may initially occupy much of a person's time when he or she is adapting to a chronic illness. Grieving can be more pronounced if the onset of the illness is abrupt and if the losses interfere directly with a major source of pleasure. The older person may begin to memorialize the "perfect" self that no longer exists.

Nursing interventions for loss and grief should focus on encouraging the person to talk about his or her losses, providing support through active listening, and recognizing the stages of grief that may be occurring. Clearly, the reaction to loss and grief will depend on the significance of the loss to the person and the number of additional losses with which he or she is attempting to cope. It is important to come to know the person, what is most meaningful in the person's life, and the impact of the losses on that person. The number of losses, and any other recent losses in the person's life, may have depleted his or her psychic reserves (see Chapter 25).

There often seems to be a subversive sense of failure or weakness in people who have developed a chronic disorder. The suffering that a chronic illness entails is compounded by a sense of responsibility for remaining healthy, especially in the current climate of wellness. There is often the persistent thought that hard work and compliance with a strict treatment regimen will bring about a cure, and when that does not occur, a sense of shame develops. This may affect an older person's willingness to seek and accept help.

Fostering Self-Care

In the day-to-day life of a person with chronic illness, self-care skills are of the greatest importance. Nurse theorist Orem provided a useful language and taxonomy for both understanding and responding to persons with self-care needs (Orem, 1980, 1995).

According to Orem, each person has self-care needs, called "universal self-care requisites." Each person also develops self-care capacity, or the ability to meet these requisites. However, under some circumstances, the needs exceed the person's capacity to meet them, and a self-care deficit ensues. These deficits can be the result of pathophysiological disorders, but they can also have a psychological or spiritual origin.

Nursing interventions include assessments of self-care abilities and deficits. The appropriate approach is highly individualized and may involve changing the environment, modifying the treatment, or teaching the person strategies to compensate for the changes caused by the chronic illness. It may also involve teaching others how to provide the needed care or teaching the older person how to direct the provision of care by others.

Rehabilitation and Restorative Care

Many individuals experiencing chronic illness will require short- or long-term rehabilitation and restorative care. The goal of rehabilitation and restorative care is to capitalize on the individual's needs and strengths in a manner that will help him or her achieve the highest practicable level of function. Rehabilitation seeks to restore or maintain physical functioning and strives to recover a person's ability to perform ADLs and improve his or her quality of life (Glenny et al., 2010).

Rehabilitation and restorative services take place in acute care settings, outpatient clinics, rehabilitation and skilled-care facilities, and the home. The rehabilitation plan often begins in the acute care setting and can continue into long-term care settings, the community, and people's homes. The following issues should be considered in rehabilitation planning:

1. The person is often in a crisis when admitted to acute care, and personal strengths are not always evident or easily assessed.
2. Interprofessional discharge planning must begin upon admission, and a nurse or case manager should be assigned to each person.
3. Rehabilitation focuses on abilities, not disabilities; it maximizes strengths and supports limitations.

Comprehensive interprofessional assessment is critical to the rehabilitation plan, which involves working alongside the older person, family, and significant others. The total assessment includes a comprehensive biopsychosocial history, functional and cognitive assessment, and a plan of care having long- and short-term goals. Weekly joint conferences of the interprofessional team, the older person, and the older person's family are held to evaluate the person's progress, revise goals as needed, and develop discharge plans. (See Chapter 26 for additional information on rehabilitative and restorative care and transitional care.)

Prevention of Iatrogenic Disturbances

While health care providers are aiming at reducing the complications of chronic illnesses, a secondary risk, that of **iatrogenesis,** increases. Iatrogenesis is defined as a complication or by-product of a health care intervention or of the environment (Box 15.6). Sometimes, the treatment of an

BOX 15.6 Common Iatrogenic Problems Associated With Hospitalization

- Loss of mobility because of insufficient ambulation
- Incontinence caused by inattention, immobility, or both
- Confusion or delirium caused by medications, treatments, anaesthesia, and/or translocation
- Pressure injury caused by immobility and reduced sensation
- Dehydration caused by limited access to fluids
- Fluid overload caused by improper use of intravenous fluids
- Health care–associated infections caused by infectious agents in surroundings
- Urinary-tract infections caused by catheter use
- Upper respiratory-tract infections caused by immobility, shallow breathing, and aspiration of oral secretions
- Fluid and electrolyte imbalances caused by medications and treatments
- Falls because of unfamiliar environment, weakness, positional instability, or medications
- Impaired sleep due to treatments and environment
- Malnutrition caused by anorexia and insufficient assistance with eating

illness can be more devastating than the illness itself.

The older person may become incontinent not because of a new physiological problem but because of a prescribed diuretic, and the person may consequently experience an increase in urinary frequency but have no increased access to toilet facilities. A new medication can cause depression, poor appetite, or fatigue while it is improving control of the underlying illness. Nurses have to be vigilant for a negative change occurring after an intervention or medication administration. Working proactively, the older person and the care team can identify the potential or actual effect of a treatment, and the treatment can be reassessed from a benefit-versus-burden perspective. The goal is to treat the illness-related problems without compromising function and quality of life. (See Chapter 2 for a discussion of some models used to prevent iatrogenesis in hospitalized older persons.)

Assistive Technology

Advances in all types of technology hold promise for improving quality of life, reducing the need for personal care services, and enhancing independence and the ability to live safely at home or in another environment. *Assistive technology* refers to any device or system that allows a person to perform a task independently or that makes the task easier and safer to perform. Health care technologies, telehealth, mobility and ADL aids, and environmental control systems (such as "smart" houses) are some examples of assistive technology. (See Chapter 12 for a discussion of mobility and ADL aids.) *Gerotechnology* (assistive technologies for older people) is expected to significantly influence how older persons live in the future.

A new technology is the growing field of telemedicine, including the remote diagnosing and electronic monitoring of people (Martin-Khan et al., 2010). In rural areas, telemedicine offers several possibilities in the home or in other settings—reducing health care costs, eliminating the need for transportation for people who need specialized health care services, and promoting the self-management of illness. For example, a home health nurse may see a person discharged home after an acute exacerbation of heart failure. The nurse completes a thorough assessment, records it on a handheld computer, and transmits it to other health care providers. The older person is instructed to sit on a specialized chair each morning; blood pressure, pulse, and weight are measured by automation at the preset times; and the information is sent over the patient's phone line directly to the visiting nurse's office and the physician's or primary care office. The home health nurse is quickly alerted to potential problems, and the physician or nurse practitioner can make changes to the medical plan as needed. Telemedicine offers exciting possibilities for nursing at both the generalist and advanced practice levels.

Some of the devices being used in hospital and in LTC homes are wireless pendants that track people's movements, load cells built into beds to alert caregivers when a person gets out of bed, devices to monitor sleep and weight patterns, and bed lifts that help the person to go from lying down to standing up with the push of a button. Electronic health records improve care and are particularly important for people with chronic illnesses that require multiple care providers across settings.

As each new generation ages, its comfort with technology increases, and people seek opportunities for better, safer, and more independent living in ways not yet imagined.

MODELS OF CHRONIC ILLNESS CARE

Many efforts are under way to improve care for persons with chronic illness by providing cost-effective and care-efficient services that improve outcomes and quality of life. The traditional medical care model and public health models have not been effective in dealing with the complexity of chronic illness. Although not all people with a chronic illness have high care needs, the cost of care for those who do is increasingly **exorbitant.** The costs accrued by chronic illness (more than 75% of total medical expenditures), access to care, quality outcomes, and patient satisfaction remain issues of concern.

People with chronic illnesses often have to navigate a system that requires them to coordinate several disparate financing and delivery systems by themselves, making it more difficult for them to obtain the full range of appropriate services. People who need access to different programs are likely to find that each program has different eligibility criteria and sets of care providers and that there is little communication or coordination among health care providers. As a result, the health care delivery system is complex and confusing, and care is often fragmented, less effective, and more costly. A summary of the challenges in care for the older person with chronic illness is presented in Box 15.7.

BOX 15.7	Challenges in Caring for the Older Person With Chronic Illness

- The long-term and uncertain nature of the illness
- Costs associated with care
- Little coordination of care across the continuum
- Inadequate funding for preventive and long-term care
- Lack of health care providers with expertise in gerontology and in the care of persons with chronic conditions
- Acute and episodic focus in medical care
- The need for active partnership between the person, his or her family and significant others, and the health care provider

Managed care, **case management,** disease management, evidence-informed protocols for illness management, **care coordination,** and collaborative models of self-management are all care models to support an integrated system that ensures that the services needed by people with chronic illness are provided in a cost-effective manner. Elements essential to new models of care include coordination of care, identification of risk, improved access, prevention and health promotion, use of evidence-informed protocols to manage illness, holistic approaches, interprofessional focus, management of transitions across the continuum, and a collaborative approach encouraging self-management of the illness in a partnership of health care providers and the person living with the chronic illness (Holroyd-Leduc et al., 2016) (see Box 15.2).

The results of a randomized controlled trial of a collaborative care model for older persons with Alzheimer's disease (Callahan et al., 2006) indicated a significant improvement in the quality of care and in the behavioural and psychological symptoms of dementia among primary care patients and their caregivers without a significant increase in the use of antipsychotics or sedative-hypnotic medications. The model used care management by an interprofessional team led by an advanced-practice nurse. Nurses, both at the generalist and advanced practice level, are particularly well suited to take lead roles in the care of people with chronic illness.

Small-Group Approaches to Chronic Illness

Early affiliation with a group of persons who are confronting similar issues may help some older persons who have chronic illnesses adapt to the altered role requirements and may also provide shared strategies for coping. Small-group meetings are among the most effective and economical ways of helping individuals meet informational and psychosocial needs. These groups can also be designed to provide family support and counselling. Self-help groups can be seen as support systems, consumer participant systems, advocacy–social influence groups, or homogeneously identified therapeutic groups. Support groups provide the opportunity to obtain information and share similar experiences and perspectives. Facilitating persons' adjustments to new roles and activities and facilitating the redefinition of self constitute a large part of working in these groups.

Many support services and opportunities for group work are available from organizations that are devoted to particular chronic illnesses (e.g., the Alzheimer Society of Canada, the Heart and Stroke Foundation of Canada, and Parkinson Canada), as well as many Internet websites.

SUMMARY

Managing chronic illness in late life is aimed toward achieving a healthier old age and enhancing health and wellness for those already in late life. Nurses must work with older persons to maximize those persons' assets and abilities and minimize their limitations and disabilities.

This kind of nursing requires a different focus from that of acute care nursing, where the emphasis is on attention to immediate and life-threatening needs and on attempts to cure. Chronic illnesses, on the other hand, are illnesses to live with, and nursing's response is one of long-term caring. Progress is not measured by attempts to achieve cure, but rather in the maintenance of a steady state or regression of the condition, all the while remembering that the condition does not define the person. Understanding the meaning of the experience of chronic illness from the older person's perspective, adopting a holistic approach, and working collaboratively with the person are of utmost importance.

KEY CONCEPTS

- Declines in mortality, increasing medical expertise, and sophisticated technological developments have resulted in a great increase in the survival of older people with multiple chronic disorders.
- The effects of chronic illness range from mild to life limiting, each person responding to circumstances in a highly individual manner.
- The Chronic Illness Trajectory and the Shifting Perspectives Model of Chronic Illness offer useful frameworks for understanding chronic illness and designing nursing interventions.
- People with chronic illnesses can achieve wellness, and the role of the nurse is critical in its promotion.

- The goals of healthy aging include minimizing the risk for disease; encouraging health promotion; and, in the presence of disease, alleviating symptoms, delaying or avoiding the development of complications, and maximizing function and quality of life.
- Loss and grief are common in chronic illness. Nursing interventions include encouraging the person to talk about his or her losses, providing support through active listening, and recognizing the grief process that may be occurring.
- New models of cost-effective care that increase access and improve outcomes and quality of life for persons with chronic illness are needed. Nurses are particularly well prepared to assume major roles in chronic illness care.
- The overall goal of rehabilitation for the older person is to achieve the highest practicable level of functioning.

ACTIVITIES AND DISCUSSION QUESTIONS

1. What type of education and counselling might the nurse provide to a 40-year-old person to promote health and prevent chronic illness in his or her later life?
2. Discuss possible ways of modifying the living situation of a person whose energy is limited owing to chronic disorders.
3. What would be the most devastating loss in ADLs?
4. What are some nursing interventions to help a person with chronic illness deal with loss? Practice or role-play various ways in which this issue can be addressed.
5. How would you encourage a person toward maximal participation in self-care?
6. What would be the measures of wellness during chronic illness?

RESOURCES

Age in Place. Imagine the future of aging
http://ageinplace.com/technology/imagine-future-aging-technology-video/

Canadian Study of Health and Aging
http://www.csha.ca

Chronic Disease Prevention Alliance of Canada
http://www.cdpac.ca

Improving Chronic Illness Care
http://www.improvingchroniccare.org

Independence, Activity and Good Health: Ontario's Action Plan for Seniors
https://dr6j45jk9xcmk.cloudfront.net/documents/215/ontarioseniorsactionplan-en-20130204.pdf

Public Health Agency of Canada. Aging & seniors
https://www.canada.ca/en/public-health/services/health-promotion/aging-seniors.html

Public Health Agency of Canada. Healthy aging in Canada: A new vision, a vital investment, from evidence to action
http://www.health.gov.bc.ca/library/publications/year/2006/Healthy_Aging_A_Vital_latest_copy_October_2006.pdf

Registered Nurses' Association of Ontario (RNAO). Strategies to support self-management in chronic conditions: Collaboration with clients
http://rnao.ca/bpg/guidelines/strategies-support-selfmanagement-chronic-conditions-collaboration-clients

The LeadingAge Center for Aging Services Technologies (CAST)
http://www.leadingage.org/center-aging-services-technologies

World Health Organization (WHO). Chronic diseases and health promotion
http://www.who.int/chp/en/

For additional resources, please visit *http://evolve.elsevier.com/Canada/Ebersole/gerontological/*

REFERENCES

Bauer, U. E., Briss, P. A., Goodman, R. A., et al. (2014). Prevention of chronic disease in the 21st century: Elimination of the leading preventable causes of premature death and disability in the USA. *The Lancet, 384*(9937), 45–52. doi:10.1016/S0140-6736(14)60648-6.

Callahan, C., Boustani, M., & Unverzagt, F. W. (2006). Effectiveness of collaborative care for older adults with Alzheimer's disease in primary care. *Journal of the American Medical Association, 295*(18), 2148–2157. doi:10.1001/jama.295.18.2148.

Canadian Institute for Health Information (CIHI). (2011). *Seniors and the health care system: What is the impact of multiple chronic conditions?* Retrieved from https://secure.cihi.ca/free_products/air-chronic_disease_aib_en.pdf.

Canadian Institute for Health Information (CIHI). (2016). *Health spending*. Retrieved from https://www.cihi.ca/en/spending-and-health-workforce/spending.

Clegg, A., Young, J., Iliffe, S., et al. (2013). Frailty in elderly people. *The Lancet, 381*(9868), 752–762.

Corbin, J. M., & Strauss, A. (1988). *Unending work and care: Managing chronic illness at home.* San Francisco: Jossey-Bass.

Corbin, J. M., & Strauss, A. (1992). A nursing model for chronic illness management based upon the trajectory framework. In P. Woog (Ed.), *The chronic illness framework: The Corbin and Strauss nursing model.* New York: Springer.

Curtin, M., & Lubkin, I. (2006). What is chronicity? In I. Lubkin & P. Larsen (Eds.), *Chronic illness: impact and interventions.* Sudbury, MA: Jones & Bartlett.

Donnelly, G. F. (1993). Chronicity: Concept and reality. *Holistic Nursing Practice, 8*(1), 1–7. Retrieved from http://journals.lww.com/hnpjournal/pages/articleviewer.aspx?year=1993&issue=10000&article=00003&type=Citation.

Fazio, S. B., Demasi, M., Farren, E., et al. (2016). Blueprint for an undergraduate primary care curriculum. *Academic Medicine: Journal of the Association of American Medical Colleges, 91*(12), 1628–1637. doi:10.1097/ACM.0000000000001302.

Glenny, C., Stolee, P., Husted, J., et al. (2010). Comparison of the responsiveness of the FIM and the interRAI post acute care assessment instrument in rehabilitation of older adults. *Archives of Physical Medicine and Rehabilitation, 91*(7), 1038–1043. doi:10.1016/j.apmr.2010.03.014.

Hao, Q., Song, X., Yang, M., et al. (2016). Understanding risk in the oldest old: Frailty and the metabolic syndrome in a Chinese community sample aged 90+ years. *The Journal of Nutrition, Health & Aging, 20*(1), 82–88. doi:10.1007/s12603-015-0553-5.

Health Canada. (2006). *Healthy Aging and Wellness Working Group. Healthy Aging in Canada: A New Vision, A Vital Investment, From Evidence to Action—A Background Paper.* Retrieved from http://www.phac-aspc.gc.ca/seniors-aines/publications/pro/healthy-sante/haging_newvision/vison-rpt/index-eng.php.

Health Canada. (2010). *Canada Health Act Annual Report 2008-2009.* Retrieved from https://www.canada.ca/en/health-canada/services/health-care-system/reports-publications/canada-health-act-annual-reports/report-2008-2009.html.

Holroyd-Leduc, J., Resin, J., Ashley, L., et al. (2016). Giving voice to older adults living with frailty and their family caregivers: Engagement of older adults living with frailty in research, health care decision making, and in health policy. *Research Involvement and Engagement, 2*(23). doi:10.1186/s40900-016-0038-7.

Hodges, H. F., Keeley, A. C., & Grier, E. C. (2001). Masterworks of art and chronic illness experiences in the elderly. *Journal of Advanced Nursing, 36*(3), 389–398.

Hwang, W., Weller, W., Ireys, H., et al. (2001). Out of pocket medical spending for care of chronic conditions. *Health Affairs, 20*(6), 268–269. Retrieved from https://www.ncbi.nlm.nih.gov/pubmed/11816667.

Jevne, R. (1993). Enhancing hope in the chronically ill. *Human Medicine, 9*(2), 121–130. Retrieved from http://hdl.handle.net/10822/1036886.

Martin-Khan, M., Wootton, R., & Gray, L. (2010). A systematic review of the reliability of screening for cognitive impairment in older adults by use of standardized assessment tools administered via the telephone. *Journal of Telemedicine and Telecare*, *16*(8), 422–428. doi:10.1258/jtt.2010.100209.

Kitwood, T. (1997). *Dementia reconsidered: The person comes first*. Berkshire, UK: Open University Press.

Koh, H. K., Graham, G., & Glied, S. A. (2011). Reducing racial and ethnic disparities: The action plan from the department of health and human services. *Health Affairs*, *30*(10), 1822–1829. doi:10.1377/hlthaff.2011.0673.

Larsen, P., Lewis, P., & Lubkin, I. (2006). Illness behavior and roles. In I. Lubkin & P. Larsen (Eds.), *Chronic illness: Impact and interventions* (6th ed.). Sudbury, MA: Jones & Bartlett.

Lee, L., Heckman, G., & Molnar, F. J. (2015). Frailty: Identifying elderly patients at high risk of poor outcomes. *Canadian Family Physician*, *61*(3), 227–231. Retrieved from http://www.cfp.ca/content/61/3/227.full.

Lindqvist, O., Widmark, A., & Rasmussen, B. (2006). Reclaiming wellness—living with bodily problems, as narrated by men with advanced prostate cancer. *Cancer Nursing*, *29*(4), 327–337. doi:10.1097/00002820-200607000-00012.

Mokraoui, N. M., Haggerty, J., Almirall, J., et al. (2016). Prevalence of self-reported multimorbidity in the general population and in primary care practices: A cross-sectional study. *British Medical Council Research Notes*, *9*(1), 314. doi:10.1186/s13104-016-2121-4.

Morse, J. M., Stern, P. N., Stern, P. N., et al. (2016). *Developing grounded theory: The second generation*. New York: Routledge.

Mueller-Schotte, S., Bleijenberg, N., van der Schouw, Y. T., et al. (2016). Fatigue as a long-term risk factor for limitations in instrumental activities of daily living and/or mobility performance in older adults after 10 years. *Clinical Interventions in Aging*, *11*, 1579. doi:10.2147/CIA.S116741.

Muscedere, J., Andrew, M. K., Bagshaw, S. M., et al. (2016). Screening for frailty in Canada's health care system: A time for action. *Canadian Journal on Aging*, *35*(03), 281–297. doi:10.1017/S0714980816000301.

Nierenberg, B., Mayersohn, G., Serpa, S., et al. (2016). Application of well-being therapy to people with disability and chronic illness. *Rehabilitation Psychology*, *61*(1), 32. doi:10.1037/rep0000060.

Orem, D. (1980). *Nursing: Concepts of practice* (2nd ed.). New York: McGraw-Hill.

Orem, D. (1995). *Nursing: Concepts of practice* (5th ed.). St Louis, MO: Mosby.

Paterson, B. L. (2001). The shifting perspectives model of chronic illness. *Journal of Nursing Scholarship*, *33*(1), 21–26. doi:10.1111/j.1547-5069.2001.00021.x.

Ploeg, J., Matthew-Maich, N., Fraser, K., et al. (2017). Managing multiple chronic conditions in the community: A Canadian qualitative study of the experiences of older adults, family caregivers and healthcare providers. *BMC Geriatrics*, *17*(1), 40. doi:10.1186/s12877-017-0431-6.

Public Health Agency of Canada (PHAC). (2009). *Executive summary: The chief public health officer's report on the state of public health in Canada 2009*. Retrieved from https://www.canada.ca/en/public-health/corporate/publications/chief-public-health-officer-reports-state-public-health-canada/report-on-state-public-health-canada-2009/executive-summary.html.

Public Health Agency of Canada (PHAC). (2012). *Chapter 4: The chief public health officer's report on the state of public health in Canada 2010—Setting conditions for healthy aging*. Retrieved from https://www.canada.ca/en/public-health/corporate/publications/chief-public-health-officer-reports-state-public-health-canada/annual-report-on-state-public-health-canada-2010/chapter-4.html.

Roach, S. (1992). *The human act of caring*. Ottawa, ON: Canadian Hospital Association.

Salem, B. E., Nyamathi, A., Brecht, M. L., et al. (2014). Constructing and identifying predictors of frailty among homeless adults—A latent variable structural equations model approach. *Archives of Gerontology and Geriatrics*, *58*(2), 248–256.

Schulman-Green, D., Jaser, S., Martin, F., et al. (2012). Processes of self-management in chronic illness. *Journal of Nursing Scholarship*, *44*(2), 136–144. doi:10.1111/j.1547-5069.2012.01444.x.

Statistics Canada. (2015). *Health at a glance – disparities in life expectancy at birth*. Retrieved from http://www.statcan.gc.ca/pub/82-624-x/2011001/article/11427-eng.htm.

Strauss, A., & Glaser, B. (1975). *Chronic illness and the quality of life*. St Louis, MO: Mosby.

Touhy, T., & Ebersole, J. K. (2014). *Hess' gerontological nursing & healthy aging*. St. Louis, MO: Mosby.

Umegaki, H. (2016). Sarcopenia and frailty in older patients with diabetes mellitus. *Geriatrics & Gerontology International*, *16*(3), 293–299. doi:10.1111/ggi.12688.

Warner, C. B., Roberts, A. R., Jeanblanc, A. B., et al. (2017). Coping resources, loneliness, and depressive symptoms of older women with chronic illness. *Journal of Applied Gerontology*, 733464816687218. doi:10.1177/0733464816687218.

Woog, P. (1992). *The chronic illness trajectory framework: The Corbin and Strauss nursing model*. New York: Springer.

World Health Organization. (2005). *Preparing a health care workforce for the 21st century: The challenge of chronic conditions*. Geneva, Switzerland: Author. Retrieved from http://www.who.int/chp/knowledge/publications/workforce_report.pdf.

World Health Organization (WHO). (2012) *Preventing chronic diseases: A vital investment*. Retrieved from www.who.int/chp/chronic_disease_report/en/.

Xue, Q. L. (2011). The frailty syndrome: Definition and natural history. *Clinics in Geriatric Medicine*, *27*(1), 1–15. doi:10.1016/j.cger.2010.08.009.

Zalai, D. M., Gottschalk, R., & Shapiro, C. M. (2016). Fatigue in chronic medical conditions: A psychosomatic perspective. In S. R. Pandi-Perumal, M. Narasimhan, & M. Kramer (Eds.), *Sleep and psychosomatic medicine* (2nd ed., pp. 41–56). Boca Raton, FL: CRC Press.

Pain and Comfort

LEARNING OBJECTIVES

Upon completion of this chapter, the reader will be able to:

- Define the concept of pain and recognize the older person's interpretation of pain.
- Differentiate acute from persistent pain.
- Identify data to include in a pain assessment.
- Describe pharmacological and nonpharmacological measures to promote comfort for the person in pain.
- Discuss the goals of pain management for the older person.
- Develop a nursing care plan for an older person in acute or persistent pain.

GLOSSARY

Adjuvant A medication that has a primary use other than pain relief (e.g., an antidepressant or anticonvulsant) but is also used to enhance the effects of traditional pain medication.

Titration The adjustment of the dosage of a given medication until the desired effect is produced.

THE LIVED EXPERIENCE

Ms. S. had cancer of the stomach and was in pain most of the time. She was referred to the local hospice, and the nurse worked with her and her physician to make Ms. S. comfortable. First the nurse assessed potential causes for the pain, the level of pain, the type of pain, and what level of relief was desired. After a careful titration of her medications, it was found that only a long-acting morphine provided her with comfort and an improved quality of life. However, at the dose needed she also hallucinated, seeing several puppies in the room. When asked if she wanted to reduce the dosage to eliminate this side effect, she responded, "No—I'll keep the puppies, I know they are not real and they don't hurt anything. I'd rather have them with me than the pain."

  Helen, RN

Comfort is a personal and intrinsic balance of the most basic physiological, emotional, social, and spiritual needs. Comfort is uniquely defined, experienced, and expressed by each person as a member of a family, community, and culture. A person comes to later life with many learned ways of promoting self-comfort and comforting loved ones. Without some level of comfort, wellness is beyond reach.

Pain, on the other hand, is a sensation of distress and can occur at a physical, psychological, and spiritual level. Pain is a multidimensional phenomenon, and usually one type of pain is intertwined with another. Physical pain and several chronic diseases (e.g., Parkinson's disease) can evoke the psychological pain of depression. Any type of pain can result in reduced socialization, impaired mobility, and a reconsideration of the meaning of life and self (Linton & Shaw, 2011). This chapter will describe acute and persistent pain, and will explore assessments, interventions, and strategies to address pain and discomfort in older persons.

COMMUNICATION OF PAIN AND DISCOMFORT

How pain is expressed is highly influenced by the history of the individual and the meaning ascribed to pain. It is not uncommon to express spiritual and psychological pain in somatic terms of "not feeling well." It is also important to realize that an individual responds in a way that reflects his or her own cultural expectations and understanding of acceptable behaviour. Very simply, pain is whatever a person says it is.

For those with cognitive and communication impairments (e.g., dementia or aphasia), pain is a particular challenge. Health care providers must interpret the person's expression of pain through subtle cues. Understanding what the person is trying to communicate through his or her behaviour is an essential skill in caring for older people with and without communication difficulties (see Chapter 21). Other factors affecting the communication of pain include hearing loss, depression, sedating medications (which do not necessarily ease pain), the individual's personality, and the way discomfort is acceptably expressed. Nurses cannot assume that those individuals who cannot or will not verbalize their pain do not have pain. Instead, nurses must be alert to the cues that suggest that pain and discomfort are present and then initiate assessments and interventions that are appropriate and acceptable to the older person.

Pain is now considered the fifth vital sign, which means that a pain assessment is part of any evidence-informed assessment (Morone & Weiner, 2013). Providing comfort to persons in pain is a quality indicator, that is, a marker of quality care. Yet, even when Best Practice Guidelines are followed, inadequate assessment and undertreatment of pain still occurs, especially when the patient is an older person, a member of a minority group, or in a long-term care (LTC) home (Inelman et al., 2012).

Nurses have their own definitions and expectations of the expression of pain. These perceptions are drawn from nurses' personal and professional experiences, culture, and so on. Myths, stereotypes, and generalizations about aging influence the nurse's response (Box 16.1). Unfortunately. these beliefs makes the undertreatment of pain more prevalent.

Nurses have a responsibility to set aside their own expectations and promote comfort for those who are suffering, regardless of the cause and manner of expression. Nurses should do so nonjudgementally and with the goals of understanding the person's pain and developing interventions to relieve, not just lessen, pain of all kinds. Gerontological nurses' skills in assessment and intervention are especially important.

ACUTE AND PERSISTENT PAIN

There are two main categories of pain: acute and persistent. Each category has subtypes (such as neuropathic and nociceptive pain).

ACUTE PAIN

Acute physical pain is temporary pain and includes postoperative, procedural, and traumatic pain. Acute physical pain is usually easily controlled by analgesic medications. In the acute care hospital setting, patients can use a self-controlled analgesic pump for a restricted period. Acute pain is a universal experience for older persons because of lifespan, opportunities for traumatic injury, and pain-producing illnesses. At the same time, an older person is more likely to have an adverse reaction to pain medication (see Chapter 14). For example, most analgesics cause sedation. Although use of the medication may be necessary, this adverse effect increases the risk for falls and delirium.

Acute pain may also be psychological or spiritual in nature, as in, for example, early bereavement or a major depressive episode. Because of the many losses in the lives of older persons (see Chapters 23 and 25), the risk for such acute pain is high.

PERSISTENT PAIN

It is estimated that 55% of the Canadian population report persistent pain (Reitsma et al., 2011). The prevalence of persistent pain is higher in females and

BOX 16.1   Facts and Myths About Pain in the Older Person

Myth	Fact
Pain is a normal part of aging.	Pain is not part of the normal changes in aging; however, its occurrence increases with age.
Pain sensitivity and perception decrease with aging.	Not true. However, some older people may have a greater tolerance for pain because of their adjustment to inadequate pain relief of longstanding pain.
If people don't complain of pain, they do not have pain.	People may not report pain for a variety of reasons; they may nonetheless have pain. Some persons feel that it is culturally inappropriate to complain of pain. Some feel that they are burdensome to those around them, including their nurses.
A person who has no functional impairment or who appears occupied is not in significant pain.	People have a variety of reactions and responses to pain. Some people are stoic and refuse to give in to their pain.
Narcotic medications are inappropriate unless used for short periods.	Opioid analgesics are often the best treatment for moderate to severe persistent pain in order to help restore the person's ability to function and quality of life.
Potential side effects of narcotic medication make these medications too dangerous to use with older people.	Narcotics are safe to use with older persons.

older persons (Reitsma et al., 2011). Lapane and colleagues (2012) report that between 33% and 83% of LTC residents experience persistent pain.

Persistent pain may be a sequela of an episode of acute pain, is not time limited, and may vary in intensity throughout the day or with changes in activity. For example, persons with dysthymia (chronic mild depression) usually feel the most sadness in the morning; however, their mood lifts as the day progresses (see Chapter 24). Higher age also creates a higher risk of developing health problems associated with persistent pain and iatrogenic side effects of treatment. Adverse iatrogenic events include falls and changes in cognitive function; these events are often the effect of different medications taken at the same time. Furthermore, loneliness and emotional pain from loss (see Chapter 25) decrease the ability to cope with physical pain. These psychosocial aspects of an older person's pain experience are rarely or superficially assessed by nurses or included in the plan of care. Older persons may under-report their pain or "undertreat" themselves because of the cost of the medications, belief in an associated stigma, attribution of the pain to the normal burdens of "old age," or fear of addiction.

Conditions that are degenerative (e.g., osteoarthritis) or pathological (e.g., herpes zoster, stroke, or peripheral neuropathy) are a common cause of pain.

Osteoarthritis

By 50 years of age, most adults have some level of degenerative abnormalities of the lower spine (see Chapter 18). One of the most typical abnormalities is the loss of support of the spinal column from osteoarthritis. Osteoarthritis is the destruction of the inner joint surfaces and is the most common form of joint disease. It is the most common joint disorder in the world and one of the most common sources of pain and disability in advanced age (Anderson & Loeser, 2010). Joint pain and stiffness in osteoarthritis are initially intermittent and then become persistent. The pain is characterized by aching and stiffness in the joints with inactivity and by discomfort or acute pain with activity.

Relief from pain requires the skilful use of both nonpharmacological and pharmacological measures. Nonpharmacological pain management of osteoarthritis includes joint care and the application of moist heat to relieve pain, spasm, and stiffness. Joint care may include the use of orthotic devices such as braces and splints to support joints, weight reduction if necessary, physiotherapy, and the avoidance of overusing the affected joint. Complementary and alternative and cognitive-behavioural measures may also be useful adjuncts.

Acetaminophen (Tylenol) remains the medication of choice for mild osteoarthritic pain. However, most people report better relief with nonsteroidal anti-inflammatory drugs (NSAIDs), such as naproxen or ibuprofen (Advil). These frequently used medications pose a considerable risk for interactions and adverse events (Canadian Institute for Health Information [CIHI], 2013). Severe arthritis with unrelieved pain and extensive disability may necessitate the use of a local anaesthetic, such as a corticosteroid injected into the affected joints. Injections of hyaluronic acid have been found to improve joint lubrication in some persons. Both treatments are limited to three to five injections (McArthur et al., 2012). In cases of extreme persistent pain, surgical intervention such as joint replacement may be performed. Long-acting narcotic pain relievers are also effective.

Herpes Zoster

Nearly 130,500 new cases of herpes zoster (HZ), or shingles, are diagnosed each year in Canada (Boivin et al., 2010). This disorder occurs most often in persons between the ages of 50 and 70 years. About one in five people who have had chicken pox will develop shingles at some time in their lives (Boivin et al., 2010; Health Link BC, 2017). A viral infection of the nerves (see Chapter 11), HZ is characterized by itching, stinging, burning pain along the pathway of the affected nerve (dermatome) and then erupting into serous vesicles. An acute episode lasts from days to weeks, whereas a chronic episode can last much longer (National Institute on Aging, 2015). Involvement in the eye is considered a medical emergency, owing to a high risk of blindness and brain involvement.

Although HZ causes acute pain, the pain may become persistent with what is diagnosed as postherpetic neuralgia (PHN), which is persistent pain from the damaged nerves after a case of HZ. The condition is difficult to treat once established; often, narcotics are necessary for pain relief. A combination of antiviral medications, steroids, Aspirin, and topical anaesthetics may be effective as well. Antiviral drugs such as acyclovir and famciclovir can shorten the duration of an acute outbreak and may prevent PHN when given promptly. Medications used to treat HZ and prevent PHN include Lyrica and gabapentin. Low doses of tricyclic antidepressants (e.g., desipramine and Elavil) have been used to treat PHN; however, some of these medications are contraindicated for use with older persons because of their anticholinergic effects (see Chapter 14).

IMPLICATIONS FOR GERONTOLOGICAL NURSING AND HEALTHY AGING

As always, care of the older person in pain starts with an assessment and continues through to the evaluation of the interventions. Nurses are usually most attuned to the needs of older people and are in a key position to work with the person until the pain is relieved. An advanced-practice nurse or nurse practitioner with expertise in pain management can be consulted or requested to assist.

ASSESSMENT

A comprehensive assessment of pain includes a complete history and physical assessment, as well as an assessment specific to pain. Several organizations offer best practice guidelines for the assessment and management of pain. The Registered Nurses' Association of Ontario (http://www.rnao.ca) has developed Best Practice Guidelines and a self-directed learning package for the assessment and management of pain in older people. The Hartford Institute for Geriatric Nursing provides an evidence-informed guide in its Try This Series, available on its website (https://consultgeri.org/tools/try-this-series). The Canadian Pain Society also offers guidelines for the management of persistent neuropathic pain.

A number of factors should be considered when caring for older persons (Box 16.2). Assessment can be particularly challenging if the person has a cognitive or communication impairment.

When possible, assessment begins with a person's self-report of pain. Many times, older persons will not report pain unless directly asked specific questions, such as "do you have pain now?"; "where is your pain?"; "do you have pain every day?"; and "does

Factors to Consider When Assessing Pain in Older Persons

Function: How is the pain affecting the older person's ability to perform activities of daily living and instrumental activities of daily living?

Expression of pain: Have there been recent changes in cognitive ability or behaviour, such as increased pacing, grimacing, or irritability? Have the number of complaints increased? Are the complaints vague and difficult to respond to? Has there been a change in sleep–wake patterns? Is the person resisting certain activities, movements, or positions?

Social support: What resources are available to help the person cope and tolerate treatment? How is pain affecting the person's usual social role? How is pain affecting his or her relationships with others?

Pain history: How have previous experiences with pain been managed? What does the person perceive to be the meaning of the past and present pain? What cultural factors affect the person's belief in the meaning of the pain and the ability to express pain and receive relief?

pain keep you from sleeping at night?" In some cases, alternate words such as "ache," "hurt," or "discomfort" are necessary. Assessment includes a history of pain and detailed descriptions of pain intensity, frequency, quality, location, and aggravating and alleviating factors. Medication history includes prescribed medications, herbs and supplements, over-the-counter medications, and street medications. Figs. 16.1 and 16.2 present a brief pain inventory and a standard pain assessment tool commonly used in hospitals and LTC homes.

For the person who is unable to express himself or herself, assessment begins with the nurse's careful observation for any potential indicators of discomfort (Box 16.3). Written or visual analogue scales (Fig. 16.3) have also been found useful; most can be used cross-culturally or with individuals who have limited English proficiency. Visual analogue scales have been clinically tested and have shown to be an accurate and reliable tools in various health care settings (Bird et al., 2016). However, their use for persons with dementia has varying results. Specific pain assessment tools such as the Pain Assessment in Advanced Dementia

(PAINAD) scale can be used to assess people with cognitive impairments. (See website address in the Resources section).

INTERVENTIONS

The goals of pain management for the older person are to promote comfort and maintain the highest level of functioning and well-being possible. Careful use of nonpharmacological and pharmacological approaches helps to achieve both of these goals. To provide optimal care for the person in pain, attention needs to be given to the psychological and social consequences of physical pain. Reducing suffering calls for careful listening, unconditional positive regard, ongoing support, and mobilization of resources. Pillows for support or body positioning, appropriate and comfortable seating and mattresses, frequent rest periods, and pacing of activities to balance activity and rest are important for providing comfort.

Nurses should encourage older people and their significant others to take an active role in their pain management. The person can keep a personal journal or pain diary that notes the times, types, and doses of medication taken; its effect; the duration of its benefit; and which activities increase or decrease the pain. This information helps establish patterns that may improve pain management by adjusting activities, providing medications at the right times, and helping the person feel in control of some aspect of care. An example of a pain diary can be found at the Canadian Pain Coalition website (http://www.canadianpaincoalition.ca). The diary should be reviewed with the health care provider and used to adjust dosages or timing for optimal relief.

Nurses should also encourage older people to stay as active as possible within their comfort range. When a person experiences pain with a necessary activity (e.g., rehabilitation), anticipation anxiety may increase the pain. In this case, the plan of care should include both nonpharmacological and pharmacological interventions before the recommended activity. Administering an effective short-acting medication 20 to 30 minutes before the specific activity may lessen or eliminate the fear of discomfort and can greatly enhance the individual's capacity for that activity. Nurses should learn the older person's ability to cope with pain and work within those parameters.

Brief Pain Inventory

Date _____ / _____ / _____   Time: _____

Name: _____ _____ _____
            Last   First   Middle Initial

1) Throughout our lives, most of us have had pain from time to time (such as minor headaches, sprains, and toothaches). Have you had pain other than these everyday kinds of pain today?
   1. Yes   2. No

2) On the diagram, shade in the areas where you feel pain. Put an X on the area that hurts the most.

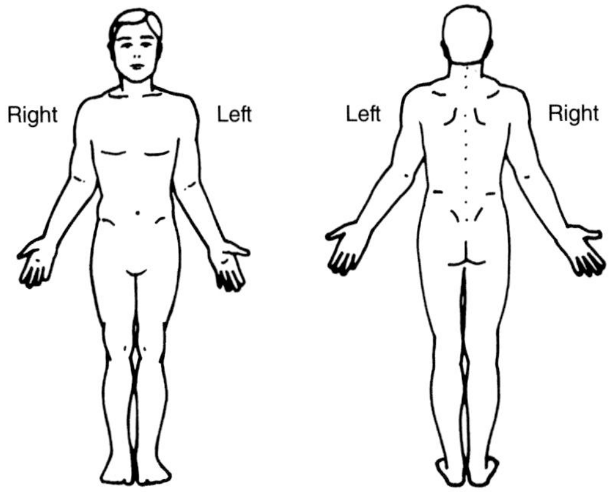

Right   Left   Left   Right

3) Please rate your pain by circling the one number that best describes your pain at its **worst** in the past 24 hours.

0	1	2	3	4	5	6	7	8	9	10
No pain								Pain as bad as you can imagine		

4) Please rate your pain by circling the one number that best describes your pain at its **least** in the past 24 hours.

0	1	2	3	4	5	6	7	8	9	10
No pain								Pain as bad as you can imagine		

5) Please rate your pain by circling the one number that best describes your pain on the **average.**

0	1	2	3	4	5	6	7	8	9	10
No pain								Pain as bad as you can imagine		

6) Please rate your pain by circling the one number that tells how much pain you have **right now.**

0	1	2	3	4	5	6	7	8	9	10
No pain								Pain as bad as you can imagine		

7) What treatments or medications are you receiving for your pain?

_____

_____

8) In the past 24 hours, how much **relief** have pain treatments or medications provided? Please circle the one percentage that most shows how much relief you have received.

0%	10	20	30	40	50	60	70	80	90	100%
No relief										Complete relief

9) Circle the one number that describes how, during the past 24 hours, pain has **interfered** with your:
   A. General activity

0	1	2	3	4	5	6	7	8	9	10
Does not interfere									Completely interferes	

   B. Mood

0	1	2	3	4	5	6	7	8	9	10
Does not interfere									Completely interferes	

   C. Walking ability

0	1	2	3	4	5	6	7	8	9	10
Does not interfere									Completely interferes	

   D. Normal work (includes both work outside the home and housework)

0	1	2	3	4	5	6	7	8	9	10
Does not interfere									Completely interferes	

   E. Relations with other people

0	1	2	3	4	5	6	7	8	9	10
Does not interfere									Completely interferes	

   F. Sleep

0	1	2	3	4	5	6	7	8	9	10
Does not interfere									Completely interferes	

   G. Enjoyment of life

0	1	2	3	4	5	6	7	8	9	10
Does not interfere									Completely interferes	

May be duplicated for use in clinical practice.

FIGURE 16.1 Brief pain inventory. Copyright Charles S. Cleeland, PhD, Houston.

Pain Assessment Tool

Addressograph

Reason for assessment:
☐ New admission   ☐ Readmission   ☐ Further assessment
☐ Change in condition   ☐ Quarterly

1. Location of pain:

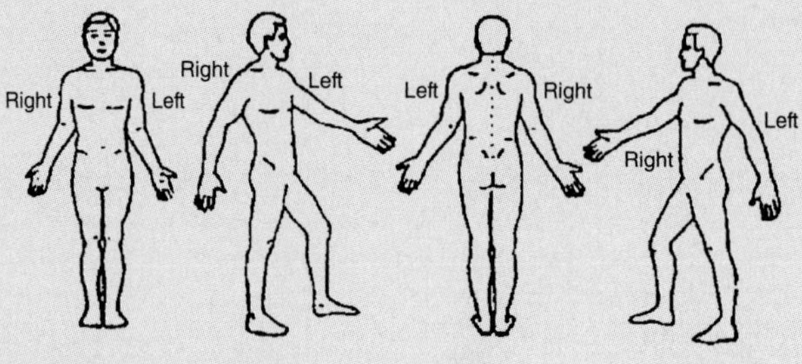

Right   Left   Right   Left   Left   Right   Left   Right

2. Severity of pain:

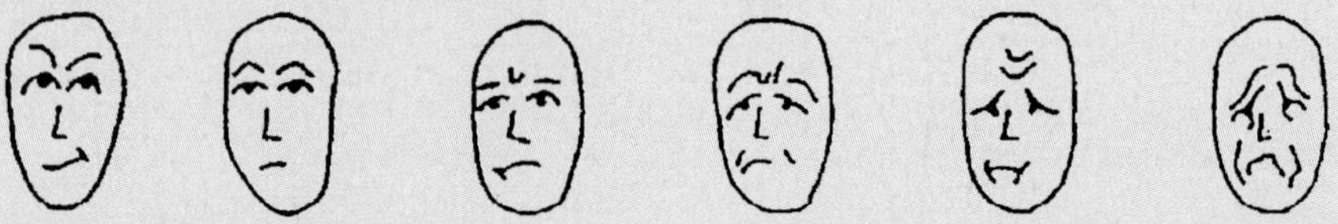

| 0 | 2 | 4 | 6 | 8 | 10 |
| No pain | Mild | Discomforting | Distressing | Horrible | Excruciating |

QUESTIONS	COMMENTS
What is the present level of pain? **(if no pain is present complete sections 6 and 7)**	
What is the rate when the pain is at its least?	
What makes the pain better?	
What is the rate when the pain is at its worst?	
What makes the pain worse?	
Is the pain continuous or intermittent?	
When did the pain start?	
What do you think is the cause of this pain?	
What level of pain are you satisfied with? (if 0 is unattainable)	

3. Quality: Indicate the words that describe the pain

☐ Aching	☐ Throbbing	☐ Shooting	☐ Stabbing	☐ Gnawing	☐ Sharp
☐ Burning	☐ Tender	☐ Exhausting	☐ Tiring	☐ Penetrating	☐ Numb
☐ Nagging	☐ Hammering	☐ Pins and needles	☐ Unbearable	☐ Tingling	☐ Stretching
☐ Pulling	☐ Other:				

FIGURE 16.2 Pain assessment tool. *Source:* Brignell, A. (Ed). (2000). *Guideline for developing a pain management program: A resource guide for long-term care facilities* (3rd ed.). Owen Sound, ON: Grey Bruce Palliative Care Hospice Association. Reprinted with permission.

4. Effects of pain on <u>activities of daily living</u>

Activities of daily living	Yes	No	COMMENTS
Sleep and rest			
Social activities			
Appetite			
Physical activity and mobility			
Emotions			
Sexuality/intimacy			

5. Effects of pain on <u>quality of life</u>

What would you like to do now that you can't do because of the pain **or** What activity would improve your quality of life?

_____

_____

6. Symptoms: What other symptoms are being experienced?

☐ Constipation	☐ Nausea	☐ Vomiting	☐ Fatigue	☐ Insomnia	☐ Depression	☐ Drowsy
☐ Sore mouth	☐ Weakness	☐ Short of breath	☐ Other:			

7. Behaviours: What behaviours are present that may be a result of pain or treatment?

☐ Calling out	☐ Restlessness	☐ Disorientation	☐ Not eating	☐ Pacing
☐ Not sleeping	☐ Withdrawn	☐ Groaning/moaning	☐ Rocking	☐ New immobility
☐ Tense	☐ Distressed	☐ Distracted	☐ Crying	☐ Inexpressive
☐ Fists clenched	☐ Striking out	☐ Knees pulled up	☐ Frowning	☐ Facial grimacing
☐ Resistant to movement	☐ Pulling or pushing away	☐ Sad	☐ Frightened	☐ Other:

8. Past pain management

Has a significant degree of pain been experienced in the past? How was that managed?

_____

_____

Past use of pharmacological and nonpharmacological pain management?

_____

_____

9. Support system: _____

10. Other concerns related to pain _____

11. Nursing pain diagnosis:

☐ Visceral	☐ Somatic (muscle or bone)	☐ Raised intracranial pressure
☐ Naturopathic	☐ Mixed	☐ Unknown

Date Care Plan updated: _____

Signature: _____ **Assessment date:** _____

FIGURE 16.2, cont'd

BOX 16.3 Pain Cues in the Person With Communication Difficulties

Behavioural Changes
Restlessness, agitation (or both), or reduction in movement
Repetitive movements
Physical tension, such as clenching teeth or hands
Unusually cautious movements, guarding

Activity Changes
Sudden resistance to help from others
Decreased appetite
Decreased sleep

Vocalization Changes
Groaning, moaning, or crying for unknown reasons
Increases or decreases in the usual vocalizations

Physical Changes
Pleading expression
Grimacing
Pallor or flushing
Diaphoresis (sweating)
Increased pulse, respirations, or blood pressure

Nonpharmacological Measures for Pain Relief

Nurses have a long history of comforting patients through nonpharmacological measures that may be in the form of a caring and supportive relationship or the form of specific techniques. A combination of pharmacological and nonpharmacological interventions appears to be most effective in the relief of both acute and persistent pain (Schulenburg, 2015). The basic approach to pain control is to encourage whatever strategies have been effective in the past without causing harm. This applies particularly to older persons with a lifetime of experience managing their own pain. In some cases, what is now referred to as complementary and alternative medicine is actually the formalization of approaches that people have used for years.

Physical Approaches

The methods of pain reduction briefly reviewed here are only a small sample of what is available.

Touch. Touch is a natural way of providing comfort, although its therapeutic properties are still not clearly understood (Kumar et al., 2014). Touch is now placed into the category of "energy medicine," which includes approaches such as reiki. The approaches in this category are reportedly very effective. When combined with purposeful relaxation, touch may lessen anxiety, reduce muscle tension, and help relieve pain. See the National Center for Complementary and Integrative Health website (https://nccih.nih.gov) for more information.

Cutaneous Nerve Stimulation. Deep and superficial stimulation of nerves for the purpose of pain relief has been practised for centuries. The Chinese practices of acupuncture, acupressure, and moxibustion are good examples of this approach. Scientific evidence of the effectiveness of acupuncture and acupressure in the treatment of persistent pain is growing (Vas et al., 2006; Vickers et al., 2012; Witt et al., 2006). Nurses have long used massage, vibration, heat, cold, and ointments. Heat and cold temporarily interrupt the transmission of pain impulses to the cerebral pain centre (Durham et al., 2015). However, caution must be used in consideration of the cause of the pain. Heat is effective for some pain, such as the deep pain of inflammatory musculo-skeletal conditions (e.g., rheumatic arthritis). On the other hand, heat increases circulation to the area and therefore is contraindicated in occlusive vascular disease and in nonexpansive tissue such as bursae (at some joints), where it may increase pain. At the same time, intermittent application of cold packs helps with low back pain and some instances of nerve irritation. Care must be taken when applying heat and cold to an older person's skin to prevent skin damage due to normal age-related thinning (see Chapter 6).

Transcutaneous Electrical Nerve Stimulation. Other methods of cutaneous stimulation are transcutaneous electrical nerve stimulation (TENS), low-level laser therapy, and percutaneous electrical nerve stimulation (PENS). Electrodes taped to the skin over the pain site or on the spine emit a mild electrical current that is felt as a tingling, buzzing, or vibrating sensation. The electrical impulses are expected to prevent pain signals from reaching the brain. Both PENS and TENS have been helpful in treating phantom limb pain, postherpetic neuralgia (PHN), and low back pain (Schestatsky et al., 2014).

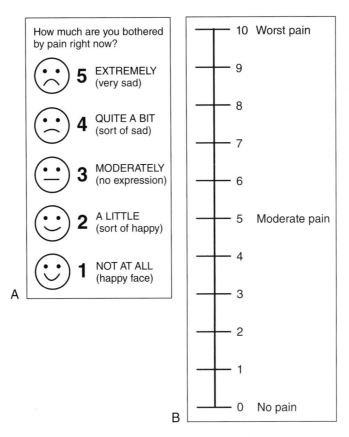

How much are you bothered by pain right now?

5 EXTREMELY (very sad)

4 QUITE A BIT (sort of sad)

3 MODERATELY (no expression)

2 A LITTLE (sort of happy)

1 NOT AT ALL (happy face)

A

10 Worst pain
9
8
7
6
5 Moderate pain
4
3
2
1
0 No pain

B

May be duplicated for use in clinical practice.

FIGURE 16.3 Visual analogue scales. **(A)** Example of a visual analogue scale. **(B)** Example of a numeric rating scale.

Cognitive-Behavioural Approaches

Some of the cognitive-behavioural approaches that can help relieve pain for older persons are biofeedback, distraction, relaxation, meditation, and imagery.

Biofeedback. In the biofeedback approach, a person can learn voluntary control over some body processes and alter them by changing the physiological correlates appropriate to them. Training and equipment of some type are needed to learn how to alter one's body response through biofeedback. Biofeedback requires full cognitive functioning and manual dexterity for self-treatment.

Distraction. Distraction is a behavioural strategy that lessens the perception of pain by drawing the person's attention away from the pain and relegating it to peripheral awareness. In some instances the individual is completely unaware of the pain; in others, the intensity of pain is significantly diminished. Pain messages are more slowly transmitted to the pain centre in the brain, and thus less pain is felt.

Mild to moderate pain responds well to distraction. At times, if an individual concentrates intently on another subject, the acute pain may be relieved. The most common forms of distraction are slow rhythmical breathing, slow rhythmical massage, rhythmical singing or tapping, active listening, guided imagery, and humour (Steele & Steele, 2009).

Relaxation, Meditation, and Imagery. The behavioural strategy of relaxation enables the quieting of the mind and the muscles, providing the release of tension and anxiety. Relaxation should be adjunctive to all pharmacological interventions.

Meditation and imagery promote relaxation. Imagery uses the person's imagination to focus on settings full of happiness and relaxation rather than on stressful situations. Studies of guided imagery and other complementary therapies showed that these therapies decreased pain perception in cases of pain related to fibromyalgia and cancer (Nash & Tasso, 2010; Carson et al., 2016).

Pharmacological Interventions for Pain Relief

Pharmacological pain relief is accomplished by using medication to alter sensory transmission to the cerebral cortex. This approach is most effective when the treatment regimen involves teamwork between the person, health care providers, family members, and significant others. In some cultures, tribal elders, the oldest son, or others must be consulted first, with permission of the older person (see Chapter 4).

A variety of pharmacological interventions are available for pain management. The World Health Organization recommends a "pain ladder" for managing analgesia for persistent pain and provides guidelines for selecting the kind of analgesia and for stepping up the amount of it.

Non-narcotics, such as paracetamol (acetaminophen), and NSAIDs (e.g., ibuprofen) are used for mild pain. For mild to moderate pain, paracetamol and NSAIDs in combination with a weak opioid (e.g., hydrocodone) can be used.

The combination of long-acting medications and short-acting analgesics has been particularly effective. To relieve moderate to severe pain, narcotics (e.g., morphine, OxyContin) and **adjuvant** medications should be used. Adjuvant medications were originally developed to treat other medical conditions but have been found to have pain-relieving qualities. Some of the more frequently used adjuvant medications are antidepressants (to relieve nerve pain and insomnia), anticonvulsants (to relieve neuropathic pain), corticosteroids (to reduce inflammation), and bisphosphonates (to relieve bone pain).

The general principles of controlling pain in older persons are the same as those for controlling pain in younger adults. However, older persons may experience more medication side effects that are related to age-associated changes in the absorption, distribution, metabolism, and excretion of medication (see Chapter 14). Meperidine (Demerol), frequently given for postoperative or post-traumatic injury pain, is absolutely contraindicated for use in older persons. A guideline for the management of pain in older persons has been developed by the Registered Nurses' Association of Ontario (http://rnao.ca/bpg/guidelines/resources/assessment-and-management-pain-elderly-learning-package-longterm-care).

In gerontological nursing, it is essential that pain medications be started at the lowest dose possible. However, it is equally important for the dosages to be **titrated** to the point that pain is relieved and relief is continuous. Too often, a low dose is started but increases are delayed, unnecessarily prolonging the patient's suffering. The goal of pain management—particularly the management of persistent pain—is to prevent the pain, not simply relieve it.

Non-narcotic Analgesics. Acetaminophen is often adequate for mild to moderate pain. However 4 g (4,000 mg) is the maximum that can be taken every 24 hours. This maximum dose is reduced for persons with renal or hepatic dysfunction or who drink alcohol.

If acetaminophen is not effective or tolerated, one of the many available NSAIDs (e.g., Aspirin or ibuprofen) may be used. Commonly used over-the-counter NSAIDs must be used with caution because of the increased risk of negative side effects or death due to acute gastro-intestinal bleeding and cardiovascular events (Al-Saeed, 2011).

Narcotic Analgesics. Narcotic medications, especially the opioids, treat both acute and persistent pain effectively. Opiates produce a greater analgesic effect, a higher peak, and a longer duration of effect in older persons when compared with younger adults. This is partly due to the prolonged half-lives of the medications (see Chapter 14). The recommendation to start with the lowest anticipated effective dose, monitor response frequently, and titrate slowly to the desired effect is especially applicable to the use of narcotic pain relievers. Pain relief should be planned for an "around the clock" approach, with a combination of long-acting or sustained-release analgesics and as-needed (PRN) medications. Breakthrough medication use that is needed on a regular basis is an indication that the dosage of the long-acting medication should be adjusted.

Opioids used for persistent pain control over a long period should be convenient and easy to administer or take. The simplest medication regimen is the one most likely to be effective and easiest to follow. The side effects of opioids include gait disturbance, dizziness, sedation, falls, nausea, pruritus, and constipation. Several of these effects will resolve on their own as the body becomes adjusted to the medication. The side effects may be lessened or prevented when the prescribing care provider works closely with the older person and the nurses to slowly titrate the dosage to the point at which the best relief is obtained with the fewest side effects. Sedation and impaired cognition do occur when opioid analgesics are started or when dosages are increased, which is often of great concern to older persons and their families. Both the older person and his or her family should be cautioned about the potential for falls, and appropriate safety precautions should be taken.

Nurses should take careful note of the person's responses and needs in order to prevent and promptly treat side effects or negative drug reactions. Since constipation is almost universal when opioids are used, nurses need to ensure that an appropriate bowel regimen starts at the same time opioid administration starts. A daily dose of a combination stool softener and mild laxative may help, along with adequate fluid intake and exercise.

EVALUATION

Evaluation of pain relief outcomes requires a reassessment of the older person's status. Re-evaluation of the frequency and intensity of pain; behavioural signs and symptoms that suggest pain; response to pharmacological and nonpharmacological interventions; and the impact of pain on mood, activities of daily living, sleep, function, and other measures of quality of life are all included in the ongoing reassessment. Adjustments of treatment regimens and interventions are based on reassessment findings. Active involvement of the older person, his or her family, and the interprofessional team is essential for the comprehensive assessment, management, and evaluation of pain.

SUMMARY

Pain should not be considered a normal part of aging. Gerontological nurses need to be able to accurately assess and manage pain for their patients. Implementing and evaluating interventions to treat pain in older persons poses several challenges. Special considerations need to be taken for older persons with communication or cognitive difficulties, as they may express pain differently from those who are able to verbally describe their pain. Gerontological nurses also need to be able to accurately evaluate the effectiveness of their interventions and assess for complications.

KEY CONCEPTS

- The absence of expressed pain does not necessarily imply comfort. Comfort is a state of ease and the satisfaction of body needs, as well as freedom from pain and anxiety.
- Pain is not limited to pain of physical origin. Pain from psychological or spiritual factors can have the same effect and is often combined with pain from physical causes.
- The assessment of pain is influenced by many misconceptions, myths, and stereotypes about pain. Inadequate treatment of pain is a major concern for older persons.
- Culture, ethnicity, family, and personal characteristics all influence a person's tolerance and expression of pain.
- Older people with various degrees of cognitive impairment may demonstrate pain by increased levels of confusion, restlessness, or withdrawal.
- The nursing goal is to assist in pain relief. Some pain medications are more appropriate than others to use with older persons.
- Acute pain and persistent pain necessitate different therapeutic approaches. Persistent pain predominates in the lives of many older persons.
- Various combinations of pharmacological and nonpharmacological pain control can be effective but must be individually designed with the older person's involvement in the decision making.

ACTIVITIES AND DISCUSSION QUESTIONS

1. What is pain?
2. Compare the features of acute and persistent pain.
3. List data necessary for an accurate pain assessment.
4. What are the barriers that interfere with the assessment and treatment of pain for all adults? What barriers are associated with pain management in older people?
5. How might pain be expressed in cognitively impaired older people? How does the assessment of pain in cognitively impaired older people differ from the assessment of pain in other people?
6. What pharmacological and nonpharmacological therapies are available?

RESOURCES

Arthritis Society
http://www.arthritis.ca

Canadian Pain Coalition
http://www.canadianpaincoalition.ca

Canadian Skin Patient Alliance
http://www.skinpatientalliance.ca

The Hartford Institute for Geriatric Nursing
(evidence-informed practice guidelines in its Try This Series)
https://hign.org/

National Center for Complementary and Integrative Health
https://nccih.nih.gov/

Pain Assessment in Advanced Dementia scale (PAINAD)
http://www.healthcare.uiowa.edu/igec/tools/pain/PAINAD.pdf

Registered Nurses' Association of Ontario (RNAO).
Assessment and management of pain in the elderly – Learning package long-term care
http://rnao.ca/bpg/guidelines/resources/assessment-and-management-pain-elderly-learning-package-longterm-care

The Canadian Pain Society
http://www.canadianpainsociety.ca

For additional resources, please visit *http://evolve.elsevier.com/Canada/Ebersole/gerontological/*

REFERENCES

Al-Saeed, A. (2011). Gastrointestinal and cardiovascular risk of nonsteroidal anti-inflammatory drugs. *Oman Medical Journal*, 26(6), 385–391. doi:10.5001/omj.2011.101.

Anderson, A. S., & Loeser, R. F. (2010). Why is osteoarthritis an age-related disease? *Best Practice & Research. Clinical Rheumatology*, 24(1), 15–26. doi:10.1016/j.berh.2009.08.006.

Bird, M., Callisaya, M. L., Cannell, J., et al. (2016). Accuracy, validity and reliability of an electronic visual analog scale for pain on a touch screen tablet in healthy older adults: A clinical trial. *Interactive Journal of Medical Research [Electronic Resource]*, 5(1), e3. doi:10.2196/jmr.4910.

Boivin, G., Jovey, R., Elliott, C. T., et al. (2010). Management and prevention of herpes zoster: A Canadian perspective. *The Canadian Journal of Infectious Diseases & Medical Microbiology*, 21(1), 45–52.

Canadian Institute for Health Information (CIHI). (2013). *Adverse drug reaction-related hospitalizations among seniors, 2006 to 2011*. Retrieved from https://secure.cihi.ca/free_products/Hospitalizations%20for%20ADR-ENweb.pdf.

Carson, J. W., Carson, K. M., Jones, K. D., et al. (2016). Mindful yoga pilot study shows modulation of abnormal pain processing in fibromyalgia patients. *International Journal of Yoga Therapy*, 26(1), 93–100. doi:10.17761/1531-2054-26.1.93.

Durham, C. O., Fowler, T., Donato, A., et al. (2015). Pain management in patients with rheumatoid arthritis. *The Nurse Practitioner*, 40(5), 38–45. doi:10.1097/01.NPR.0000463784.36883.23.

Health Link B.C. (2017). *Shingles*. Retrieved from https://www.healthlinkbc.ca/health-topics/hw75433.

Inelman, E. M., Mosele, M., Sergi, G., et al. (2012). Chronic pain in the elderly with advanced dementia: Are we doing our best for their suffering? *Aging Clinical and Experimental Research*, 24(3), 207–212. doi:10.3275/8020.

Kumar, S. P., Adhikari, P., Jeganathan, P. S., et al. (2014). Efficacy of therapeutic touch and Reiki therapy for pain relief in disease conditions: A systematic review. *Journal of Psychiatric Nursing*, 3(1), 1–40. Retrieved from http://rfppl.co.in/subscription/upload_pdf/KUMAR%20SENTHIL_1464.pdf.

Lapane, K. L., Quilliam, B. J., Chow, W., et al. (2012). The association between pain and measures of well-being among nursing home residents. *Journal of the American Medical Directors Association*, 13(4), 344–349. doi:10.1016/j.jamda.2011.01.007.

Linton, S. J., & Shaw, W. S. (2011). Impact of psychological factors in the experience of pain. *Physical Therapy*, 91(5), 700–711. doi:10.2522/ptj.20100330.

McArthur, B. A., Dy, C. J., Fabricant, P. D., et al. (2012). Long term safety, efficacy, and patient acceptability of hyaluronic acid injection in patients with painful osteoarthritis of the knee. *Patient Preference and Adherence [Electronic Resource]*, 6, 905–910. doi:10.2147/PPA.S27783.

Morone, N. E., & Weiner, D. K. (2013). Pain as the 5th vital sign: Exposing the vital need for pain education. *Clinical Therapeutics, 35*(11), 1728–1732. doi:10.1016/j.clinthera.2013.10.001.

Nash, M. R., & Tasso, A. (2010). The effectiveness of hypnosis in reducing pain and suffering among women with metastatic breast cancer and among women with temporomandibular disorder. *The International Journal of Clinical and Experimental Hypnosis, 58*(4), 497–504. doi:10.1080/00207144.2010.499353.

National Institute on Aging. (2015). *Frequently asked questions.* Retrieved from https://nihseniorhealth.gov/shingles/faq/faq15.html.

Reitsma, M. L., Tranmer, J. E., Buchanan, D. M., et al. (2011). The prevalence of chronic pain and pain-related interference in the Canadian population from 1994 to 2008. *Chronic Diseases and Injuries in Canada, 31*(4), 157–164.

Schestatsky, P., Vidor, L., Winckler, P. B., et al. (2014). Promising treatments for neuropathic pain. *Arquivos de Neuro-Psiquiatria, 72*(11), 881–888. Retrieved from http://www.scielo.br/scielo.php?pid=S0004-282X2014001100881&script=sci_arttext.

Schulenburg, J. (2015). Considerations for complementary and alternative interventions for pain. *AORN Journal, 101*(3), 319–326. doi:10.1016/j.aorn.2015.01.013.

Steele, L. L., & Steele, J. R. (2009). Chronic pain. In P. D. Larsen & I. M. Lubkin (Eds.), *Chronic illness: Impact and intervention* (7th ed., pp. 295–412). Jones & Barlett.

Vas, J., Perea-Milla, E., Mendex, C., et al. (2006). Efficacy and safety of acupuncture for chronic uncomplicated neck pain: A randomized controlled study. *Pain, 126*(1–3), 245–255. Retrieved from https://www.researchgate.net/profile/Camila_Mendez/publication/6854894_Efficacy_and_safety_of_acupuncture_for_chronic_uncomplicated_neck_pain_A_randomised_controlled_study/links/00b4951f79fae4b6e2000000.pdf.

Vickers, J., Cronin, A. M., Maschino, A. C., et al. (2012). Acupuncture for chronic pain: Individual pain data meta-analysis. *Archives of Internal Medicine, 172*(19), 1444–1453. doi:10.1001/archinternmed.2012.3654.

Witt, C. M., Jena, S., Brinkaus, B., et al. (2006). Acupuncture in patients with osteoarthritis of the knee or hip: A randomized, controlled trial with an additional nonrandomized arm. *Arthritis and Rheumatism, 54*(11), 3485–3493. doi:10.1002/art.22154.

Diabetes Mellitus

LEARNING OBJECTIVES

Upon completion of this chapter, the reader will be able to:

- Explain the risks for and complications of diabetes in the older person.
- Identify the unique aspects of diabetes management in older persons.
- Describe the assessment necessary in the screening and monitoring of individuals with diabetes.
- Explain the important components of diabetes management.
- Discuss the nurse's role in diabetes management.
- Develop a nursing care plan for an older person with diabetes.
- Discuss the evidence and rationale for a high rate of diabetes among those over 75 years of age.

GLOSSARY

Autoimmune A term applied to the condition when the immune system sees a part of the body as a foreign object and produces antibodies to attack it.

Glycosylated hemoglobin (HgB A1c) test A blood test that measures the amount of glucose in the hemoglobin of red blood cells averaged over the 90-day lifespan of the cells.

Hyperosmolar nonketotic syndrome A metabolic complication of diabetes, often during periods of physiological stress, characterized by a rise in blood glucose (hyperglycemia), dehydration, hyperosmolar plasma, and an altered level of consciousness.

Insulin resistance Insensitivity of the body cells to the insulin produced by the pancreas, thus impairing glucose metabolism.

Intertriginous area An area where two skin areas may touch or rub together. Examples are the axilla of the arm, the anogenital region, the nares, and the skinfolds of the breasts.

Macrovascular Term referring to the larger, more prominent blood vessels in the body, such as the coronary arteries and the aorta.

Microvascular Term referring to the smaller blood vessels in the body.

Polydipsia Feelings of excessive thirst, often associated with diabetes.

Polyphagia Feelings of excessive hunger, often associated with diabetes.

Polyuria Abnormally excessive urine production and excretion, often associated with diabetes.

THE LIVED EXPERIENCE

I can see that Rita is going to need a lot of help learning to manage her diabetes. I know I overwhelmed her with brochures and information right off. She just looked frightened to death. I will call her tomorrow and see if she is less anxious.

Anna, gerontological clinical nurse specialist

DIABETES

Diabetes mellitus (DM), type 1 or type 2, is a syndrome of disorders of glucose metabolism resulting in hyperglycemia. Although no direct genetic influence has been found in connection with the development of type 2 DM, genes that are related to the risk for type 1 DM have been identified. Type 1 DM (formerly called *insulin-dependent diabetes mellitus*) develops in early life and is a result of **autoimmune** destruction of the insulin-producing beta cells of the pancreas. The resulting absence of insulin is incompatible with life; without replacement of the insulin, the person will die.

Type 2 DM (formerly called *non–insulin-dependent diabetes mellitus*) develops later in life, when the pancreas makes insulin but not enough to keep up with the needs of the body. This inadequate supply of naturally occurring insulin is combined with the **insulin resistance** that is characteristic of type 2 DM. The onset is usually insidious, and up to one-half of all persons with type 2 DM may be undiagnosed (Box 17.1). These persons may go a number of years without treatment while they are developing serious complications.

The number of persons with diabetes and the risk for diabetes vary by ethnicity, place of residence, and age (Box 17.2). In 2011, about 2.7 million (1 in 10) Canadians 20 years of age and older were living with diabetes (Government of Canada, 2016). People from some populations (e.g., people of South Asian, Asian, African, Latin American, or Indigenous descent) are at a higher risk for type 2 diabetes (Diabetes Canada, 2017a). Rates of diabetes in the Indigenous population are at least three times higher than those in the general population (Diabetes Canada, 2017a). Various studies conducted throughout Canada reported extremely high rates of diabetes in some Indigenous communities; the prevalence in some communities is as high as 48%.

The question remains whether diabetes is a primary or secondary event when there is a coexisting illness. Coexisting illnesses, such as hypertension and dyslipidemia, are associated with a decrease in insulin sensitivity. Alcohol and drugs such as diuretics, glucocorticoids, and nonsteroidal anti-inflammatory drugs may also contribute to insulin resistance or the body's failure to utilize the insulin that is present. Persons

---

BOX 17.1 Signs and Symptoms Suggestive of Diabetes in the Older Person

1. General symptoms are **polyphagia, polyuria, polydipsia,** and weight loss. (As these symptoms are rarely seen in older persons, the nurse should also focus on additional, vague symptoms, such as fatigue, and varied or recurrent infections.)
2. Recurrent infections (particularly those of bacterial or fungal origin) that involve the skin, **intertriginous areas,** or genito-urinary tract, and sores or wounds that tend to heal slowly.
3. Neurological dysfunction, including paresthesia, dysesthesia, or hyperesthesia; muscle weakness and pain (amyotrophy); cranial nerve palsies; autonomic dysfunction of the gastro-intestinal tract (diarrhea), cardiovascular abnormalities (orthostatic hypotension, dysrhythmias), reproductive system problems (erectile dysfunction), or bladder abnormalities (atony, overflow incontinence).
4. Arterial disease (macroangiopathy) involving the cardiovascular, cerebrovascular, or peripheral vasculature structures.
5. Small-vessel disease (microangiopathy) involving the kidneys (proteinuria, glomerulopathy, uremia) and eyes (macular disease, exudates, hemorrhages).
6. Lesions of the skin (Dupuytren's contracture, facial rubeosis, diabetic dermopathy).
7. Endocrine-metabolic complications (dyslipidemia, obesity, history of thyroid or adrenal insufficiency [Schmidt's syndrome]).

BOX 17.2 Risk Factors for Diabetes Mellitus

- Ethnicity
- Increasing age
- Blood pressure ≥140/90 mm Hg
- First-degree relative (parent, sibling, or child) with diabetes mellitus (DM)
- History of impaired glucose tolerance or impaired fasting plasma glucose
- Obesity (>120% of desirable weight, or body mass index >30 kg/m^2)
- Previous gestational DM or having had a child with a birth weight of >4.1 kg (9 lb)
- Undesirable lipid levels (high-density lipoproteins <0.90 mmol/L [35 mg/dL] or triglycerides >2.82 mmol/L [250 mg/dL])

with diabetes often have other health problems as well, including problems metabolizing lipids and proteins. Diabetes is the leading cause of end-stage renal disease and blindness and is especially prevalent among persons over 65 years of age.

COMPLICATIONS

Complications occur over the long course of the disease and are **microvascular**, **macrovascular**, or both. The microvascular problems are loss of vision (diabetic retinopathy) and end-stage renal failure from diabetic nephropathy. Delayed wound healing, when combined with peripheral neuropathy, may necessitate amputation.

Macrovascular complications include myocardial infarction, stroke, peripheral vascular disease, and neuropathy. Combined macro- and microvascular damage can lead to erectile dysfunction as a result of reduced vascular flow, peripheral neuropathy, and uncontrolled circulating blood glucose. Persons with diabetes commonly have problems with their feet, which can have a considerable impact on their functional status (see Chapter 12). Warning signs of foot problems derive from different body systems and include cold feet and intermittent pain from claudication (vascular); burning, tingling, hypersensitivity, or numbness (neurological); a gradual change in shape or a sudden, painless change without trauma (musculo-skeletal); and infections, changes of skin colour and texture, and slow-healing painful or painless wounds (dermatological) (Diabetes Canada, 2017b; Registered Nurses' Association of Ontario [RNAO], 2013).

Diabetes is often associated with a number of other health problems. Between 2009 and 2010, 22.7% of Canadians with diabetes reported having heart disease (Public Health Agency of Canada [PHAC], 2011). The number of hospitalizations for cardiovascular disease in persons with diabetes is three times higher than that in persons without diabetes (PHAC, 2011). Persons with diabetes most often die of heart disease. Approximately 80% of people who have diabetes in Canada will die as a result of heart disease or stroke (Diabetes Canada, 2013a). Other common health problems associated with diabetes are chronic kidney disease, heart failure, stroke, and lower-limb amputations (PHAC, 2011).

Some of the barriers to the delivery of effective care for diabetes are related to the patient's access to primary health care practitioners, especially in rural and remote areas. Also, the cost of test supplies is often an issue for people who do not have private health care insurance coverage. The gerontological nurse needs to collaborate with colleagues in the community, the diabetes educator, and social workers to find the best solution in these situations.

TREATMENT AND GOALS

Diabetes is a chronic disease that causes damage to the body's organs even in the best of circumstances. When diabetes is untreated or undertreated, complications develop more quickly and are more severe. Therefore, holding back the progression of the disease is the major goal.

For younger adults (aged 18–60), the main goal of treatment focuses on maintaining glycemic control most of the time, aiming for a blood sugar level of 4.4–6.1 mmol/L (82–110 mg/dL) and **glycosylated hemoglobin (Hgb A1c)** at or below 7.0% (Diabetes Canada, 2008). However, a consensus report on diabetes management of older persons asserted that tight glycemic control, especially for those older persons with ischemic heart disease, is not always preferred (Kirkman et al., 2012). Based on the results of several large studies, the American Diabetes Association modified its recommendations in 2011 for glycemic control in older persons (American Diabetes Association [ADA], 2011). It is now recommended that the degree of glycemic control be based on the condition of the person rather than on a universal number. For healthy older persons with a reasonably long life expectancy, the same evidence-informed practice as for younger adults should be followed. However, for those who are medically fragile and whose life expectancy is limited, some flexibility may be more appropriate, along with an emphasis on quality of life rather than length of life. Tight control of glucose levels in these circumstances may lead to life-threatening hypoglycemia. A goal of a hemoglobinA1c greater than 8% for the very frail may be adequate (Zarowitz, 2011).

As might be expected, anxiety, depression, and poor perceptions of one's health are often associated with diabetes, and these emotional states may reduce the person's motivation for self-management. Social support has a positive effect on the depression and anxiety surrounding the diagnosis of diabetes and living with diabetes (Wu et al., 2013). A holistic approach and more depth and breadth in nursing practice in the care of the diabetic patient facilitates improved health maintenance and adherence to recommended therapies.

IMPLICATIONS FOR GERONTOLOGICAL NURSING AND HEALTHY AGING

Gerontological nurses have great potential for helping individuals with diabetes, ranging from conducting screenings to educating and coaching the patient and his or her family. Nurses can participate in early detection through public screenings or pay attention to the need for the screening of persons residing in communal settings such as long-term care (LTC) homes and assisted-living facilities. Furthermore, nurses should promote healthy aging by helping people reach or maintain an ideal body weight, eat a healthy diet that provides adequate protein without excessive carbohydrates, exercise regularly, and keep cholesterol levels and blood pressure under control, all of which reduce the risk for diabetes.

For persons at higher risk for diabetes, especially those with impaired fasting glucose or impaired glucose tolerance, attention should be directed at reducing their risks for both diabetes and heart disease. This means education and the carrying out of interventions to help the older person reach the following goals:

- No smoking
- Blood pressure ≤130/80 mm Hg
- Cholesterol <5.18 mmol/L (200 mg/dL)
- Low-density lipoprotein <2.56 mmol/L (100 mg/dL)
- High-density lipoprotein >1.03 mmol/L (40 mg/dL)
- Triglycerides <1.69 mmol/L (150 mg/dL)
- Fasting blood glucose <7 mmol/L (<126 mg/dL)

Screening for diabetes by fasting plasma and random blood glucose testing is important for the early identification of potential or actual disease. Annual screening of fasting plasma glucose measurements is recommended for all persons in high-risk groups, which includes all persons over 65 years of age.

ASSESSMENT

The nurse begins with an assessment for risk factors and a subjective report of signs and symptoms, including an evaluation of the presence or absence of hyperglycemia, polydipsia, polyuria, or polyphagia. Because these symptoms are rarely seen in older persons, it is important to also focus on symptoms that are more vague, such as fatigue, change in weight, and varied or recurrent infections. When there are symptoms, their duration and character of should be described. Family history is important because of genetic influence. Nutrition, weight, and exercise history can identify eating patterns, an active or sedentary lifestyle, and weight control measures, all of which can provide clues for realistic education. Assessing economic resources helps establish the person's ability to purchase equipment, materials, and foods that may be needed to maintain diabetes control. This is important for older persons who may have limited incomes. A history of alcohol and tobacco use provides information about the person's risk for complications.

The nursing assessment also includes the careful measurement of blood pressure, visual acuity, and gross neurological function. Distance vision can be checked with a Snellen chart, and near vision can be checked with a newspaper. The skin and feet should be thoroughly inspected for any injury, such as corns, calluses, blisters, cracks, or fungal infections. The use of the Semmes-Weinstein monofilament instrument is recommended to test for peripheral neuropathy.

MANAGEMENT

Promoting healthy aging in persons with diabetes requires an array of interventions and usually involves people from a number of professions working together with the person and his or her significant others. Management of diabetes requires support for the person and expertise in medication use, diet and exercise, and counselling. The interprofessional team may include nurses as well as dietitians, pharmacists, podiatrists, ophthalmologists, physicians, nurse practitioners, certified diabetic educators, and counsellors. If the disease is hard to control, endocrinologists are involved; as complications develop, more specialists (such as nephrologists, cardiologists, and wound care specialists) are called in.

Diabetes self-management, diabetes self-management education, and patient empowerment are now the cornerstones of disease management (Kirkman et al., 2012; Murray & Shah, 2016). The skills needed for self-management include a knowledge about nutrition, the development of an exercise plan, the safe use of medication, what to do during periods of other illness, attention to the psychological aspects of dealing with a chronic illness, the ability to use personal glucose monitors, optimal care of the feet, and knowledge about the disease. The nurse is highly instrumental in the teaching of self-management skills, encouraging patient empowerment, and supporting the person.

Standards of Care

Diabetes Canada has developed a set of clinical practice guidelines for the prevention and management of diabetes in Canada (Diabetes Canada, 2013b). The first and perhaps most important recommendation is that the care of the older person with diabetes must be individually planned to consider the relative costs and benefits for the person. Among those recommendations are the following:

- When collecting the person's health history, the nurse should include smoking history, dietary habits, weight patterns, previous treatment programs, current treatment regimen, exercise and activity levels, infections, illnesses, and complications of diabetes. Information about the approaches that worked and those that failed will help the nurse design programs specific to the older person.
- Annual physical examination includes blood pressure measurement; dilated eye examination; thyroid palpation; palpation of pulses; foot, periodontal, and skin examination; and neurological examination. Testing fine sensation with a monofilament is recommended.
- Laboratory tests should include both a fasting plasma glucose test and an Hgb A1c test; fasting lipid profile; serum creatinine if proteinuria is present; urinalysis (including microalbuminuria) and urine culture if indicated; assessment of thyroid function (thyroxine [T_4] or thyroid-stimulating hormone); and an electrocardiogram (ECG).

Gerontological nurses have an important educational role in the treatment of diabetes and must encourage and help older adults obtain care that can delay or minimize complications. One of the most significant skills for the older person to master is the technique for the self-monitoring of blood glucose (SMBG), including how to obtain a blood sample with glucose-monitoring equipment, troubleshoot when results indicate an error, and record the values from the machine. Older persons with arthritis, low vision, or peripheral neuropathy will have difficulties with the mechanics of SMBG and will require creative teaching and perhaps the help of others with the tasks that are necessary. New technologies and medication delivery systems (e.g., nasal sprays) are being designed to address some of these issues.

Daily foot care and foot examination should be discussed and demonstrated (RNAO, 2013). A person who is not particularly flexible will have difficulty reaching and inspecting the feet; a family member or a friend can be asked to do this. As long as the person's vision is adequate, she or he can place a mirror on the floor to reflect the sole of the foot for examination. Attention to foot care can reduce the risk of amputation. Also it is essential that the person be aware of the need for shoes that fit well (see Chapter 11).

Knowing about diabetes and its effects includes knowing what affects the blood sugar. The older person should have a list of warning signs for high and low blood sugar levels and know that extra SMBG is necessary any time he or she feels clammy or cold, sweaty, shaky, or confused—all signs of low blood sugar. Hypoglycemia is the most common problem for older people with diabetes, especially for those taking sulphonylureas. Sulphonylureas are antidiabetic medications that act by increasing the release of insulin from pancreatic beta cells. An identification bracelet is highly recommended, especially because of possible misdiagnosis if the person is found to be confused.

Experiential teaching, encouragement, and reinforcement of mastery are important factors that promote successful self-management. Some of the factors affecting diabetes control in older persons are identified in Box 17.3.

BOX 17.3 Interaction Between Diabetes and the Aging Process

1. A decline in visual acuity can affect the individual's ability to see printed educational material, medication labels, markings on a syringe, and the screen on blood glucose monitoring devices.
2. Auditory impairments can lead to difficulty hearing instructions.
3. Altered taste can affect food choices and nutritional status.
4. Poor dentition or changes in the gastro-intestinal system can lead to difficulties with food ingestion and digestion.
5. Altered ability to recognize hunger and thirst may lead to weight loss, dehydration, and increased risk for **hyperosmolar nonketotic syndrome.**
6. Changes in hepatic or renal function can affect the ability to absorb or excrete medications.
7. Arthritis or tremors can affect the ability to self-administer medications and use monitoring devices.
8. Polypharmacy complicates medication choices.
9. Depression affects motivation for self-management.
10. Cognitive impairment and dementia decrease self-care ability.
11. Inadequate education and poor literacy call for modifications in the method of teaching about diabetes care.
12. Level of income can affect the level of care sought or obtained.
13. Living alone without a resource person can have a negative effect on the person with diabetes.
14. A sedentary lifestyle and obesity can result in decreased tissue sensitivity to insulin.

Nutrition

Adequate and appropriate nutrition is a key factor in the control of diabetes. An initial nutrition assessment with a 24-hour recall will provide some clues to the person's dietary habits, intake, and style of eating. If the person is a member of a specific minority ethnic group, the nurse will need to learn about that group's usual food ingredients and methods of food preparation in order to be able to give reasonable instructions. Particular foods of such groups will need to be considered. It is generally recommended that people with diabetes follow the healthy balanced diet presented in *Eating Well with Canada's Food Guide* (Diabetes Canada, 2013b) (see Chapter 8). Ideally, all persons with diabetes should have annual medical nutrition therapy by a registered dietitian who is a certified diabetic educator. Diabetes Canada provides information, resources, and guidelines for a healthy diet, with attention to an adequate variety of foods, macronutrients, and low–glycemic index foods (Diabetes Canada, 2013b). The recommended daily caloric intake ranges from 1,600 calories for women to a maximum of 2,200 calories for men. The goal is to keep the glucose level under control by balancing exercise with eating, weight loss if overweight, and limiting saturated fats. Carbohydrates are included on the diabetes food pyramid but are restricted to whole grains. For details about all aspects of diet and diabetes, see the Diabetes Canada website at http://www.diabetes.ca/diabetes-and-you/healthy-living-resources/diet-nutrition.

It is part of the nurse's responsibility to learn if there is difficulty with access to food (including fresh fruit and vegetables), shopping for food, and food preparation. Working with older persons, whose dietary habits have been formed over a lifetime, can be difficult but is not impossible.

Exercise

Exercise is an important aspect of therapy for type 2 DM because it increases insulin production and decreases insulin resistance. Walking is an inexpensive and beneficial way to exercise, and daily exercise is recommended. For older persons whose mobility is limited, chair exercises or exercise machines that permit sitting and holding on for support can be helpful.

In some cases, exercise in conjunction with an appropriate diet may be sufficient to maintain blood glucose within normal levels. A more intensive exercise program should not be started until the older person has had a physical examination, including a stress test and an ECG. A physician or nurse practitioner and a diabetic educator will then have the information necessary to develop a safe exercise plan for and with the person. If the person is using insulin, exercise must be done on a regular rather than an erratic basis. To avoid hypoglycemia, blood glucose should be tested before and after exercise.

TABLE 17.1   Types of Insulin

INSULIN TYPE/ACTION (APPEARANCE)	BRAND (GENERIC) NAMES	DOSING SCHEDULE
Rapid-acting analogue (clear) • Onset: 10–15 min • Peak: 60–90 min • Duration: 3–5 hr	Apidra (insulin glulisine) Humalog (insulin lispro) NovoRapid (insulin aspart)	Usually taken right before eating, or to lower high blood glucose
Short-acting (clear) • Onset: 30 min • Peak: 2–3 hr • Duration: 6.5 hr	Humulin-R Novolin GE Toronto	Taken about 30 min before eating, or to lower high blood glucose
Intermediate-acting (cloudy) • Onset: 1–3 hr • Peak: 5–8 hr • Duration: up to 18 hr	Humulin-N Novolin GE NPH	Often taken at bedtime, or twice a day (morning and bedtime)
Long-acting analogue (clear and colourless) • Onset: 90 min • Peak: none • Duration: up to 24 hr (Lantus, 24 hr; Levemir, 16–24 hr)	Lantus (insulin glargine) Levemir (insulin detemir)	Usually taken once or twice a day
Premixed (cloudy) A single vial or cartridge contains a fixed ratio of insulin (the numbers refer to the percent of rapid- or fast-acting insulin to the percent of intermediate-acting insulin)	**Premixed Regular Insulin–NPH** • Humulin (30/70) • Novolin GE (30/70, 40/60, 50/50) **Premixed Insulin Analogues** • Humalog Mix25 and Mix50 • NovoMix 30	Depends on the combination

Source: Adapted from Diabetes Canada. (2013). Clinical practice guidelines for the prevention and management of diabetes in Canada. *Canadian Journal of Diabetes, 37*(1)(Suppl. 1), S1–S212 (p. S47, Table 1). Retrieved from http://guidelines.diabetes.ca/app_themes/cdacpg/resources/cpg_2013_full_en.pdf.

Medications

Antihyperglycemics include oral drugs (including the new inhalant insulin). Oral medications are prescribed according to the identified insulin deficit—insulin resistance, or inadequate or no secretion of insulin. The sulphonylureas (e.g., glyburide) and meglitinides (e.g., repaglinide and nateglinide) increase insulin secretion. Biguanides (e.g., metformin) or thiazolidinediones (e.g., glitazones) enhance insulin sensitivity by decreasing insulin resistance.

The mainstay of the treatment of type 2 DM in later life is oral medication. However, when the blood sugar is greater than 11.11 mmol/L (200 mg/dL) and is difficult to control, additional insulin may be necessary. It is important to note that the use of insulin by someone with type 2 DM does not "convert" the person to a type 1 diabetic, because the diagnosis is made on the basis of the type of disorder rather than on the treatment. Common types of insulin prescribed for older persons are rapid-acting insulin and long-acting insulin (Table 17.1). Most people need two or more types of insulin to reach their blood glucose targets. Insulin can be administered through subcutaneous injections (needle or insulin pen), an insulin pump, or an insulin jet injector, which sends a fine spray of insulin through the skin with high-pressure air).

If other medications are prescribed, they must be carefully reviewed. The effect of medications on blood glucose must be given serious consideration, because a number of medications commonly used for older patients adversely affect blood glucose levels (Box 17.4). Therefore, older persons who have diabetes

| BOX 17.4 | Medications Affecting Blood Sugar |

Medications That Increase Blood Glucose Levels
- Corticosteroids
- Diazoxide
- Estrogens
- Furosemide and thiazide diuretics
- Glucagon
- Lithium
- Phenytoin
- Rifampin
- Sympathomimetics (antihistamines, decongestants, bronchodilators)
- Thyroid-replacement preparations
- Atypical antipsychotics (risperidone, olanzapine)

Medications That Decrease Blood Glucose Levels
- Alcohol
- Anabolic steroids
- Beta blockers (antihypertensives)
- Salicylates (high doses)

Medications That Interact With Sulphonylureas (Oral Hypoglycemics)
Increased Effects (Blood Glucose Levels Further Lowered)
- Allopurinol
- Beta blockers
- Clofibrate
- Histamine antagonists
- Imidazole antifungals
- Low-dose salicylates
- Monoamine oxidase inhibitors
- Probenecid
- Tricyclic antidepressants

Medications Not to Be Taken in Combination With Sulphonylureas
- Chloramphenicol
- Salicylates (high dose)
- Sulphonamides

Medications That Have Decreased Effects (i.e., Hinder Hypoglycemic Action)
- Barbiturates
- Corticosteroids
- Diuretics
- Estrogens
- Rifampin

Source: Adapted from Diabetes in Control.com. (2016). *Drugs that can affect blood glucose levels.* Retrieved from http://www.diabetesincontrol.com/drugs-that-can-affect-blood-glucose-levels/; and Diabetes Monitor. (2012). *Diabetes information, education and resources.* Retrieved from http://www.diabetesmonitor.com.

should be advised to ask if a particular prescribed medication affects their therapy and should check with their primary care provider before taking any over-the-counter medications.

Long-Term Care and the Older Person With Diabetes

Many persons cared for by gerontological nurses in LTC homes have diabetes. According to data from the Continuing Care Reporting System maintained by the Canadian Institute for Health Information, the prevalence of diabetes in Ontario LTC homes is about 25% (in 2011); approximately 90 to 95% of diabetes cases are cases of type 2 diabetes (Bronskill et al., 2011; Osman et al., 2016).

In LTC homes, nurses are responsible for many of the activities that would otherwise fall to the older person, a significant other, or a home caregiver to carry out. Meals, nutritional status, intake and output, and exercise and activity are monitored. The nurse assesses the resident for signs of hypoglycemia and hyperglycemia, as well as evidence of complications, and ensures that the standards of care are met. Having effective working relationships within the nursing team and ensuring that unregulated workers who provide care for residents with dementia know the signs of hypoglycemia and hyperglycemia are essential in providing the best care to residents with diabetes. The nurse monitors the effect and side effects of diet, exercise, and medication use; encourages self-care whenever possible; and administers medications or supervises their administration.

Box 17.5 presents an intervention to improve outcomes in patients with diabetes.

SUMMARY

Given the numerous complications and comorbidities associated with diabetes, gerontological nurses play an essential role in the prevention, early detection, and management of this disease. Nurses must be able to assess and identify older persons who are most at risk of developing diabetes or complications associated with it. In addition, gerontological nurses help educate patients about relevant health matters and provide accurate information about healthy lifestyle

BOX 17.5	Research for Evidence-Informed Practice: Effectiveness of a Behaviour Modification Program for Older People With Uncontrolled Type 2 Diabetes

Problem: Diabetes mellitus is a chronic disease and a major health problem around the world. Older persons often need support in adopting health-related behaviours—eating a healthy diet, taking appropriate medication, and exercising—to try to improve glycemic levels. Previous studies have demonstrated the relationship between self-efficacy and behaviour modification (BM) for diabetes. However, the effects of BM on older persons with uncontrolled type 2 diabetes and the impact of those effects on quality of life are not well understood.

Methods: A quasi-experimental study with an intervention and control group was designed to evaluate the effectiveness of a BM program, including activities in relation to group counselling, group discussions, and encouragement to enhance a healthy diet and exercise. Fifty-nine older adults from two neighbouring communities in a large urban area participated in the study. All participants had recently been diagnosed with type 2 diabetes (during the previous 6 months). The intervention group received four 2-hour group BM sessions over a 3-month period. The BM sessions focused on encouraging the patient to, set goals to control diabetes, enhance self-efficacy in maintaining a healthy diet, consume medication, use exercise and relaxation techniques, plan actions for glycemic control, and discuss the prevention of the complications of diabetes. The control group received the usual care, including individual health education from their health care providers for 3–4 months.

Findings: Participants in the intervention group exercised more frequently and did a wider range of exercise than did participants of the control group. In addition, the intervention group had improved scores of knowledge, self-efficacy, changed behaviours toward a healthy diet, exercise, and medication consumption. All scores were significantly higher than those in the control group.

Application to Nursing Practice: Nurses can assist in implementing BM programs in diabetes clinics, hospitals, and primary care settings. Nurses play an important role in strengthening older persons' confidence and ability to self-care and to optimize health behaviours related to diabetes.

Source: Ounnapiruk et al. (2014). Effectiveness of a behavior modification program for older people with uncontrolled Type 2 Diabetes. *Nursing and Health Sciences, 16*, 216–23.

choices that would help slow the progression of diabetes and its associated conditions.

KEY CONCEPTS

- The signs and symptoms of diabetes in the older person may be vague or suggestive of other medical conditions. They may be considered part of aging rather than symptoms of polyuria, polydipsia, and polyphagia.
- Close monitoring of blood glucose levels is the most effective way to prevent, delay, or slow the progression of macrovascular, microvascular, and neurological complications of the disease.
- The management of diabetes is a comprehensive team effort and should include the older person as much as possible. If this is not possible, the health care provider will need to ensure that the medical regimen is effective.
- Preventive foot care is essential for the prevention of future problems.

ACTIVITIES AND DISCUSSION QUESTIONS

1. What are the risks and complications of diabetes for the older person?
2. State the components of diabetes management, and explain what each component entails.
3. Describe the nurse's role in the management of diabetes.
4. Develop a nursing care plan for an older person with type 2 DM in each of the following settings: the community, an acute care hospital, and a LTC home.

RESOURCES

Diabetes Canada
http://www.diabetes.ca

Diabetes Canada. *Clinical guidelines for the prevention and management of diabetes in Canada*
http://guidelines.diabetes.ca/app_themes/cdacpg/resources/cpg_2013_full_en.pdf

Diabetes in Control.com. **Drugs that can affect blood glucose levels** http://www.diabetesincontrol.com/drugs-that-can-affect-blood-glucose-levels/

Heart and Stroke Foundation of Canada
http://www.heartandstroke.ca

Public Health Agency of Canada. Type 2 diabetes info sheet for seniors
http://www.wrha.mb.ca/community/seniors/files/CMP-44.pdf

Registered Nurses' Association of Ontario (RNAO). *Assessment and Management of Foot Ulcers for People with Diabetes* **(Second Edition)**
http://rnao.ca/bpg/guidelines/assessment-and-management-foot-ulcers-people-diabetes-second-edition

Registered Nurses' Association of Ontario (RNAO). *Best Practice Guideline for the Subcutaneous Administration of Insulin in Adults with Type 2 Diabetes*
http://rnao.ca/sites/rnao-ca/files/BPG_for_the_Subcutaneous_Administration_of_Insulin_in_Adults_with_Type_2_Diabetes.pdf

For additional resources, please visit *http://evolve.elsevier.com/Canada/Ebersole/gerontological/*

REFERENCES

American Diabetes Association (ADA). (2011). Standards of medical care in diabetes–2011. *American Diabetes Care Diabetes Care, 34*(1), S11–S61. doi:10.2337/dc11-S011.

Bronskill, S. E., Grunier, A., Ho, M. M., et al. (2011). Older adults newly placed in longterm care system, in use by frail Ontario seniors. In S. E. Bronskill, X. Camacho, A. Gruneir, et al. (Eds.), *Health system use by frail Ontario seniors: An in-depth examination of four vulnerable cohorts.* Toronto, ON: Institute for Clinical Evaluative Sciences (ICES).

Diabetes Canada. (2008). Canadian Diabetes Association 2008 clinical practice guidelines for the prevention and management of diabetes in Canada. *Canadian Journal of Diabetes, 32*(1).

Diabetes Canada. (2013a). *Diabetes and your heart.* Retrieved from http://guidelines.diabetes.ca/cdacpg/media/documents/patient-resources/heart-disease-and-stroke-2014.pdf.

Diabetes Canada. (2013b). Clinical practice guidelines for the prevention and management of diabetes in Canada. *Canadian Journal of Diabetes, 37*(1)(Suppl. 1), S1–S212.

Diabetes Canada. (2017a). *Diabetes statistics in Canada.* Retrieved from http://www.diabetes.ca/how-you-can-help/advocate/why-federal-leadership-is-essential/diabetes-statistics-in-canada.

Diabetes Canada. (2017b). *Signs of foot problems.* Retrieved from http://www.diabetes.ca/diabetes-and-you/healthy-living-resources/foot-care/signs-of-foot-problems.

Government of Canada. (2016). *Health status of Canadians 2016: Report of the chief public health officer—How are we unhealthy?—Diabetes.* Retrieved from https://www.canada.ca/en/public-health/corporate/publications/chief-public-health-officer-reports-state-public-health-canada/2016-health-status-canadians/page-18-how-are-we-unhealthy-diabetes.html.

Kirkman, M. S., Jones Briscoe, V., Clark, N., et al. (2012). Diabetes in older adults: A consensus report. *Journal of the American Geriatrics Society, 60*(12), 2342–2356. doi:10.1111/jgs.12035.

Murray, C. M., & Shah, B. R. (2016). Diabetes self-management education improves medication utilization and retinopathy screening in the elderly. *Primary Care Diabetes, 10*(3), 179–185. doi:10.1016/j.pcd.2015.10.007.

Osman, O., Sherifali, D., Stolee, P., et al. (2016). Diabetes management in long-term care: An exploratory study of the current practices and processes to managing frail elderly persons with type 2 diabetes. *Canadian Journal of Diabetes, 40*(1), 17–30. doi:10.1016/j.jcjd.2015.10.005.

Public Health Agency of Canada (2011). *Highlights: Diabetes in Canada: Facts and figures from a public health perspective.* Ottawa, ON: Health Canada. Retrieved from https://www.canada.ca/en/public-health/services/chronic-diseases/reports-publications/diabetes/diabetes-canada-facts-figures-a-public-health-perspective/report-highlights.html.

Registered Nurses' Association of Ontario (RNAO) (2013). *Assessment and management of foot ulcers for people with diabetes* (2nd ed.). Toronto, ON: Author.

Wu, S. F., Young, L. S., Yeh, F. C., et al. (2013). Correlations among social support, depression, and anxiety in patients with type-2 diabetes. *Journal of Nursing Research, 21*(2), 129–138. doi:10.1097/jnr.0b013e3182921fe1.

Zarowitz, B. J. (2011). The ADA focus on diabetes. *Geriatric Nursing, 32*(2), 119–122. doi:10.1016/j.gerinurse.2011.01.003.

Bone and Joint Health

LEARNING OBJECTIVES

Upon completion of this chapter, the reader will be able to:

- Describe the most common bone and joint problems affecting the older person.
- Discuss the potential risks of osteoporosis.
- Recognize postural changes that suggest the presence of osteoporosis.
- Explain effective ways of preventing or slowing the progression of osteoporosis.
- Relate the differences between osteoarthritis, rheumatoid arthritis, and gout.
- Describe the nurse's responsibility in care for the person with osteoarthritis, rheumatoid arthritis, and gout.
- Name several methods of managing older persons' pain and disability resulting from joint and bone disorders.

GLOSSARY

Bone mineral density The mineral content of the bones.

Crepitus The sound or feel of bone rubbing on bone.

Osteopenia Loss of bone mineral density and structure at a mild to moderate level.

Osteophyte Excessive bone growth.

Osteoporosis Loss of bone mineral density and structure to a great degree.

Resorption The loss of a substance or bone by physiological or pathological processes.

THE LIVED EXPERIENCE

Halfway through the mall I had to sit because I couldn't go any further. I was just in agony with the pain; I was in agony. And so I just sat there and I had sunglasses on and I think tears were rolling out of my eyes because I couldn't—I just couldn't—go for a walk, and ugh, now I have to go back to the van. Can I drive back home? I had to call my daughter and I said, look, I'm not feeling good. So that's being dependent. You know, always not knowing, not trusting, that you can do something.

Source: Maly, M. R. & Krupa, T. (2007). Personal experience of living with knee osteoarthritis among older persons. *Disability and Rehabilitation, 29*(18), 1423–1433.

MUSCULO-SKELETAL SYSTEM

A healthy musculo-skeletal system allows the human body to be upright and is necessary for comfortably carrying out the basic activities of daily living. For some older persons, later life is an opportunity to explore the limits of their ability and become more athletic. For others, later life is a time of significant restriction in movement. However, in both cases, older persons may have to deal with the challenges of one or more of the musculo-skeletal problems commonly encountered in later life. Gerontological nurses attend to the needs of older persons to promote healthy bones and joints. This chapter will discuss osteoporosis and the different forms of arthritis and their implications for nursing interventions. For a discussion of activity and exercise to maintain musculo-skeletal health, see Chapter 10.

OSTEOPOROSIS

During the normal process of bone growth, bones build up mass (formation) and strength; at the same time, bones are losing mass and strength through **resorption.** In a healthy adult, formation and resorption are balanced, and peak bone mass is reached at 30 years of age. After that, the loss of **bone mineral density** (BMD) is minimal at first but then speeds up with age. For women, the period of the fastest overall loss of BMD is 5 to 7 years immediately following menopause. Severe loss of BMD is called **osteoporosis.**

Osteoporosis means "porous bone" and is characterized by reduced BMD, disrupted bone microarchitecture, and an altered amount and variety of proteins in the bone. Primary osteoporosis is sometimes thought to be a part of the normal aging process, especially in women. *Secondary osteoporosis* is the term used for porous bones caused by another disease, such as Paget's disease, or by medication, such as long-term steroids. Both types of osteoporosis are characterized by low BMD and subsequent deterioration of bone structure, as well as changes in posture. Approximately two million Canadians have osteoporosis (Osteoporosis Canada, 2012a). A negative consequence of osteoporosis is a high risk of fractures when a fall occurs. One in three women and one in five men will have an osteoporotic fracture in their lifetime (Osteoporosis Canada, 2017a). Approximately 28% of women and 37% of men with a hip fracture die within the following year (Osteoporosis Canada, 2017a).

Osteoporosis is a silent disorder. A person may have no symptoms of any kind for many years; another person may never show any symptoms. With the treatments and interventions now available, some osteoporosis can be prevented or can be treated and

stabilized to some extent. Osteoporosis is diagnosed through a dual energy x-ray absorptiometry (DEXA) scan, but is presumed to be present in older persons who have nontraumatic fractures, a loss of 7.5 cm (3 inches) or more in height, or kyphosis (pathological curvature of the upper spine) (Fig. 18.1) (Osteoporosis Canada, 2012a). The Scientific Advisory Council of the Osteoporosis Society of Canada (Brown & Josse, 2002) recommends that all persons aged 65 years and older individuals with at least one major or two minor risk factors should have their BMD measured with a DEXA scan. If the screening is positive, nurses can advocate that the older person receive appropriate treatment.

A number of other factors increase or decrease a person's risk for both **osteopenia,** a condition in persons whose BMD is lower than normal, and osteoporosis. Some of these factors cannot be changed (e.g., gender, race, or ethnicity), but others (e.g., calcium intake and exercise) are amenable to change (Box 18.1).

REDUCING OSTEOPOROSIS-RELATED RISKS AND INJURY

Measures to prevent osteoporosis-related injury or the progression of the disease include exercise, proper nutrition, and lifestyle changes. One major risk factor that can be changed is smoking. To prevent falls and fall-related injuries, home safety inspection and education regarding injury prevention strategies are essential (see Chapter 12). (An assortment of print and interactive educational materials for both a lay and professional audience can be found at https://www.osteoporosis.ca).

Weight-bearing physical activity and exercises help maintain bone mass. Brisk walking and working out with light weights apply mechanical force to the spine and long bones (see Chapter 10). Muscle-building exercises help maintain skeletal architecture by improving muscle strength and flexibility. Tai chi has been used successfully to strengthen the muscles and bones of older persons (Hui et al., 2015). Tai chi and exercise have the added advantage of improving balance and stamina, which may prevent falls or limit the damage if a fall should occur.

Teaching for patients includes teaching the key aspects of the prevention and treatment of

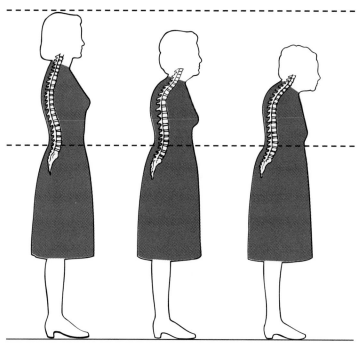

FIGURE 18.1 Osteoporosis spine alignment.

BOX 18.1 Risk Factors for Osteoporosis

Nonmodifiable Factors
Female gender
White race
Northern European ancestry
Advanced age
Family history of osteoporosis

Modifiable Factors
Low body weight (underweight)
Low calcium intake
Estrogen deficiency
Low testosterone
Inadequate exercise or activity
Use of steroids or anticonvulsants
Excessive coffee or alcohol intake
Current cigarette smoking

---

osteoporosis. Information about the sites that are most vulnerable to injury through accidents, falls, back strain, and poor posture is important. Changes in the upper spine that occur when vertebrae are weakened should be explained, as should the pain that results from strain on the lower spine caused by the effort to compensate for changes of balance and height. Education also includes teaching the appropriate way to take medications and how to manage their side effects.

Fall prevention is especially important for decreasing the morbidity and mortality associated with osteoporosis. The nurse should emphasize the importance of living safely in the home (e.g., wearing shoes with good support, and using handrails) and the risks of walking in poorly lighted areas. Several fracture prevention strategies, such as wearing hip protectors and performing exercises for balance and agility, are listed on the Osteoporosis Canada website (www.osteoporosis.ca). Basic body mechanics, such as the mechanics of lifting heavy objects, can be discussed. The use of stepstools or chairs to reach things in high places should be discouraged. Walkways should be kept free of obstacles, and loose rugs and electrical cords should be arranged so that they do not cause falls (see Chapter 12).

Pharmacological Interventions. In the last decade, considerable progress has been made in the development of pharmacological interventions for both the prevention and the treatment of osteoporosis.

Adequate intake of calcium and vitamin D supplements is recommended for persons at all ages, and these should be taken with all of the prescribed treatments currently available (Weaver et al., 2016).

Ideally, optimal nutrition in late life follows a lifetime of good eating habits (see Chapter 8). Several common foods have high calcium content, such as cheese (between 400 and 500 mg of calcium per 50 g), plain yogurt (between 260 and 270 mg of calcium per ¾ cup), milk (between 290 and 320 mg of calcium per 1 cup), and other foods, including canned sardines and beans, tofu, almonds, and spinach. Calcium can be obtained from combined dietary and supplementary sources. If supplements are used, combined calcium and vitamin D (e.g., Caltrate-D) is recommended. The doses are best spread over the course of the day; for example, 400 mg of calcium is taken in the morning, 400 mg during the day, and another 400 mg before bed. However, this regimen might be difficult for older persons to keep track of (see Chapter 14). The current recommendation calls for 400 to 1 000 international units (IU) of supplemental vitamin D for adults under the age of 50 years without osteoporosis or conditions affecting vitamin D absorption, and 800 to 2 000 IU for those 50 years of age and older (Osteoporosis Canada, 2017b).

Nurses are also responsible for educating patients about factors that inhibit calcium absorption (e.g., excess alcohol, protein, or salt) and enhance calcium excretion (e.g., caffeine; excess fibre; and phosphorus in meats, sodas, and preserved foods) and about the influence of the body's response to stress (decreased calcium absorption and increased excretion of calcium in the urine). Constipation is worsened by calcium supplements and may reduce the person's willingness to take them. Good nursing care includes developing, with the patient, a preventive plan including extra fluid intake (if not contraindicated) and the use of stool softeners. Neither calcium nor calcium-enriched products can be taken at the same time thyroid preparations are taken. Instead, calcium or calcium-enriched products should be taken at least 4 hours before or after thyroid preparations are taken (Gaitonde et al., 2012).

Estrogen has long been the medication of choice for increasing the BMD of women. However, estrogen also increases the rate of breast cancer, colon cancer, and heart disease, and thus it is no longer recommended (Black & Rosen, 2016).

Currently available medications include bisphosphonates, selective estrogen receptor modulators (SERMs), and parathyroid hormone. All increase bone mass, reduce bone turnover, or both. Bisphosphonates (e.g., Fosamax and Actonel) are often prescribed in daily, weekly, or monthly formulations. However, owing to the seriousness of the risk for esophageal erosion, the person must take them on an empty stomach, with a full glass of water, and must stay completely upright for half an hour after ingestion. Bisphosphonates are not appropriate for a person with memory loss or for anyone who cannot comply with directions. Some intravenously delivered bisphosphonates (e.g., Aclasta, Zometa) are being considered for use with older persons but are quite costly (Osteoporosis Canada, 2012b).

Evista, a type of SERM, is used as a substitute for estrogen and decreases the risk for breast cancer. It is approved for both prevention and treatment of bone loss, but it can cause hot flashes and coagulation disorders and is contraindicated for anyone who has a history of deep venous thrombosis or who is taking blood thinners.

The newest treatment for osteoporosis is daily injections of parathyroid hormone in the commercial form of teriparatide (Forteo). It is used for men and women at risk for fractures; however, its use is also associated with an increased risk of developing osteosarcoma. Because of this, teriparatide is typically considered a second line of therapy, and even then, it is not used for longer than 2 years (Meier et al., 2014).

Another useful medication is calcitonin (Miacalcin), which is used to slow bone loss and increase spinal BMD in women who are at least 5 years past menopause; it is not indicated for men. Calcitonin has been found to incidentally reduce back pain in some women. It is given either subcutaneously or as a nasal spray.

ARTHRITIS

The term *arthritis* refers to more than 100 diseases that involve damage to the joints of the body, affecting 4.2 million persons of all ages in Canada (Public Health Agency of Canada [PHAC], 2010). The number of

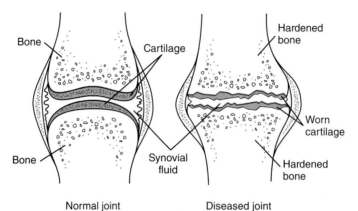

Bone

Cartilage

Hardened bone

Bone

Synovial fluid

Worn cartilage

Hardened bone

Normal joint   Diseased joint

FIGURE 18.2 A normal joint and a diseased joint.

people older than 15 years who are affected by arthritis is expected to increase to seven million by the year 2031 (PHAC, 2010). Arthritis is the number-one reason for activity limitations in older persons. The most common forms of the disease are osteoarthritis (OA), polymyalgia rheumatica (PMR), rheumatoid arthritis (RA), and gout.

OSTEOARTHRITIS

Osteoarthritis (OA), also known as degenerative arthritis or degenerative joint disease, is a degenerative joint disorder that affects at least three million (one in ten) Canadians (MacDonald et al., 2015). Risk factors include age, obesity, a family history of OA, repetitive use of the joint, and trauma to the joint. It is likely that persons over 65 years of age will have radiographic evidence of OA even if they are asymptomatic. It should be noted that although OA is more common with increased age, it affects younger persons as well. The prevalence of OA is significantly higher in Indigenous populations (Barnabe et al., 2017).

In an osteoarthritic joint, the normal soft and resilient cartilaginous lining becomes thin and damaged. This causes the joint space to narrow and the bones of the joint to rub together, causing joint and bone destruction, pain, swelling, and loss of motion. **Osteophytes** (bone spurs) may develop in the spaces, causing deformation and deterioration (Fig. 18.2). OA results from a complex interplay of many factors, including genetic predisposition, local inflammation, joint integrity, mechanical forces, and cellular

and biochemical processes. Treatment is available to lessen pain and increase function (see Chapter 16).

Osteoarthritis presents with stiffness with inactivity, which is relieved by activity, and pain with activity, which is relieved by rest. The stiffness can be greater in the morning after disuse during sleep but normally resolves within 30 minutes of arising, but the pain is associated with the use of the joints. As the disease advances, there is pain at rest as well, and more joints become involved. There may be joint instability, and **crepitus** may be felt or heard, indicating the deterioration of the joint. The joint enlarges, and range of motion is reduced. The most common locations for OA are the knees, hips, neck (cervical spine), lower back (lumbar spine), fingers, and thumbs (Fig. 18.3).

At this time, OA cannot be "cured" without a joint replacement. Many older people elect to undergo this procedure for hips and knees when the pain becomes unbearable and the effect on function and quality of life becomes severe. The nurse is involved in the preoperative and perioperative periods and during rehabilitation (while the person is learning to use the new joint) and focuses on the treatment of pain.

POLYMYALGIA RHEUMATICA

Polymyalgia rheumatica (PMR) is one of the more common inflammatory diseases seen in older persons. It may occur at the same time as OA, and the two diseases may be difficult to distinguish from each other. The classic presentation of PMR is acute-onset pain beginning in the neck and upper arms and possibly spreading to the pelvic and pectoral girdles. The

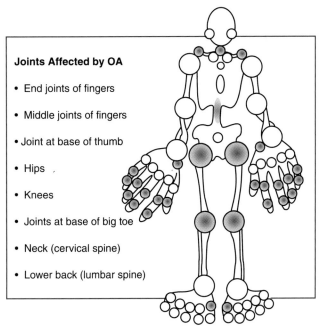

Joints Affected by OA

- End joints of fingers

- Middle joints of fingers

- Joint at base of thumb

- Hips

- Knees

- Joints at base of big toe

- Neck (cervical spine)

- Lower back (lumbar spine)

FIGURE 18.3 Common locations for osteoarthritis. *Source:* The Arthritis Society. (2007). *Osteoarthritis: Know your options.* Retrieved from http://www.arthritis.ca/local/files/pdf%20documents/Types%20of%20 Arthritis/TAS_OA_eBROCH_ENG.pdf.

person may have a low-grade fever and feel fatigued. Pain is usually greatest at night and in the early morning.

This disorder causes stiffness, which occurs especially in the morning and lasts more than 1 hour, as well as severe stiffness and pain in the muscles (rather than the joints) of the neck, shoulders, lower back, buttocks, and thighs. The onset may be sudden or slow. Unlike OA, PMR resolves in 1 to 2 years and necessitates a different treatment. Symptoms may be quickly relieved by small doses of corticosteroids (Dejaco et al., 2011).

PMR rarely occurs in people under the age of 50 years, and women are at higher risk than men (Kermani & Warrington, 2013). It is thought that PMR is the result of the inflammation of blood vessels (Yamashita et al., 2012). Its cause is unknown, but it is thought that genetic factors play a role (Kermani & Warrington, 2013).

RHEUMATOID ARTHRITIS

Rheumatoid arthritis is a chronic, systemic, inflammatory joint disorder. It is considered an autoimmune disease in which products from the inflamed lining of the joint invade and destroy the cartilage and bone within the joint. The cause is unknown. Rheumatoid arthritis affects approximately twice as many women as men—about 1% of the Canadian adult population (330,000 people). It most often starts in midlife, between the ages of 20 and 50 years, although it can occur at any age, including the childhood years (Statistics Canada, 2006).

Rheumatoid arthritis (RA) is characterized by pain and swelling in multiple joints in a symmetrical pattern; for example, both hands will be affected at the same time. It generally affects the small joints of the wrist, knee, ankle, and hand, although it can affect large joints as well. Whereas morning stiffness from OA lasts less than 30 minutes, that from RA lasts much longer. Since RA is a systemic disease, the person may feel generalized fatigue and malaise and have occasional fevers. The joints are warm and tender. Weight loss is common. The natural course of RA is highly variable, with good and bad days. The disease may last a few months or years or may become a chronic condition with progressive damage

Purpose: To determine the relationship between the different forms of arthritis, osteoporosis, and fractures.

Sample: Almost 147,000 women who participated in the Women's Health Initiative supported by the National Institute of Arthritis and Musculoskeletal and Skin Diseases.

Method: A statistical comparison of reports of fractures occurring over an 8-year period.

Results: Those participants who had either osteoarthritis (OA) or rheumatoid arthritis (RA) had significantly more fractures than those who did not have OA or RA. Those with RA had greater risk for all types of fractures, whereas those with OA had a modest overall risk for spine fractures but no increased risk for hip fractures.

Implications for Nursing Practice: The results indicate the importance of effective fall and injury preventive strategies that are particularly geared to persons who already have arthritis.

Source: National Institute of Arthritis and Musculoskeletal and Skin Diseases. (2011). *Spotlight on research: Study further elucidates role of arthritis in fracture risk.* Retrieved from https://www.niams.nih.gov/newsroom/spotlight-on-research/study-further-elucidates-role-arthritis-fracture-risk.

BOX 18.3	Examples of Foods High in Purines

Asparagus
Beef kidneys
Cow, pig, or sheep brains
Sweetbread
Dried beans and peas
Gravy
Herring, mackerel, and sardines
Mushrooms
Scallops

to the joints and increase the risk for fractures (Box 18.2). Risk elements include environmental and genetic factors.

In the past, nonsteroidal anti-inflammatory drugs were used for treatment early in the disease, and the use of RA-specific medications was "saved" for later. However, prompt efforts may halt or slow the damage (Arthritis Society, 2015). Persons diagnosed with RA usually come under a rheumatologist's care, which involves aggressive therapy using disease-modifying antirheumatic drugs (DMARDs), such as methotrexate, sulfasalazine, and cyclosporine (Singh et al., 2012). Biological DMARDs (e.g., Enbrel and Remicade) are the newest class of medications that stimulate or restore the ability of the immune system to fight RA. Ongoing care of the person with RA includes monitoring the progression of the disease and effectiveness of treatment, as well as providing pain relief, comfort, and support. Support groups specifically for persons with RA may help to empower older persons, which in turn may improve their quality of life.

GOUT

Gout is a common form of inflammatory arthritis that appears to result from the accumulation of uric acid crystals in a joint (Arthritis Society, 2016). Uric acid is produced when purines found in food break down.

Gout typically starts with an acute attack. The person complains of exquisite pain in the affected joint, often starting in the middle of the night during sleep. The joint is bright purple—red, hot, and too painful to touch. The proximal joint of the great toe is the most typical site, although the ankle, knee, wrist, or elbow is sometimes involved. The development of gout and the body's response to uric acid accumulation differ from person to person. It is important to note that some people have elevated levels of uric acid and do not get gout, a condition called asymptomatic hyperuricemia.

After an acute attack, gout may become chronic, with periodic acute attacks. Risk factors include high blood pressure, a diet high in purines (Box 18.3), and the following medications: thiazide diuretics, salicylates (e.g., aspirin), and cyclosporines (Singh et al., 2011).

The medical goal after the first acute attack is to prevent another attack, prevent the systemic spread of the disease, and prevent the development of chronic gout. This may be accomplished the patient's avoidance of alcohol and high-purine foods. Medications can be used to either decrease uric acid production (e.g., allopurinol, colchicine) or increase uric acid excretion (e.g., probenecid). Nurses need to ensure that the person takes in enough fluids to help flush the uric acid through the kidneys (2 L per day if not contraindicated).

The nurse's roles include educating the person about the side effects of medications, how to decrease the likelihood of another attack, and care of the joint. In administering medications for treating gout, the nurse will pay close attention to renal function and notify the physician or nurse practitioner of any change, so that the dosage can be adjusted promptly.

IMPLICATIONS FOR GERONTOLOGICAL NURSING AND HEALTHY AGING

ASSESSMENT

When assessing the musculo-skeletal system, the nurse examines the joints and muscles for tenderness, swelling, warmth, and redness. With a person with OA, crepitus is felt or heard in the affected joints. The hands are examined for osteophytes. If osteophytes appear in the distal joints as deformities of the fingers, they are called Heberden's nodes; if in the proximal joints, they are called Bouchard's nodes. The nurse has an important role in evaluating both passive and active range of motion. How far can the person reach, and bend all joints without assistance, and what are the person's reach, flexion, and extension when assisted? The testing of range of motion must go only to the point of discomfort and never to that of inducing pain. The functional ability of the arms is tested by asking the person to touch the back of the head and the midback with both hands. A referral to a physiotherapist might be needed. A pain assessment should always be included.

INTERVENTIONS

The goals of intervention and management of the different forms of arthritis are to obtain treatment as soon as possible for inflammatory conditions, control pain, and minimize disability. Nurses are patients' primary advocates for adequate and prompt treatment, pain control, medication administration, evaluation, and education. (See Chapter 16 for a discussion of the pharmacological treatment of arthritis pain.)

Another pharmacological drug that may be used for pain control is capsaicin cream, made from pepper plants and available over the counter. Capsaicin cream is an effective and safe medication for reducing pain in persons with arthritis (Chhabra et al., 2012). Menthol and aspirin creams are also useful and are preferred by many older people. Pain management and the minimization of disability are interconnected. To minimize disability for persons with OA and RA, the affected joint must be used, strengthened, and protected; the nurse has an important teaching role in this regard.

It cannot be overstated that ongoing physiotherapy is necessary for persons with OA and RA to retain joint use. Nurses and physiotherapists should collaborate in tailoring exercises for the patient. Nurses should assist with range-of-motion activities. Weight loss (if necessary) and muscle building are highly recommended. For severe and disabling pain in the knees and hips from OA, surgical replacement of the joint (arthroplasty) may be highly successful in restoring the person's previous level of functioning. Nearly twice as many women as men have joint replacements. Surgical replacements are recommended for even very old persons in select cases. Outcomes of joint replacement depend on the timing of the surgery, the experience of the surgeon performing this surgery, the nursing care received, the patient's medical status before the surgery, and his or her ability to participate in rehabilitation.

For persons with OA or RA, exercise is the cornerstone of maintaining function and promoting physical functioning post fracture. Regular exercise can improve flexibility and muscle strength, which in turn help to support the affected joints, reduce pain, and reduce falls. Walking, swimming, and water aerobics are preferred by many; the last is often available at seniors' centres, public swimming pools, and YMCAs in many communities.

Attention should also be given to diet, and a referral to a dietitian may be necessary (see Chapter 8). With the reduced activity associated with pain in all forms of arthritis, it is easy for the person to gain weight. Excess weight significantly increases the pressure and wear and tear on the body, leading to less activity and more weight gain. Weight reduction should be considered for all persons who are overweight. The nurse and registered dietitian can work with the person to identify realistic weight and caloric goals and develop meal plans that are personally and culturally acceptable but still balanced and healthy.

The therapeutic use of local heat and cold application in the management of pain in OA and RA patients is well known. The older person's preference is important, but cold usually works best for an acute process—for example, to decrease muscle spasm, decrease swelling, and relieve inflammatory pain. Heat may be applied superficially or deeply. Ultrasound provides deep heat; hot packs, hydrotherapy, and radiant heat provide superficial heat. Liquid paraffin baths for submerging the hands to provide deep heat and temporary relief can be purchased in most pharmacies. A physiotherapist can determine the best course of therapy for each individual.

Devices are available to relieve some of the pressure to the joints and possibly decrease pain and improve balance and function. Canes, crutches, walkers, collars, shoe orthotics, and corsets are such devices that can help persons with of OA or RA. A cane can reduce hip pressure by 60%; a shoe lift can improve lumbar pain. A knee brace is useful, especially in the case of lateral instability. If the hands are affected, the person can avoid carrying packages with the fingers and can use household equipment and utensils that have larger rather than small grips. Not exposing the affected joints to cold temperatures may also help. The person is encouraged to wear leggings, gloves, or scarves as necessary when out of doors. An occupational therapist may be of help in identifying each individual's needs.

COMPLEMENTARY AND ALTERNATIVE INTERVENTIONS FOR OSTEOARTHRITIS

A number of complementary and alternative interventions may provide pain relief for persons with arthritis. Among the most popular are the dietary supplements glucosamine and chondroitin sulphate, along with acupuncture and massage. While glucosamine and chondroitin have been used for some time for self-treatment, research has found that their effect on pain is no better than that of placebos (Fransen et al., 2015).

Increasingly accepted in Canada is the centuries-old Chinese technique of acupuncture—the insertion of very fine needles into the body along what are called "meridians" in locations specific to a problem. Acupuncture can stimulate the natural pain-relieving endorphins produced by the nervous system, thereby temporarily relieving the pain caused by arthritis. Research has confirmed the effectiveness of acupuncture for the treatment of pain in persons with OA (Manyanga et al., 2014). (For information about these and other techniques, see Chapter 16 and the Arthritis Society website (http://www.arthritis.ca).

SUMMARY

Older persons often have to deal with chronic bone and joint problems that affect their mobility, physical and emotional health, and overall quality of life. Gerontological nurses' assessment and interventions are necessary components of the management of these diseases. In caring for the person with osteoarthritis, rheumatoid arthritis, or gout, the nurse focuses on prevention (if possible), early detection, the optimization of mobility and function, and effective pain management. The nurse will use a number of approaches to teach and support the older person and empower the person to participate in achieving the highest level of wellness possible.

KEY CONCEPTS

- Osteoporosis is a crippling problem for many older people, especially women. Although it cannot be prevented, it can be minimized by early interventions, such as exercise, weight bearing exercise, and calcium and vitamin D intake.
- The most serious outcomes of osteoporosis are fractures, which are associated with high mortality.
- Most older people will have some osteoarthritis, even though it may be asymptomatic.
- Rheumatoid arthritis produces swelling, inflammation, intense pain, and distortion of the joints.
- Gout is both an acute and a chronic condition. One of the goals of the treatment of gout is to minimize a future attack.
- Some complementary and alternative interventions are very helpful for individuals with joint disorders and persistent discomfort.

ACTIVITIES AND DISCUSSION QUESTIONS

1. What are the most effective ways of preventing osteoporosis?
2. What lifestyle issues would you discuss with a person with advanced osteoporosis?
3. What are the differences in the appearance of osteoarthritis and rheumatoid arthritis?
4. What advice would you give someone who is experiencing joint pain and limited mobility?
5. Discuss your thoughts and experiences in regard to alternative methods of dealing with chronic pain.

RESOURCES

Arthritis Society
http://www.arthritis.ca

Osteoporosis Canada
http://www.osteoporosis.ca/

Public Health Agency of Canada
https://www.canada.ca/en/public-health.html

Scientific Advisory Council of Osteoporosis in Canada: Clinical practice guidelines
https://www.ncbi.nlm.nih.gov/pmc/articles/PMC2988535/

For additional resources, please visit *http:// evolve.elsevier.com/Canada/Ebersole/gerontological/*

REFERENCES

Arthritis Society. (2015). *Arthritis medications: A reference guide.* Retrieved from http://arthritis.ca/getmedia/dccf0bdc-7ff0-4b3c-aa0c-fd2b36729fff/Arthritis-Medications-A-Reference-Guide-2015.pdf.

Arthritis Society. (2016). *Gout.* Retrieved from https://arthritis.ca/understand-arthritis/types-of-arthritis/gout.

Barnabe, C., Jones, C. A., Bernatsky, S., et al. (2017). Inflammatory arthritis prevalence and health services use in the First Nations and non–First Nations populations of Alberta, Canada. *Arthritis Care & Research, 69*(4), 467–474. doi:10.1002/acr.22959.

Black, D. M., & Rosen, C. J. (2016). Postmenopausal osteoporosis. *The New England Journal of Medicine, 374,* 254–262. doi:10.1056/NEJMcp1513724.

Brown, J. P., & Josse, R. G. (2002). 2002 Clinical practice guidelines for the diagnosis and management of osteoporosis in Canada. *Canadian Medical Association Journal, 167*(10), S1–S34.

Chhabra, N., Aseri, M. L., Goyal, V., et al. (2012). Capsaicin: A promising therapy—A critical reappraisal. *International Journal of Nutrition, Pharmacology, Neurological Disease, 2*(1), 8–15. doi:10.4103/2231-0738.93124.

Dejaco, C., Duftner, C., Cimmino, M. A., et al. (2011). Definition of remission and relapse in polymyalgia rheumatica: Data from a literature search compared with a Delphi-based expert consensus. *Annals of the Rheumatic Diseases, 70*(3), 447–453. doi:10.1136/ard.2010.133850.

Fransen, M., Agaliotis, M., Nairn, L., et al. (2015). Glucosamine and chondroitin for knee osteoarthritis: A double-blind randomised placebo-controlled clinical trial evaluating single and combination regimens. *Annals of the Rheumatic Diseases, 74*(5), 851–858. doi:10.1016/j.joca.2014.02.868.

Gaitonde, D. Y., Rowley, K. D., & Sweeney, L. B. (2012). Hypothyroidism: An update. *South African Family Practice, 54*(5), 384–390. doi:10.1080/20786204.2012.10874256.

Hui, S. S., Xie, Y. J., Woo, J., et al. (2015). Effects of tai chi and walking exercises on weight loss, metabolic syndrome parameters, and bone mineral density: A cluster randomized controlled trial. *Evidence-based Complementary and Alternative Medicine, 2015,* doi:10.1155/2015/976123. (Online: Article ID: 976123).

Kermani, T. A., & Warrington, K. J. (2013). Polymyalgia rheumatica. *The Lancet, 381*(9860), 63–72. doi:10.1016/S0140-6736(12)60680-1.

MacDonald, K. V., Sanmartin, C., Langlois, K., et al. (2015). *Symptom onset, diagnosis and management of osteoarthritis.* Retrieved from http://www.statcan.gc.ca/pub/82-003-x/2014009/article/14087-eng.htm.

Manyanga, T., Froese, M., Zarychanski, R., et al. (2014). Pain management with acupuncture in osteoarthritis: A systematic review and meta-analysis. *BMC Complementary and Alternative Medicine, 14,* 312. doi:10.1186/1472-6882-14-312.

Meier, C., Lamy, O., Krieg, M. A., et al. (2014). The role of teriparatide in sequential and combination therapy of osteoporosis. *Swiss Medical Weekly, 4*(144), w13952. doi:10.4414/smw.2014.

Osteoporosis Canada. (2012a). *Diagnosis: The importance of a comprehensive fracture risk assessment.* Retrieved from http://www.osteoporosis.ca/multimedia/pdf/publications/Diagnosis_EN.pdf.

Osteoporosis Canada. (2012b). *Canadians living with osteoporosis have access to a new treatment option: Provincial governments list Aclasta on public drug plans.* Retrieved from http://www.osteoporosecanada.ca/nouvelles/communiques-de-presse/canadians-living-with-osteoporosis-have-access-to-a-new-treatment-option/.

Osteoporosis Canada. (2017a). *Osteoporosis facts & statistics.* Retrieved from http://www.osteoporosis.ca/osteoporosis-and-you/osteoporosis-facts-and-statistics/.

Osteoporosis Canada. (2017b). *Vitamin D: An important nutrient that protects you against falls and fractures.* Retrieved from http://www.osteoporosis.ca/osteoporosis-and-you/nutrition/vitamin-d/.

Public Health Agency of Canada (PHAC). (2010). *Arthritis.* Retrieved from https://www.canada.ca/en/public-health/services/chronic-diseases/arthritis.html.

Singh, J. A., Furst, D. E., Bharat, A., et al. (2012). 2012 Update of the 2008 American College of Rheumatology recommendations for the use of disease-modifying antirheumatic drugs and biologic agents in the treatment of rheumatoid arthritis. *Arthritis Care & Research, 64*(5), 625–639. doi:10.1002/acr.21641.

Singh, J. A., Reddy, S. G., & Kundukulam, J. (2011). Risk factors for gout and prevention: A systematic review of the literature. *Current Opinion in Rheumatology, 23*(2), 192. doi:10.1097/BOR.0b013e3283438e13.

Statistics Canada (2006). *Rheumatoid arthritis.* Retrieved from http://www.statcan.gc.ca/pub/82-619-m/2006003/4053552-eng.htm.

Weaver, C. M., Alexander, D. D., Boushey, C. J., et al. (2016). Calcium plus vitamin D supplementation and risk of fractures: An updated meta-analysis from the National Osteoporosis Foundation. *Osteoporosis International, 27*(1), 367–376. doi:10.1007/s00198-015-3386-5.

Yamashita, H., Kubota, K., Takahashi, Y., et al. (2012). Whole-body fluorodeoxyglucose positron emission tomography/computed tomography in patients with active polymyalgia rheumatica: Evidence for distinctive bursitis and large-vessel vasculitis. *Modern Rheumatology, 22*(5), 705–711. doi:10.1007/s10165-011-0581-x.

Visual and Auditory Changes

LEARNING OBJECTIVES

Upon completion of this chapter, the reader will be able to:

- Identify and discuss visual and auditory changes that may occur in older persons.
- Describe the importance of assessment, health education, and treatment of eye ailments or disorders to prevent unnecessary vision loss in older persons.
- Increase awareness of the resources available to assist older persons with visual and auditory impairments and changes.

GLOSSARY

Drusen Yellow deposits under the retina, often found in people over the age of 60 years.

Funduscopy Ophthalmoscopic examination of the fundus of the eye.

Keratoconjunctivitis sicca Diminished tear production with age.

Lipofuscin An age-related fatty brown pigment found in the liver, retina, kidneys, adrenals, nerve cells, and heart tissue.

Prelingual deafness Deafness that occurs before the acquisition of spoken language.

Tonometry The procedure used by eye care professionals to determine the intraocular pressure of the eye.

THE LIVED EXPERIENCE

My Eyes Are Failing

For quite a while now, I've been pretending. That I was tired. That the light was bad. But my eyes are really getting worse. I'm afraid to go to the doctor because I'm afraid of what he'll say. Which is silly. Either there is something to be done. Or there is not. If it's glasses, hallelujah, and help me find the money. If it's an operation, see me through. If I am going blind, hold me. Help me put down the terror that rises in my gut at the word. Blind. There. I've said it. The ghost word that has been haunting me. Help me remember, if I have to walk in the dark, that I have had a lot of years of seeing clean and clear. I know the slender shape of a birch tree. I have seen thousands and thousands of things in my life. I can conjure them in my mind's eye. No matter what happens, I shall not be without beautiful sights. It is just that I may have to settle for the ones I have already seen.

Maclay, E. (1977). *Green winter: Celebrations of old age.* **New York, NY: McGraw-Hill. (Copyright 1977, Elise Maclay)**

This chapter discusses illnesses that affect vision and hearing in older persons. Because visual and hearing impairments affect daily activities such as driving, reading, dressing, cooking, and engaging in social activities, it is important to assess the effect of these changes on functional abilities, safety, and quality of life. Nurses need to know about age-related changes in vision and hearing as opposed to losses caused by disease or illness; conduct appropriate assessments; provide health teaching to help prevent or cope with diseases and illnesses that affect vision and hearing; provide appropriate referrals for treatment; and help the older person compensate for sensory losses by supplementing the remaining senses and abilities. The main focus is to augment and maximize sensory experiences when the senses are diminished and to help design a colourful, rewarding environment that fits the needs and abilities of the individual.

See Chapter 6 for a more detailed discussion of age-related changes in vision and hearing; see Chapter 13 for information about the assessment of vision and hearing; see Chapter 3 for a discussion of communication adaptations for older people with vision and hearing loss; and see Chapter 12 for information on safety precautions in the environment.

AGE-RELATED CHANGES IN VISION

It is important to distinguish between normal age changes and vision-related illness when assessing older persons. **Keratoconjunctivitis sicca,** or dry eyes, is a frequent complaint among older people and is due to diminished tear production associated with age. The etiology is unclear, but researchers suspect that there may be age-related changes in the mucin-secreting cells that are necessary for surface wetting, changes in the lacrimal glands, or changes in the meibomian glands that secrete surface oil; all of these changes may occur at the same time. Vitamin A deficiency or certain medications (such as antihistamines, diuretics, beta-blockers, and some sleeping pills) can also cause dry eyes. The condition occurs most commonly in women after menopause. Symptoms include a dry, scratchy feeling in mild cases (xerophthalmia) and discomfort and decreased mucus production in severe cases. The problem is diagnosed by an ophthalmologist using Schirmer's test, in which filter paper strips are placed under the lower eyelid to measure the rate of tear production. Dry eyes are commonly treated with artificial tears; however, the eyes may be too sensitive to tolerate the preservatives in artificial tears. Other management methods include keeping the air in the living environment moist with humidifiers, avoiding wind and the use of hair dryers, and using artificial tear ointments at bedtime.

DISEASES AFFECTING VISION

Several diseases can affect the vision of the older population and result in blindness. An estimated one in nine Canadians over the age of 65 years will develop irreversible vision loss, as will one in four of those aged 75 years or older (The National Coalition for Vision Health, 2011).

A diagnosis of blindness does not equate to complete vision loss. The person may have some retained vision, and the nurse should be mindful and respectful of this. For older people with visual impairment, the consequences for functional ability, safety, and quality of life can be profound. Therefore, it is important to identify older persons who have visual impairment and to provide appropriate assessment and treatment. Certain signs and behaviours that may indicate visual problems should prompt the nurse to action (Box 19.1).

The major diseases affecting the vision of older persons are glaucoma, cataracts, diabetic retinopathy, and macular degeneration.

GLAUCOMA

Glaucoma is a major public health problem. It is estimated that more than 250,000 Canadians are living with glaucoma (Canadian National Institute for the Blind [CNIB], 2017a). The etiology of glaucoma is variable and often unknown. However, the progression of glaucoma indicates a process by which the natural fluids of the eye are blocked by ciliary muscle rigidity, causing a gradual build-up of intraocular pressure (IOP) and damage to the optic nerve.

Normal IOP is between 12 mm Hg and 22 mm Hg (Glaucoma Research Society of Canada, n.d.). Age, diabetes, steroid use, past eye injuries, and a family history of glaucoma are risk factors for the development of glaucoma. Age is the single most important

BOX 19.1 Signs and Behaviours That May Indicate Vision Problems

Reported by Individuals

Squinting, greater sensitivity to light, or both

Choosing bright-coloured over dull-coloured objects or clothing

Misjudging where items are, resulting in spills

Having difficulty copying written texts

Having difficulty threading a needle or buttoning a shirt

Seeing flashes of light or rapid movement from the corners of the eyes

Having difficulties with driving at night

Experiencing uncontrolled eye movement

Making driving mistakes, such as missing street or traffic signs

Falling because of a missed step or an unseen object on the floor

Noticed by Health Care Providers

Mis-stepping

Mis-sitting

Walking into objects

Changes in ability to perform activities of daily living (e.g., brushing teeth)

Sources: Adapted from Health Canada. (2017). *Seniors and aging— vision care.* Retrieved from http://www.hc-sc.gc.ca/hl-vs/iyh-vsv/life-vie/ seniors-aines_vc-sv-eng.php#sy; Kumar Dev, M., Paudel, N., Dev Joshi, N., et al. (2013). Impact of visual impairment on vision-specific quality of life among older persons living in nursing home. *Current Eye Research, 39*(3), 232–238. doi:10.3109/022713683.2013.838.973

predictor, and older women are affected twice as frequently as older men are. People of African, Asian, or Latin American ancestry have an increased risk of developing glaucoma (Glaucoma Research Society of Canada, n.d.).

Among the several types of glaucoma are primary open-angle glaucoma, acute angle-closure glaucoma, and low-tension or normal-tension glaucoma. Glaucoma can be bilateral but occurs more commonly in only one eye.

Primary open-angle glaucoma accounts for about 80% of glaucoma cases. It is asymptomatic until very late in the disease, when there is noticeable loss in vision fields. This vision loss is irreversible; however, if detected early, glaucoma can be treated and blindness or severe vision loss can be prevented (CNIB, 2017a). Signs of open-angle glaucoma include headaches, poor vision in dim lighting, increased sensitivity to

glare, "tired eyes," impaired peripheral vision, a fixed and dilated pupil, and frequent changes in prescriptions for corrective lenses (Miller, 2008). Fig. 19.1B illustrates the effects of glaucoma on vision.

Acute angle-closure glaucoma is characterized by a rapid rise in IOP, accompanied by redness and acute pain in and around the eye, severe headache, nausea and vomiting, and blurred vision. These symptoms occur when the path of the aqueous humour (the thick, watery substance filling the space between the lens and the cornea) is blocked and the IOP builds up to more than 50 mm Hg. If the disease is untreated, blindness can occur within 2 days. Iridectomy, the surgical removal of part of the iris, can ease pressure. Risk factors for acute angle-closure glaucoma include female sex, increased age, Inuit or Asian ethnicity, a shallow anterior chamber, and shorter axial length (Marchini et al., 2015; Harasymowycz et al., 2016). Many medications with anticholinergic properties, such as antihistamines, stimulants, vasodilators, clonidine, and sympathomimetics, are particularly dangerous for patients who are predisposed to angle-closure glaucoma. Older people with glaucoma should be counselled to review all medications (both over-the-counter and prescribed) with their primary care provider.

Low-tension or normal-tension glaucoma is a third type of glaucoma occurring in older persons. In this type of glaucoma, the IOP is within normal range (12–22 mm Hg), but there is damage to the optic nerve and a narrowing of the visual fields. The cause of this type of glaucoma is unknown, but its risk factors include a family history of any kind of glaucoma, Japanese ancestry, and cardiovascular disease. Management consists of the same medications and surgical interventions that are used to manage chronic glaucoma (Glaucoma Research Foundation, 2011).

Assessment

When caring for an older person in hospital or in a long-term care setting, the nurse must obtain a medical history to determine if the person has glaucoma and to ensure that eye drops are given according to the person's treatment regimen. Without the eye drops, eye pressure can rise and cause an acute exacerbation of glaucoma (Boltz et al., 2016). Persons over the age of 65 years need annual eye examinations, and

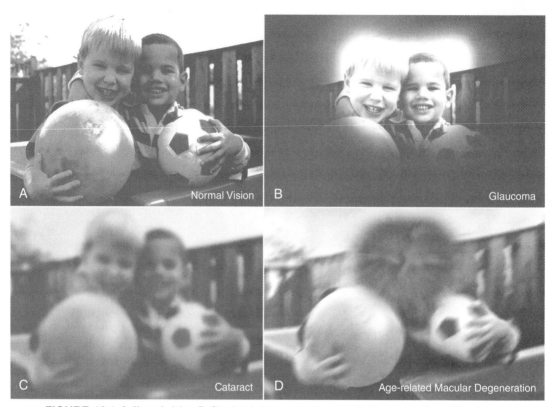

FIGURE 19.1 A, Normal vision. B, Simulated vision with glaucoma. C, Simulated vision with cataracts. D, Simulated vision with age-related macular degeneration (AMD). *Source:* National Eye Institute. (2012). *Age-related macular degeneration.* Retrieved from https://nei.nih.gov/photo/amd.

those with medication-controlled glaucoma should schedule follow-up appointments every 6 months. Annual screening is also recommended for persons of African, Asian, or Latin American ancestry, as well as persons who are older than 40 years and have a family history of glaucoma (Glaucoma Research Society of Canada, n.d.). The examination consists of a dilated-eye examination and **tonometry,** a procedure that measures IOP. These procedures can be performed by an optometrist, who will then refer the person to an ophthalmologist if glaucoma is suspected. Most provinces and territories cover the cost of annual eye examinations for older persons (Unite for Sight, 2015).

Interventions

Glaucoma is managed with medications (i.e., oral medications or topical eye drops), laser surgery, or both. Eye drops and oral medications lower the IOP

either by decreasing the amount of aqueous fluid produced within the eye or by improving the flow through the drainage angle.

Beta-blockers are the first-line therapy for glaucoma, and some people need combinations of several types of eye drops. Usually, medications can control glaucoma, but laser surgery (trabeculoplasty) may be recommended for some types of glaucoma. Surgery is usually recommended to prevent further damage to the optic nerve.

Some nonpharmacological or nonsurgical interventions that might be helpful for all types of vision loss are illumination, glare control, appropriate levels of magnification, and the use of colour contrast to identify or find objects.

CATARACTS

A second major disease affecting the vision of older persons is cataracts, which are caused by oxidative damage to the lens protein and by fatty deposits **(lipofuscin)** in the ocular lens. Cataracts are a prevalent disorder among older persons; more than 2.5 million Canadians are living with cataracts (http://www.cnib.ca).

The most common causes of cataracts are heredity and advanced age. Cataracts may occur more frequently and at an earlier age in individuals who have been exposed to excessive sunlight or who have poor dietary habits, diabetes, hypertension, kidney disease, previous eye trauma, or a history of alcohol and tobacco use. Cataracts are also more likely to occur after surgery for glaucoma and after other types of eye surgery. There is evidence that a high dietary intake of lutein and zeaxanthin (compounds found in yellow or dark leafy vegetables), as well as vitamin C, vitamin E, copper, and zinc from food and supplements, lowers the risk for cataracts (McCusker et al., 2016).

Assessment

Cataracts are recognized by the clouding of the ordinarily clear ocular lens. The principal symptom of cataracts is the appearance of halos around objects. Other common symptoms include blurring, decreased perception of light and colour (giving a yellow tint to most things), and sensitivity to glare. Fig. 19.1C illustrates the effects of a cataract on vision.

When lens opacity reduces visual acuity to 20/30 or less in the central axis of vision, the vision impairment is considered a cataract. Cataracts are categorized according to their location within the lens and are usually bilateral.

Interventions

When visual acuity decreases to 20/50 and the cataract affects the person's safety or quality of life, surgery is recommended (Casparis et al., 2017). Cataract surgery is the most commonly performed surgical procedure in developed countries. Most often, cataract surgery involves only local anaesthesia on an outpatient basis, and 95% of patients report excellent vision after surgery. The surgery involves the removal of the lens and the placement of a plastic intraocular lens. If the person has bilateral cataracts, surgery is performed on one eye first; surgery on the other eye is performed at least a month later to ensure healing (Gothwal et al., 2011). Persons who have cataracts or

have had recent cataract surgery or trauma can have a detached retina; in some cases, the detachment occurs spontaneously. A detached retina manifests as a curtain coming down over the person's line of vision. It necessitates immediate emergency treatment.

Nursing interventions when caring for the person who will be undergoing cataract surgery include teaching and preparing the person for significant changes in vision and adaptation to light, discussing realistic postsurgical expectations, and rigorously assessing potential postsurgery delirium. Postsurgical teaching includes teaching the patient to avoid heavy lifting, straining, and bending at the waist. Eye drops may be prescribed to aid healing and prevent infection.

MACULAR DEGENERATION

Age-related macular degeneration (AMD) is a degenerative eye disease that affects the macula, the central part of the eye responsible for clear central vision. The disease causes a progressive loss of central vision, leaving only peripheral vision intact. It usually starts in one eye but may affect the other eye later on (National Eye Institute, 2015). There are few symptoms in the early stages of AMD, and intermediate AMD may cause some vision loss (National Eye Institute, 2015). Therefore, it is important for adults to have their eyes examined regularly. Fig. 19.1D illustrates the effects of AMD on vision.

Two million Canadians are affected by AMD; the majority are over the age of 50 years (Devenyi et al., 2016). The prevalence of AMD increases drastically with age, and its incidence is higher among women. Other nonmodifiable risk factors include genetic factors; the risk of developing AMD is greater if an immediate family member has the disease, and White persons are at higher risk than are others (National Eye Institute, 2015). As the number of older persons affected is projected to increase over the next 20 years, AMD is considered a growing epidemic (Devenyi et al., 2016).

Although its etiology is unknown, AMD results from systemic changes in circulation, an accumulation of cellular waste products, tissue atrophy, and the growth of abnormal blood vessels in the choroid layer beneath the retina. Fibrous scarring disrupts the nourishment of photoreceptor cells, causing the death

BOX 19.2	Stages of Dry Age-Related Macular Degeneration

1. Early age-related macular degeneration (AMD): Several small drusen or a few medium-sized drusen; no symptoms; no vision loss
2. Intermediate AMD: Several medium-sized drusen, or one or more large drusen; blurred spot in the centre of vision; more light required for reading and other tasks
3. Advanced AMD: In addition to drusen, a breakdown of light-sensitive cells and supporting tissues in the central retinal area; expanding blurred spot in the centre of vision; difficulty reading or recognizing faces until they are very close

Source: National Eye Institute. (2014). *Facts about age-related macular degeneration.* Retrieved from https://nei.nih.gov/health/maculardegen/armd_facts.

of the cells and the loss of central vision. Risk factors include genetic predisposition, smoking, obesity, family history, and excessive exposure to sunlight.

There are two forms of macular degeneration: dry AMD and wet AMD. Dry AMD accounts for 85 to 90% of all cases of AMD. This type of AMD has three stages, which may occur in one or both eyes (Box 19.2). Dry AMD occurs when the light-sensitive cells in the macula slowly break down and cause blurring in the central vision of the affected eye. As dry AMD gets worse, the person may see a blurred spot in the centre of vision. One of the most common early signs of dry AMD is the presence of **drusen,** yellow deposits under the retina that are often found in people over the age of 60 years. The relationship between drusen and AMD is not clear, but an increase in the size or number of drusen increases the risk of developing advanced or wet AMD (National Eye Institute, 2015).

Wet AMD occurs when abnormal blood vessels begin to grow under the macula and leak fluid or blood, which raises the macula from its normal place at the back of the eye. When the fluid or blood begins to accumulate in the macula, light-sensing cone cells degenerate and die. Damage to the macula occurs rapidly, sometimes within months, resulting in blurred or even lost central vision. Peripheral vision usually remains normal, but the person will have difficulty seeing at a distance or doing detailed work such as sewing or reading. Faces may begin to blur, and it becomes harder to distinguish colours. An early sign

may be distortion that causes edges or lines to appear wavy.

Assessment

There is no cure for AMD, and treatment options are limited to slowing the progression of the disease. Therefore, the focus is on screening, early detection, and prevention. People in the early stage of dry AMD may attribute their vision problems to normal aging or to cataracts. Early diagnosis is the key, and individuals over the age of 40 years should have an eye examination at least every 2 years.

People diagnosed with AMD should check their eyes daily, using an Amsler grid (Canadian National Institute for the Blind [CNIB], 2017b). The Amsler grid is used to determine the clarity of central vision (Fig. 19.2). The perception of wavy lines is diagnostic of a beginning macular degeneration.

The National Eye Institute Age-Related Eye Disease Study (http://www.nei.nih.gov) found that a high-dose formulation of antioxidants and zinc significantly reduced the risk of advanced AMD and associated vision loss. Individuals with intermediate AMD in one or both eyes or with advanced wet AMD in one eye but not the other should consider taking the National Eye Institute's formulation (Box 19.3) (National Eye Institute, 2015). Because of some toxicity risks, these supplements are initiated by a physician or a nurse practitioner, and people cannot start these on their own as a preventive measure.

Interventions

Treatment of wet AMD includes photodynamic therapy and laser photocoagulation. The most common medications for the treatment of advanced AMD include Lucentis and Avastin, both of which prevent vascular endothelial growth factor (VEGF) from binding to its receptors. The binding of VEGF to its receptors results in cell proliferation and increased vascularization, including vascular leakage, which contribute to the progression of AMD.

Abnormally high levels of a specific growth factor occur in eyes with wet AMD, promoting the growth of abnormal blood vessels. Anti-VEGF therapy blocks the effect of the growth factor. These medications are injected into the eye as often as once a month and can help slow vision loss from AMD and improve sight

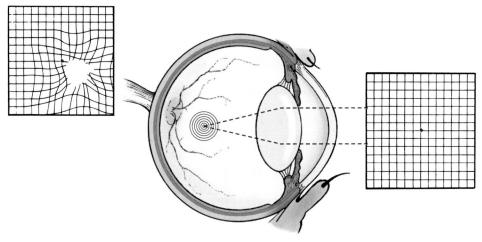

FIGURE 19.2 Macular degeneration: distortion of centre vision; normal peripheral vision. Illustration by Harriet R. Greenfield, Newton, MA.

BOX 19.3 Age-Related Eye Disease Study (AREDS) Recommended Formulation

- Vitamin C 500 mg
- Vitamin E 400 IU
- Beta-carotene 15 mg (often labelled as equivalent to vitamin A 25,000 IU)
- Zinc oxide 80 mg
- Copper (cupric oxide) 2 mg

Sources: National Eye Institute. (2015). *Facts about age-related macular degeneration.* Retrieved from https://nei.nih.gov/health/maculardegen/armd_facts; The Age-Related Eye Disease Study Research Group. (2001). A randomized placebo-controlled, clinical trial of high-dose supplementation with vitamins C and E, beta carotene, and zinc for age-related macular degeneration and vision loss. *Archives of Ophthalmology, 119*(10), 1417–1436.

---

in some cases. Other treatments being researched are gene therapy, stem cell therapy, and retinal transplantation (Solinis et al., 2015; Olmos et al., 2015; Marazova & Sahel, 2016).

DIABETIC RETINOPATHY

The deleterious effects of elevated blood sugar due to diabetes can cause a visual impairment called diabetic retinopathy. Diabetic retinopathy is a disease of the retinal microvasculature and is characterized by increased vessel permeability. Blood and lipid leakage leads to macular edema and hard exudates (composed

of lipids). Because of the vascular and cellular changes accompanying diabetes, other pathological vision conditions often worsen rapidly.

Diabetic retinopathy is the third leading cause of blindness in Canada, following macular degeneration and glaucoma. Approximately 500,000 Canadians live with diabetic retinopathy (Canadian National Institute for the Blind [CNIB], 2017c). Most diabetic patients develop diabetic retinopathy within 20 years of diagnosis.

Assessment

There is little to no evidence of retinopathy until 3 to 5 years or more after the onset of diabetes. Early signs, which include microaneurysms, flame-shaped hemorrhages, cotton wool spots, hard exudates, and dilated capillaries, can be seen through **funduscopy.** Annual dilated funduscopic examination of the eye, beginning 5 years after diagnosis of type 1 diabetes and at the time of the diagnosis of type 2 diabetes, is recommended.

Interventions

Continuous, strict control of blood glucose, cholesterol, blood pressure, and laser photocoagulation treatments can halt the progression of the disease (Ham et al., 2007). Laser treatment can reduce vision loss in 50% of patients, and recent evidence indicates that treatment with various drugs may deliver a better outcome (U.S. Department of Health and Human Services [USDHHS], 2012).

AUDITORY IMPAIRMENT AND LOSS

Hearing impairments can have severe consequences for an older person's quality of life, well-being, and socialization, and may even be perceived as a social stigma. Two common auditory impairments that nurses caring for older people will need to take into consideration are tinnitus and prelingual deafness. (See Chapter 3 for a discussion of presbycusis, a form of sensorineural hearing loss related to aging.)

TINNITUS

Tinnitus is the perception of sound in the absence of acoustic stimuli. It is characterized by ringing in the ear and may also manifest as buzzing; hissing; whistling; cricketlike chirping; bell sounds; and roaring, clicking, pulsating, humming, or swishing sounds. The sounds may be constant or intermittent and are more acute at night or in quiet surroundings. The most common type of tinnitus is high pitched with sensorineural loss; the root cause lies in the vestibulo-cochlear nerve, the inner ear, or the central processing centres of the brain. A less common type of tinnitus is low pitched and is associated with conduction loss—that is, loss of sound conductivity through the small, bony structures in the ear.

Tinnitus generally increases over time. It affects many older people and can interfere with hearing, as well as become extremely irritating. Tinnitus affects 10 to 15% of the population (Canadian Hearing Society [CHS], 2013). Of those affected with tinnitus, 5% of the population report that the tinnitus affects the carrying out of daily activities (CHS, 2013). The incidence of tinnitus peaks between the ages of 65 and 74 years and is higher in men than in women. (In men, the incidence seems to decrease after this period of age.) Tinnitus can be caused by loud noises, excessive cerumen (earwax) or other obstructions of the auditory canal, disorders of the cervical vertebrae or the temporomandibular joint, allergies, an underactive thyroid, cardiovascular disease, tumours, conductive hearing loss, anxiety, depression, degeneration of the bones in the middle ear, infections, and trauma to the head or ear. In addition, more than 200 prescription and nonprescription medications list tinnitus as a potential side effect. (Aspirin is the most common of these medications.)

Assessment

Tinnitus may be subjective (i.e., audible only to the affected person) or objective (i.e., audible to the examiner as well). The Tinnitus Handicap Questionnaire developed by Newman, Wharton, and Jacobsen (1995) measures the physical, emotional, and social consequences of tinnitus. It also can be used to assess the changes the individual experiences with treatment. The Tinnitus Functional Index is another measure of the effects of tinnitus (Henry et al., 2016). The cause of tinnitus in some persons is never found. For some persons, the problem may arbitrarily disappear.

Interventions

Hearing aids can be prescribed to amplify environmental sounds to obscure tinnitus, and there is a device that combines the features of a masker and a hearing aid and emits a competitive but pleasant sound that distracts from head noise. Some of the therapeutic modes of treating tinnitus are transtympanal electrostimulation, iontophoresis (use of a small electric charge to deliver local anaesthesia through the skin), biofeedback, tinnitus masking with alternative sound production (i.e., "white noise"), dental treatment, cochlear implants, and hearing aids. Hypnosis, acupuncture, and chiropractic, naturopathic, allergy, or medication treatment are effective for some people.

Nursing actions include having discussions with the person about times when the noises are most irritating and having the person keep a diary to identify patterns. There is some evidence that caffeine, alcohol, cigarettes, stress, and fatigue may exacerbate the problem. The nurse assesses medications for possibly contributing to the problem and discusses lifestyle changes and alternative methods that are effective.

PRELINGUAL DEAFNESS

Prelingual deafness in older persons is rarely addressed, because it is assumed that individuals who have been deaf since childhood learned to communicate early in life through the use of hearing aids and sometimes sign language. Until 50 years ago, deaf children were commonly placed in a school for the deaf to develop within a culture of their own; hence, many older people with prelingual deafness will have had an entirely different childhood from those with normal hearing. Persons with prelingual deafness often learn audible speech, sign language, or both, as well as lip reading. However, their reading and writing skills may be impaired even though their intelligence is normal. For those who depend on visual cues, communication can also be compromised when vision changes occur. Often, older persons with prelingual deafness use signing as their first language and English as their second. Subtleties of verbal communication may be lost to them, although they often compensate and become extremely alert to nonverbal cues and feelings. At times, a certified and experienced interpreter will be needed.

IMPLICATIONS FOR GERONTOLOGICAL NURSING AND HEALTHY AGING

The older person whose vision or hearing is impaired is deprived of major sensory input, which has a direct effect on everyday life. Sensory losses can lead to potential isolation, depression, withdrawal, and loss of self-esteem; raise personal safety issues; affect health; and (in some cases) influence the risk for or the experience of delirium. Nurses should take a leadership role in education related to visual and auditory diseases. To promote healthy aging and quality of life, gerontological nurses must be knowledgeable about regular screening for vision and auditory function, the impact of hearing and vision changes on the functional abilities and quality of life of older persons, vision and hearing assessment, prevention and treatment of diseases affecting vision and hearing, effective communication techniques, and ways to help the older person adapt to these losses and compensate for them.

In the assessment of vision and hearing losses, it is important that the nurse include the impact of losses on functional ability, mood, and quality of life. A recent study found that depression frequently develops within a few months after AMD is diagnosed in both eyes. A study reviewing problem-solving skills found that problem-solving interventions on emotional distress improved vision-related functioning;

yet, no improvements were noted in depressive symptoms (Holloway et al., 2015). The problem-solving sessions, led by a nurse or counselor in the patient's home, focused on identifying problems caused by loss of eyesight and on finding ways to compensate.

It is important that the nurse be considerate of potential vision or hearing loss when working with older persons. Care must be adapted to the person's needs, and environmental changes need to ensure the highest possible safety for the older person (see Chapter 6). Especially in a health care setting where the environment is unfamiliar and constantly changing, close attention to environmental safety and the person's mobility is warranted. Ensuring that individuals with vision impairment have access to visual aids (i.e., appropriate eyeglasses, books on tape, or a variety of devices available through the Canadian National Institute for the Blind) and that persons with hearing impairment have access to their hearing aids will promote independence and social engagement.

SUMMARY

Hearing and vision impairments can contribute to challenges at all levels of the hierarchy of needs, from biological integrity needs (such as activity, safety, and security) to higher-level needs (such as self-esteem, self-actualization, and a sense of belonging). These impairments severely affect the person's quality of life. They also predispose the person to having negative health and quality-of-life outcomes. Whatever the person's age or impairments, both the task of aging and the continued growth and development toward self-actualization require interactions and environments in which the older person is assured that basic needs are being met, compensations for losses are being made, and meaningful and satisfying experiences will continue to be part of life.

KEY CONCEPTS

- Vision and hearing impairment can significantly affect the functional ability, safety, and quality of life of older persons.
- Vision loss from an eye disease is a global concern; the screening, prevention, and treatment of eye

diseases are important priorities for nurses and other health care providers.

- The major diseases and disorders that affect vision are glaucoma, macular degeneration, diabetic retinopathy, and the presence of cataracts, all of which can be identified through proper screening and appropriately treated. All persons over the age of 65 years should have annual eye examinations.
- Hearing impairment often has severe consequences for a person's quality of life and socialization.
- Tinnitus is a common condition among older people and can interfere with hearing and become extremely irritating. It is characterized by ringing in the ear and may also manifest itself by buzzing, hissing, whistling, clicking, pulsating, or swishing sounds.
- To promote healthy aging and a good quality of life, nurses must be knowledgeable about the following: the impact of hearing and vision changes on the functional abilities and quality of life of older persons, vision and hearing assessment, the prevention and treatment of diseases that affect vision and hearing, effective communication techniques, and ways to help persons adapt to and compensate for these changes and losses.

ACTIVITIES AND DISCUSSION QUESTIONS

1. How can nurses enhance awareness and education in regard to vision and hearing disorders?
2. What is the role of a nurse in community, acute care, or residential care settings in screening for and assessing eye and ear diseases?
3. Develop a teaching plan for an older person with glaucoma.
4. What type of resources could a nurse in any setting offer to an older person with vision or hearing loss?
5. Develop a plan of care for an older person with diabetic retinopathy.
6. What are your local community resources for supporting older persons with low vision or hearing impairment?
7. What hearing and vision adaptive supports can be found on the Internet and used for free?

RESOURCES

Canadian National Institute for the Blind (CNIB). EyeSimulator
http://www.cnib.ca/en/your-eyes/eye-conditions/eye-connect/Pages/EyeSimulator.aspx

Canadian Ophthalmological Society
http://www.cos-sco.ca

Eye care coverage in Newfoundland and Labrador
http://www.health.gov.nl.ca/health/mcp/healthplancoverage.html

Eye care coverage in Ontario
http://www.health.gov.on.ca/en/public/publications/ohip/eyecare.aspx

Eye care coverage in Quebec
http://www4.gouv.qc.ca/EN/Portail/Citoyens/Evenements/aines/Pages/services-optometriques-couverts.aspx

Health care coverage in Manitoba
http://www.gov.mb.ca/health/mhsip/

Health-related services in Saskatchewan
https://www.saskatchewan.ca/residents/health/accessing-health-care-services

Health services in Alberta
http://www.albertahealthservices.ca/default.aspx

Healthy Aging and Wellness Working Group. *Healthy aging in Canada: A new vision, a vital investment from evidence to action*
http://www.health.gov.bc.ca/library/publications/year/2006/Healthy_Aging_A_Vital_latest_copy_October_2006.pdf

Medical and health benefits in British Columbia
http://www2.gov.bc.ca/gov/content/health/health-drug-coverage/msp

New Brunswick Provincial Health Plan
http://ucm.greatwestlife.com/web5/groups/group/@public/documents/web_content/s6_000282.pdf

Simulation of glaucoma, cataracts, macular degeneration, and diabetic retinopathy
http://vision-simulator.tripod.com/screenshots.html

Unite for Sight. (2015). *Eye care policy in Canada*
http://www.uniteforsight.org/eye-care-policy/module2

World Health Organization. (2007). *Vision 2020: The Right to sight: Global initiative for the elimination of avoidable blindness* http://www.who.int/blindness/Vision2020_report.pdf

For additional resources, please visit *http://evolve.elsevier.com/Canada/Ebersole/gerontological/*

REFERENCES

Boltz, M., Capezuti, E., Fulmer, T. T., et al. (2016). *Evidence-based geriatric nursing protocols for best practice* (5th ed.). New York, NY: Springer.

Canadian Hearing Society (CHS). (2013). *Tinnitus and hyperacusis.* Retrieved from http://www.chs.ca/tinnitus-and-hyperacusis.

Canadian National Institute for the Blind (CNIB). (2017a). *Glaucoma.* Retrieved from http://www.cnib.ca/en/your-eyes/eye-conditions/Glaucoma/Pages/default.aspx.

Canadian National Institute for the Blind (CNIB). (2017b). *Check your vision: The Amsler grid.* Retrieved from http://www.cnib.ca/en/your-eyes/eye-conditions/amd/diagnosing/amsler-grid/Pages/default.aspx.

Canadian National Institute for the Blind (CNIB). (2017c). *Eye connect: Diabetic retinopathy.* Retrieved from http://www.cnib.ca/en/your-eyes/eye-conditions/eye-connect/DR/Pages/default.aspx.

Casparis, H., Lindsley, K., Kuo, I. C., et al. (2017). Surgery for cataracts in people with age-related macular degeneration. *The Cochrane Database of Systematic Reviews*, 13(6), CD006757. doi:10.1002/14651858.CD006757.pub3.

Devenyi, R., Maberley, D., Sheidow, T. G., et al. (2016). Real-world utilization of ranibizumab in wet age-related macular degeneration patients from Canada. *Canadian Journal of Opthalmology*, 51(2), 55–57. doi:10.1016/j.jcjo.2015.11.008.

Glaucoma Research Foundation. (2011). *Are you at risk for glaucoma?* Retrieved from http://www.glaucoma.org/glaucoma/are-you-at-risk-for-glaucoma.php.

Glaucoma Research Society of Canada. (n.d.). *Learning about glaucoma.* Retrieved from http://www.glaucomaresearch.ca/en/about/about_glaucoma.shtml.

Gothwal, V. K., Wright, T. A., Lamoureux, E. L., et al. (2011). Improvements in visual ability with first-eye, second-eye, and bilateral cataract surgery measured with the visual symptoms and quality of life questionnaire. *Journal of Cataract & Refractive Surgery*, 37(7), 1208–1216. doi:10.1016/j.jcrs.2011.01.028.

Ham, R., Sloane, P., & Warshaw, G. (2007). *Primary care geriatrics* (5th ed.). St Louis: Mosby.

Harasymowycz, P., Birt, C., Gooi, P., et al. (2016). Medical management of glaucoma in the 21st century from a Canadian perspective. *Journal of Ophthalmology (2016)*, (Online: Article ID 6509809.). doi:10.1155/2016/6509809.

Henry, J. A., Griest, S., Thielman, E., et al. (2016). Tinnitus functional index: Development, validation, outcome research, and clinical application. *Hearing Research*, 334, 58–64. doi:10.1016/j.heares.2015.06.004.

Holloway, E. E., Xie, J., Sturrock, B. A., et al. (2015). Do problem-solving interventions improve psychosocial outcomes in vision impaired adults: A systematic review and meta-analysis. *Patient Education and Counseling*, 98(5), 553–564. doi:10.1016/j.pec.2015.01.013.

Maclay, E. (1977). *Green winter: Celebrations of old age.* New York: McGraw-Hill.

Marazova, K., & Sahel, J. A. (2016). Macular dystrophies: management and interventions. In *Macular dystrophies* (pp. 101–116) (e-book). Switzerland: Springer International Publishing. doi:10.107/978-3-319-26621-3_11.

Marchini, G., Chemello, F., Berzaghi, D., et al. (2015). Chapter 10: New findings in the diagnosis and treatment of primary angle-closure glaucoma. *Progress in Brain Research*, 221, 191–212. doi:10.1016/bs.pbr.2015.05.001.

McCusker, M. M., Durrani, K., Payette, M. J., et al. (2016). An eye on nutrition: The role of vitamins, essential fatty acids, and antioxidants in age-related macular degeneration, dry eye syndrome, and cataract. *Clinics in Dermatology*, 34(2), 276–285. doi:10.1016/j.clindermatol.2015.11.009.

Miller, C. (2008). *Nursing for wellness in older adults* (5th ed.). Philadelphia: Wolters Kluwer/Lippincott Williams & Wilkins.

National Eye Institute. (2015). *Age-related macular degeneration.* Retrieved from https://nei.nih.gov/health/maculardegen/armd_facts.

Newman, C. W., Wharton, J. A., & Jacobsen, G. P. (1995). Retest stability of the tinnitus handicap questionnaire. *Annals of Otology, Rhinology, & Laryngology*, 104(9 Pt. 1), 718–723. doi:10.1177/000348949510400910.

Olmos, L. C., Nazari, H., Rodger, D. C., et al. (2015). Stem cell therapy for the treatment of macular degeneration. *Current Opthalmology Reports*, 3(1), 16–25. doi:10.1007/s40135-014-0058-0.

Solinis, M. A., Pozo-Rodriguez, A., Apaolaza, P. S., et al. (2015). Treatment of ocular disorders by gene therapy. *European Journal of Pharmaceutics and Biopharmaceutics*, 95(B), 331–342. doi:10.1016/j.ejpb.2014.12.022.

The National Coalition for Vision Health. (2011). *Vision loss in Canada.* Retrieved from http://www.cos-sco.ca/wp-content/uploads/2012/09/VisionLossinCanada_e.pdf.

Unite for Sight. (2015). *Eye care policy in Canada.* Retrieved from http://www.uniteforsight.org/eye-care-policy/module2.

U.S. Department of Health and Human Services [USDHHS]. (2012). *Healthy people 2020.* Retrieved from http://www.healthypeople.gov/2020/default.aspx.

LEARNING OBJECTIVES

Upon completion of this chapter, the reader will be able to:

- Identify common types of cardio-vascular and respiratory diseases occurring in later life.
- Discuss assessment of and intervention for cardio-vascular and respiratory diseases in the older population.
- Suggest ways to prevent cardio-vascular and respiratory diseases to the extent possible.
- Differentiate infectious, obstructive, and restrictive lung disease.
- Discuss the signs and symptoms of pneumonia and influenza.
- Develop a tuberculosis surveillance plan for a long-term care home.

GLOSSARY

Arterio-sclerosis Thickening and loss of elasticity of the arterial wall.

Comorbid Pertaining to a disease or other pathological process that occurs simultaneously with another.

Dyspnea The subjective report of shortness of breath.

Health care–associated infection An infection whose source is related to a particular setting or treatment.

Morbidity Disability as the result of a health condition.

Mortality Death as a result of a health condition or event.

THE LIVED EXPERIENCE

When I first had that heart attack, I was so frightened it seemed I would die just from the fear. It was the first time I realized how comforting, calm, and efficient nurses could be.

Jerry, age 63 years

When Dad had that heart attack, it really scared us all, and I know we were afraid we would say or do something that would bring on another. I think he was also afraid of everything. I'm so grateful for the nurses at the hospital. They seem to give him lots of attention and information about the things he needs to know. He seems quite relaxed with himself now.

Ruth, Jerry's youngest daughter

Caring for older persons means caring for persons with cardio-vascular disease (CVD), respiratory problems, or both. These two systems are interconnected. When the nurse is helping a patient with a cardiac problem, such as heart failure, the patient's respiratory system must be assessed as well; for example, pneumonia may trigger heart failure. Conversely, a patient who has a problem with the respiratory system can experience some consequences at a cardiac level. Therefore, nursing interventions frequently overlap. One carefully planned action can address several systems at the same time and achieve goals of homeostasis, energy conservation, and meeting basic physiological needs, and therefore reducing **mortality** and **morbidity.**

CARDIO-VASCULAR DISORDERS

Although the number of deaths from heart disease has decreased, heart disease remains the leading cause of death in Canada (Public Health Agency of Canada, 2015) (see Fig. 15.1). The rate of deaths per 100,000 persons increases dramatically with age, owing to a combination of normal changes with aging (see Chapter 6) and the presence of risk factors (Box 20.1). Older persons also undergo the majority of cardio-vascular–related procedures, but treatment approaches are highly variable by ethnicity and sex.

The Public Health Agency of Canada (2010) defines cardio-vascular disease as a disease that affects the circulatory system, including the heart and blood vessels. These diseases could affect organs such as the lungs, brain, kidneys and liver. In 2011, the major cardio-vascular–related causes of death in those aged 65 years and older included heart disease (21%) and stroke (6%) (Statistics Canada, 2015a). Table 20.1 gives information about cardio-vascular disease in Canada.

Risk factors of CVD are often part of a metabolic syndrome—namely, a combination of medical disorders that increase the risk of developing CVD and diabetes. Heart disease affects one in five people, and its prevalence increases with a person's age.

HYPERTENSION

Hypertension is the most common chronic risk factor for CVD. Hypertension Canada has provided guidelines for the assessment, diagnosis, and treatment of hypertension (http://www.hypertension.ca) (Box 20.2). Hypertension (HTN) is diagnosed whenever the diastolic blood pressure (BP) is consistently ≥90 mm Hg or the systolic BP is consistently

---

BOX 20.1 Risk Factors for Heart Disease

- Older age (>55 years for men; >65 years for women)
- Family history of premature CHD (<55 years for men; <65 years for women)
- Microalbuminuria or estimated GFR <60 mL/min
- Hypertension*
- Cigarette smoking
- Central obesity
- Physical inactivity
- Dyslipidemia*
- Diabetes, IGT, or IFG*

*Components of metabolic syndrome.
CHD, Coronary heart disease; *GFR*, glomerular filtration rate; *IGT*, impaired glucose tolerance; *IFG*, impaired fasting glucose.

TABLE 20.1 Heart Disease in Canada

DEATH RATE	MEN VS. WOMEN	RISK-REDUCING FACTORS
Three times higher among adults aged 20 years and over with diagnosed heart disease, compared with those without	Men are two times more likely than women to have a heart attack.	Smoking cessation Physical activity Healthy, balanced diet
Four times higher among adults aged 20 years and over who have had a heart attack, compared with those who have not	Men are newly diagnosed with heart disease 10 years younger than women.	Healthy weight Limited alcohol intake
Six times higher among adults aged 40 years and over with diagnosed heart failure, compared with those without		

Source: Government of Canada. (2017). *Heart disease in Canada.* Retrieved from https://www.canada.ca/en/public-health/services/publications/diseases-conditions/heart-disease-canada.html.

- The BP of all adults should be assessed at all appropriate visits, to determine cardio-vascular risk and for monitoring antihypertensive treatment.
- If systolic BP is ≥140 mm Hg, diastolic BP is ≥90 mm Hg, or both, a follow-up is needed to assess for HTN. If systolic BP is between 130 mm Hg and 139 mm Hg, diastolic BP is between 85 mm Hg and 89 mm Hg, or both, annual follow-up is recommended.
- Global cardio-vascular risk, including both modifiable and nonmodifiable risk factors, should be assessed.
- Home BP monitoring should be encouraged for hypertensive adults, especially if they have diabetes mellitus, chronic kidney disease, suspected nonadherence to antihypertensive therapy, masked hypertension, or demonstrate white-coat effect.
- Thiazide diuretics should be the initial medication therapy, either alone or combined with other types of medication, unless compelling reasons to do otherwise are present. Hypokalemia should be carefully monitored when treating with thiazide diuretic monotherapy.
- Most patients require two or more antihypertensive medications to achieve the goal BP. The combination of an angiotensin-converting enzyme inhibitor and angiotensin II receptor blockers is not recommended.
- If BP is >20/10 mm Hg above goal, initiate therapy with two agents, one of which usually should be a diuretic of the thiazide type.

BP, Blood pressure; *HTN,* hypertension.
Source: Adapted from Leung, A. A., Nerenberg, K., Daskalopoulou, S. S., et al. (2016). Hypertension Canada's 2016 Canadian Hypertension Education Program Guidelines for blood pressure measurement, diagnosis, assessment of risk, prevention, and treatment of hypertension. *Canadian Journal of Cardiology, 32*(5), 569–588. doi:10.1016/j.cjca.2016.02.066.

- Cigarette smoking or tobacco use
- Excessive alcohol intake
- Sedentary lifestyle
- Inadequate stress management, anger management, or both
- High-sodium diet
- High-fat diet

TABLE 20.2   Blood Pressure Classification

CLASSIFICATION	BLOOD PRESSURE
Normal	<120 systolic and <80 diastolic
Prehypertension	120–139 systolic or 80–89 diastolic
Stage 1 HTN	140–159 systolic or 90–99 diastolic
Stage 2 HTN	>160 systolic or >100 diastolic

HTN, Hypertension.

recommendations, based on up-to-date research, for improving the care of people with HTN.

Hypertension is often treatable and is preventable in some cases. In 2013, approximately 5.3 million Canadians (i.e., 17.7% of the population) aged 12 years and older were diagnosed with HTN (Statistics Canada, 2015b). As indicated by the Canadian Community Health Survey, there are significant disparities between White, South Asian, Chinese, and Black groups (Chiu et al., 2015). Although a person's race, ethnicity, and family history of HTN cannot be changed, other factors are within the person's control to reduce the risk for HTN (Box 20.3).

Most HTN is discovered during screening or examination for another problem, when related complications may have already developed. The most important complication of HTN is long-term effects resulting in end-organ damage, especially to the heart. Older persons with HTN have an absolute higher risk for cardiac disease, such as coronary heart disease (CHD), atrial fibrillation, and heart failure, as well as acute cardio-vascular and cerebro-vascular events such as myocardial infarction, stroke, and sudden death. Poorly controlled HTN is also implicated in chronic renal insufficiency, end-stage renal disease,

≥140 mm Hg (Lee et al., 2011) (Table 20.2). Older persons often have isolated systolic HTN, unlike younger people, who are more likely to have an elevation of just the diastolic BP or elevation indicated by both systolic and diastolic BP readings. The goals of therapy for HTN are to treat modifiable risk for persons with diabetes and other chronic diseases and to maintain a systolic BP <140 mm Hg and a diastolic BP <90 mm Hg (Leung et al., 2016). (It is important to note that the Canadian guidelines for HTN are different, depending on whether or not the person has diabetes.) The guidelines also provide annual

and peripheral vascular disease (American College of Cardiology Foundation/American Heart Association [ACCF/AHA], 2011).

CORONARY HEART DISEASE

Like all other muscles, the heart receives its oxygen from arteries within it; CHD is caused by a blockage of these vessels and may be referred to as **arterio-sclerosis,** or "hardening of the arteries." Coronary artery disease develops when cholesterol and other fats are deposited in the layers of the arteries, narrowing the channel through which blood flows and, combined with arterio-sclerosis, limiting the amount of oxygen reaching the tissue (a process known as *ischemia*). Coronary artery disease is in part a direct consequence of chronic, untreated, or inadequately treated HTN (Buttaro et al., 2012). Seventy-five percent of all cardiac-related deaths each year are attributed to CHD.

The symptoms of gripping chest pain, radiation to the shoulder, etc., that are usually thought to indicate acute ischemia caused by myocardial infarction are not usually seen in older persons. Instead, the older person is more likely to have what is called a "silent myocardial infarction." Discomfort may be mild and be localized to the back, abdomen, shoulders, or one or both arms. Nausea and vomiting or merely a sensation like heartburn may be the only symptoms. Older women often present with weakness or lethargy as a sign of a myocardial infarction. More often, there are no noticeable signs or symptoms at all, and the event is only noticed at the time of death or when an electro-cardiogram (ECG) is performed for some other purpose. These vague symptoms are often not brought to the attention of a medical provider.

HEART FAILURE

The damage to the heart from CHD may lead to heart failure, which is the most frequent cause for the hospitalization of older persons. Approximately 600,000 Canadians are living with heart failure (Heart and Stroke Foundation, 2016). As the population ages, it is expected that hospitalization rates will also increase (Heart and Stroke Foundation, 2016).

Heart failure (HF) is a progressive disorder of the heart muscle in which the muscle is damaged, malfunctions, and can no longer pump enough blood to meet the needs of the body. The severity of malfunctioning depends on whether the abnormality is mechanical or functional. Some causes of HF are previous myocardial infarction, HTN, excessive use of alcohol and drugs, diabetes, obesity, infection, high cholesterol, and other medical conditions (Heart and Stroke Foundation, 2017). Over time, the heart is further damaged because of poor control of the underlying problem (e.g., arterio-sclerosis, HTN, or CHD), leading to more and more severe HF. An unhealthy diet, smoking, and a lack of exercise aggravate the development of heart disease and the extent of damage, especially for those who have a family (genetic) history of heart disease. There is no cure for HF, only the management of symptoms and the attempt to prevent worsening (Moe et al., 2015). About 50% of persons with HF will die within 5 years; most die within 10 years, depending on the severity of symptoms and other factors (Heart and Stroke Foundation, 2016).

Clinical HF is categorized as a left-sided, right-sided, or biventricular (i.e., both sides) failure. It can also be described as either systolic or diastolic dysfunction (American Heart Association, 2017). Left-sided and diastolic failures are the most common types of HF found in the older population. McKelvie et al. (2013) of the Canadian Cardiovascular Society provided recommendations for the assessment, diagnosis, and management of HF, and discussed the New York Heart Association functional classifications (Box 20.4).

Common signs and symptoms of HF in older persons include fatigue and **dyspnea** (shortness of breath) with exertion, an inability to lie flat without getting short of breath (orthopnea), waking up at night gasping for air, weight gain, and swelling in the lower extremities. Dyspnea may occur at rest or with exertion, or it may appear intermittently at night (paroxysmal nocturnal dyspnea). The dyspnea may be relieved by sitting up or by sleeping on multiple pillows or with the head of the bed elevated. If a cough is present, it is worse at night.

In addition, the nurse should be alert for the atypical clinical presentation of exacerbations of HF in the older person. The person may appear confused or delirious; begin falling; or complain of insomnia or urinary frequency at night (nocturia). He or she may

BOX 20.4   Classification of Heart Failure

Class I: Asymptomatic
Cardiac disease is present without resulting limitations of physical activity.

Class II: Mild Heart Failure
Physical activity is slightly limited.
The person is comfortable at rest.
An increase in activity may cause fatigue, palpitations, dyspnea, or anginal pain.

Class III: Moderate Heart Failure
Physical activity is markedly limited.
The person is comfortable at rest.
Ordinary walking or climbing stairs can quickly bring on fatigue, palpitations, dyspnea, or anginal pain.
Substantial periods of bed rest are required.

Class IV: Severe Heart Failure
Patient is almost permanently confined to bed.
Patient is unable to carry out any physical activity without discomfort or severe symptoms.
Some symptoms occur when patient is at rest.
Chronic shortness of breath is common.

Source: New York Heart Association Functional Class. (1982). Retrieved from http://www.lb7.uscourts.gov/documents/INSD/112-cv-851.pdf.

also complain of dizziness or may have syncope (i.e., may faint). More often, the nurse will notice that the person has "droops," or malaise and a subtle decline in activity tolerance or in functional or cognitive abilities.

One major way in which cardiac conditions differ from other chronic problems is that they can become acute problems very rapidly and often necessitate acute hospitalization and intensive treatment followed by rehabilitation. Many other chronic disorders are managed at home.

 IMPLICATIONS FOR GERONTOLOGICAL NURSING AND HEALTHY AGING

ASSESSMENT

A pertinent history of the events leading up to and including the presentation of cardio-vascular problems is essential. Monitoring of vital signs, laboratory results, and kidney function; assessing the cardiac and respiratory function; and conducting a mental status examination are essential (see Chapters 13 and 21). The University of Iowa Gerontological Nursing Intervention Center offers an evidence-informed assessment tool that can be used as a basic assessment measure as well as one that indicates change in older patients with HF in any setting (Harrington, 2008). The tool can be used to document status in the three following categories: activities of daily living, quality of sleep, and dyspnea (https://nursing.uiowa.edu/sites/default/files/documents/hartford/EBP%20Guideline%20Catalog.pdf).

INTERVENTIONS

The goals of interprofessional treatment of persons with CVD are to provide relief of symptoms, improve quality of life, reduce mortality and morbidity, and slow or stop the progression of dysfunction through the use of aggressive medication therapy. Additional goals are to maximize the person's function and quality of life and, when appropriate, provide expert palliative care. Concurrent and supportive therapies include diet modification by reducing the intake of fat, cholesterol, and sodium; exercise; education; and family and social supports (American College of Cardiology Foundation/American Heart Association, 2011). Collaboration with other professionals on the team (such as physiotherapists, dietitians, respiratory therapists, and social workers) is crucial.

Several nursing interventions that help the person accomplish his or her goals are highly effective (Heckman et al., 2016; Moe et al., 2014). Which specific interventions are used will depend on the person, the severity of disease, and the person's desire for either palliative or aggressive care. Nursing actions range from teaching the older person about lifestyle changes in diet, activity, and rest (see Chapter 10) to taking acute measures, such as the administration of oxygen and medications. In general, the nurse needs be knowledgeable about interventions related to the following:

- Noting responses to prescribed exercise
- Administering medication and evaluating medication effects
- Watching for signs and symptoms of CHF
- Monitoring diet and fluid intake and output
- Monitoring weight (either daily, biweekly, or weekly)

BOX 20.5	Minimizing Risk for Heart Disease

Blood pressure ≤130/80
Total cholesterol <5.18 mmol/L (200 mg/dL)
LDL <2.56 mmol/L (100 mg/dL)
HDL >1.03 mmol/L (40 mg/dL)
Triglycerides <1.69 mmol/L (150 mg/dL)

LDL, Low-density lipoprotein; *HDL,* high-density lipoprotein.

BOX 20.6	Benefits of Controlling Blood Pressure: Average Reduced Risk for New Events

- 35–40% decreased risk for stroke
- 20–25% decreased risk for myocardial infarction
- 50% decreased risk for heart failure

- Auscultating heart and lung sounds
- Monitoring laboratory values
- Educating the patient about all of the above
- Providing comfort (see Chapter 25)

The goal of the management of HTN is to minimize the risk of complications and reduce or eliminate modifiable risk factors. This means keeping the blood pressure at less than 140/90 mm Hg in otherwise healthy adults and less than 130/80 mm Hg in persons with diabetes. By doing so, many long-term complications (e.g., HF) can be avoided, minimized, or delayed (Boxes 20.5 and 20.6). To accomplish this, nurses have a responsibility to work with older persons and their families comprehensively. Frail older persons with CVD and who reside in LTC homes or at home require appropriate treatment and a careful risk–benefit analysis regarding treatment and outcomes (Heckman et al., 2016). Limited food choices and the significant side effects of some medications may result in an unnecessary reduced quality of life for a person with a limited life expectancy. When aggressive treatment is no longer effective, a referral to hospice or palliative care services in the community may be a possibility.

The potential for wellness of older persons after a major cardiac event or procedure is increased when they participate fully in any available cardiac rehabilitation program. Otherwise, disability can progress rapidly, especially if the person believes that any exertion overtaxes the heart and will cause acute CHF, another myocardial infarction, or death. To prevent this, cardiac-exercise rehabilitation programs are designed to address the physical, mental, and spiritual needs and overall health of the person and his or her family. Typical programs are prescribed by the physician or nurse practitioner and begin with self-managed education and light activity, progressing to moderate activity under the supervision of a rehabilitation nurse and physiotherapist. If the person is more physically compromised, it is necessary to identify energy-conserving measures applicable to his or her daily tasks.

Nurses and the person with CVD must be cautious with exercise. With a person who has had a myocardial infarction, exercise-related orthostatic hypotension is more likely to occur. This hypotension is a result of age-related decreases in baroreceptor responsiveness, which controls the body's ability to respond to the need for changes in blood pressure (see Chapter 6). Because the person's thermoregulation is also impaired, the intensity of exercise must be reduced in hot, humid climates (see Chapter 12). A healthy alternative is "mall walking" in local, covered, and climate-controlled shopping centres. In some locations, this becomes a social event as well as a safe way to exercise.

Risk-reduction programs should be instituted with a clear understanding of the difficulties involved in attempts to alter harmful lifestyle practices such as smoking, overeating, habitual anger or irritation, and a sedentary lifestyle. These practices may have been going on for all of the person's life and are not easily changed by education. The nurse's role in these instances is to discuss these practices in a nonjudgemental manner, providing acceptance, encouragement, resources, knowledge, and affirmation of both the difficulty of making lifestyle changes and the person's right to choose.

RESPIRATORY DISORDERS

The normal physical changes from aging (see Chapter 6) result in a higher risk for respiratory problems; when such problems occur, older persons have a higher risk for death than younger persons have. Diseases of the respiratory system involve the upper or lower respiratory tract and are identified as infectious, acute, or chronic. Infections are further defined as either obstructive (preventing airflow out as a result of obstruction or narrowing of the respiratory structures) or restrictive (causing a decrease in total lung capacity as a result of limited expansion). Almost all chronic obstructive pulmonary diseases that occur in late life arise from tobacco use or exposure to tobacco and other environmental pollutants earlier in life. Although asthma may be triggered by environmental factors, strong genetic and allergic factors contribute to its occurrence. In addition to being vigilant for signs of infection, the nurse should focus on helping the person maintain function and quality of life.

CHRONIC OBSTRUCTIVE PULMONARY DISEASE

Chronic obstructive pulmonary disease consists of a group of conditions that affect airflow, including asthma, bronchitis, and emphysema. This group of disorders is the fourth leading cause of death for older men and women; however, it is expected to be the third leading cause of death by 2020. Chronic obstructive pulmonary disease (COPD) affects 6.7% of men and 7.2% of women who are between 65 and 74 years of age (Public Health Agency of Canada [PHAC], 2012); the percentages increase to 11.8% and 7.5%, respectively, for men and women who are 75 or more years of age. While the overall death rate from COPD has decreased, the age-adjusted death rate for women over 79 years of age has increased from approximately 210 per 100,000 persons in 1989 to approximately 380 in 2004; the death rate for men during this same time period decreased from slightly over 900 per 100,000 persons to approximately 720 (PHAC, 2012). Cigarette smoking is the underlying cause of approximately 80 to 90% of COPD cases (Public Health Agency of Canada [PHAC], 2013).

COPD contributes to severe activity limitations. The 2009–2010 Canadian Community Health Survey (CCHS) found that 45% of Canadians with self-reported COPD reported their health as "fair or poor" (PHAC, 2013).

The type of signs and symptoms seen varies with the type of COPD. For example, persons with emphysema have little sputum production, and they appear pink because they are receiving adequate oxygen. On the other hand, persons with bronchitis have chronic sputum production, frequent cough, and are pale and somewhat cyanotic. Thorough discussions of these symptoms can be found in medical–surgical nursing and pathophysiology texts. What is crucial to gerontological nursing is the need to watch the person with COPD very closely for signs of worsening infection and aggravation of any underlying heart disease.

When respirations exceed 30 breaths per minute, the person with COPD is having a worsening of his or her illness, and prompt response is necessary. An acute episode of emphysema or bronchitis is characterized by significantly worsened dyspnea and increased volume and change in the colour of sputum (Esherick, 2012). An acute episode of asthma is characterized by shortness of breath and wheezing. A number of factors—for example, viral or bacterial infections, exposure to polluted air or other environmental pollution, or changes in the weather—may trigger a change in the person's respiratory health. Persons with advanced COPD, as seen in most older persons with the disease, can expect to have periods of worsening of symptoms and functioning between periods of control. During periods of illness, medication changes are usually needed. Persons with well-developed skills in self-management often will begin to deal with the changes before consulting a health care provider. Hospitalization is always a possibility with COPD exacerbations, especially when the person has or is suspected of having an acute infection.

PNEUMONIA

Pneumonia is a bacterial or viral lower respiratory-tract infection that causes inflammation of the lung tissue. Pneumonia and influenza are the seventh and eighth leading causes of death for men and women, respectively, over the age of 65 years (Statistics Canada, 2015c). Particularly susceptible are older people with **comorbid** conditions (such as alcoholism, asthma, COPD, or heart disease) and older persons who live in institutional settings. Older persons residing in LTC homes (for any reason) have a ten-fold greater incidence of pneumonia. Other factors that increase the risk of acquiring pneumonia are related to normal age-related respiratory system changes, such as a diminished cough reflex, increased residual volume, and decreased chest compliance (see Chapter 6). Many cases of pneumonia can be either prevented by immunization or treated effectively. The pneumococcal vaccine is a one-time vaccine that can prevent pneumonia and other infections and is recommended for people who are at high risk or who are older than 65 years or who are both. More information can be found on the Health Canada website (http://www.hc-sc.gc.ca).

Pneumonia is classified as either a community-acquired infection or a **health care–associated infection;** that is, it is acquired either as a consequence of living in the community or as a result of medical treatment or hospitalization. In LTC homes, the most frequent causes of aspiration pneumonia are reflux of colonized oral secretions either from an enteral tube or from simply eating.

The usual signs and symptoms of pneumonia, such as cough, fatigue, and dyspnea, may easily be attributed initially to something else, such as medications or underlying COPD. In older persons, other signs of pneumonia may be seen, such as falling, mental status changes or signs of confusion, general deterioration, weakness, anorexia, rapid pulse, and rapid respirations. When a person appears to have pneumonia, an abnormal chest X-ray, fever, and an elevated white blood count are expected. However, these signs may be delayed in an older person, and treatment that is not started until they are present may be too late, and the result may be death. For the best possibility of survival of a frail older person with pneumonia, very prompt interventions are necessary. For the frail and medically compromised, interventions may be necessary as soon as an infection is determined to be a reasonable explanation for a sudden change.

One of the most important questions a nurse needs to consider is whether recommendation and advocacy for hospitalization are appropriate. Fortunately, several evidence-informed indicators help the nurse make this decision (Box 20.7).

For the older person, especially a person who is frail or decompensated, the decision to hospitalize or not will be determined by the person's wishes regarding aggressive treatment. It is always imperative to make sure that the person and the person's significant others realize the severity of the situation

---

BOX 20.7 Indicators of Pneumonia-Related Death

The indicators of an increased likelihood of pneumonia-related death for persons in the community are the following: (1) aggravation of another health condition at the same time, (2) respiratory rate >25, and (3) elevated C-reactive protein (if known).

The indicators of an increased risk for death within 30 days for persons residing in LTC homes are the following: respiratory rate >30, pulse >125, altered mental status, and history of dementia.

TABLE 20.3 Seasonal Influenza in Canada

INFLUENZA SEASON	NUMBER OF CASES
1999–2000	7,027
2000–2001	4,154
2006–2007	8,133
2007–2008	12,256
2008–2009*	23,376
2009–2010*	38,980
2010–2011	17,535
2011–2012	12,194
2012–2013	31,737
2013–2014	28,778
2014–2015	43,510
2015–2016	33,559
2016–2017 (to date)	22,110

*Increased cases due to pandemic (H1N1) 2009 influenza virus.
Source: Data from Infection Prevention and Control Canada. (2017). *Seasonal influenza, avian influenza and pandemic influenza.* Retrieved from https://ipac-canada.org/influenza-resources.php.

---

and that there are always options, such as treatment in the facility (e.g., intravenous antibiotics or oxygen per cannula) and comfort measures. The decision will always be a personal one.

INFLUENZA

In Canada, influenza causes 500 to 1,500 deaths and thousands of hospitalizations each year (Table 20.3). The greatest morbidity and mortality occur in those aged 65 years and older, owing to comorbid conditions and complications (Government of Canada, 2017). In addition to medical complications, an older person can experience a significant decline in functional ability as a result of a bout with the flu (Noazzami et al., 2014).

The influenza vaccine remains the cornerstone of prevention. In Canada, the National Advisory Committee on Immunization (NACI) suggests that everyone older than 6 months of age get a flu vaccine once a year. A yearly flu vaccine is especially important for certain people who are more likely to have complications from the flu, such as people who are 65 years and older, people who are living in a home or a residential facility, people with CVD or respiratory disease, and people with a health condition that requires regular medical care or hospitalization (National Advisory Committee on Immunization [NACI], 2010). If used accordingly, the vaccine could prevent 70% of hospitalizations and 80% of deaths due to influenza among older individuals living in the community. The NACI provides important guidelines on immunization strategies, surveillance, and the early identification and isolation of persons with influenza.

 ## IMPLICATIONS FOR GERONTOLOGICAL NURSING AND HEALTHY AGING

ASSESSMENT

The nursing assessment of the person with respiratory problems focuses on (1) objective observations of oxygen saturation, sputum production, and coughing and (2) subjective reports of dyspnea and its effect on functional status and quality of life. Only persons experiencing a problem can really tell us what it is like for them. Visual analogue scales and numerical rating scales similar to those used to assess pain may be helpful (see Chapter 16). Persons can be asked how they would rate their breathing from 1 (no dyspnea) to 10 (worst dyspnea possible), and so on.

When an infection is suspected, a "wait and see" approach is never appropriate; elevations in temperature or white blood cell count may not occur until the person is in a septic state, and chest X-ray examinations in chronically ill persons are often falsely negative at the beginning of the infection or

when dehydration is present. Patients and their families should be told about the seriousness of this or any infection in older persons. More timely diagnosis calls for sensitive clinical assessments by both the nurse and the other health care providers.

Assessment includes detailed information about a cough. When did it start? How long are the episodes of coughing? Is there any associated pain? What seems to make it better, and what makes it worse? Is the person using anything to treat the cough? Is the person smoking (and how much) or exposed to smoke or other respiratory irritants? If the cough is productive, what is the colour, texture, and odour of the mucus? Does the colour change according to the time of the day?

The remaining physical examination is the same as that for persons with cardiac disease, since it is not always clear whether symptoms such as fatigue and shortness of breath are cardiac or respiratory in nature. Observation of airway clearance, breathing patterns, and mobility; measurement of pulse oximetry; mental status examination; and functional assessment can provide a clear picture of the person's health status. Pulmonary function testing is most definitive in terms of lung capacity; along with a chest X-ray examination, such testing can show the extent of respiratory damage from acute or chronic conditions. Box 20.8 presents the key components of a respiratory assessment.

INTERVENTIONS

For pneumonia and influenza, the focus of intervention is on prevention and vaccination. As with heart failure, many respiratory diseases in later life cannot be cured. Nursing interventions are based on palliative goals; namely, stabilizing the disease, reducing the risk of exacerbations and hospitalizations, promoting maximal functional capacity, and preventing premature disability. Education always includes teaching smoking cessation, secretion clearance techniques, the identification and management of exacerbations, breathing retraining, management of depression and anxiety, nutritional support, the proper use and administration of medications, and dealing with supplemental oxygen therapy if and when necessary (Esherick, 2012). Except in severe cases, treatment can be done at home or in an LTC home, as long as

BOX 20.8   Performing a Respiratory Assessment

Obtain the Following Histories:
Family
Past medical
Symptoms

Assess the Following:
Overall body configuration (e.g., posture, chest symmetry, shape)
Respirations, including ease of ventilation, use of accessory muscles, and so forth
Level of dyspnea per activity, in detail
Oxygenation (pulse oximetry, skin colour, capillary refill, and pallor)
Sputum (colour, amount, and consistency)
Palpation, percussion, and auscultation
Functional status
Cognitive status (if indicated)
Mood (if indicated)
Advance planning and patient's wishes for treatment
Presence or absence of a living will and a designated health care surrogate

BOX 20.9   Instructions for Persons With Chronic Obstructive Pulmonary Disease

Nutrition
Eat small, frequent meals with a high protein and caloric content.*
Select foods that do not require a lot of chewing, or cut the food into bite-size pieces to conserve energy.
Drink 2–3L of fluid daily.*
Weigh yourself at least twice each week.

Activity Pacing to Conserve Energy
Plan exertion during the best periods of the day.
Arrange regular rest periods.
Allow plenty of time to complete activities.
Schedule sex around the best-breathing time of day.
Use prescribed bronchodilators 20 to 30 minutes before sexual activity.
During sex, use a position that does not call for pressure on the chest or for the support of the arms.

General Instructions
Participate in regular exercise.*
Select and wear clothing and shoes that are easy to put on and remove.
Avoid indoor and outdoor pollutants.
Avoid exposure to others who are ill.
Obtain an annual flu shot if not allergic to the vaccine.
Obtain pneumococcal immunization, as appropriate.
Notify the health care provider of any temperature elevation, changes in the colour or amount of sputum, and increased shortness of breath.

*As prescribed.

oxygen therapy, parenteral fluids, and antibiotics can be administered by nursing staff.

If someone is available to assume a caregiver role, the older person's care and treatment can be carried out in his or her home with temporary home health service support. If the older person fails to improve or deteriorates, then hospitalization is often necessary, unless this is against the wishes of the older person. A change to active palliative care may be appropriate at any time. If the person is hospitalized, a prolonged rehabilitation may be necessary, either at home or in a rehabilitation facility or both (see Chapter 26). Pharmacological and mechanical interventions for the treatment of infection are based on the health status of the person before the infection, the expected outcomes of treatment, where treatment will be provided, and the wishes of the patient (as noted above).

Interdisciplinary Care

Education is a part of every aspect of pulmonary care (Box 20.9). The person is taught to recognize the signs and symptoms of respiratory infection; how to maintain adequate nutrition; how to use and clean an inhaler, nebulizer, and peak flow meter; how to use oxygen safely; how to tell which type of exercise is beneficial; how to pace activities; and how to use coping strategies. Each of these areas (and any other issues, such as sexual function) calls for teaching and indicates specific interventions that will help older persons participate in their management.

Diet education should address the reasons for monitoring weight and the signs of malnutrition. Weight loss can occur rapidly because of the energy expenditure needed to breathe while eating. A sense of being full early in the meal is caused by congestion in the abdomen because of a flattened diaphragm.

Anorexia or decreased appetite occurs as a result of sputum production and gastric irritation from the use of bronchodilators and steroids.

Activity and exercise tolerance should be assessed by the occupational and respiratory therapists, and activities should be prescribed to increase endurance and improve respiratory status. Exercise may be done with or without oxygen as a supplement to control symptoms so that the older person can spend enough time in exercise to benefit from it. The person should be informed that sexual activity is still possible, and education and counselling should be provided, either by the rehabilitation nurse or a professional counsellor.

Medications are used to treat infection and control dyspnea, cough, and sputum production. When teaching about any medication, the nurse needs to make sure that the person knows the purpose and correct dosage and regimen of any medication he or she is taking, its side effects, and what to do if these side effects occur (see Chapter 14). Inhalers are difficult to use for persons with limited manual dexterity, strength, or both (such as people with arthritis in their hands). Special adaptive devices are available if needed.

Rehabilitation is an important aspect of maximizing quality of life for the person with respiratory problems, as it is for those with cardio-vascular problems. An older person with COPD would be considered a candidate for pulmonary rehabilitation as long as he or she has pulmonary reserve and as long as any heart disease is stable. Rehabilitation programs for the older person with COPD consist of medication therapy, reconditioning exercises, and counselling. A multiprofessional team of health care providers works to help the older person do the following:

- Increase the level of independence
- Maintain individuality and autonomy
- Improve function in his or her environment
- Decrease the number of hospitalizations and the need for hospitalization
- Increase exercise tolerance
- Increase self-esteem and self-care skills
- Improve quality of life and comfort

The number of these goals that are achieved depends on many factors, including the extent of illness and coexisting conditions. Rehabilitation may be prolonged for persons recovering from pneumonia.

Economic issues are always a concern for persons with chronic disease (see Chapter 15). Not all prescription medication costs are covered by the health system, and the amount of coverage varies among provinces and territories. Medications can be very expensive, especially when needed for an indefinite period of time.

Mouth care is very important, especially for people who are receiving supplemental oxygen and those who are medically or physically debilitated. Inadequate mouth care leads to the propagation of bacteria, which compounds an already serious situation and may lead to aspiration pneumonia. Sputum is considered potentially infectious and must be handled appropriately.

Monitoring nutrition and obtaining nutritional consultation as necessary are the responsibility of the nurse in all settings. The nurse will also ensure that the person recovering from pneumonia or influenza is adequately nourished and—while monitoring fluid volume—is adequately hydrated. Overload is a risk for persons with coexisting heart disease. As soon as the condition allows, the older person should be mobilized and referred for physiotherapy and occupational therapy to prevent or stop functional decline.

TUBERCULOSIS

Tuberculosis (TB) is a communicable and infectious disease caused by *Mycobacterium tuberculosis*, a bacterium that affects one-third of the world's population (Centers for Disease Control and Prevention, 2015). *Tuberculosis infection* is identified by a positive TB skin test result with no evidence of active disease. The term "tuberculosis disease" refers to cases in which a person has a positive acid-fast smear or culture for *M. tuberculosis* or has radiographic and clinical evidence of TB.

M. tuberculosis was considered to be conquered in the 1950s with the development of the isoniazid. Many older persons were treated following infections contracted during the Second World War; many others were infected as children. However, if older persons become immunocompromised as a result of chemotherapy, extreme old age, or human immunodeficiency virus (HIV) infection, the bacterium could be reactivated.

The number of cases of TB in Canada has steadily decreased, with a drop from approximately 6.7 per 100,000 in 1995 to 0.7 per 100,000 in 2010 (Public Health Agency of Canada [PHAC], 2014). However, foreign-born individuals still have higher rates of TB, (around 13.3 per 100,000 in 2010), and Indigenous people have the highest rates in Canada, peaking at 200 cases per 100,000 for the Inuit population (PHAC, 2014).

Gerontological nurses working in areas where TB rates are high must be particularly knowledgeable about this potentially life-threatening disease and must protect themselves and others. Persons who are immunosuppressed, persons who are from areas with high infection rates, and persons who live in group settings are at particular risk. Older residents in congregate living settings are more likely to acquire the disease than those who live in the community (Dhaolakia & Mistry, 2017).

The symptoms of TB, regardless of age group, include unexplained weight loss or fever and a cough lasting more than 3 weeks. The person may experience night sweats and generalized anxiety. In more advanced stages, the person will also experience dyspnea, chest pain, and hemoptysis. Laboratory results for older persons may show an increased sedimentation rate and lymphocytopenia. Because these signs and symptoms are associated with many disorders common in older persons, diagnosis is often made during a health screening (Tierney et al., 2011). For persons with positive skin test results, it is necessary to confirm the diagnosis with a chest X-ray and a sputum culture (National Library of Medicine [NLM], 2012a).

IMPLICATIONS FOR GERONTOLOGICAL NURSING AND HEALTHY AGING

In promoting healthy aging in the context of TB, the nurse has a responsibility to both the public and the patient. The nurse must be proactive in the prevention of contagious disease and in the prompt treatment of persons who are ill or become ill; this responsibility is especially important in a residential care setting, where older persons are at higher risk for TB because of the communal living situation and a high rate of

---

BOX 20.10 Surveillance Guidelines for Tuberculosis in the Long-Term Care Setting

- Each LTC home should have an individual responsible for tuberculosis (TB) infection control and an infection prevention and control plan.
- Each LTC home should conduct regularly scheduled TB risk assessments that consider the residents and health care workers.
- Determine the need for TB screening as indicated by the results of the risk assessments. Most LTC homes are low-risk settings.
- Screen all new residents on admission and employees on hire for symptoms, and consider using the two-step tuberculin skin test for *Mycobacterium tuberculosis*. Repeat the tests annually.
- For persons who test positive or have had a positive test result in the past, perform one chest X-ray examination, then review the symptoms annually.
- No person with a diagnosis of TB should remain in an LTC home unless adequate administrative and environmental controls and a respiratory protection program are in place.

Source: Public Health Agency of Canada (PHAC), Canadian Lung Association/Canadian Thoracic Society. (2014). *Canadian tuberculosis standards* (7th ed.). Retrieved from http://www.phac-aspc.gc.ca/tbpc-latb/pubs/tb-canada-7/tb-standards-tb-normes-ch1-eng.php#a6_.

---

medical frailty. The Ontario Lung Association (2015) has described how residents in LTC homes and the staff that cares for them are at the highest risk of developing TB. To ensure the prompt identification of persons with TB and to limit its spread, especially in LTC or residential care facilities, nurses should develop and implement an appropriate surveillance plan (Box 20.10). If need be, the Public Health Agency of Canada and the Canadian Lung Association are excellent sources of guidance and assistance in developing such a plan.

TB is a reportable condition, which means that all suspected and confirmed cases are reported to the appropriate health authorities (National Library of Medicine [NLM], 2012b). The local public health nurses usually conduct investigations to ensure that all potentially infected people have been tested and that all persons with the disease receive treatment. The nurse actively participates in health screenings that may include TB testing. As a health care provider,

BOX 20.11 Research for Evidence-Informed Practice: Tuberculosis Outbreak in a Long-Term Care Home

Problem: Tuberculosis (TB) is re-emerging and is a high-risk disease for older persons in Canada.

Method: The researchers completed a case finding study in Ontario. Three rounds of tuberculin screening tests were completed at 8- to 12-week intervals. Public Health Ontario Laboratories conducted the laboratory analysis. The researchers also conducted an indoor air quality assessment to determine if inadequate air quality is a risk factor for TB.

Results: At the home, there was one active case of pulmonary TB (in one staff member). Approximately 6 months later, there were 3 additional active cases and 24 latent tuberculosis cases among staff and residents. Four cases were infected by an identical strain. Nine of 15 locations in the LTC home had air exchange rates that were below those called for by the published guidelines.

Implications for nursing practice: TB outbreaks are still an issue of concern in LTC homes. Nurses should be aware of this and value the importance of annual tuberculin testing.

Source: Khalil, N. J., Kryanowski, J. A., Mercer, N. J., et al. (2013). Tuberculosis outbreak in a long-term care facility. *Canadian Journal of Public Health, 104*(1), e28–e32. doi:10.17269/cjph.104.3504.

the nurse is also at risk for acquiring the infection and needs to be screened regularly to keep from becoming a carrier (Box 20.11).

In regard to persons with TB, nurses have a role in monitoring laboratory values, assessing any medication side reactions, and monitoring medication adherence in persons with TB, all of which are crucial to the treatment's effectiveness and the person's well-being. The gerontological nurse participates in screening, educating the person about the seriousness of the infection, and helping the person obtain the appropriate treatment.

KEY CONCEPTS

- Heart disease is the most common cause of death for persons in Canada.
- The underlying cause for the majority of cardio-vascular and pulmonary disease is smoking; therefore, assisting persons in smoking cessation can have a significant impact on improving their health.

- Pneumonia and influenza are particularly important health problems for persons over 65 years of age and are significantly more so for persons who are frail or immunocompromised, have HIV infection, or are otherwise decompensated.
- The mortality associated with pneumonia and influenza can be minimized through vaccination.
- The goal of therapy for cardiac and respiratory disorders is to relieve symptoms, improve quality of life, reduce mortality, stabilize and slow the progression of the disease, reduce the risk of exacerbation, and maximize functional capacity.
- Continued careful attention to the early detection and prompt treatment of TB is necessary to the attempt to completely eradicate this communicable disease.

ACTIVITIES AND DISCUSSION QUESTIONS

1. What is heart failure?
2. Compare and contrast the types of heart failure (HF) and COPD.
3. Discuss the assessment and interventions for older people with a diagnosis of HF, COPD, or pneumonia.
4. Discuss why pneumonia and influenza are so dangerous to the older person.
5. What preventive measures can be instituted to prevent or lessen the severity of pneumonia, influenza, and TB among the older population?
6. Develop a nursing care plan for an older person with HF or a respiratory condition.
7. Discuss the implications of cardio-vascular disease and respiratory illness for an older person's ability to live independently.

RESOURCES

Canadian Cardiovascular Society (CCS).
Recommendations for the assessment, diagnosis, and management of cardio-vascular disease
http://www.ccs.ca

Canadian Heart Failure Network (CHFN). A resource for health care providers, patients, and the general public
http://www.chfn.ca

Canadian Hypertension Education Program (CHEP). Educational tools for patients and families
http://guidelines.hypertension.ca

Canadian Lung Association
http://www.lung.ca

Health Canada. Information on vaccinations and immunization policy for pneumonia and influenza
http://www.hc-sc.gc.ca

Heart and Stroke Foundation
http://www.heartandstroke.ca

Hypertension Canada
http://www.hypertension.ca

For additional resources, please visit *http:// evolve.elsevier.com/Canada/Ebersole/gerontological/*

REFERENCES

American College of Cardiology Foundation/American Heart Association (ACCF/AHA). (2011). Expert consensus document on hypertension in the elderly. *Journal of the American College of Cardiology, 57*(20), 2037–2114.

American Heart Association. (2017). *Types of heart failure.* Retrieved from http://www.heart.org/HEARTORG/Conditions/ HeartFailure/AboutHeartFailure/Types-of-Heart-Failure_UCM _306323_Article.jsp#.WMvgwxIrJmA.

Buttaro, T. M., Trybulski, J., Polgar-Bailey, P., et al. (2012). *Primary care: A collaborative approach* (4th ed.). St. Louis, MO: Mosby.

Centers for Disease Control and Prevention. (2015). *Tuberculosis: Data and statistics.* Retrieved from https://www.cdc.gov/tb/ statistics/default.htm.

Chiu, M., Maclagan, L. C., Tu, J. V., et al. (2015). Temporal trends in cardiovascular disease risk factors among white, South Asian, Chinese and black groups in Ontario, Canada, 2001 to 2012: A population-based study. *BMJ Open, 5*(8), e007232. doi:10.1136/ bmjopen-2014-007232.

Dhaolakia, Y., & Mistry, N. (2017). Tuberculosis in congregate settings: Policies and practices in various facilities in Mumbai, India. *Indian Journal of Tuberculosis, 64*(1), 10–13. doi:10.1016/ j.ijtb.2016.11.006.

Esherick, J. S. (2012). *Tarascon medical procedures pocketbook.* Sudbury, MA: Jones & Bartlett Learning.

Government of Canada. (2017). *Flu Watch report: January 8 to January 14, 2017 (Week 2).* Retrieved from http://www .healthycanadians.gc.ca/publications/diseases-conditions -maladies-affections/fluwatch-2016-2017-02-surveillance -influenza/index-eng.php.

Harrington, C. C. (2008). Evidence-based guideline: Assessing heart failure in long-term care facilities. *Journal of Gerontological Nursing, 34*(2), 9–14. Retrieved from https:// www.ncbi.nlm.nih.gov/pubmed/18286787.

Heart and Stroke Foundation. (2016). *The burden of heart failure.* Retrieved from https://www.heartandstroke.ca/-/media/pdf-files/ canada/2017-heart-month/heartandstroke-reportonhealth-2016.ashx ?la=en.

Heart and Stroke Foundation. (2017). *Heart failure.* Retrieved from https://www.heartandstroke.ca/heart/conditions/heart-failure.

Heckman, G. A., Boscart, V. M., D'Elia, T., et al. (2016). Managing heart failure in long-term care: Recommendations from an interprofessional stakeholder consultation. *Canadian Journal on Aging, 35*(4), 447–464. doi:10.1017/S071498081600043X.

Lee, C. T., Williams, G. H., & Lilly, L. S. (2011). Hypertension. In L. S. Lilly (Ed.), *Pathophysiology of heart disease* (pp. 301–323). Philadelphia, PA: Lippincott Williams & Wilkins.

Leung, A. A., Nerenberg, K., Daskalopoulou, S. S., et al. (2016). Hypertension Canada's 2016 Canadian Hypertension Education Program Guidelines for blood pressure measurement, diagnosis, assessment of risk, prevention, and treatment of hypertension. *Canadian Journal of Cardiology, 32*(5), 569–588. doi:10.1016/j.cjca.2016.02.066.

McKelvie, R. S., Moe, G. W., Ezekowitz, J. A., et al. (2013). The 2012 Canadian cardiovascular society heart failure management guidelines update: Focus on acute and chronic heart failure. *Canadian Journal of Cardiology, 29*, 168–181. doi:10.1016/ j.cjca.2012.10.007.

Moe, G. W., Ezekowitz, J. A., O'Meara, E., et al. (2015). The 2014 Canadian cardiovascular society heart failure management guidelines focus update: Anemia, biomarkers and recent therapeutic trial implications. *Canadian Journal of Cardiology, 31*(1), 3–16. doi:10.1016/j.cjca.2014.10.022.

Moe, G. W., Ezekowitz, J. A., O'Meara, E., et al. (2014). The 2013 Canadian Cardiovascular Society Heart Failure Management Guidelines Update: Focus on rehabilitation and exercise and surgical coronary revascularization. *Canadian Journal of Cardiology, 30*(3), 249–263. doi:10.1016/j.cjca.2013.10.010.

National Advisory Committee on Immunization (NACI). (2010). Statement on seasonal trivalent inactivated influenza vaccine (TIV) for 2010–2011. *Canada Communicable Disease Report, 36*(ACS-6), 1–49. Retrieved from http://www.phac-aspc.gc.ca/ publicat/ccdr-rmtc/10pdf/36-acs-6.pdf.

National Library of Medicine (NLM). (2012a). *PPD skin test.* Retrieved from http://www.nlm.nih.gov/medlineplus/ency/ article/003839.htm.

National Library of Medicine (NLM). (2012b). *Pulmonary tuberculosis.* Retrieved from http://www.nlm.nih.gov/medlineplus/ ency/article/000077.htm.

Noazzami, K., McElhaney, J. E., & Rezaei, N. (2014). Influenza infection in the elderly. In A. Massoud & N. Rezaei (Eds.), *Immunology of Aging.* Berlin Heidelberg: Springer-Verlag.

Ontario Lung Association. (2015). *Tuberculosis: Let's end the story.* Retrieved from https://www.on.lung.ca/tb.

Public Health Agency of Canada. (2015). *Cardiovascular disease.* Retrieved from https://www.canada.ca/en/public-health/services/ diseases/heart-health/heart-diseases-conditions.html.

Public Health Agency of Canada (PHAC). (2014). *Canadian Tuberculosis Standards* (7th Edition). Retrieved from https://www .canada.ca/en/public-health/services/infectious-diseases/

canadian-tuberculosis-standards-7th-edition/edition-13.html #a6_0.

Public Health Agency of Canada (PHAC). (2013). *Chronic obstructive pulmonary disease (COPD)*. Retrieved from https://www.canada.ca/en/public-health/services/chronic-diseases/chronic-respiratory-diseases/chronic-obstructive-pulmonary-disease-copd.html.

Public Health Agency of Canada (PHAC). (2012). *Life and breath: Respiratory disease in Canada*. Retrieved from https://www.canada.ca/en/public-health/services/reports-publications/2007/life-breath-respiratory-disease-canada-2007.html.

Public Health Agency of Canada (PHAC). (2010). *Six types of cardiovascular disease*. Retrieved from https://www.canada.ca/en/public-health/services/chronic-diseases/cardiovascular-disease/six-types-cardiovascular-disease.html.

Statistics Canada. (2015a). *Percentage distribution for the 5 leading causes of death in Canada, 2011*. Retrieved from http://www.statcan.gc.ca/pub/82-625-x/2014001/article/11896/c-g/c-g01-eng.htm.

Statistics Canada. (2015b). *High blood pressure, 2013*. Retrieved from http://www.statcan.gc.ca/pub/82-625-x/2014001/article/14020-eng.htm.

Statistics Canada. (2015c). *The 10 leading causes of death, 2011*. Retrieved from http://www.statcan.gc.ca/pub/82-625-x/2014001/article/11896-eng.htm.

Tierney, L. M., Saint, S., & Whooley, M. A. (2011). *Current essentials of medicine* (4th ed.). New York, NY: Lange.

Cognitive Impairment and Neurological Disorders

LEARNING OBJECTIVES

Upon completion of this chapter, the reader will be able to:

- Differentiate between dementia, delirium, and depression.
- Discuss the different types of dementia and appropriate diagnosis.
- Explain the differences between hemorrhagic and ischemic stroke.
- Describe the effects of Parkinson's disease and the appropriate nursing interventions.
- Describe nursing models of care for persons with dementia and cognitive impairment.
- Discuss common concerns in caring for persons with dementia.
- Develop a nursing care plan for a person with delirium.
- Develop a nursing care plan for a person with dementia.

GLOSSARY

Affect A person's prevailing emotion, as observed by an interviewer or assessor.

Agnosia Inability to recognize common objects, familiar faces, or sounds, despite intact sensory abilities.

Aphasia Loss of the ability to use and understand spoken and written language.

Apraxia Impaired ability to manipulate objects or perform purposeful acts.

Ataxia Impaired ability to coordinate movement, typified by a staggering gait.

Cognitive functioning "Comprises perception, memory, and thinking. The processes by which an individual perceives, stores, retrieves, and uses information" (Heeren et al., 2016).

Computed tomography An X-ray technique that produces an image representing a detailed cross-section of tissue; used primarily to diagnose space-occupying lesions.

Dysarthria A speech disorder caused by a weakness or incoordination of the muscles used for speech.

Electro-encephalogram A recording of the electrical activity of the brain by means of electrodes attached to the scalp.

Hallucinations Perceptions of sensory experiences with no external stimuli.

Magnetic resonance imaging A noninvasive technology that uses magnets (not radiation) and radio-frequency current to produce an image of the soft tissues of the body, including the brain.

Milieu Environment or setting.

Perseveration Persistent repetition of an activity, phrase, or set of ideas.

Subarachnoid space The space under the arachnoid membrane and above the pia mater; it may fill with blood during a cerebral hemorrhage.

THE LIVED EXPERIENCE

Comments by participants in a research study about living with early stages of dementia:

"I have dementia and I'm going to reach a stage whereby I can no longer think as a logical person or do things in a logical way."

"Dementia also includes, as I say, organizational skills, erm, coordination skills, and memory skills, and I never used to use, consider these."

"I'll stand my ground and fight it at the moment, in my own way on my own."

"You can't do anything about it."

"I'm giving up various activities because I have the onset of Alzheimer's disease."

"I'm misconstrued and misunderstood until I … blow."

"If I'm a patient, nobody seems to care."

"People tend to talk about them behind your back rather than to your face."

Source: Harman, G., & Clare, L. (2006). Illness representations and lived experience in early-stage dementia. *Qualitative Health Research, 16*, 484–502. doi:10.1177/1049732306286851.

This chapter focuses on cognitive impairment and neurological diseases that affect cognition and discusses delirium, Alzheimer's disease, and other dementias. Stroke and Parkinson's disease are also discussed, since they can affect **cognitive functioning.** The chapter also presents nursing interventions for people experiencing delirium and dementia, as well as caregiving for persons with dementia. See Chapter 7 for a discussion of cognitive function in aging; see Chapter 13 for a discussion of instruments for cognitive assessment; and see Chapter 3 for a discussion of communication with persons experiencing cognitive impairment.

COGNITIVE IMPAIRMENT

The term "cognitive impairment" describes a range of disturbances of cognitive functioning, including disturbances in memory, orientation, attention, and concentration. Other disturbances of cognition may affect intelligence, judgement, learning ability, perception, problem solving, psychomotor ability, reaction time, and social intactness.

THE THREE D'S

Delirium, dementia, and depression, which occur frequently in older persons, have been called the "three D's of cognitive impairment." These important geriatric syndromes are not normal consequences of aging,

although their incidences increase with age. Because cognitive and behavioural changes characterize all three "D's," it can be difficult to diagnose delirium, delirium superimposed on dementia, or depression. The inability to concentrate, along with the resulting memory impairment and other cognitive dysfunction, can occur in late-life depression (see Chapter 24).

Delirium is characterized by a relatively rapid onset, usually over hours or days, with symptoms that fluctuate throughout the day. The other key features of delirium are disturbances in consciousness and attention, and changes in cognition (memory deficits and perceptual disturbances). Perceptual disturbances are often accompanied by delusional (paranoid) thoughts and behaviour and by disturbances of the sleep-wake cycle, psychomotor behaviour, and emotions. In contrast, dementia typically has a gradual onset and a slow, steady pattern of decline without alterations in consciousness (Voyer et al., 2012; Inouye et al., 2014).

Dementia, delirium, and depression are manifestations of serious pathology and require urgent assessment and intervention (Heeren et al., 2016). However, changes in the cognitive function of older persons are often seen as "normal" and are thus not investigated. Any change in mental status in an older person requires appropriate assessment. Knowledge about cognitive function in aging and appropriate assessment and evaluation are the keys to differentiating

TABLE 21.1 Differentiating Delirium, Depression, and Dementia

CHARACTERISTIC	DELIRIUM	DEPRESSION	DEMENTIA
Onset	Sudden, abrupt	Recent, may relate to life change	Insidious, slow (over years), often unrecognized until deficits are obvious
Course over 24 hours	Fluctuating, often worse at night	Fairly stable, may be worse in the morning	Fairly stable, may change with stress
Consciousness	Disturbed	Clear	Clear
Alertness	Increased, decreased, or variable	Normal	Generally normal
Psychomotor activity	Increased, decreased, or mixed	Variable, agitated or retarded	Normal, may have apraxia or agnosia
Duration	Hours to weeks	Variable, at least 2 weeks and may be chronic	Years
Attention	Disordered, fluctuates	Little impairment	Generally normal but may have trouble focusing
Orientation	Usually impaired, fluctuates	Usually normal; may answer "I don't know" to questions, or may not answer	Often impaired
Thinking	Disorganized, rambling, illogical, or incoherent	May be slow; hopelessness, helplessness	Difficulty finding words, **perseveration,** impoverished thoughts, difficulty with abstraction, delusions in severe cases
Perception	Disturbed; illusions, hallucinations, misperceptions	Misperception usually absent	Intact, hallucinations in severe cases
Affect	Variable but may look disturbed, frightened	Flat	Slowed response, may be labile

Source: Adapted from Heeren, P., Flamaing, J., Tournoy, J., et al. (2016). Assessing cognitive function. In M. Boltz, E. Capezuti, T. Fulmer, et al. (Eds.). *Evidence-based geriatric nursing protocols for best practice* (5th ed.). New York: Springer Publishing Company; Sendelbach, S., Guthrie, P. F., & Schoenfelder, D. P. (2009). Acute confusion/delirium. *Journal of Gerontological Nursing, 35*(11), 11–18. doi:10.3928/00989134-20090930-01.

the three syndromes. Table 21.1 presents the clinical features and differences in cognitive and behavioural characteristics in delirium, dementia, and depression.

COGNITIVE ASSESSMENT

An older person with a change in cognitive function needs a thorough assessment to identify the presence of specific pathological conditions, as well as to rule out potentially reversible causes of cognitive impairment. Pathological conditions causing impairment of cognition include delirium, dementia, depression, Parkinson's disease, and stroke. During the assessment,

the physical environment should be comfortable and free from distractions that could affect the older person's performance.

Cognitive assessment is a component of the mental status examination conducted by nurses and other health care providers (see Chapter 24). Mental status is assessed through observation and careful interviewing, and the examination may also include standardized assessments. Screening instruments provide some information about cognitive status and may indicate a need for a more comprehensive cognitive assessment.

The components of a cognitive assessment are level of consciousness; orientation to person, place, and time; immediate, short-term, recent, and long-term memory; attention and concentration; abstract reasoning; and problem solving. In addition, **aphasia, apraxia,** and **agnosia** are assessed when there is an indication of cognitive disturbance.

The literature reveals that both nurses and physicians in all settings routinely fail to appropriately assess an individual's cognitive functioning. Pathological conditions are often undiagnosed, reversible causes are not identified, and opportunities for early intervention are missed. As a result, the affected person experiences greater impairment and functional decline (Heeren et al., 2016). There are a number of excellent resources to assist nurses in assessing cognition (Box 21.1). Many of these resources are available on streaming video or as e-learning instructions.

Screening for Cognitive Impairment

Screening can determine if cognitive impairment exists, but basic screening methods are insufficient to diagnose specific pathological conditions. If impairment is identified through screening, the person should be referred for a more comprehensive evaluation to confirm a diagnosis of dementia, delirium, depression, or some other health problem (Heeren et al., 2016). Screening for depression should be conducted with instruments such as the Geriatric Depression Scale (see Chapter 13). A comprehensive evaluation includes a complete assessment, including a laboratory workup, to rule out any medical causes of cognitive impairment. Formal cognitive testing, neuro-psychological examination, interview (of family and patient), observation, and functional assessment are additional components of a comprehensive assessment. **Computed tomography** (CT), **magnetic resonance imaging** (MRI), and an **electro-encephalogram** (EEG) may be indicated in the diagnostic process. Several evidence-informed guidelines are available for the assessment of changes in cognition, including the Registered Nurses' Association of Ontario Best Practice Guideline *Delirium, Dementia, and Depression in Older Adults: Assessment and Care* (http://www.rnao.org).

The Short Portable Mental Status Questionnaire, the Mini-Cog, the Confusion Assessment

---

BOX 21.1   Resources for Assessment of Cognition

Try This Series (ConsultGeri.org)
Issue 3: Mental status assessment of older persons: The Mini-Cog (article and video)
Issue 13: Confusion Assessment Method (CAM) (article and video)
Issue 25: The Confusion Assessment Method for the Intensive Care Unit (CAM-ICU)
Issue D3: Brief evaluation of executive dysfunction—an essential refinement in the assessment of cognitive impairment
Issue D8: Assessing and managing delirium in persons with dementia (article and video)

Other Resources
Canadian Coalition for Seniors' Mental Health. National guidelines: The assessment and treatment of delirium; Clinician's Pocket Card: Delirium: Assessment & treatment for older adults: Interactive, case-based tutorial (http://www.ccsmh.ca.)
Hospital Elder Life Program (HELP) (http://www.hospitalelderlifeprogram.org/for-clinicians/clinician-resources/.)
BC Guidelines. Cognitive impairment - recognition, diagnosis and management in primary care (http://www2.gov.bc.ca/gov/content/health/practitioner-professional-resources/bc-guidelines/cognitive-impairment.)
Montreal Cognitive Assessment (MoCA) (http://www.mocatest.org.)
Registered Nurses' Association of Ontario (RNAO). Best Practice Guideline: Delirium, dementia, and depression in older adults: Assessment and care and e-learning course (http://www.rnao.ca.)
Tullmann, D. F., Fletcher, K., & Foreman, M. D. (2012). Nursing Standard of Practice Protocol: Delirium (https://consultgeri.org/geriatric-topics/delirium.)

Method, the Neecham-Champagne Confusion Scale (NEECHAM), and the Montreal Cognitive Assessment are examples of screening instruments (see Chapter 13). These instruments may also be used to monitor and evaluate cognitive status. Box 21.1 presents other suggestions for the assessment and screening of cognitive impairment.

Considerations in Cognitive Assessment

Cognitive functioning assessments are often stressful experiences for older persons. Many older persons worry about developing memory problems or dementia. Cognitive tests and poor performance on memory tests often cause great anxiety. Assessment of cognitive functioning can be perceived by the person as "intrusive, intimidating, fatiguing, and offensive; characteristics that can seriously and negatively affect performance" (Heeren et al., 2016, p. 81). Too often, assessments are done when a person is not wearing his or her hearing aids or eyeglasses, or the person is rushed through a series of questions in a noisy, distracting environment, without any preparation or explanation.

It is important to attend to these concerns by establishing rapport and developing a therapeutic relationship, ensuring comfort (pain relief), accommodating physical impairments such as hearing and vision loss, creating an environment free of distractions, and putting the person in the best environment to ensure that performance is truly reflective of ability. The challenge is to stress the importance of the assessment without creating undue anxiety for the person. Heeren et al. (2016) warn that "it is essential to avoid counterproductive statements that describe the assessment as consisting of 'simple,' 'silly,' or 'stupid' questions. These tend to diminish motivation to perform and heighten anxiety when errors are committed."

Timing is also important; cognitive assessments should not be conducted immediately upon the person's awakening from sleep or immediately before or after meals or medical diagnostic and therapeutic procedures (Heeren et al., 2016). What seems to be a routine procedure to health care providers can be very intimidating for an older person, especially one who is ill or frail.

DELIRIUM

ETIOLOGY

Delirium is most often a result of complex interactions among predisposing factors (e.g., vulnerability due to predisposing conditions, such as cognitive impairment, severe illness, and sensory impairment) and precipitating factors or insults (e.g., medications, procedures, restraints, iatrogenic events) (Inouye,

2006). Although a single factor, such as an infection, can trigger an episode of delirium, several coexisting factors are also likely to be present. A highly vulnerable older person requires fewer precipitating factors to develop delirium (Inouye, 2006; Voyer et al., 2010).

The exact patho-physiological mechanisms involved in the development and progression of delirium remain uncertain, and further research is needed to understand its neuro-pathogenesis. Delirium is thought to be related to disturbances in the neurotransmitters in the brain—such as acetylcholine deficiency or dopamine excess (Inouye et al., 2014). These neurotransmitters modulate the control of cognitive function, behaviour, and mood, and their imbalance results in the cognitive changes of delirium. The causes of delirium are in most cases reversible; therefore, accurate assessment and diagnosis are critical. Delirium is given many labels, among which are *acute confusional state, acute brain syndrome, confusion, reversible dementia, metabolic encephalopathy,* and *toxic psychosis.* The correct term is "delirium."

INCIDENCE AND PREVALENCE

Delirium is a prevalent, serious, and often preventable disorder that occurs in older persons across the continuum of care. Delirium may affect more than half of hospitalized older persons and as many as 87% of older persons in Critical Care Units (CCUs) (Dahlke & Phinney, 2008) and intensive care units (Sweeny et al., 2008). Older people who have undergone surgery and those with dementia are particularly vulnerable to delirium. The prevalence of delirium is as high as 65% after orthopedic surgery, particularly hip fracture repair (Rigney, 2006). At the time of discharge from the hospital, approximately 30 to 90% of patients who experienced delirium continue to show symptoms. In a study of older persons admitted to a home care agency after hospital discharge, 46% had delirium at the time of admission. Of even greater significance, 50% of that group lived alone (Marcantonio et al., 2003). Delirium can significantly affect functional outcomes and mortality in long-term care (LTC) homes, where prevalence of delirium is between 6 and 40% (Canadian Coalition for Seniors' Mental Health [CCSMH], 2006a).

The incidence of delirium superimposed on dementia ranges from 22 to 89% (Tullmann et al.,

2016). A Canadian investigation of the prevalence of delirium in an acute care facility found that 68% of older patients with pre-existing dementia had delirium at the time of admission (Voyer et al., 2006). In a study of LTC residents with dementia, the same research group identified delirium in 26.5 to 45.8% of residents, depending on which diagnostic criteria were applied (Voyer et al., 2009). Older patients with dementia are three to five times more likely to develop delirium, and delirium is less likely to be recognized and treated than is delirium without dementia (Fick & Mion, 2005). Delirium superimposed on dementia is associated with high mortality among hospitalized older people (Bellelli et al., 2007). Changes in the mental status of older people with dementia are often attributed to underlying dementia, or "sundowning," and are thus not investigated. This is particularly significant, because about 25% of all older patients in acute care settings may have Alzheimer's disease or another dementia (Voelker, 2008).

RECOGNITION OF DELIRIUM

Delirium is a medical emergency and one of the most significant geriatric syndromes (Waszynski, 2007). However, it is often not recognized by nurses and other health care providers. Studies indicate that delirium is unrecognized in 34 to 90% of patients and residents in acute and LTC settings (Barron & Holmes, 2013; Voyer et al., 2012). Failure to recognize delirium, identify the underlying causes, and implement timely interventions contribute to higher mortality and worse outcomes (CCSMH, 2006a).

Factors that contribute to the lack of recognition of delirium by health care providers include inadequate education about delirium, a lack of formal assessment methods, and ageist attitudes (Waszynski, 2007). A Canadian study investigated interventions nurses use to assess, prevent, and treat delirium, as well as the challenges and barriers nurses face in this work (Dahlke & Phinney, 2008). The authors concluded that cognitive changes in older people are often labelled "confusion" by nurses and physicians; frequently accepted as part of normal aging; and rarely questioned. If nurses believe that confusion is normal in older persons, they are less likely to recognize symptoms of delirium as a medical emergency necessitating their attention and intervention. Confusion in

a child or younger adult is recognized as a medical emergency, but confusion in older persons is often accepted as a natural occurrence, "part of the older person's personality" (Dahlke & Phinney, 2008, p. 46).

In Dahlke and Phinney's study, nurses reported that caring for patients with delirium was seen as "annoying, frustrating and not interesting" (Dahlke & Phinney, 2008, p. 45). Nurses reported that the care of older patients with delirium interfered with what was perceived as the "real work" of caring for a medical or surgical patient. Insufficient knowledge, inadequate time, and lack of resources also influenced appropriate care. The authors concluded that nurses are faced with the predicament of fitting care for older persons into a system that does not recognize the unique needs of this population. Clearly, health care providers' education and attitudes about older people must be addressed to improve care outcomes for the growing number of older persons who need care.

RISK FACTORS FOR DELIRIUM

Identification of risk factors, prompt and appropriate assessment, and continued surveillance are the cornerstones of delirium prevention. The model presented by Inouye and Charpentier (1996) explains the interaction between baseline vulnerability factors for delirium (i.e., factors present at the time of admission) and precipitating factors for delirium (i.e., things that happen to patients while hospitalized). This model has been used to refine screening instruments and to design hospital environments and systems that minimize delirium risk through a program called the Hospital Elder Life Program (HELP) (Inouye, 2003, 2007). Predisposing risk factors and precipitating risk factors are listed in Box 21.2. Unrelieved or inadequately treated pain significantly increases the risk of delirium (Inouye et al., 2014). Medications account for 22 to 39% of all deliriums, and all medications, particularly those with anticholinergic effects and any new medications, should be considered suspect. Invasive equipment such as nasogastric tubes, intravenous (IV) lines, catheters, and restraints also contribute to delirium by interfering with the normal feedback mechanisms of the body. Persons with multiple predisposing factors are more vulnerable to delirium; for such persons, "a seemingly benign insult—e.g., a dose of a sedative-hypnotic drug—may be enough to

---

BOX 21.2	Predisposing and Precipitating Risk Factors for Delirium

Predisposing Risk Factors

- Demographic characteristics (age 65 years or older, male sex)
- Cognitive status (dementia, cognitive impairment, history of delirium, depression)
- Functional status (dependence, immobility, low level of activity, history of falls)
- Sensory impairment (visual, hearing)
- Decreased oral intake (dehydration, malnutrition)
- Medications (multiple psychoactive medications, many medications, alcohol abuse)
- Coexisting medical conditions (severe illness, multiple coexisting conditions, chronic renal or hepatic disease, history of stroke, neurological diseases, metabolic derangements, fracture or trauma, terminal illness, human immunodeficiency virus infection)

Precipitating Risk Factors

- Medications (sedative-hypnotic, narcotic, anticholinergic medications; multiple medications; alcohol or medication withdrawal)
- Primary neurological diseases (stroke, intracranial bleeding, meningitis or encephalitis)
- Intercurrent illnesses (infections, iatrogenic complications, severe acute illness, hypoxia, shock, fever or hypothermia, anemia, dehydration, poor nutritional status, low serum albumin level, metabolic derangements [e.g., electrolyte or acid–base])
- Surgery (orthopedic, cardiac, prolonged cardiopulmonary bypass, noncardiac)
- Environmental (admission to Critical Care Unit, physical restraints, bladder catheter, multiple procedures)
- Pain
- Emotional stress
- Prolonged sleep deprivation

Source: Adapted from Inouye, S. (2006). Delirium in older persons. *New England Journal of Medicine, 354*(11), 1157–1165 (Tables 2 & 3).

BOX 21.3	Risk Factors for Delirium Severity in LTC Homes

Absence of the following:
- Reading eyeglasses
- Aids to orientation
- Family member
- Glass of water

Presence of the following:
- Bed rails
- Other restraints

Source: McCusker, J., Cole, M. G., Voyer, P., et al. (2013). Environmental factors predict the severity of delirium symptoms in long-term care residents with and without delirium. *Journal of the American Geriatrics Society, 61,* 502–511. doi:10.1111/jgs.12164.

---

precipitate delirium" (Inouye et al., 2014, p. 912). For those with low or no vulnerability, delirium "develops only after exposure to a series of noxious insults, such as general anaesthesia, major surgery, several psychoactive medications, a stay in an ICU, or sleep deprivation" (Inouye et al., 2014, p. 912).

Among residents of LTC homes, predisposing factors may be more predictive of delirium than precipitating factors are (Voyer et al., 2010). Environmental factors that are associated with worsening delirium symptoms among LTC residents are presented in Box 21.3. The effects of these factors were more significant for residents with dementia than for other residents (McCusker et al., 2013).

CLINICAL SUBTYPES OF DELIRIUM

Delirium is categorized into three clinical subtypes, according to the level of the person's alertness and psychomotor activity—hyperactive, hypoactive, and mixed. *Hyperactive delirium* is characterized by agitation, vigilance, **hallucinations,** restlessness, and hyperactivity. *Hypoactive delirium* is characterized by lethargy and decreased motor activity. *Mixed delirium* comprises alternating features of hyperactive and hypoactive delirium. In settings other than Critical Care Units (CCUs), approximately 30% of delirium is hyperactive, 24% is hypoactive, and 46% is mixed. Because of the increased severity of illness and the use of psychoactive medications, hypoactive delirium may be more prevalent in the CCU. Although the negative consequences of hyperactive delirium are serious, the hypoactive subtype is missed more often and is associated with a worse prognosis because of the development of complications such as aspiration, pulmonary embolism, pressure ulcers, and pneumonia. Hypoactive delirium is associated with increased hospital stays, a longer duration of delirium, and higher mortality.

CONSEQUENCES OF DELIRIUM

Delirium has serious consequences, and nurses play a key role in preventing these (Tullmann et al., 2016). Delirium results in significant distress for the person experiencing it, the person's family and significant others, and health care providers. Delirium during hospitalization is associated with high morbidity and mortality, functional decline, increased postoperative complications, increased length of hospital stay and hospital re-admissions, increased services after discharge, long-term cognitive decline, and high rates of institutionalization (Inouye et al., 2014; Tullmann et al., 2016).

Although delirium is considered a reversible cause of altered mental status, a significant number of older persons with delirium never return to their baseline cognitive status, especially in the presence of pre-existing dementia (Inouye et al., 2014). Several studies reported that older persons with delirium continue to manifest symptoms up to 6 months after discharge, along with persistent memory deficits of particular significance (Inouye et al., 2014).

 IMPLICATIONS FOR GERONTOLOGICAL NURSING AND HEALTHY AGING

ASSESSMENT

To detect changes in cognition, it is important to determine the usual mental status. If the older person cannot convey this to the nurse, family members or other caregivers who are with the person can be asked to provide this information. In hospital, if the patient is alone, the responsible party or the institution transferring the patient can provide this information by phone. Nurses cannot assume that the person's current mental status represents his or her usual state and cannot attribute altered mental status to age or assume that dementia is present. All older persons, regardless of their current cognitive function, should have a formal assessment to identify possible delirium when admitted to hospital (see Box 21.1). Several instruments can be used to assess the presence and severity of delirium.

The following instruments can be used to assess the presence and severity of delirium: the Confusion Assessment Method (CAM) (Inouye et al., 1990), the NEECHAM Confusion Scale (Neelon et al., 1996), and the Delirium Index (see Chapter 13). A Canadian practice guideline (CCSMH, 2006a) recommends the CAM for screening and as a diagnostic aid in hospital medical, surgical, and emergency settings and recommends the CAM-ICU (Ely et al., 2001) for nonverbal CCU patients. Training is necessary for the valid use of the CAM. A video demonstrating its use is available at http://www.consultgeri.org, and a training manual and scoring guide are also available (Inouye, 2003).

Persons with dementia are at high risk of delirium superimposed on dementia and of having their delirium overlooked or misidentified by nurses (Voyer et al., 2008; Voyer et al., 2009). The assessment of these patients must involve a person or persons who know the patient's baseline cognitive functioning, such as a family or staff member who has worked with the person at home or at an LTC home. In an LTC home, health care aides are often the first to identify subtle changes in a resident's behaviour that may indicate delirium; nurses in this setting must investigate any health care aide reports of changes in a person's behaviour. For all older patients who are at risk for delirium, assessment with the CAM should be integrated into routine assessments, upon admission to hospital or an LTC home, in the first assessment by the home care nurse, and during every shift in hospital or routinely in LTC and community settings (Tullmann et al., 2016). When a patient is identified as having delirium, a reassessment should be conducted as frequently as every 2 hours.

Documenting specific objective indicators of alterations in mental status rather than using the global nonspecific term "confusion" will lead to more-appropriate prevention, detection, and management of delirium and its negative consequences. Findings from assessments using a validated instrument should be combined with observation, chart review, and physiological findings. Delirium often has a fluctuating course and can be difficult to recognize, so assessment must be ongoing and include multiple data sources.

INTERVENTIONS

Effective care for delirium must include vigilant prevention efforts, as well as treatment to target the root

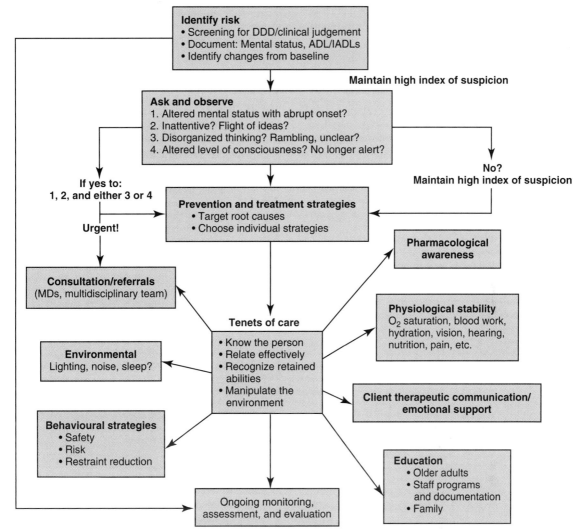

FIGURE 21.1 Flow-of-care diagram of caregiving strategies for delirium. *Source:* Registered Nurses' Association of Ontario (RNAO). (2004). *Caregiving strategies for older persons with delirium, dementia, and depression* [p. 33, Fig. 2]. Toronto, ON: Author.

cause of delirium that cannot be prevented. This care includes risk screening, ongoing assessment, and the implementation of prevention and treatment strategies (Fig. 21.1).

Nonpharmacological

Intervention for delirium begins with prevention. Prevention requires the identification of the person's risk factors for delirium and a formal assessment of the person's mental status. Nurses play a pivotal role

in the identification of delirium, and it is imperative that they accurately report patients' mental status to the medical team so that potential causative factors can be identified and treated (Tullmann et al., 2016). Prevention should be targeted to the person's individual risk factors (RNAO, 2016).

Interprofessional, multicomponent approaches to delirium prevention have the best evidence of effectiveness. One such approach, the well-researched Hospital Elder Life Program (HELP), focuses on managing the following six risk factors for delirium: cognitive impairment, sleep deprivation, immobility, visual impairments, hearing impairments, and dehydration. Standardized intervention protocols target each risk factor (Hospital Elder Life Program, 2017; Inouye, 2006; Inouye et al., 1999). The elements of the program are daily visitors, therapeutic activities, early mobilization, nonpharmacological sleep protocol, hearing and vision protocol, oral volume repletion and mealtime assistance, interdisciplinary care, transition assistance, and staff education (Hospital Elder Life Program, 2017). Patient outcomes with the use of this model include a 40% reduction in the incidence of delirium and a decrease in the number of days and episodes of delirium. There is a demonstrated cost effectiveness in hospitals and LTC homes when this model is applied (Inouye, 2006).

Most HELP interventions could be considered part of good nursing care. The interventions are at the system level (e.g., keeping the unit quiet at night by using vibrating beepers instead of paging systems, having volunteers be with restless patients, implementing fall risk reduction interventions such as low beds and bed and chair alarms) and at the level of the health care provider (e.g., offering herbal tea or warm milk instead of sleeping medications, removing catheters and other devices that hamper movement as soon as possible, assessing and managing pain, encouraging mobilization, and correcting hearing and vision deficits).

The family HELP program, an adaptation and extension of the original HELP program, trains family caregivers in selected protocols (e.g., orientation, therapeutic activities, use of vision and hearing aids). The active engagement of family members in preventive interventions for delirium is feasible and supports a culture of family-centred care (Rosenbloom & Fick, 2014). (Further information on the HELP can be found at http://elderlife.med.yale.edu/public/public-main.php).

When delirium is present, strategies used to prevent it should be maintained or implemented. In addition, identifying and treating the root cause of the delirium is vital. Because delirium is so complex, with multifactorial causes, effective treatment is often multifactorial and dependent on interprofessional collaboration. Caring for patients with delirium can be a challenging experience. They can be difficult to communicate with and can exhibit disturbing behaviours, such as pulling out IV lines or attempting to get out of bed. They may disrupt medical treatment and compromise safety. It is important for nurses to realize that the patient's behaviour is an attempt to communicate and express needs such as pain or anxiety. The patient with delirium feels frightened and out of control. The more the nurse is calm and reassuring, the safer the patient will feel. Box 21.4 presents suggested interventions for delirium prevention and treatment, including effective communication strategies.

A commonly used intervention for older persons with delirium in acute care is the use of "sitters" or "constant observers." The costs associated with this practice can be very high, and data indicate that the use of sitters or constant observers does not consistently improve safety when delirium is present. Nor does this practice assist in identifying the causes of delirium or identifying appropriate interventions (Sweeny et al., 2008).

Pharmacological

Benzodiazepines and (at times) other psychotropic medications are used in the treatment of delirium associated with alcohol withdrawal (Mirijello et al., 2015). Clinical trials of the use of sedatives and antipsychotics in the treatment of delirium due to causes other than alcohol withdrawal show either no effect or worse outcomes for patients receiving them. Thus, pharmacological treatment of delirium is not recommended (Inouye et al., 2014).

OVERVIEW OF DEMENTIA

In contrast to delirium, which is usually a reflection of an acute physiological disturbance, dementia is an irreversible state that progresses over years and causes memory impairment and loss of other intellectual abilities severe enough interfere with daily life. Other key features of dementia are the following:

- Aphasia—loss of the ability to express and understand spoken and written language
- Apraxia—inability to carry out purposeful movements, although motor and sensory abilities are intact

BOX 21.4	Multicomponent Care Strategies for Delirium

Consultation and Referral

- Initiate prompt consultation to specialized services when symptoms develop or worsen, for assessment and possible treatment of a causative condition.

Physiological Stability/Reversible Causes

- Maintain ongoing assessment, interpretation, management, documentation, and communication of physiological status to interprofessional team.
- Ensure adequate hydration, nutrition, mobilization, and sleep.
- Avoid restraints.
- Provide hearing aids and eyeglasses.
- Assess and manage pain.
- Remove unnecessary catheters and IV lines (see Chapter 9).

Pharmacological

- Maintain—in collaboration with interprofessional team—an awareness of medications that contribute to delirium, and review patients' medication profiles for potential deliriogenic medications (see Beers Criteria for Potentially Inappropriate Medication Use in Older Adults at http://www.consultgeri.org).
- Limit use of psychoactive medication to the treatment of specific symptoms; use as a last resort.
- Discontinue nonessential medications when delirium is present.

Environmental

- Identify, reduce, or eliminate environmental factors that may contribute to delirium.

- Ensure adequate sensory stimulation (provide light during the day, and reduce light at night).
- Introduce one task at a time; provide structure and predictable routine.
- Implement noise-reduction strategies.
- Foster a familiar environment (familiar objects are in sight of the patient; encourage family or friends to stay with the patient; consistent caregivers; minimal relocation).

Education

- Provide delirium education to the patient and family (see relevant Registered Nurses' Association of Ontario [RNAO] Health Education Fact Sheet at http://www.rnao.org/bestpractices.
- Provide postdelirium support and education.

Communication and Emotional Support

- Identify yourself.
- Establish and maintain a therapeutic relationship.
- Provide orientation and support.
- Communicate clearly and speak slowly.
- Tell the patient what you want him or her to do, not what you do not want him or her to do.
- Provide explanations.
- Provide one-step directions; use gestures and demonstrations.
- Allow time for responses.

Behavioural Interventions

- Avoid the use of restraints.
- Monitor safety regularly.

Sources: Adapted from Registered Nurses' Association of Ontario (RNAO). (2016). *Delirium, dementia, and depression in older adults: Assessment and care.* Toronto, ON: Author; Tullmann, D. F., Blevins, C., & Fletcher, K. (2016). Delirium: Prevention, early recognition, and treatment. In M. Boltz, E. Capezuti, T. Fulmer, et al. (Eds.), *Evidence-based geriatric nursing protocols for best practice* (5th ed., pp. 251–261). New York, NY: Springer Publishing Co.

- Agnosia—inability to recognize common objects or faces of familiar people despite intact sensory abilities
- Disturbances in executive functioning—difficulty in planning, organizing, sequencing, and abstracting

TYPES OF DEMENTIA

Degenerative dementias include Alzheimer's disease, Parkinson's disease dementia, dementia with Lewy bodies, and frontotemporal lobe dementias. Alzheimer's disease (AD) accounts for 50 to 70% of all dementia cases. Vascular cognitive impairment encompasses several syndromes—vascular dementia; primary neurodegenerative disease mixed with vascular dementia; and cognitive impairment of vascular origin that does not meet the dementia criteria.

Less commonly occurring dementias are Creutzfeldt-Jakob disease (subacute spongiform encephalopathy), human immunodeficiency virus (HIV)–related dementia, and Korsakoff syndrome.

Normal pressure hydrocephalus causes a dementia characterized by **ataxia,** incontinence, and memory impairment. This disease is reversible and is treated with a shunt that diverts cerebrospinal fluid away from the brain. Many dementias in old age can be described as mixed dementia, produced by a number of primary and secondary causes. For example, dementia can be caused by a combination of AD, vascular brain changes, and prior alcoholism (two primary causes and one secondary cause). Many dementias manifest symptoms of cognitive impairment. However, associated features and the age of onset vary among the different types of dementia syndromes (Table 21.2).

INCIDENCE AND PREVALENCE

Approximately 564,000 Canadians (1% of the population) and 35.6 million people worldwide have dementia (Chambers et al., 2016).

The prevalence of AD increases with age, doubling approximately every 5 years for persons between the ages of 60 and 95 years. An estimated 35% of people older than 85 years have AD. If current trends continue, by the year 2031 the increasing prevalence of AD will mean that 937,000 Canadians will be affected (Chambers et al., 2016). The direct health care cost of dementia is over $10.4 billion (Chambers et al., 2016), not including the cost ($1.2 billion) of almost 20 million hours of caregiving time by informal caregivers (Chambers et al., 2016). Research in Alberta found a higher prevalence of dementia among First Nations people, along with a younger age of onset. This may be explained by increased vulnerability associated with social determinants of health (Jacklin et al., 2013) (see Chapter 1).

Accurate diagnosis is important, since treatment and prognosis vary. However, dementia is difficult to diagnose, and the rate of diagnosis of dementia in primary care is low (Parmar et al., 2014). The complexity of dementia, diagnostic uncertainty (there are no diagnostic tests, and the symptoms overlap those of other disorders), and a tendency to rely on specialists rather than family physicians for diagnosis mean that reaching a diagnosis can take a long time (Drummond et al., 2016; Parmar et al., 2014). Furthermore, the period from the time persons first notice symptoms to the time they talk to a physician about the symptoms is typically a long one. More timely diagnoses and treatment will require appropriate education for the public and for health care providers.

ALZHEIMER'S DISEASE

First described in 1906 by Dr. Alois Alzheimer, AD is a cerebral degenerative disorder of unknown origin. The disease destroys the proteins of nerve cells of the cerebral cortex by diffuse infiltration with nonfunctional tissue called neurofibrillary tangles and plaques. The tangles and plaques represent the death of nerve cells throughout the brain, which shrinks to about one-third of its normal weight. The tangles consist of a protein called tau protein, which "clogs" the insides of brain cells and their connections. Deposits of beta-amyloid accumulate abnormally in the brains of people with AD. The disease is progressive and is accompanied by increasing memory loss, inability to concentrate, personality deterioration, and impaired judgement.

The course of AD ranges from 1 to 20 years. The typical life expectancy is 8 to 9 years after the onset of symptoms; usually, death occurs as a result of pulmonary infections, urinary tract infections, pressure ulcers, or iatrogenic disorders. The most important risk factor is age. About 8% of Canadians aged 65 years and older have dementia. Among those aged 65 to 74 years, the prevalence is 2.5%, increasing to 11% among 75- to 84-year-old persons and 35% among those aged 85 years and older (Canadian Study of Health and Aging, 2002).

There are two types of AD: early-onset dementia and late-onset dementia. Early-onset dementia is rare, affecting only 5% of all people who have AD, and develops between the ages of 30 and 60 years. It has a stronger genetic component than late-onset dementia has (Box 21.5).

The focus of AD research is on the interaction between risk-factor genes and lifestyle or environmental factors (Table 21.3). In regard to the pathogenesis and clinical manifestations of dementia (especially AD and vascular dementia), increasing evidence strongly points to the potential risk roles of vascular disorders (e.g., obesity, dyslipidemia, hypertension, cigarette smoking, and cerebrovascular lesions) and the potential protective roles of psychosocial factors (e.g., higher education, regular exercise, healthy diet, intellectually challenging leisure activity, and active socially integrated lifestyles). Head trauma is also a risk factor, as is a history of clinical depression (Alzheimer Society of Canada, 2015).

TABLE 21.2	Types of Dementia and Typical Characteristics
TYPE OF DEMENTIA	**CHARACTERISTICS**
Alzheimer's disease (AD)	Most common type of dementia, accounting for 60–80% of cases. Hallmark abnormalities are deposits of the protein fragment beta-amyloid (plaques) and twisted strands of the protein tau (tangles). Difficulty remembering names and recent events; difficulty expressing oneself with words; spatial cognition problems; impaired reasoning and judgement; apathy; and depression are often early symptoms. Language disturbances may also be a presenting symptom. Later symptoms include impaired judgement, disorientation, behaviour changes, and difficulty speaking, swallowing, and walking.
Vascular dementia (also known as multi-infarct or poststroke dementia or vascular cognitive impairment)	Second most common type of dementia. Impairment is caused by decreased blood flow to parts of the brain, due to a series of small strokes that block arteries. Symptoms often overlap with those of AD, although memory may not be as seriously affected.
Mixed dementia	Characterized by the hallmark abnormalities of AD and another type of dementia (most commonly vascular dementia, but also other types, such as dementia with Lewy bodies). More common than previously thought. Neurodegenerative changes occur along with vascular changes.
Parkinson's disease dementia	Later onset of dementia (at least 1 year after onset of parkinsonian features). Hallmark abnormality is Lewy bodies (abnormal deposits of the protein alpha-synuclein) that forms inside the nerve cells of the brain.
Dementia with Lewy bodies	Pattern of decline is similar to that of AD, including problems with memory and judgement as well as behaviour changes. Alertness and severity of cognitive symptoms may fluctuate daily. Visual hallucinations, muscle rigidity, and tremors are common. Exhibits a sensitivity to neuroleptic drugs, so these medications should be avoided.
Creutzfeldt-Jakob disease and variant Creutzfeldt-Jakob disease (vCJD) (transmissible bovine spongiform encephalopathy [mad cow disease])	A rapidly fatal and rare form of dementia, characterized by tiny holes that give the brain a "spongy" appearance under microscope. May be hereditary, occur sporadically, or be transmitted from infected individuals. Failing memory, behavioural changes, lack of coordination, visual disturbances. vCJD occurs in younger patients; may be caused by contaminated cattle feed.
Frontotemporal dementia	Involves damage to brain cells, especially in the front and side regions of the brain. Symptoms include change in personality and behaviour and difficulty with language. Pick's disease, characterized by Pick's bodies in the brain, is one form of frontotemporal dementia.
Normal-pressure hydrocephalus	Caused by buildup of fluid in the brain without corresponding increase in cerebrospinal fluid pressure. Symptoms include difficulty walking (ataxic gait), memory loss, and incontinence. Can sometimes be corrected with surgical installation of a shunt to drain excess fluid.

Source: Data from Alzheimer's Association. (2010). 2010 Alzheimer's disease facts and figures. *Alzheimers and Dementia, 6*(2), 158–194.

BOX 21.5   Genetics in Alzheimer's Disease

Genetic Basis

Early Onset (Familial) (<60 years old at onset)
- Autosomal dominant disorder.
- Various mutations in the following genes:
  - Amyloid precursor protein *(APP)* gene on chromosome 21
  - Presenilin-1 *(PSEN1)* gene on chromosome 14
  - Presenilin-2 *(PSEN2)* gene on chromosome 1

Late Onset (Sporadic) (>60 years old at onset)
- Genetically more complex than early-onset form.
- Apolipoprotein E-4 *(ApoE-4)* allele on chromosome 19 increases the likelihood of developing Alzheimer's disease (AD).
- Presence of *ApoE-2* allele is associated with a lower risk of AD.

Incidence

Early Onset
- Rare form of AD, accounting for <5% of cases.
- Fifty percent risk of disease for children of affected parents.
- May occur in people as young as 30 years old.

Late Onset
- *ApoE-4* is present in about 40% of people with late-onset AD. (It is present in 25–30% of the normal population.)
- Many *ApoE-4*–positive people do not develop AD, and many *ApoE-4*–negative people do.

Genetic Testing

Early Onset
- Genetic screening is available for mutations on chromosomes 1, 14, and 21.

Late Onset
- Blood test can identify which *ApoE* allele a person has but cannot predict who will develop AD.
- *ApoE* testing is mainly used in research to identify people who may have an increased risk of developing AD.

Clinical Implications
- Genetic testing and counselling for family members of patients with early-onset AD may be appropriate.
- A positive test result for *ApoE-4* does not mean that the person will develop AD.

Source: Lewis, S. L., Dirksen, S .R., Heitkemper, M. M., et al. (2017). *Medical-surgical nursing: Assessment and management of clinical problems* (p. 1446). St. Louis, MO: Mosby.

Diagnosis of Alzheimer's Disease

The diagnostic guidelines for AD that are published by the National Institute on Aging and by the Alzheimer's Association (Hyman et al., 2012) are endorsed by the Fourth Canadian Consensus Conference on the Diagnosis and Treatment of Dementia (Moore et al., 2014). These guidelines describe three stages of AD—the preclinical stage, mild cognitive impairment, and dementia due to AD pathology. The only way to confirm a diagnosis of AD is to perform a brain biopsy after the person dies. Clinically, the diagnosis of AD is based on the history of the affected person and his or her family and on testing to rule out other disorders that may mimic the disease. Neuroimaging is not required in most cases but is indicated "if the presence of unsuspected cerebrovascular disease would change clinical management" (Moore et al., 2014, p. 436).

Preclinical Stage. In the preclinical stage, measurable changes in the brain, cerebrospinal fluid, or blood markers (or all three) are the earliest signs of the disease, but the person has not yet developed symptoms (such as memory loss). This preclinical, presymptomatic stage reflects the current view that AD begins causing changes in the brain up to 20 years before symptoms appear. Further research on biomarkers may make possible the prediction of who is at risk for mild cognitive impairment and AD and who would benefit most from interventions (Alzheimer's Association, 2012).

Mild Cognitive Impairment. A change in the level of cognition, in comparison to the prior level, signals mild cognitive impairment. The cognitive changes in this stage are more than would be expected for the person's age and educational background. Memory problems are enough to be noticed and measured but do not compromise a person's functioning. People with mild cognitive impairment may or may not progress to AD.

Alzheimer's Disease. In addition to memory loss, the early symptoms of AD may include declines in other aspects of cognition such as word-finding problems, vision or spatial issues, and impaired reasoning or judgement. The symptoms of AD are often present several years before a diagnosis is made. Apathy and depression may be the first and earliest signs of AD, occurring up to 3 years before diagnosis. The history

TABLE 21.3   Risk Factors and Protective Factors for Alzheimer's Disease: Potential Mechanisms

FACTOR	RISK	POTENTIAL MECHANISMS
Advanced age	Increased	Possible decreased brain reserves
Sex	Increased for females	Living longer, loss of neuroprotective effects of estrogen
Family history	Increased	Mutations of APP, presenilin-1, and presenilin-2 may result in oversecretion of beta-amyloid in familial AD; ApoE-4 allele increases risk of sporadic (late-onset) AD
Depression	Increased	May decrease brain reserves/transmitters
High-fat, high-cholesterol diet	Increased	Increased neuroinflammation; possible increased substrate for APP
CRP	Increased	Increased neuroinflammation
Homocysteine	Increased	Increased oxidative stress, free radical toxicity, increased atherosclerotic sequelae
Smoking	Increased	Accelerated cerebral atrophy, perfusional decline, white-matter lesions
Diabetes mellitus	Increased	Impaired glucose uptake in neuronal cells, decreased blood supply due to small-vessel disease
Hyperlipidemia	Increased	Increased beta-amyloid accumulation
Genetic	Increased	Mutations of presenilin-1, presenilin-2, APP
Hypertension	Increased	Decreased cerebral blood flow/cerebral ischemia, white matter lesions
Head trauma	Increased	Not fully understood—possible blood-brain barrier disruption
Obesity	Increased	Hyperlipidemia and hypertension and via their mechanisms described earlier
Mediterranean diet	Decreased	Decreased neuroinflammation, decreased oxidative stress, decreased $A\beta_{42}$ toxicity
Increased education	Decreased	May increase neural connections
Increased mental activity	Decreased	Cognitive reserve model—people cope better and can generate more neurons during lifetime
Increased physical activity	Decreased	Increased cerebral blood flow, increased brain-derived neurotrophic factor

AD, Alzheimer's disease; *ApoE-4,* apolipoprotein E-4; *APP,* amyloid precursor protein; *CRP,* C-reactive protein.
Source: Kamat, S., Kamat, A., & Grossberg, G. (2010). Dementia risk prediction: are we there yet? *Clinics in Geriatric Medicine, 26*(1), 113–123. doi:10.1016/j.cger.2009.12.001.

given by the affected person and the family is another important part of assessing and diagnosing probable AD. However, it often takes a long time for people who have dementia or their family members to recognize the early symptoms as something other than normal aging, and periods of up to 4 years from the emergence of the first symptom to the person's seeking of help are common (McCleary et al., 2013). Stigma associated with dementia also contributes to the delay in seeking help (Koehn et al., 2016). A delayed

diagnosis means that the affected person has been without critical support, resources, and treatment.

Cultural Differences

Research on the influence of culture and ethnicity on the recognition and interpretation of cognitive changes and on the assessment, diagnosis, and treatment of AD and other dementias is limited. Further research is needed to understand how various ethnocultural groups view dementia and how cultural beliefs about disease etiology and symptoms influence diagnosis, treatment, and help-seeking behaviours (Williams et al., 2010).

Research indicates that some minority ethnic groups are underrepresented in regard to seeking and receiving services for dementia. This underrepresentation may be related to specific cultural beliefs about mental illness and the causes of dementia. However, the following other factors also affect these persons' access to services: language, stigmatization, lack of knowledge about dementia and available resources, hesitancy to use services viewed as culturally incongruent, and barriers to physically accessing services (Koehn et al., 2016; Sayegh & Knight, 2013). The development of culturally and linguistically appropriate sources of information about dementia is important.

Pharmacological Treatment

Medication therapy with cholinesterase inhibitors offer hope for enhanced function and reduction of the speed of decline of AD. Cholinesterase inhibitors (ChEIs) that are approved to treat AD include donepezil (Aricept), rivastigmine (Exelon), and galantamine (Reminyl). Memantine (Ebixa), an N-methyl-D-aspartate antagonist, is indicated for the treatment of moderate to severe AD. Unlike the ChEIs, which increase the amount of acetylcholine in the brain, memantine blocks the effect of abnormal glutamate activity that may lead to neuronal cell death and cognitive dysfunction. Memantine may be used alone or in combination with a ChEI. The Fourth Canadian Consensus Conference on Diagnosis and Treatment of Dementia recommended the use of a ChEI for treatment of mild to severe AD, mixed AD and vascular dementia, and dementia associated with Parkinson's disease (Gauthier et al., 2012). The Conference's experts concluded that there is insufficient evidence for or against the use of ChEI for vascular dementia.

These medications may also be prescribed for MCI. Therapy should be long term, even if the person shows slight decline, provided that function is better than it would have been without treatment. These medications are usually well-tolerated, but adverse effects include gastrointestinal disturbances (nausea, vomiting, diarrhea, anorexia), sleep disturbances, and sedation (Fletcher, 2016). An initial low dose with slow

titration is recommended to minimize side effects. Rivastigmine (Exelon) is available in a patch that may be more convenient, has fewer adverse effects, and provides a consistent day-long dose. There is no evidence that one ChEI is more effective than another. Because the medications work in similar ways, it is not expected that switching from one to another will produce significantly different results. However, a person may respond better to one medication than to another, and there is evidence that galantamine (Reminyl) may be better tolerated (Fisher et al., 2017; Gauthier et al., 2012).

Cholinesterase inhibitors are associated with increased risk of bradycardia and syncope (and associated falls) (Hogan, 2014). The bradycardia may be transient and therefore difficult to detect in diagnostic investigations. The high mortality risk associated with falls for persons with dementia should be considered when the decision regarding whether to initiate ChEI therapy is made. Cardiac evaluation and careful monitoring are necessary.

Medication therapy is directed toward the symptoms of AD and does not affect the neuronal decline that will eventually produce severe disability. However, medications are likely to produce a plateau of brain function and functional abilities and delay the progression of AD. Delaying both disease onset and progression would significantly reduce the burden of AD, particularly in the late stages of the disease. Therapy with ChEIs has positive effects on the behavioural manifestations of AD.

VASCULAR DEMENTIA

Vascular dementia—also known as multi-infarct, post-stroke dementia, or vascular cognitive impairment—consists of a group of heterogeneous disorders arising from cerebrovascular insufficiency or ischemic or hemorrhagic brain damage. Vascular dementia (VaD) often coexists with AD (a combination known as mixed dementia). Memory may not be impaired or may be more mildly impaired than in AD (Fletcher, 2016). Apathy, mood changes, anxiety, and agitation are more common in VaD than in AD (Fletcher, 2016). Dementia after stroke is thought to occur in one-quarter to one-third of stroke cases. Hypertension, cardiac disease, diabetes, smoking, alcoholism, and dyslipidemia are risk factors for VaD.

The management of diabetes, hypertension, and dyslipidemia is important for the primary prevention of VaD. Secondary prevention includes treatments (e.g., the use of antihypertensives and antiplatelet medications) to prevent the recurrence of a vascular stroke.

LEWY BODY DEMENTIA

Lewy body dementia, widely underdiagnosed, is the second most common form of degenerative dementia. Lewy body dementia (LBD) is not a single disorder but rather a spectrum of disorders including dementia with Lewy bodies and Parkinson's disease dementia. Many individuals with LBD are erroneously diagnosed as having other types of dementia, most commonly AD, or Parkinson's disease if they present with movement problems. The presence of Lewy bodies, which are protein deposits in the nerve cells, characterizes LBD, and its presentation is different from that of AD; memory impairment is milder, and impaired executive function is common. Symptoms include cognitive fluctuations, unpredictable changes in concentration and attention, visual hallucinations, parkinsonian symptoms, rapid eye movement sleep behaviour disorder (see Chapter 10), and severe sensitivity to neuroleptics (Lewy Body Dementia Association, 2016).

No medications are approved specifically for the treatment of LBD, but ChEIs may offer symptomatic benefits. Early and accurate diagnosis of LBD is essential, because neuroleptics can cause a severe worsening of movement and a fatal condition known as neuroleptic malignant syndrome, which causes severe fever and muscle rigidity and can lead to kidney failure. Anticholinergics and some antiparkinsonian medications can worsen these symptoms. For more information on LBD, see https://www.lbda.org.

FRONTOTEMPORAL DEMENTIA

Frontotemporal dementia is a clinical syndrome associated with shrinkage of the frontal and temporal anterior lobes of the brain. Frontotemporal dementia (FTD) is linked to chromosomal abnormalities, and 30 to 40% of people with FTD have family members with a neuro-degenerative disease. Mean age at onset is between 52 and 56 years, but the disease has been found in younger and older persons as well. The disease progresses rapidly, and the prognosis is poor. As with LBD, FTD is often not accurately diagnosed. Its early symptoms are different from those of AD and are more often related to changes in personality and to inappropriate or bizarre social behaviour. There are no approved medications that slow the progress of FTD. Medications for which there is some evidence of effectiveness for depression associated with FTD include trazodone (Desyrel) and selective serotonin reuptake inhibitors. However, evidence of their effectiveness is mixed (Kirshner, 2014). Treatments are aimed at managing behavioural symptoms, compensating for functional decline, and supporting family caregivers (Barton et al., 2016). Evidence of the effectiveness of treatments for behavioural symptoms is limited.

 IMPLICATIONS FOR GERONTOLOGICAL NURSING AND HEALTHY AGING

PERSON-CENTRED CARE

Dementias such as AD have no cure, and although medications offer hope for improved function, the most important treatment for the disease is competent and compassionate person-centred care. Person-centred care looks beyond the disease and the tasks nurses must perform, to the person within and the nurse's relationship with that person. The focus is not on what nurses need to "do to persons" but rather on the persons themselves and how to enhance their well-being and quality of life.

Gerontological nurses know that the person, not the disease, is the focus of care, and they practise in the belief that a person with dementia is still a whole person, someone who can think, feel, learn, grow, and be in a relationship (RNAO, 2016). Person-centred care fosters abilities, supports limitations, ensures safety, enhances quality of life, prevents excess disability, and offers hope. The culture-change movement in LTC homes is grounded in the concept of person-centred care and quality of life (McGreevy, 2016).

Despite a growing body of evidence on the importance of person-centred care and therapeutic work with people with dementia, the emphasis in the literature and in practice continues to be on the care of the body (e.g., bathing and feeding) and the management of behavioural symptoms and "problem" behaviour. A focus on behaviour management can distract nurses from recognizing these behaviours as responses to the environment and indicators of unmet needs. Special skills and attitudes are required to nurse the person with dementia, and caring is paramount. It is not an area of nursing that "just anyone can do" (Splete, 2008, p. 11).

Quality of life, meaningful engagement, nutrition, activities of daily living (ADLs), maintenance of health and function, safety, communication, and caregiver needs and support are major care concerns for persons with dementia, their families, and staff members who care for them. The overriding goals in caring for older persons with dementia are to create a therapeutic **milieu** that nurtures the personhood of the individual and maintains quality of life, to maintain function and prevent excess disability, to structure the environment and relationships to maintain stability, and to compensate for the losses associated with the disease. Box 21.6 presents general nursing interventions in the care of persons with dementia.

BOX 21.6   General Nursing Interventions in Care of Persons With Dementia

- Create meaningful moments and activities.
- Structure daily living to maximize remaining abilities.
- Monitor the general health and impact of dementia on the management of the person's acute and chronic medical conditions, paying careful attention to the person's experience of pain and mental health.
- Create opportunities for social engagement, freedom of choice, self-expression, spirituality, and creativity.
- Support advance care planning and advanced directives.
- Educate caregivers in the areas of problem solving, resources access, long-range planning, emotional support, and respite.

Source: Adapted from Aselage, M. B. *Complex care needs in older adults with common cognitive disorders.* Retrieved from https://consultgeri.org/complex-care-needs-older-adults-dementia; McKeown, J., Fortune, D., & Dupuis, S. (2015). "It is like stepping into another world": Exploring the possibilities of using appreciative participatory action research to guide culture change work in community and long-term care. *Action Research, 14*(3), 318–334. doi:10.1177/1476750315618763.

Three common care concerns for people with moderate- to late-stage dementia are behaviour, ADLs, and wandering. (See Chapter 8 for a discussion of nutrition, see Chapter 3 for a discussion of communication, and see Chapter 23 for an in-depth discussion of family care for persons with dementia. The Hartford Institute for Geriatric Nursing's Try This Series lists many excellent resources for the care of persons with dementia, as does the Resources section at the end of this chapter.)

BEHAVIOUR CONCERNS AND NURSING MODELS OF CARE FOR PERSONS WITH DEMENTIA

Several nursing models of care are useful in guiding practice and assisting families and staff in providing care to people with dementia. The models share a common focus on understanding the importance of the meaning of behaviour of the person with dementia. Using these models, nurses can avoid labelling the behaviour of persons with dementia as aggressive (Cohen-Mansfield, 2000; Dupuis & Luh, 2005). The term "responsive behaviours" describes reactions that result from unmet needs or environmental stress (Dupuis & Luh, 2005). Whereas responsive behaviours are disruptive and distressing to people with dementia and their caregivers, using terms such as "aggressive" draws attention away from the perspective of the person (Talerico & Evans, 2000).

Four models—the Progressively Lowered Stress Threshold model, the need-driven dementia-compromised behaviour model, the recognition of retained abilities model, and the relating well model—describe the behaviour of the person with dementia as an interaction between the person's abilities and impairments and the physical and social environment. To understand these behaviours and provide care to a particular person with dementia, nurses and other care providers need to understand the person's experiences, abilities, and personality and how they align with the physical and social environment. The Alzheimer Society of Canada's *Guidelines for Care: Person-Centred Care of People with Dementia Living in Care Homes* presents extensive evidence-informed guidelines and instructions (Alzheimer Society of Canada, 2011).

BOX 21.7	Conditions Precipitating Responsive Behaviours in Persons With Dementia

- Communication deficits
- Pain or discomfort
- Acute medical problems
- Sleep disturbances
- Perceptual deficits
- Depression
- Need for social contact
- Hunger, thirst, need to toilet
- Loss of control
- Misinterpretation of the situation or environment
- Crowded conditions
- Changes in environment or people
- Noise, disruption
- Being forced to do something
- Fear
- Loneliness
- Psychotic symptoms
- Fatigue
- Environmental overstimulation or understimulation
- Depersonalized, rushed care
- Restraints
- Psychoactive drugs

BOX 21.8	Principles of Care Derived From the Progressively Lowered Stress Threshold Model

1. Maximize functional abilities by supporting all losses in an assistive manner.
2. Establish a caring relationship with the patient, and provide unconditional positive regard.
3. Use the patient's behaviour and anxiety and avoidance to determine the appropriate limits of activity and stimuli.
4. Teach caregivers to observe and listen to the person; try to determine the causes of behaviour.
5. Identify triggers related to discomfort or stress reactions (e.g., factors in the environment, caregiver communication).
6. Modify the environment to support losses and promote safe function.
7. Evaluate care routines and responses on a 24-hour basis, and adjust the plan of care accordingly.
8. Provide as much control as possible—encourage self-care, offer choices, explain all actions, and do not force the person to do something.
9. Keep the environment stable and predictable.
10. Provide ongoing education, support, care, and problem solving.

Source: Adapted from Hall, G. R., & Buckwalter, K. C. (1987). Progressively lowered stress threshold: A conceptual model for care of adults with Alzheimer's disease. *Archives of Psychiatric Nursing, 1*(6), 399–406.

Progressively Lowered Stress Threshold Model

The Progressively Lowered Stress Threshold (PLST) model was one of the first models used to plan and evaluate care for people with dementia (Hall & Buckwalter, 1987; Hall, 1994). The person with dementia is seen to experience a progressive lowering of the stress threshold. Behavioural symptoms such as agitation are a result of a progressive loss of the person's ability to cope with demands and stimuli in the environment that exceed the person's stress threshold. Box 21.7 lists common stressors and conditions that may trigger these behavioural symptoms.

With the PLST model, the social and physical environment and nursing care are structured to reduce stressors and provide the person with a safe and predictable environment. Behaviours are monitored as an indicator of the patient's stress tolerance. Box 21.8 presents the principles of care derived from the PLST model in long-term care settings. Reported outcomes include increased sleep, socialization, food intake, and caregiver satisfaction, along with reductions in

night-time awakening, psychoactive medication use, psychotic symptoms, repetitive questions, wandering, agitation, and staff and family stress (Smith et al., 2004).

Need-Driven Dementia-Compromised Behaviour Model

The Need-Driven Dementia-Compromised Behaviour model proposes that the behaviour of a person with dementia indicates need that can be addressed appropriately if the person's history and habits, physiological status, and physical and social environment are carefully evaluated (Kolanowski, 1999). Behaviour is viewed as having meaning and expressing needs. Behaviour reflects the interaction between background factors (gender, ethnicity, culture, education, personality, response to stress, and cognitive changes resulting from dementia) and proximal factors (physiological needs [such as hunger or pain], mood, physical environment, and social environment) (Richards et al., 2000).

Optimal care is provided by identifying the meaning of the behaviour, manipulating the proximal factors that precipitate that behaviour, and maximizing strengths and minimizing the limitations of the background factors. For instance, sleep disruptions are common. If the person with dementia is not getting adequate sleep at night, agitation during the day may signal the need for more rest. Interventions to modify proximal factors interfering with sleep, such as noise, frequent awakenings during the night, and daytime boredom, can help meet the need for rest and sleep and decrease agitation.

Developed and widely disseminated in Ontario, the Gentle Persuasive Approaches model trains health care providers to understand, minimize, accommodate, and manage responsive behaviours. It is based on the principles of person-centred care and the Need-Driven Dementia-Compromised Behaviour model. Staff learn to reframe behaviours typically labelled as aggressive as "self-protective and an attempt to exert control over a life that has become unfamiliar and frightening" (Speziale et al., 2009, p. 572). Staff training was shown to increase self-reported competence and to reduce "physical aggression" (Schindel Martin et al., 2016).

Recognition of Retained Abilities Approach

The recognition of retained abilities approach, developed by Canadian researchers, emphasizes the importance of focusing on abilities rather than disabilities (Dawson et al., 1993; Wells & Dawson, 2000). Careful assessment of the person's abilities allows the nurse to assist with care in ways that compensate for lost abilities and enhance remaining abilities. An environment that supports retained abilities is important. Education about this approach results in nurses' and health care aides' increased use of abilities-focused interventions and in patients' decreased agitation, increased engagement in morning care, and increased independence in dressing and grooming (Sidani et al., 2012).

This approach may prevent or reverse excess disability, which is "a discrepancy between existing and potential functional capacity which is greater than warranted by any co-existing, irreversible cognitive,

physical, or affective impairments" (Slaughter & Bankes, 2007, p. 41). Excess disability is rarely recognized in dementia care; care providers assume that a lack of capacity for performing ADLs means a lack of ability. Iatrogenic excess disability occurs when patients do not use existing abilities because of the way nursing care is provided; for example, when care providers "do for" rather than assist or facilitate participation in ADLs. Reducing excess disability includes providing supportive environments, using cognitive enhancer medications, and preventing or treating depression and the adverse effects of antidepressants (Slaughter et al., 2011).

Relating Well

In LTC homes, care provider–resident relationships enhance the quality of life of residents and enrich the work experience of care providers (McGilton et al., 2012). A therapeutic relationship is achieved when a care provider is reliable, empathetic, and consistent in interactions with the person with dementia. Three kinds of nursing actions soothe residents who have dementia: "(1) staying with the resident during the care episode; (2) altering the pace of care by recognizing the person's rhythm and adapting to it; and (3) focusing the care beyond the task" (Hillberg et al., 1995 [as cited in McGilton et al., 2012, p. 507]). These actions are associated with better outcomes for residents with dementia, including lower levels of anxiety, sadness, and agitation during care.

 IMPLICATIONS FOR GERONTOLOGICAL NURSING AND HEALTHY AGING

ASSESSMENT

It is essential to view all behaviour as meaningful and an expression of needs. The focus must be on understanding that behavioural expressions communicate distress, and the response is to investigate the possible sources of distress and intervene appropriately. There are many possible reasons for behavioural and psychological symptoms of dementia. After medical problems (e.g., pneumonia, dehydration, impaction, infection, fractures, pain, and depression) are ruled out as causes of the behaviour, continued assessment to identify why distressing symptoms are occurring is important (RNAO, 2016). Conditions such as constipation or urinary-tract infections can cause great distress that may not be readily communicated by the person with later-stage dementia. These conditions may lead to marked changes in behaviour (e.g., agitation or resistance to care), so careful assessment is important. Pain is common among persons with dementia and is a frequent cause of agitation; after careful assessment of other possible causes, treatment with a trial of analgesics should be considered (RNAO, 2016) (see Chapter 16).

Nurses must use appropriate assessment to understand the meaning of behaviours and determine what interventions would be most helpful to meet the needs being expressed. Yet, behaviours are frequently treated without appropriate assessment. Trying to see the world from the viewpoint of the person with dementia will help the nurse understand the person's behaviour. The questions *what, where, why, when, who,* and *what now* are important components of the assessment of behaviour. Box 21.9 presents a framework for asking questions about the possible meanings and messages behind observed behaviour. Using a behavioural log for 2–3 days to track when the behaviour occurs, the circumstances under which it occurs, and the response to interventions is recommended.

INTERVENTIONS

All evidence-informed guidelines endorse an approach that begins with the comprehensive assessment of the behaviour and its possible causes, followed by nonpharmacological interventions as the first line of treatment. Despite this recommendation, psychotropic medications are often the first-line treatment of the behavioural and psychological symptoms of dementia. In Canada, 39% of older persons living in LTC homes are prescribed an antipsychotic (Canadian Institute for Health Information [CIHI], 2016). The overuse of antipsychotic medications to treat behavioural responses is of serious concern in light of the adverse drug events and risks associated with such medications, including sedation and associated orthostatic hypotension, falls and fractures, stroke, extrapyramidal symptoms, worsening cognition, infections, and death (CIHI, 2016; Steinberg & Lyketsos, 2012).

BOX 21.9 Framework for Asking Questions About the Meaning of Behaviour of Persons With Dementia

What?
What is being sought? What is happening? Does the behaviour have a physical component, an emotional component, or both? What are the person's responses? What would be done if the person were 20 years old instead of 80 years old? What is the behaviour saying? What emotion is being expressed?

Where?
Where is the behaviour occurring? Are there environmental triggers?

When?
When does the behaviour most frequently occur? For example, does it occur after performing activities of daily living, during family visits, at mealtimes, at other times?

Who?
Who is involved? (Other residents, caregivers, family?)

Why?
What happened before the behaviour? Poor communication? Tasks too complicated? Physical or medical problems? Being rushed or forced to do something? Has this happened before, and if so, why?

What Now?
Approaches and interventions (physical, psychosocial)? Changes needed? Implemented by whom? Who else might know something about the person or the behaviour and approaches to it? Is everyone who is involved communicated with and included in the plan of care?

Sources: Adapted from Hellen, C. (2000). Can you provide care for residents with difficult behaviors? *Alzheimer's Care Quarterly, 14*(4), 4–7; Ortigara, A. (2000). Understanding the language of behaviors. *Alzheimer's Care Quarterly, 1*(4), 89–92.

Several authors suggest that the following contribute to less than optimal practice: insufficient staffing in LTC homes, time constraints, an emphasis on controlling residents rather than understanding them, lack of interdisciplinary team approaches and family involvement, and inadequate education about behaviours and the use of nonpharmacological interventions (Kolanowski et al., 2010). The rate of antipsychotic use in LTC homes in Canada has been stable over the past decade, except in Manitoba, where the rate decreased from 38.2% to 31.5%. This reduction is due to an initiative to reduce inappropriate antipsychotic use by improving staff knowledge about behaviours, patient-centred care, and interdisciplinary approaches to caring for people with dementia (CIHI, 2016).

Pharmacological approaches may be considered in addition to nonpharmacological approaches if there has been a comprehensive assessment of causes of behaviour, the person presents a danger to self or others, nonpharmacological interventions have not been effective, and the risk–benefit profiles of medications have been considered (Canadian Coalition for Seniors' Mental Health [CCSMH], 2006b). Risperidone is the only medication approved for this use in Canada (Health Canada, 2015, ¶2). Appropriate medication must be carefully monitored and evaluated for tapering and discontinuation.

Nonpharmacological Approaches

The approaches recommended in the PLST, Need-Driven Dementia-Compromised Behaviour, recognition of retained abilities, and relating well models described previously allow nurses to identify and address the underlying causes of behaviours. All health care providers who work in any setting with people with dementia need the knowledge and skills to effectively provide person-centred care and avoid the inappropriate use of medication. A team approach to care of persons with dementia is necessary.

A large amount of literature is concerned with nonpharmacological interventions, and these interventions are recommended in the culture change movement. In general, these interventions have shown promise for improving quality of life for persons with dementia, despite a lack of rigorous evaluation. The most effective approaches are the following: individualizing activities, music therapy, sensory interventions (e.g., touch, massage, and multisensory interventions), exercise (see Chapter 10), reminiscence, simplifying tasks, enhancing communication, group activities (e.g., animal-assisted therapy, dance, and cooking), and art therapy (Cabrera et al., 2015; Kales et al., 2014; Livingston et al., 2014; RNAO, 2016). Other interventions include environmental design (e.g., supportive care units, homelike environments, gardens, and safe walking areas), changes in

mealtime and bathing environments, and consistent staffing assignments (Kales et al., 2014). Combined multiple interventions for the person with dementia are often more beneficial than are single interventions (Olazarán et al., 2010).

Activities of Daily Living

The losses associated with dementia interfere with the person's communication patterns and ability to understand and express thoughts and feelings. Perceptual disturbances and misinterpretations of reality often contribute to fear and misunderstanding. People with dementia sometimes struggle to understand the world and make their needs known. Often, bathing and the provision of other ADL care such as dressing, grooming, and toileting are the cause of much distress for both the person with dementia and the caregiver.

Bathing. Bathing and assistance with ADLs, particularly in LTC homes, can be perceived as attacks by persons with dementia, who may attempt to protect themselves by screaming or striking out. A rigid focus on tasks or institutional care routines (such as showering 2 days a week) can contribute to the person's distress and precipitate distressing behaviours. Being touched or bathed against one's will violates one's trust in the caregiver and can be considered a major affront (Rader & Barrick, 2000). The resulting behaviours that may be exhibited by a person with dementia are not deliberate attacks on caregivers by a violent person. The message is, "Please find another way to keep me clean, because the way you are doing it now is intolerable" (Rader & Barrick, 2000, p. 49).

Person-centred care is vital when persons with dementia are assisted with bathing. The following relates this experience from the person's perspective: *You are asleep in the chair at home when suddenly you are awakened by a person you have never seen before trying to undress you. Then he or she puts you naked into a hard, cold chair and wheels you down a hallway. Suddenly, cold water hits you in the face and the person is touching your private areas. You don't understand why the person is trying to do this to you. You are embarrassed, frightened, cold, and angry. You hit and scream at this person and try to get away.*

Family members and nurses caring for people with dementia must understand that they are the ones who must change their behaviours, reactions, and approaches in order to avoid or minimize the person's agitation and self-protective behaviours. Using appropriate communication strategies, explaining all actions before doing, not pushing or forcing the person, providing positive feedback, paying attention to body posture and facial expressions, using gestures and demonstration, giving one-step directions, staying calm and pleasant, providing warmth and comfort, and allowing appropriate time for response are some of the ways the person's ADL care can be enhanced.

Rader and Barrick (2000) provided comprehensive guidelines for bathing people with dementia in ways that are pleasurable and that decrease their distress. The answer to the question "What is the easiest, most comfortable, least frightening way for me to bathe the person right now?" guides the choice of interventions (Rader & Barrick, 2000, p. 42). The following are important for the nurse who bathes a person who has dementia: knowing the person's lifetime bathing routines and preferences; ensuring the person's privacy and providing care only when the person is receptive; respecting refusals to participate in care; explaining all actions; realizing that a bath is not an essential intervention; encouraging self-care to the extent possible; making bathrooms and shower areas warm, comfortable, and safe; keeping the person warm with towels; being attentive to the person's pain and discomfort; reassuring residents that they are safe; providing distractions; playing preferred music; and using alternative bathing methods such as towel baths, thermal baths, and no-rinse cleaners. Individualized bathing care plans are helpful.

Research indicates that the actions listed above result in less physical responsive behaviour, verbal outbursts, and agitation (Konno et al., 2013; Gozalo et al., 2014). Staff training, policies that support a person-centred approach to bathing as a pleasant experience, and support from supervisors are important to achieve these outcomes (Konno, et al., 2013).

Wandering. Wandering associated with dementia is one of the most difficult management problems encountered in home and institutional settings. One in five people with dementia wander (Cipriani et al., 2014). Wandering is a complex behaviour and is not well understood. Risk factors for wandering include visuospatial impairments, anxiety and depression, poor sleep patterns, unmet needs, delusions, depression, more-severe cognitive impairment, and a more socially active and outgoing premorbid lifestyle (Lester et al., 2012; Cipriani et al., 2014). There is a need for more research on wandering as well as interventions for this behaviour.

Wandering presents safety concerns in all settings. Wandering affects sleep, eating, safety, and the caregiver's ability to provide care; it also interferes with the privacy of others. It can lead to falls, elopement (i.e., leaving the home or LTC home), injury, and death (Futrell et al., 2010; Rowe et al., 2010). The stimulus for wandering arises from many internal and external sources. Wandering can be considered an intrinsically and extrinsically driven rhythm. The following excerpts from a book by a man with dementia provide insight into wandering from the person's perspective. *"Very often, I wander around looking for something which I know is very pertinent, but then after awhile I forget all about what it was I was looking for. When I'm wandering around, I'm trying to touch base with— anything, actually. If anything appeared I'd probably enjoy it, or look at it or examine it and wonder how it got there. I feel very foolish when I'm wandering around not knowing what I'm doing and I'm not always quite sure how to do any better. It's not easy to figure out what the heck I'm looking for."* (Henderson, 1998, p. 24)

Wandering behaviours can be predicted through careful observation and knowing the person's patterns. For example, if the person with dementia starts wandering or trying to leave the home around dinnertime every day, meaningful activities such as music, exercise, and refreshment can be provided at this time. There are also several instruments with which to assess risk for wandering; Futrell et al. (2010) developed an evidence-informed protocol for wandering. Wandering may be less likely to occur when the person is involved in social interaction. Environmental interventions such as camouflaging doorways, providing enclosed outdoor gardens and paths for walking, and providing electronic bracelets that activate alarms at exits are also used. There are a number of assistive technology devices and programs that can enhance the safety of persons who wander. Box 21.10 presents suggestions for additional interventions, but further research is needed to determine the nature

BOX 21.10 Interventions for Wandering or Exiting Behaviours

- Face the person and make direct eye contact (unless this is interpreted as threatening).
- Gently touch the person's arm, shoulders, back, or waist if he or she does not move away.
- Call the person by his or her formal name (e.g., Mr. Jones).
- Listen to what the person is communicating verbally and nonverbally; listen to the feelings being expressed.
- Identify the agenda, the plan of action, and the emotional needs the agenda is expressing.
- Respond to the feelings expressed, staying calm.
- Repeat specific words or phrases, or state the need or emotion (e.g., "You need to go home; you're worried about your husband").
- If such repetition fails to distract the person, accompany him or her and continue talking calmly, repeating back phrases and the emotion you identify in the person.
- Provide orienting information only if it calms the person. If such information increases the person's distress, stop talking about the present situation. Do not "correct" the person or belittle his or her agenda.
- At intervals, redirect the person toward the home by suggesting, "Let's walk this way now," or "I'm so tired, let's turn around."
- If orientation and redirection fail, continue to walk, allowing the person control but ensuring his or her safety.
- Make sure you have a backup person. However, he or she should stay out of the patient's eyesight.
- Have someone call for help if you are unable to redirect the person. Usually, the behaviour is time limited because of the person's attention span and the security and trust between you and the person.

Source: Adapted from Rader, J., Doan, J., & Schwab, M. (1985). How to decrease wandering, a form of agenda behavior. *Geriatric Nursing, 6*(4), 196–199.

of wandering and appropriate evidence-informed interventions.

Wandering behaviour in a person with dementia may also result in the person's going outside and getting lost. This phenomenon was studied by Rowe (2003), who conducted a retrospective review of the records of a US system that is similar to the Alzheimer Society of Canada Safely Home program (http://www.safelyhome.ca/en/safelyhome/

aboutsafelyhome.asp) and is designed to help identify, locate, and return people with dementia to safety. Rowe advised caregivers to prevent people with dementia from leaving homes or LTC homes unaccompanied, register the person in a program such as Safely Home, and have a plan of action in case the person does become lost. Rowe also suggested that police must respond rapidly to requests for searches and that the general public should be informed about how to recognize and assist people with dementia who may be lost. The Alzheimer Society of Canada Safely Home program website (http://www.safelyhome.ca/en/) has information for caregivers about wandering and how to manage it.

 FAMILY CAREGIVING FOR PERSONS WITH DEMENTIA

Most Canadians with dementia live in the community; 85% of them rely on family and friends for assistance, and 41% rely solely on care from family and friends (Wong et al., 2016). Informal caregivers such as family and friends provide 20 million hours of caregiving, valued at $1.2 billion, and spend $1.4 billion on care-related expenses (Chambers et al., 2016). Family caregivers are usually spouses (46%) or adult children (44%) (Wong et al., 2016).

These caregivers provide more hours of help than caregivers of persons who do not have dementia provide, and they experience more adverse consequences to their physical and mental health. Caregivers of persons with dementia have lower self-rated health scores; display fewer health-promoting behaviours; and have higher depression and anxiety rates, higher morbidity and mortality rates, higher numbers of illness-related symptoms, and sleep problems (Elliott et al., 2010; Richardson et al., 2013). Factors that influence the stress of caregiving include grief over the multiple losses that occur, the physical demands and duration of caregiving (up to 20 years), and resource availability. The negative effects of caring for persons with dementia are intensified when the care recipient demonstrates behavioural disturbances and impairments in performing ADLs and instrumental activities of daily living, activities that allow a person to function independently, such as shopping, managing money, and preparing meals.

Most research on the care of persons with dementia has focused on the late stages of dementia and on the "burden" of caregiving. However, this is a simplification of the complex process of caregiving and a negation of the positive aspects and outcomes of family caregiving. Positive outcomes include role satisfaction (which is common among caregivers); emotional rewards; personal growth (such as increased self-awareness and humility); new skills; spiritual growth; strengthened family relationships; and the rewards of having a sense of duty and being able to give back to the person with dementia (Lloyd et al., 2016).

The most effective caregiver intervention programs include bundled interventions, such as individual and group interventions for both the person with dementia and the caregiver, as well as combined groups, education, counselling, support group participation, care management, and the continuous availability of telephone support. Teaching caregivers about AD and training them in the skills needed to manage behaviours, maintain social support, reframe negative emotions, manage stress, and enhance their own healthy behaviours appear to be most effective in reducing the caregiver's depression and burden and improving his or her quality of life (Elliott et al., 2010; Mittelman et al., 2007). It is important that caregiver support start in the early stages of dementia.

Family caregiving continues after a person with dementia moves to an LTC home. Family caregiving in an LTC home involves not only providing personal care but also monitoring the quality of care; providing companionship; preserving the individuality, dignity, and self-esteem of the resident; and communicating the family member's unique knowledge of the resident to the staff (Baumbusch & Phinney, 2014). Positive relationships between staff in LTC homes and family caregivers of residents are important. These relationships depend on staff members establishing their trustworthiness; listening to family caregivers' views, including their complaints about care; and encouraging appropriate family involvement in the home and in care (Bauer et al., 2014) (Box 21.11).

To date, most research and intervention programs have been directed toward persons in the later stages of dementia and toward those persons' families. More research is needed to develop interventions

---

BOX 21.11 Research for Evidence-Informed Practice: The Role of Family Members Within Long-Term Residential Care

Problem: Compared to family care at home and in the community, the role of families and the care they provide in long-term care (LTC) homes is less known and acknowledged.

Method: A critical ethnographic study examined the role of highly involved family members in two LTC homes in British Columbia, Canada. Eleven family members who were regularly present at the LTC homes were interviewed, the researchers observed the participants, and a thematic analysis was conducted.

Findings: About half of the participants spent much of the day with their relatives. They provided personal care to their relatives, assisted staff, and monitored the care provided to their relative by the staff. These participants were integrated into routines at the LTC homes and were socially engaged with other residents and staff. They communicated with health care aides but were frustrated by being left out of decisions made by regulated staff members, whom they were less likely to encounter. Participants described tension in their relationships with managers and felt that their input was seen as interference and was unwelcome. They reported having their criticisms of managers silenced by threats, a particularly challenging response because of how important it was to the participants to monitor their relative's conditions and to notice and report any changes in those conditions.

Application to nursing practice: The researchers noted that staff relied on families to provide care. Families contributed to the well-being of their relatives and other residents. However, the absence of policies and philosophies that supported family involvement in care contributed to families being left out or silenced. True partnership with relatives of residents of LTC homes is important.

Source: Baumbusch, J., & Phinney, A. (2014). Invisible hands: The role of highly involved families in long-term residential care. *Journal of Family Nursing, 20*(1), 73–97. doi:10.1177/107484071350777.

---

for the growing numbers of individuals experiencing early-onset dementia, MCI, and early to mild stages of dementia, persons whose needs are quite different from persons who are in later stages of disease. See Chapter 23 for additional information on care for persons with dementia.

CEREBRO-VASCULAR DISEASE

Cerebro-vascular disease, a group of pathological processes in cerebral blood vessels that results in brain injury, is the most commonly occurring neurological disorder. Cerebro-vascular disease is either ischemic or hemorrhagic and manifests as either a stroke (the term "cerebro-vascular accident" is discouraged) or a transient ischemic attack (TIA). Because the initial signs and symptoms of stroke and TIA are similar but the outcomes are different, diagnosis is geared toward identifying the specific cause of the symptoms and the location of the brain injury. Only when the cause is known can appropriate therapy be implemented.

Each year in Canada, about 50,000 people have a stroke, and about 14,000 die of stroke (Ontario Stroke Network, 2016). More than 75% of all strokes occur in persons older than 65 years. Premenopausal women are at lower risk than are men, and people with a family history of stroke are at higher risk. Indigenous people and people of African or South Asian descent are at higher risk because they are more likely to have high blood pressure and diabetes (Ontario Stroke Network, 2016). People who have had a stroke or TIA are at increased risk of having another. In Canada, about 246,000 people are living with the effects of a stroke (Ontario Stroke Network, 2016).

ETIOLOGY

Ischemic Events

Ischemic stroke is the death of brain cells because of an insufficient supply of blood and oxygen resulting from blockage of an artery. The four main causes of ischemic strokes are arterial disease, cardioembolism, hematological disorders, and systemic hypoperfusion. Arterial disease in the form of inflammatory arteriosclerosis is the most common cause. Cardioembolism includes ischemic events caused by a dysrhythmia such as atrial fibrillation, which is frequently seen in coronary heart disease (see Chapter 20). The use of antithrombotics (e.g., acetylsalicylic acid [ASA] and warfarin) for persons with heart disease is an attempt to reduce the risk for stroke. Hematological disorders include coagulation disorders and hyperviscosity syndromes. Systemic hypoperfusion can occur from dehydration, hypotension (as well as overtreatment of

---

BOX 21.12   Relative Risk for a Major Stroke After a Transient Ischemic Attack

Age >60 years = 1 point
Blood pressure >140/90 mm Hg = 1 point
Resulting unilateral weakness = 2 points
Speech impairment; no weakness = 1 point
Duration of deficit, 10–59 minutes = 1 point
Duration >1 hour = 2 points
Diabetes = 1 point
Risk Score
    6–7 = high risk (9.1% chance of a major stroke in 2 days)
    4–5 = moderate risk (4.1% chance)
    0–3 = low risk (1% chance)

Source: Llinas, R. (2010). Stroke. In S. C. Durso (Ed.), *Oxford American handbook of geriatric medicine* (p. 168). New York, NY: Oxford University Press. By permission of Oxford University Press, USA.

hypertension), cardiac arrest, or syncope (Graykowski, 2008).

A TIA is ischemic but clinically different from an ischemic stroke, in that the symptoms of a TIA begin to resolve within minutes, and all neurological deficits caused by it resolve within 24 hours. In some cases, a TIA is followed by a stroke, yet most strokes are not preceded by TIAs (Box 21.12).

A person who has a TIA is at high risk for stroke or another TIA in the following weeks. Each year, 15,000 Canadians are diagnosed with TIA; a large number of TIAs are unreported (Stroke Network of Southwestern Ontario, 2015). TIA is more prevalent in men than in women and is more prevalent in older persons.

Hemorrhagic Events

Hemorrhagic strokes are less frequent than ischemic strokes but are more life-threatening. They are primarily caused by uncontrolled hypertension and less often by malformations of the blood vessels (e.g., aneurysms). Although the exact mechanism is not fully understood, it appears that chronic hypertension causes thickening of the vessel wall, microaneurysms, and necrosis. When enough damage to the vessel accumulates, it is at risk for rupture. The rupture may be large and acute, or it may be small, with a slow leakage of blood into the adjacent brain tissue. In many cases, there is a rupture or seepage of blood into the ventricular system of the brain and damage to the affected tissue through necrosis (Boss & Huether, 2014). Resolution of the event can occur only with the resorption of excess blood and damaged tissue. Hemorrhagic strokes are more life-threatening than ischemic strokes but are much less frequent.

SIGNS AND SYMPTOMS OF CEREBRO-VASCULAR DISEASE

The first signs of both strokes and TIAs are acute neurological deficits consistent with the part of the brain affected. They are often heralded by a severe headache. In **subarachnoid** hemorrhages, the headache is not only sudden but also explosive, very severe, and without other neurological manifestations (Graykowski, 2008).

Some of the clinical signs and symptoms of cerebro-vascular disease are suggestive of either ischemia or hemorrhage (see Box 21.12). Persons with hemorrhage have more focal neurological changes, including seizures and a more depressed level of consciousness than persons who have an ischemic stroke. If a deep unresponsive state occurs, the person is unlikely to survive (Boss & Huether, 2014). Nausea and vomiting are suggestions of increased cerebral edema in response to an event of either type. Depending on the area of damage, neurological deficits include alterations in coordination, cognition, and language and alterations in motor, sensory, and visual function.

Diagnosis includes the determination of possible extra-cerebral causes (e.g., infection or hypoglycemia), the confirmation of stroke, and the identification of the exact location of the damage in the brain through CT or MRI.

COMPLICATIONS

After a TIA resolves, there should be no residual effect other than an increased chance of recurrence and the possible increased risk for stroke. Early complications of a simple stroke include extension of the amount of damage and recurrence. Brain edema (always a problem) can result in obstructive hydrocephalus (Graykowski, 2008).

Although the potential long-term effects of a stroke may be minimal, they may include paralysis and hemiparesis, **dysarthria,** dysphagia, and aphasia, depending on type, extent, and area affected. Post-stroke depression negatively affects rehabilitation (see Chapter 24).

Whenever paralysis results from a stroke, there is a risk of the development of spasticity in the affected limb or limbs. Spasticity can lead to contractures if it is not managed. Pain in the affected side is common and may be treated with muscle relaxants or medications specific for neuropathic pain. (See Chapter 3 for a discussion of aphasia, and see Chapter 8 for a discussion of dysphagia.) Iatrogenic complications include deep venous thrombosis in a flaccid lower limb, aspiration pneumonia, and urinary-tract infections (Llinas, 2010). Vascular dementia, discussed earlier, is more common in people who have a history of hypertension, TIAs, or stroke.

MANAGEMENT

All actual or potential cerebro-vascular events should be treated as emergencies. However, because TIAs are highly transient, they often resolve on their own before the affected person is seen by a health care provider. Instead, the person reports, "I think I had a small stroke last week," or they do not seek care at all. If the deficits and symptoms were fleeting, the diagnosis is made through the clinical interview. Management is considered preventive; its aim is to prevent recurrences and to reduce the risk factors for strokes (Manuel, et al., 2015) (Box 21.13). The person and family are also instructed in the appropriate

---

BOX 21.13 Risk Factors for Stroke

Heart disease and risk factors for heart disease
Hypertension
Arrhythmias
Hypercholesterolemia
Diabetes
Smoking
Heavy alcohol use
Physical inactivity
Diet low in fruit and vegetables
Self-perceived stress
Coagulopathies
Brain tumours
Family history

emergency response to the return of any signs or symptoms of a stroke or another TIA. Anticoagulant therapy prevents recurrent embolic strokes and TIAs. Acetylsalicylic acid (Aspirin) 81 to 325 mg per day is the mainstay of therapy for persons with TIAs, and clopidogrel (Plavix) may be used for persons who are Aspirin sensitive (Llinas, 2010). Warfarin therapy or one of the newer related medications is usually used in persons to prevent another stroke and for those with atrial fibrillation, to prevent the occurrence of the first stroke (Graykowski, 2008).

Acute management is usually accomplished in emergency departments and Critical Care Units. The acute management of the stroke requires careful attention to the accuracy of the diagnosis. Reperfusion therapy with recombinant tissue–type plasminogen activator (rt-PA) is used for ischemic strokes only if a CT scan confirms the absence of hemorrhage. The sooner rt-PA or other appropriate treatment is begun, the better the chances for recovery. If the person has had a hemorrhagic stroke and is misdiagnosed, the bleeding will be rapidly accelerated by the rt-PA, and the person will die (Box 21.14). The initial response to a hemorrhagic stroke is to find a means to stop the bleeding rather than dissolve an occlusion.

About 90% of neurological recovery occurs within 3 months of the stroke; 10% occurs more slowly, especially after a hemorrhagic stroke (Porter & Kaplan, 2010–2011). At 18 months after the stroke, there tends to be a small decline in improvement. The inverse relationship between functional improvement and advanced age, social isolation, and emotional distress is clear. Recovery from a stroke is affected by the location and extent of the brain damage. Difficulties and handicaps after stroke often involve neurological and functional deficits. Post-ischemic stroke management begins immediately with anticoagulants or antiplatelets.

The interprofessional team is essential to the care of the person after a stroke. The needs assessment after a stroke is extremely complex and requires a team coordinated by a nurse and including a neurologist, a physiatrist, a speech pathologist, an occupational therapist, a physiotherapist, an ophthalmologist, a rehabilitation specialist, a psychologist, a social worker, and a spiritual advisor. The older person's significant other, who may be involved with the day-to-day life and needs of the person after a stroke, is also included. The Canadian Heart and Stroke Foundation, the American Heart Association, and the American Stroke Association provide excellent educational resources, as well as support groups for persons affected by stroke and their families. (See Resources, later in this chapter.) Specialized stroke units improve outcomes in persons after ischemic strokes.

 ## IMPLICATIONS FOR GERONTOLOGICAL NURSING AND HEALTHY AGING

The best approach to stroke is prevention and prompt intervention. Identifying high-risk or stroke-prone persons is something nurses can do in their patient's homes, in the community, or at the health facilities where the nurses work. In a quick assessment of risk factors (see Box 21.13), the nurse can work with individuals to reduce their risk for stroke and teach them how to respond to signs or symptoms.

Smoking cessation and control of blood pressure may be the most important strategies for reducing modifiable risk factors. Maintaining a blood pressure equal to or less than 130/85 mm Hg is recommended. Additional prevention includes a healthy diet, limited salt and alcohol intake, and acetylsalicylic acid therapy unless contraindicated. Controlling lipids and diabetes and preventing atrial fibrillation are helpful, as well as regular exercise and weight-management programs.

Nursing assessment during the acute period includes general and neurological assessments (Table 21.4). Aspiration and sepsis precautions, pneumatic

---

BOX 21.14   Safety Alert

Reperfusion Therapy With Recombinant Tissue-Type Plasminogen Activator
Reperfusion therapy (using recombinant tissue plasminogen activator) can be used only for ischemic occlusive (usually embolic) strokes and only if a CT scan confirms the absence of hemorrhage and is performed within 3 hours of the onset of the event.

Source: Llinas, R. (2010). Stroke. In S. C. Durso (Ed.), *Oxford American handbook of geriatric medicine.* New York, NY: Oxford University Press.

TABLE 21.4	Assessment of Person After Stroke or TIA
GENERAL	**Neurological**
Vital signs	Level of arousal, orientation, attention
Cardiovascular	Speech (dysarthria, dysphasia)
Respiratory	Cranial nerves
Abdominal	Motor strength
	Coordination
	Sensation
	Gait (if possible)
	Reflexes

stockings, attention to bowel function, and early mobilization are necessary, and rehabilitation therapists are often involved even before the person leaves the acute care setting. Eating may be a problem; a nasogastric or semipermanent percutaneous endoscopic gastrostomy (PEG) tube may be needed.

A period of intense rehabilitation often takes place in a rehabilitation or complex continuing care facility setting and continues long after the person returns home or to an assisted living setting. An important role for the nurse is documenting clearly and in detail the functional capacities that are retained and those that are impaired. The assessment must be routinely repeated to carefully evaluate and document signs of depression and areas of progress and need.

Prevention of iatrogenic complications, such as skin breakdown, falls, and delirium, is a priority. Assessment includes monitoring mental status, respiratory functioning, sleep, and constipation. The goals of nursing care include maximizing the person's capacity for self-care and improving the person's quality of life.

PARKINSON'S DISEASE

Parkinson's disease is one of the most common neuro-degenerative diseases. It was first described in 1817 by Dr. James Parkinson, a British physician, who described "the shaking palsy" and described the major symptoms of the disease.

ETIOLOGY

Parkinson's disease (PD) is a slowly progressing disease that results from the destruction of the cells in the substantia nigra in the brain. As the nigrostriatal pathway deteriorates, it is no longer able to produce the neurotransmitter dopamine. Dopamine loss also occurs in the brainstem, thalamus, and cortex. Dopamine plays a major part in regulating movement; thus, PD is considered a movement disorder. By the time the first symptoms are seen, 80% of the specific brain cells have been lost, and 70 to 80% of the dopamine needed to control involuntary movement and the initiation of voluntary smooth movement has been lost (Boss & Huether, 2014). The average age of onset is 60 years, and the median time between diagnosis and death is 9 years (Boss & Huether, 2014).

The exact cause of PD is unknown. A systematic review of causal factors identified advancing older age as the only established causal risk factor (Keiburtz & Wunderle, 2013). Furthermore, the authors found that PD is more common in men than in women and that people who smoke or who drink coffee have a lower risk for PD. Other environmental exposures (for example, exposure to pesticides) may interact with genetic factors, but evidence of causal associations is limited (Keiburtz & Wunderle, 2013).

Parkinson's disease is classified as either primary or secondary parkinsonism. Primary parkinsonism is either idiopathic or genetic. In about 10% of people who have primary PD, the disorder appears to have a familial component (Boss & Huether, 2014). Secondary parkinsonism occurs as a secondary effect of another disorder that causes loss of or interference with the action of dopamine in the basal ganglia (e.g., head trauma, post-encephalitic parkinsonism, stroke, tumours, and toxin- and medication-induced parkinsonian syndrome).

SIGNS AND SYMPTOMS OF PARKINSON'S DISEASE

Parkinson's disease has an insidious onset and usually progresses very slowly, making it difficult to diagnose, particularly in the early stages. Diagnosis consists of ruling out other possible causes of symptoms. When there is no other explanation, a diagnosis is made on the basis of the presence of two of the four classic symptoms (Box 21.15). One of these symptoms must

BOX 21.15 Signs and Symptoms of Parkinson's Disease

Classic Signs and Symptoms
Bradykinesia (slowness of movement)
Tremor at rest (trembling in hands, arms, legs, jaw, or face)
Cogwheel rigidity (resistance of the limbs and trunk in a jerking manner)
Postural instability (impaired balance and coordination)

Other Signs
Disordered sleep
Constipation
Fatigue
Excessive salivation
Pain
Depression
Visual disturbances
Psychosis
Seborrhea
Excessive sweating
Hypertension
Soft-spoken voice
Little facial animation
Infrequent blinking
Restless legs

be either a resting tremor or bradykinesia ("paucity of movement") (Boss & Huether, 2014). Diagnosis is supported by a challenge test in which a person with symptoms is given a dose of levodopa; if there is a significant and rapid improvement, the diagnosis is thought to be confirmed. Falls early in the course of the illness, poor response to levodopa, symmetry of motor symptoms, lack of tremor, and early autonomic dysfunction (e.g., incontinence) are conditions that may be useful in distinguishing PD from other motor disorders (Boss & Huether, 2014).

The most conspicuous sign of PD is an asymmetrical, regular, rhythmic, low-amplitude tremor. It disappears briefly during voluntary movement and increases with stress and anxiety.

Tremor, however, is a minor part of the clinical picture. Other symptoms that can cause disability include rigidity and postural instability. The characteristic gait is called "festination" and consists of very short steps and minimal arm movement. Postural

reflexes are lost. The person has difficulty initiating movement. "Freezing" is a common problem and may be precipitated by trying to move, by turning, or by initiating tactile and visual contact. The person will have involuntary flexion of the head and neck, a stooped posture, and a tendency to fall backward. If the person is off balance, correction is very slow, so falls are common. A person with moderately advanced PD will typically be bent forward from the waist but with the head up, standing still and then suddenly moving forward relatively rapidly but in a shuffling manner and with small steps. The person may come to a sudden halt, only to start all over again, clearly with effort. The necessity of high-back wheelchairs is common sometime during the course of the illness.

Rigidity, a state of involuntary contractions of all striated muscles, impedes both passive and active movement. Severe muscle cramps may occur in the toes or hands. When examined, a limb may exhibit either "lead pipe" or "cogwheel" (intermittent) resistance during passive movement. All the striated muscles in the extremities, trunk, ocular area, and face are affected, including the muscles of mastication (chewing), deglutition (swallowing), and articulation. Handwriting is small (micrographia). The person with PD will sit for long periods or lie motionless with few shifts in position and few changes in facial expression (Boss & Huether, 2014). This lack of movement puts the person at high risk for pressure ulcers.

There are also a number of cognitive and affective symptoms. Half of persons with PD have signs of depression, sometimes severe. It is believed that this depression is associated with the neuropathology of the disease and not necessarily the situation. The depression may vary from day to day, but in all cases, it worsens over time (Boss & Huether, 2014). About 30% of persons with PD who are living in the community and 80% of those living in LTC homes have dementia.

The symptoms of PD grow worse over time. The symptoms vary, and their intensity also varies from person to person; some persons become severely disabled, but others experience only minor motor disturbances. The progression of symptoms may take 20 years or more. In late stages of the disease, complications such as pressure ulcers, pneumonia, aspiration, and falls can lead to death.

BOX 21.16 Safety Alert

Monoamine Oxidase Inhibitors
Monoamine oxidase inhibitors (MAOIs), sometimes used to control Parkinson's disease symptoms, have significant drug–drug and drug–food interactions and must be used with caution. The nurse must monitor the patient carefully.

BOX 21.17 Safety Alert

Sinemet
Sinemet must be taken 1 hour before or 2 hours after a meal, to minimize gastro-intestinal side effects. It must also be given routinely and on time to prevent fluctuations in symptoms.

MANAGEMENT

The management of PD focuses on relieving symptoms with medication, increasing functional ability, preventing excess disability, and reducing the risk of injury.

Medication therapy focuses on dopamine replacement, mimicking, or slowing dopamine breakdown. The choice of medication is based on specific symptoms and the person's age (Connolly & Lang, 2014). First-line approaches include the combination of carbidopa and levodopa (Sinemet) or other dopamine agonists (pramipexole [Miraplex] or ropinirole ([Requip]). The monoamine oxidase (MAO) inhibitors selegiline (Eldepryl) and rasagiline (Azitect) are also used in initial treatment (Connolly & Lang, 2014). People who are taking MAO inhibitors must avoid food or drinks that contain tyramine because of interactions causing sudden and severe rises in blood pressure, which lead to stroke or death (Box 21.16). Sinemet loses effectiveness since the amino acid levodopa competes with other amino acids for absorption at both the intestinal wall and the blood–brain barrier. It also poses a higher risk for the adverse effect, dyskinesia (involuntary movement).

Other medications useful in management are the dopamine agonists, dopaminergics, catechol-O-methyltransferase (COMT) inhibitors, antihistamines, and anticholinergics (for tremor relief). Although anticholinergics are not usually recommended for use in older persons because of their high association with falls, they are sometimes necessary for the person with PD. Amantadine may be used to reduce dyskinesia. Many of the medications may be used in combination for specific effects.

Persons who are stable on Sinemet are often followed by their primary care providers (Box 21.17). However, when this is no longer effective, such persons are more often cared for by neurologists specializing in PD.

Medication therapy is complicated and should be closely supervised. The medications used to treat PD are not without serious side effects. Hypotension, dyskinesia (involuntary movement), dystonia (lack of control of movement), hallucinations, sleep disorders, and depression are common effects of the disease and side effects of the medications used to treat it. The medications of choice for depression are the selective serotonin reuptake inhibitors (SSRIs), such as sertraline and paroxetine, and the serotonin-norepinephrine reuptake inhibitors (SNRIs), such as venlafaxine. Bupropion, which is neither an SSRI nor an SNRI, is also used. Tricyclic antidepressants have greater evidence of effectiveness for persons with depression associated with PD, but these medications are less likely to be used owing to the higher risk of adverse effects (Connolly & Lang, 2014).

Cholinesterase inhibitors may be used for cognitive impairment and dementia associated with PD. However, many patients do not benefit, and the gastro-intestinal side effects may be significant (Connolly & Lang, 2014). Deep brain stimulation may be used in patients who have not responded to drug therapy or have intractable motor fluctuations, dyskinesias, or tremor (National Institute of Neurological Disorders and Stroke [NINDS], 2012).

Nonpharmacological interventions such as exercise therapy, speech therapy (for those with dysarthria), relaxation, stress management, education, self-care management, and caregiver support should be considered.

 IMPLICATIONS FOR GERONTOLOGICAL NURSING AND HEALTHY AGING

Ongoing nursing care focuses on enhancing quality of life, increasing functional ability, preventing excess disability, and decreasing the risk of injury. Persons with PD experience great functional problems in mobility, communication, and performance of ADLs. Nursing interventions can contribute greatly to quality of life and functional ability. Comprehensive functional assessments with attention to self-care abilities in ADLs and nutritional assessment are important (see Chapter 9), as well as fall assessment and risk reduction interventions.

The goal of treatment is to preserve self-care abilities and prevent complications. Encouragement to persons in the support system and information about the disease are essential if the family and the person are to cope with the losses associated with PD (see Chapter 23). The Sickness Impact Profile is a useful tool that can be used by nurses to determine the problems that are most troublesome from the person's perspective.

Exercise—including walking, moving all of the joints, and improving balance—needs to be included early in the course of PD; physical therapy evaluation and treatment are important. Rigidity of facial muscles and bradykinesia can affect eating ability, nutrition, swallowing, and communicating. Occupational therapy can assist the person in using adaptive equipment such as weighted utensils, nonslip dinnerware, and other self-care aids. Speech therapy is beneficial for dysarthria and dysphagia (swallowing difficulty). Patients can be taught facial exercises and swallowing techniques.

Regular pain assessments and appropriate pain management are also essential to address the often unnoticed problem of pain related to rigidity, contractures, dystonia, and central-pain syndromes of the disease itself (see Chapter 16). Other important interventions are the treatments of postural hypotension, incontinence (see Chapter 9), gastro-intestinal distress, depression and anxiety (see Chapter 24), sleep disturbances (see Chapter 10), and constipation (see Chapter 9).

Because of the usually slow progression of the disease and the disability that accompanies PD, affected persons experience changes in roles, activities, and social participation. Tremors may produce embarrassing moments. The expressionless face, slowed movement, and soft, monotone speech may give the impression of apathy, depression, or disinterest and might discourage others from socializing with affected individuals. Observing these symptoms, others may think that the person is unable to participate in activities and relationships and may even think the person is cognitively impaired. A sensitive nurse is aware that the visible symptoms produce an undesired facade that may hide an alert and responsive individual who wishes to interact but is trapped in a body that no longer responds. It is important to see beyond the disease to the person and provide nursing interventions that enhance the person's hope and promote the highest quality of life despite the disease.

Many resources are available for people with PD to provide practical information about living with the disease, as well as information about new developments and treatments. (See the Resources section at the end of this chapter and *evolve.elsevier.com/Canada/Ebersole/gerontological* for more information.)

SUMMARY

Many of the interventions for preventing delirium and for caring for people with cognitive impairment are achieved by applying the principles of good gerontological nursing care. An understanding of these principles and how to adapt responses and the environment to older persons with cognitive impairment will ensure that basic needs are met and will enhance quality of care and quality of life. Some of these principles may seem like the principles of basic nursing, but too often they are not practiced, leading to iatrogenesis, distress, and excess disability. Often these consequences are more problematic than the illnesses themselves. Nursing care must not increase disability; care must be based on knowledge and research to be considered best practice.

Fig. 21.2 presents a nursing situation that one nurse experienced in caring for a person with dementia who was being admitted to an LTC home. Written from the perspective of the nurse, who knew the person, the story provides insight into important nursing responses such as person-centred care, therapeutic communication, and a meaningful relationship with the person.

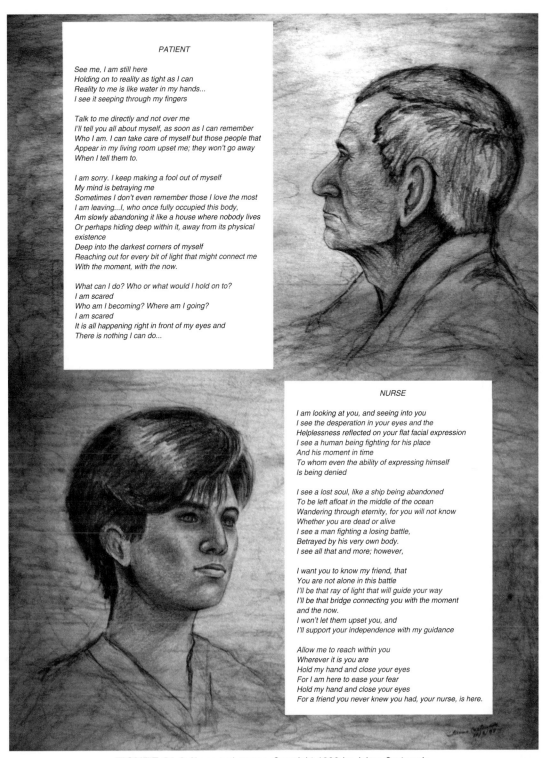

PATIENT

See me, I am still here
Holding on to reality as tight as I can
Reality to me is like water in my hands...
I see it seeping through my fingers

Talk to me directly and not over me
I'll tell you all about myself, as soon as I can remember
Who I am. I can take care of myself but those people that
Appear in my living room upset me; they won't go away
When I tell them to.

I am sorry. I keep making a fool out of myself
My mind is betraying me
Sometimes I don't even remember those I love the most
I am leaving...I, who once fully occupied this body,
Am slowly abandoning it like a house where nobody lives
Or perhaps hiding deep within it, away from its physical
existence
Deep into the darkest corners of myself
Reaching out for every bit of light that might connect me
With the moment, with the now.

What can I do? Who or what would I hold on to?
I am scared
Who am I becoming? Where am I going?
I am scared
It is all happening right in front of my eyes and
There is nothing I can do...

NURSE

I am looking at you, and seeing into you
I see the desperation in your eyes and the
Helplessness reflected on your flat facial expression
I see a human being fighting for his place
And his moment in time
To whom even the ability of expressing himself
Is being denied

I see a lost soul, like a ship being abandoned
To be left afloat in the middle of the ocean
Wandering through eternity, for you will not know
Whether you are dead or alive
I see a man fighting a losing battle,
Betrayed by his very own body.
I see all that and more; however,

I want you to know my friend, that
You are not alone in this battle
I'll be that ray of light that will guide your way
I'll be that bridge connecting you with the moment
and the now.
I won't let them upset you, and
I'll support your independence with my guidance

Allow me to reach within you
Wherever it is you are
Hold my hand and close your eyes
For I am here to ease your fear
Hold my hand and close your eyes
For a friend you never knew you had, your nurse, is here.

FIGURE 21.2 Nurse and person. Copyright 1998 by Jaime Castaneda.

KEY CONCEPTS

- Nurses must advocate for thorough assessment of any older person who appears to be experiencing cognitive decline and a reduced ability to function in important aspects of life.
- *Delirium* is sometimes the result of physiological imbalances and may be caused by a variety of biological disturbances. Delirium is characterized by acute onset, inattention, disorganized thinking, and an altered level of consciousness. It often goes unrecognized or is falsely attributed to age or dementia. People with dementia are more susceptible to delirium. Knowledge of risk factors, preventive measures, and the treatment of underlying medical problems is essential to prevent serious consequences.
- Medications and pain are frequently the causes of delirium in older people.
- Irreversible dementias follow a pattern of inevitable decline accompanied by decreased intellectual function, personality changes, and impaired judgement. The most common of these dementias is Alzheimer's disease.
- *Alzheimer's disease* (AD) has been the subject of an enormous amount of research that has attempted to understand its causes. Research is continuing in the attempt to discover ways to protect persons against AD or to halt the progress of the disease. There is no known cure, but some medications seem to slow the progress of the dementia for a time.
- *Vascular dementia* (VaD) is actually a group of heterogeneous disorders arising from cerebro-vascular insufficiency or from ischemic or hemorrhagic brain damage. It is the second most prevalent type of dementia and often coexists with AD. Hypertension, cardiac disease, diabetes, smoking, and dyslipidemia are additional risk factors for VaD. Prevention and treatment of risk factors are important.
- The assessment of cognitive impairment is complex. Nurses may do a screening assessment using any number of brief mental status examinations and must request a more thorough assessment when there is an indication of dementia.
- People with cognitive impairment respond best to calmness and patience, adaptations of communication techniques, and environments and relationships that support and enhance function, support limitations, ensure safety, and provide opportunities for a meaningful quality of life. Because cognitively impaired persons may be unable to express their feelings and needs in ways that are easily understood, the gerontological nurse must always try to understand the world from their perspective.
- There are a number of things that an individual can do to reduce risk for cerebrovascular disease.
- *Ischemic stroke* is caused by a temporary loss of oxygen to the brain, resulting in damage to the tissue.
- *Hemorrhagic stroke* results from a ruptured blood vessel in the brain. They are less common than ischemic strokes but much more deadly.
- For the best possible outcome, immediate treatment is required for the person having a stroke. The public needs to learn the signs and symptoms of stroke and how to activate the emergency response system.
- Correct diagnosis of the type of stroke is necessary before treatment can begin.
- *Parkinson's disease* is a progressive, incurable disorder that affects the voluntary control of movement.
- The signs and symptoms of Parkinson's disease may initially be mistaken for those of other common disorders that are experienced by older persons.
- Cognitive and neurological disorders frequently affect the person's ability to speak in a way that is understandable to others.
- Working with persons who have cognitive and neurological disorders requires a team approach that includes the health care providers, the patient, and the patient's significant others.

ACTIVITIES AND DISCUSSION QUESTIONS

1. What are the differences between delirium, dementia, and depression?
2. What are some of the risk factors for the development of delirium?
3. Discuss communication strategies that are useful for the person experiencing delirium.

4. Why is it important to ensure that the person experiencing any change in mental status receives a thorough assessment and evaluation?

5. What would you say to a person who reports to you that he or she has had symptoms of a transient ischemic attack?

6. How do the symptoms of Parkinson's disease affect functional abilities? What nursing interventions would be important when caring for a person with Parkinson's disease?

7. Brainstorm with fellow students about how it would feel to be bathed by a total stranger.

8. The health care aides in a long-term care home complain to you that Mr. G. hit them when they were trying to give him his required twice-weekly shower. How might you assist them in supporting Mr. G.'s care needs?

9. Describe how you would design a supportive care unit for individuals with dementia.

10. A family caregiver tells you that his or her loved one keeps trying to leave the house to find the children. What are some strategies you might share with the caregiver to help him or her deal with this situation?

RESOURCES

Alzheimer Society of Canada
http://www.alzheimer.ca/en/Home

Alzheimer Society of Canada. *Guidelines for care: Person-centred care of people with dementia living in care homes*
http://www.alzheimer.ca/sites/default/files/files/national/culture-change/culture_change_framework_e.pdf

Alzheimer Society of Canada. Safely Home program
http://www.alzheimer.ca/en/Home/Living-with-dementia/Day-to-day-living/Safety/Safely-Home

BrainXchange
http://brainxchange.ca/

Canadian Coalition for Seniors' Mental Health (CCSMH). *Tool on the assessment and treatment of behavioural symptoms of older adults living in long term care facilities (pocket tool).*
http://ccsmh.ca/wp-content/uploads/2016/03/MHI-in-LTC-Final.pdf

College of Family Physicians & P.I.E.C.E.S. Canada. Behavioural and Psychological Symptoms of Dementia (BPSD) Toolkit
https://sagelink.ca/sites/default/files/clinical-resources/bpsd_toolkit_full_pdf.pdf

Parkinson Canada
http://www.parkinson.ca

Regional Geriatric Program (RGP) Central. Resources
http://www.rgpc.ca/resources/

For additional resources, please visit *http://evolve.elsevier.com/Canada/Ebersole/gerontological/*

REFERENCES

Alzheimer Society of Canada (2011). *Guidelines for care: Person-centred care of people with dementia living in care homes.* Toronto, ON: Author. Retrieved from http://www.alzheimer.ca/sites/default/files/files/national/culture-change/culture_change_framework_e.pdf.

Alzheimer Society of Canada. (2015). *Risk factors.* Retrieved from http://www.alzheimer.ca/ns/~/media/Files/national/Research/research_Risk_Factors_e.pdf.

Alzheimer's Association. (2012). *Alzheimer's disease facts and figures, Alzheimer's and dementia.* Retrieved from http://www.alz.org/facts/overview.asp#quickfacts.

Barron, E. A., & Holmes, J. (2013). Delirium within the emergency care setting, occurrence and detection: A systematic review. *Emergency Medicine Journal, 30*(4), 263–268. doi:10.1136/emermed-2011-200586.

Barton, C., Ketelle, R., Merrilees, J., et al. (2016). Non-pharmacological management of behavioral symptoms in frontotemporal and other dementias. *Current Neurology and Neuroscience Reports, 16*(2), 14. doi:10.1007/s11910-015-0618-1.

Bauer, M., Fetherstonhaugh, D., Tarzia, L., et al. (2014). Staff–family relationships in residential aged care facilities: The views of residents' family members and care staff. *Journal of Applied Gerontology, 33*(5), 564–585. doi:10.1177/0733464812468503.

Baumbusch, J., & Phinney, A. (2014). Invisible hands: The role of highly involved families in long-term residential care. *Journal of Family Nursing, 20*(1), 73–97. doi:10.1177/1074840713507777.

Bellelli, G., Frisoni, G. B., Turco, R., et al. (2007). Delirium superimposed on dementia predicts 12-month survival in elderly patients discharged from a postacute rehabilitation facility. *Journal of Gerontology, Series A: Biological & Medical Sciences, 62*(11), 1306–1309. doi:10.1093/gerona/62.11.1306.

Boss, B., & Huether, S. E. (2014). Alterations in cognitive systems, cerebral hemodynamics, and motor function. In K. L. McCance, S. E. Huether, V. L. Brashers, et al. (Eds.), *Pathophysiology: The biologic basis for disease in adults and children* (7th ed., pp. 527–580). St. Louis, MO: Mosby.

Cabrera, E., Sutcliffe, C., Verbeek, H., et al. (2015). Non-pharmacological interventions as a best practice strategy in people with dementia living in nursing homes. A systematic review. *European Geriatric Medicine, 6*(2), 134–150. doi:10.1016/j.eurger.2014.06.003.

Canadian Coalition for Seniors' Mental Health (CCSMH). (2006a). *National guidelines for seniors' mental health: The assessment and treatment of delirium.* Toronto, ON: Author.

Canadian Coalition for Seniors' Mental Health (CCSMH). (2006b). *National guidelines for seniors' mental health: The assessment and treatment of mental health issues in long term care homes.* Toronto, ON: Author.

Canadian Institute for Health Information (CIHI). (2016). *Use of antipsychotics among seniors living in long-term care facilities, 2014.* Retrieved from https://secure.cihi.ca/free_products/LTC_AiB_v2_19_EN_web.pdf.

Canadian Study of Health and Aging (CSHA). (2002). *About the study.* Retrieved from http://www.csha.ca/about_study.asp.

Chambers, L. W., Bancej, C., & McDowell, I. (2016). *Prevalence and monetary costs of dementia in Canada: Population health expert panel.* Retrieved from http://www.alzheimer.ca/ab/~/media/Files/national/Statistics/PrevalenceandCostsofDementia_EN.pdf.

Cipriani, G., Lucetti, C., Nuti, A., et al. (2014). Wandering and dementia. *Psychogeriatrics, 14*(2), 135–142. doi:10.1111/psyg.12044.

Cohen-Mansfield, K. (2000). Nonpharmacological management of behavioral problems in persons with dementia: The TREA model. *Alzheimer's Care Quarterly, 1*(4), 22–34.

Connolly, S., & Lang, A. E. (2014). Pharmacological treatment of Parkinson Disease: A review. *JAMA: The Journal of the American Medical Association, 311*(16), 1670–1683. doi:10.1001/jama.2014.3654.

Dahlke, S., & Phinney, A. (2008). Caring for hospitalized older adults at risk for delirium: The silent, unspoken piece of nursing practice. *Journal of Gerontological Nursing, 34*(6), 41–47. doi:10.3928/00989134-20080601-03.

Dawson, P., Wells, D. L., & Kline, K. (1993). *Enhancing the abilities of persons with Alzheimer's and related dementias: A nursing perspective.* New York, NY: Springer Publishing Co.

Drummond, N., Birtwhistle, R., Williamson, T., et al. (2016). Prevalence and management of dementia in primary care practices with electronic medical records: A report from the Canadian Primary Care Sentinel Surveillance Network. *CMAJ Open, 4*(2), E177–E184. doi:10.9778/cmajo.20150050.

Dupuis, S., & Luh, J. (2005). Understanding responsive behaviours: The importance of correctly perceiving triggers that precipitate residents' responsive behaviours. *Canadian Nursing Home, 16*(1), 29–34. Retrieved from http://www.nursinghomemagazine.ca.

Elliott, A. F., Burgio, L. D., & DeCoster, J. (2010). Enhancing caregiver health: Findings from the resources for enhancing Alzheimer's caregiver health II intervention. *Journal of the American Geriatrics Society, 58*(1), 30–37. doi:10.1111/j.1532-5415.2009.02631.x.

Ely, E. W., Margolin, R., Francis, J., et al. (2001). Evaluation of delirium in critically ill patients: Validation of the Confusion Assessment Method for the intensive care unit (CAM-ICU).

Critical Care Medicine, 29(7), 1370–1379. doi:10.1097/00003246-200107000-00012.

Fick, D., & Mion, L. (2005). Assessing delirium in persons with dementia. *Hartford Geriatric Nursing Foundation Try This Dementia Series.* Retrieved from http://consultgeri.org.

Fisher, A., Carney, G., Bassett, K., et al. (2017). Tolerability of cholinesterase inhibitors: A population based study of persistence, adherence, and switching. *Drugs and Aging, 34*(3), 221–231. doi:10.1007/s40266-017-0438-x.

Fletcher, K. (2016). Dementia: A neurocognitive disorder. In M. Boltz, E. Capezuti, T. T. Fulmer, et al. (Eds.), *Evidence-based geriatric nursing protocols for best practice* (5th ed., pp. 233–250). New York, NY: Springer.

Futrell, M., Melillo, K. D., & Remington, R. (2010). Wandering. *Journal of Gerontological Nursing, 36*(2), 6–16. doi:10.3928/00989134-20100108-02.

Gauthier, S., Patterson, C., Chertkow, H., et al. (2012). Recommendations of the 4th Canadian Consensus Conference on the Diagnosis and Treatment of Dementia (CCCDTD4). *Canadian Geriatrics Journal, 15*(4), 120–126. doi:10.5770/cgj.15.49.

Gozalo, P., Prakash, S., Qato, D. M., et al. (2014). Effect of the bathing without a battle training intervention on bathing-associated physical and verbal outcomes in nursing home residents with dementia: A randomized crossover diffusion study. *Journal of the American Geriatrics Society, 62*(5), 797–804. doi:10.1111/jgs.12777.

Graykowski, J. J. (2008). Cerebrovascular events. In R. Buttaro, J. Trybulski, J. P. Bailey, et al. (Eds.), *Primary care: A collaborative practice* (3rd ed., pp. 1031–1036). St. Louis, MO: Mosby.

Hall, G. R. (1994). Caring for people with Alzheimer's disease using the conceptual model of progressively lowered stress threshold in the clinical setting. *The Nursing Clinics of North America, 29*(1), 129–141.

Hall, G. R., & Buckwalter, K. C. (1987). Progressively lowered stress threshold: A conceptual model for care of adults with Alzheimer's disease. *Archives of Psychiatric Nursing, 1*(6), 399–406.

Health Canada. (2015). *Recalls and safety alerts: Risperidone – Restriction of the dementia indication.* Retrieved from http://healthycanadians.gc.ca/recall-alert-rappel-avis/hc-sc/2015/43797a-eng.php.

Henderson, C. (1998). *Partial view: An Alzheimer's journal.* Dallas, TX: Southern Methodist Press.

Heeren, P., Flamaing, J., Tournoy, J., et al. (2016). Assessing cognitive functioning. In M. Bolz, L. Capezuti, T. T. Fulmer, et al. (Eds.), *Evidence based geriatric protocols for best practice* (5th ed., pp. 72–88). New York, NY: Springer Publishing Co.

Hogan, D. B. (2014). Long-term efficacy and toxicity of cholinesterase inhibitors in the treatment of Alzheimer Disease. *Canadian Journal of Psychiatry, 59*(12), 618–623. doi:10.1177/070674371405901202.

Hospital Elder Life Program (HELP). (2017). *What we do.* Retrieved from http://www.hospitalelderlifeprogram.org/about/what-we-do/.

Hyman, B. T., Phelps, C. H., Beach, T. G., et al. (2012). National Institute on Aging–Alzheimer's Association guidelines for the neuropathologic assessment of Alzheimer's disease. *Alzheimer's & Dementia*, 8(1), 1–13. doi:10.1016/j.jalz.2011.10.007.

Inouye, S. K. (2003). *The Confusion Assessment Method training manual and coding guide*. New Haven, CT: Yale University School of Medicine. Retrieved from http://hospitalelderlife program.org/pdf/The%20Confusion%20Assessment%20 Method.pdf.

Inouye, S. K. (2006). Delirium in older persons. *New England Journal of Medicine*, 354(11), 1157–1165. doi:10.1056/ NEJMra052321.

Inouye, S. K. (2007). *The Hospital Elder Life Program (HELP)*. Retrieved from http://elderlife.med.yale.edu/public/public-main .php?pageid=01.00.00.

Inouye, S. K., & Charpentier, P. A. (1996). Precipitating factors in delirium in hospitalized elderly persons: Predictive model and interrelationship with baseline vulnerability. *JAMA: The Journal of the American Medical Association*, 275(11), 852–857. doi:10.1001/jama.1996.03530350034031.

Inouye, S. K., Bogardus, S. T., Jr., Charpentier, P. A., et al. (1999). A multicomponent intervention to prevent delirium in hospitalized older patients. *New England Journal of Medicine*, 340(9), 669–676. doi:10.1056/NEJM199903043400901.

Inouye, S. K., van Dyck, C. H., Alessi, C. A., et al. (1990). Clarifying confusion: The confusion assessment method. A new method for detection of delirium. *Annals of Internal Medicine*, 113(12), 941–948. doi:10.7326/0003-4819-113-12-941.

Inouye, S. K., Westendorp, R. G., & Saczynski, J. S. (2014). Delirium in elderly people. *The Lancet*, 383(9920), 911–922. doi:10.1016/ S0140-6736(13)60688-1.

Jacklin, K. M., Walker, J. D., & Shawande, M. (2013). The emergence of dementia as a health concern among First Nations populations in Alberta, Canada. *Canadian Journal of Public Health*, 104(1), e39–e44. doi:10.17269/cjph.104.3348.

Kales, H. C., Gitlin, L. N., & Lyketsos, C. G. (2014). Management of neuropsychiatric symptoms of dementia in clinical settings: Recommendations from a multidisciplinary expert panel. *Journal of the American Geriatrics Society*, 62(4), 762–769. doi:10.1111/jgs.12730.

Keiburtz, K., & Wunderle, K. B. (2013). Parkinson's disease: Evidence for environmental risk factors. *Movement Disorders: Official Journal of the Movement Disorder Society*, 28(1), 8–13. doi:10.1002/mds.25150.

Kirshner, H. S. (2014). Frontotemporal dementia and primary progressive aphasia, a review. *Neuropsychiatric Disease and Treatment*, 10, 1045–1055. doi:10.2147/NDT.S38821.

Koehn, S., Badger, M., Cohen, C., et al. (2016). Negotiating access to a diagnosis of dementia: Implications for policies in health and social care. *Dementia (London)*, 15(6), 1436–1456. doi:10.1177/1471301214563551.

Kolanowski, A. M. (1999). An overview of the Need-Driven Dementia–Compromised Behavior Model. *Journal of Gerontological Nursing*, 25(9), 7–9. doi:10.3928/0098-9134-19990901 -05.

Kolanowski, A., Fick, D., Frazer, C., et al. (2010). It's about time: Use of nonpharmacological interventions in the nursing home.

Journal of Nursing Scholarship, 42(2), 214–222. doi:10.1111/j. 1547-5069.2010.01338.x.

Konno, R., Stern, C., & Gibb, H. (2013). The best evidence for assisted bathing of older people with dementia: A comprehensive systematic review. *JBI Database of Systematic Reviews and Implementation Reports*, 11(1), 123–212. doi:10.11124/ jbisrir-2013-607.

Lester, P. E., Garite, A., & Kohen, I. (2012). Wandering and elopement in nursing homes. *Annals of Long-Term Care: Clinical Care and Aging*, 20(3), 32–36. Retrieved from http:// www.managedhealthcareconnect.com/article/wandering-and -elopement-nursing-homes.

Lewy Body Dementia Association. (2016). *Lewy body update*. Retrieved from http://www.lbda.org.

Livingston, G., Kelly, L., Lewis-Holmes, E., et al. (2014). Non-pharmacological interventions for agitation in dementia: Systematic review of randomised controlled trials. *The British Journal of Psychiatry*, 205(6), 436–442. doi:10.1192/bjp.bp.113 .141119.

Llinas, R. (2010). Stroke. In S. C. Durso (Ed.), *Oxford handbook of geriatric medicine* (pp. 1072–1076). New York, NY: Oxford University Press.

Lloyd, J., Patterson, T., & Muers, J. (2016). The positive aspects of caregiving in dementia: A critical review of the qualitative literature. *Dementia (London)*, (14713012). 15(6), 1534–1561. doi:10.1177/1471301214564792.

Manuel, D. G., Tuna, M., Perez, R., et al. (2015). Predicting stroke risk based on health behaviours: Development of the Stroke Population Risk Tool (SPoRT). *PLoS ONE*, 10(12), e014342. doi:10.1371/journal.pone.0143342.

Marcantonio, E. R., Simon, S. E., Bergmann, M. A., et al. (2003). Delirium symptoms in post-acute care: Prevalent, persistent, and associated with poor functional recovery. *Journal of the American Geriatrics Society*, 51(1), 4–9. doi:10.1034/j.1601-5215.2002.51002.x.

McCleary, L., Persaud, M., Hum, S., et al. (2013). Pathways to dementia diagnosis among South Asian Canadians. *Dementia: The International Journal of Social Research and Practice*, 12(6), 769–789. doi:10.1177/1471301212444806.

McCusker, J., Cole, M. G., Voyer, P., et al. (2013). Environmental factors predict the severity of delirium symptoms in long-term care residents with and without delirium. *Journal of the American Geriatrics Society*, 61(4), 502–511. doi:10.1111/jgs .12164.

McGilton, K. S., Sidani, S., Boscart, V. M., et al. (2012). The relationship between care providers' relational behaviors and residents mood and behavior in long-term care settings. *Aging & Mental Health*, 16(4), 507–515. doi:10.1080/13607863.2011 .628980.

McGreevy, J. (2016). Implementing culture change in long-term dementia care settings. *Nursing Standard*, 30(19), 44–50. doi: 10.7748/ns.30.19.44.s43.

Mirijello, A., D'Angelo, C., Ferrulli, A., et al. (2015). Identification and management of alcohol withdrawal syndrome. *Drugs*, 75(4), 353–365. doi:10.1007/s40265-015-0358-1.

Mittelman, M. S., Roth, D. L., Clay, O. J., et al. (2007). Preserving health of Alzheimer caregivers: Impact of a spouse caregiver intervention. *The American Journal of Geriatric Psychiatry*, *15*(9), 780–789. doi:10.1097/JGP.0b013e31805d858a.

Moore, A., Patterson, C., Lee, L., et al. (2014). Fourth Canadian Consensus Conference on the Diagnosis and Treatment of Dementia: Recommendations for family physicians. *Canadian Family Physician*, *60*(5), 433–438. doi:10.1111/j.1532-5415.200 5.53221.x.

National Institute of Neurological Disorders and Stroke [NINDS]. (2012). *NINDS deep brain stimulation for Parkinson's disease information*. Retrieved from https://www.ninds.nih.gov/ Disorders/All-Disorders/Deep-Brain-Stimulation-Parkinson s-Disease-Information-Page.

Neelon, V. J., Champagne, M. T., Carlson, J. R., et al. (1996). The NEECHAM confusion scale: Construction, validation and clinical testing. *Nursing Research*, *45*(6), 324–330. doi:10.109 7/00006199-199611000-00002.

Olazarán, J., Reisberg, B., Clare, L., et al. (2010). Nonpharmaco- logical therapies in Alzheimer's disease: A systematic review of efficacy. *Dementia and Geriatric Cognitive Disorders*, *30*(2), 161–178. doi:10.1159/000316119.

Ontario Stroke Network. (2016). *Stroke stats & facts*. Retrieved from http://ontariostrokenetwork.ca/information-about-stroke/ stroke-stats-and-facts/.

Ortigara, A. (2000). Understanding the language of behaviors. *Alzheimer's Care Quarterly*, *1*(4), 89–92. Retrieved from http:// journals.lww.com/actjournalonline/pages/default.aspx.

Parmar, J., Dobbs, B., McKay, R., et al. (2014). Diagnosis and man- agement of dementia in primary care. Exploratory study. *Cana- dian Family Physician*, *60*(5), 457–465. Retrieved from http:// www.cfp.ca/.

Porter, R. S., & Kaplan, J. L. (Eds.). *The Merck manual online* (2010-2011). Retrieved from http://www.merckmanuals.com/ professional/index.html.

Rader, J., & Barrick, A. (2000). Ways that work: Bathing without a battle. *Alzheimer's Care Quarterly*, *1*(4), 35–49. Retrieved from http://journals.lww.com/actjournalonline/pages/default.aspx.

Registered Nurses' Association of Ontario (RNAO). (2004). *Nursing Best Practice Guideline: Caregiving strategies for older adults with delirium, dementia, and depression*. Toronto, ON: Author. Retrieved from http://www.rnao.org/Storage/69/6404_ FINAL_-_Caregiving_-_BPG_+_Supplement.pdf.

Registered Nurses' Association of Ontario (RNAO). (2016). *Clini- cal Best Practice Guidelines: Delirium, dementia, and depression in older adults: Assessment and care*. Toronto, ON: Author. Re- trieved from http://rnao.ca/sites/rnao-ca/files/3Ds_BPG_WEB _FINAL.pdf.

Richards, K., Lambert, C., & Beck, C. (2000). Deriving inter- ventions for challenging behaviors from the need-driven, dementia-compromised behavior model. *Alzheimer's Care Quarterly*, *1*(4), 62–76.

Richardson, T. J., Lee, S. J., Berg-Weger, M., et al. (2013). Caregiver health: Health of caregivers of Alzheimer's and other dementia patients. *Current Psychiatry Reports*, *15*(7), 367. doi:10.1007/ s11920-013-0367-2.

Rigney, T. (2006). Delirium in the hospitalized elder and recom- mendations for practice. *Geriatric Nursing*, *27*(3), 151–157. doi:10.1016/j.gerinurse.2006.03.014.

Rosenbloom, D. A., & Fick, D. M. (2014). Nurse/family caregiver intervention for delirium increases delirium knowledge and improves attitudes toward partnership. *Geriatric Nursing*, *35*(3), 175–181. doi:10.1016/j.gerinurse.2013.12.004.

Rowe, M. A. (2003). People with dementia who become lost. *Amer- ican Journal of Nursing*, *103*(7), 32–39. doi:10.1097/0000044 6-200307000-00016.

Rowe, M. A., Kairalla, J. A., & McCrae, C. S. (2010). Sleep in dementia caregivers and the effect of a nighttime monitoring system. *Journal of Nursing Scholarship*, *42*(3), 338–347. doi: 10.1111/j.1547-5069.2010.01337.x.

Sayegh, P., & Knight, B. G. (2013). Cross-cultural differences in dementia: The Sociocultural Health Belief Model. *Inter- national Psychogeriatrics*, *25*(04), 517–530. doi:10.1017/ S104161021200213X.

Schindel Martin, L., Gillies, L., Coker, E., et al. (2016). An education intervention to enhance staff self-efficacy to provide dementia care in an acute care hospital in Canada: A nonrandomized con- trolled study. *American Journal of Alzheimer's Disease & Other Dementias*, *31*(8), 664–677. doi:10.1177/1533317516668574.

Sidani, S., Streiner, D., & LeClerc, C. (2012). Evaluating the effec- tiveness of the abilities-focused approach to morning care of people with dementia. *International Journal of Older People Nursing*, *7*(1), 37–45. doi:10.1111/j.1748-3743.2011.00273.x.

Slaughter, S., & Bankes, J. (2007). The functional transitions model: Maximizing ability in the context of progressive disability asso- ciated with Alzheimer's disease. *Canadian Journal on Aging*, *26*(1), 39–48. doi:10.3138/Q62V-1558-4653-P0HX.

Slaughter, S. E., Eliasziw, M., Morgan, D., et al. (2011). Incidence and predictors of excess disability in walking among nursing home residents with middle-stage dementia: A prospective cohort study. *International Psychogeriatrics*, *23*(01), 54–64. doi:10.1017/S1041610210000116.

Smith, M., Gerdner, L. A., Hall, G. R., et al. (2004). History, devel- opment, and future of the progressively lowered stress thresh- old: A conceptual model for dementia care. *Journal of the American Geriatrics Society*, *52*, 1755–1760. doi:10.1111/j.1532 -5415.2004.52473.x.

Speziale, J., Black, E., Coatsworth-Puspoky, R., et al. (2009). Moving forward: Evaluating a curriculum for managing responsive behaviours in a geriatric psychiatry inpatient population. *The Gerontologist*, *49*(4), 570–576. doi:10.1093/geront/gnp069.

Splete, H. (2008). Nurses have special strategies for dementia. *Caring for the Ages*, *9*(6), 11.

Steinberg, M., & Lyketsos, C. G. (2012). Atypical antipsychotic use in patients with dementia: Managing safety concerns. *Ameri- can Journal of Psychiatry*, *169*(9), 900–906. doi:10.1176/appi. ajp.2012.12030342.

Stroke Network of Southwestern Ontario. (2015). *Stroke statistics*. Retrieved from: http://swostroke.ca/stroke-statistics/.

Sweeny, S. J., Bridges, E. J., Wild, L. M., et al. (2008). Care of the patient with delirium. *American Journal of Nursing*, *108*(5), 72CC–72FF. doi:10.1097/01.NAJ.0000318007.70410.27.

Talerico, K., & Evans, L. (2000). Making sense of aggressive/protective behaviors in persons with dementia. *Alzheimer's Care Quarterly*, *1*(4), 77–88. Retrieved from http://journals.lww.com/actjournalonline/pages/default.aspx.

Tullmann, D. F., Blevins, C., & Fletcher, K. (2016). Delirium: Prevention, early recognition, and treatment. In M. Boltz, E. Capezuti, T. Fulmer, et al. (Eds.), *Evidence-based geriatric nursing protocols for best practice* (5th ed., pp. 251–261). New York, NY: Springer.

Voelker, R. (2008). Programs ease hospitalization experience for patients with dementia. *CNS Senior Care*, *7*(1), 17–18. 3.

Voyer, P., Cole, M. G., McCusker, J., et al. (2006). Prevalence and symptoms of delirium superimposed on dementia. *Clinical Nursing Research*, *15*(1), 46–66. doi:10.1177/1054773805282299.

Voyer, P., Richard, S., Doucet, L., et al. (2008). Detection of delirium by nurses among long-term care residents with dementia. *BMC Nursing*, *7*, 4. doi:10.1186/1472-6955-7-4.

Voyer, P., Richard, S., McCusker, J., et al. (2012). Detection of delirium and its symptoms by nurses working in a long term care facility. *Journal of the American Medical Directors Association*, *13*(3), 264–271. doi:10.1016/j.jamda.2010.11.002.

Voyer, P., Richard, S., Doucet, L., et al. (2009). Detecting delirium and subsyndromal delirium using different diagnostic criteria among demented long-term care residents. *Journal of the American Medical Directors Association*, *10*(3), 181–188. doi:10.1016/j.jamda.2008.09.006.

Voyer, P., Richard, S., Doucet, L., et al. (2010). Examination of the multifactorial model of delirium among long-term care residents with dementia. *Geriatric Nursing*, *31*(2), 105–114. doi:10.1016/j.gerinurse.2009.12.001.

Waszynski, C. M. (2007). How to try this: Detecting delirium. *The American Journal of Nursing*, *107*(12), 50–59. doi:10.1097/01.NAJ.0000301029.87489.35.

Wells, D., & Dawson, P. (2000). Description of retained abilities in older persons with dementia. *Research in Nursing and Health*, *23*(2), 158–166. doi:10.1002/(SICI)1098-240X(200004)23:2%3C158::AID-NUR8%3E3.0.CO;2-L.

Williams, C. L., Tappen, R. M., Rosselli, M., et al. (2010). Willingness to be screened and tested for cognitive impairment: Cross-cultural comparison. *American Journal of Alzheimer's Disease & Other Dementias*, *25*(2), 160–166. doi:10.1177/1533317509352333.

Wong, S. L., Gilmour, H., & Ramage-Morin, P. L. (2016). Alzheimer's disease and other dementias in Canada. *Health Reports*, *27*(5), 11–16. Retrieved from http://www.statcan.gc.ca/pub/82-003-x/2016005/article/14613-eng.htm.

CHAPTER 22

Economic and Legal Issues

Upon completion of this chapter, the reader will be able to:

- Explain reasons for differences between Canadian provinces and territories in health insurance for out-of-hospital health care services.
- Describe the financing of the Canadian health care system.
- Compare the Old Age Security Program, the Canada Pension Plan, and the Quebec Pension Plan.
- Compare and discuss the roles of a power of attorney and a guardian.
- Explain the process of assessing mental capacity.
- Detect and assess elder abuse.
- Describe strategies for preventing and detecting the abuse of older persons.

GLOSSARY

Gross domestic product The main measure of economic activity, defined as "the total market value of all final goods and services produced within a country in a given period of time (usually a calendar year)" (Black, Hashimzade, & Myles, 2009. ¶1).

Intersectoral collaboration Health care providers working with experts in fields that are outside the health sector (e.g., housing, employment, justice).

Net income Income after deductions for certain payments and deductions specified by Revenue Canada (pensions, union dues, child care expenses, disability support, moving expenses, support payments, employment expenses, and clergy residence costs).

THE LIVED EXPERIENCE

My CPP [Canada Pension Plan] pension is so small because I worked part-time back when it started and I stopped my full-time job early because of my husband's illness. The OAS [Old Age Security] pension makes a big difference for me. Without it, I'd have just enough money to get by. There would be no extras, like going to the church supper.

A 73-year-old woman

Growing older isn't so bad if you're financially okay. There are one or two ladies here [community centre] who are worried about finances. That must be very wearing too. I mean you don't have to be rich, but as long as you know that you're not going to be financially strapped all the time.

An older participant in a study of healthy aging

From Tomlinson, R. G. (1992). *The experience of aging: A qualitative study of well elderly individuals* (Unpublished master's thesis) (p. 58). Vancouver, BC: University of British Columbia. Retrieved from https://circle.ubc.ca/bitstream/handle/2429/3120/ubc_1992_fall_tomilson_roxanne_gaye.pdf? sequence=1.

Canadians represent all levels of education, experience, and income. However, everyone has in common the potential need for health care. It is rare to meet an older person who does not have some experience with both the past and the present Canadian health care systems. The Canadian health care system is in a constant state of flux. Health care financing is a political issue and a topic of debate in Canada. It is important to have a basic understanding of how the health care system is financed and what the implications are for our aging society. Contrary to some claims, financial sustainability is possible, even with a growing number of older Canadians.

Standard V of the *Canadian Gerontological Nursing Competencies and Standards of Practice* (Canadian Gerontological Nursing Association, 2010) specifies that gerontological nurses are expected not only to advocate for the older patient and the health care system but also to identify gaps, barriers, and fragmentation in the health care system and to work to overcome them. This chapter provides an overview of the Canadian health care system, including financing and services for veterans. Social security programs for older Canadians are described, and legal issues of capacity and guardianship are discussed. The final section of the chapter deals with the abuse of older persons, a problem that is gaining recognition in Canada.

THE CANADIAN HEALTH CARE SYSTEM

The Canadian health care system has been evolving for many years. Older people who grew up in Canada have experienced dramatic changes in the way health care is funded. Prior to 1947, health care in Canada was privately delivered and funded. People paid for health care out of pocket or through private insurance; people who could not pay relied on charity. In 1947, the government of Saskatchewan introduced a provincial hospital insurance plan, and in 1957, the federal government passed legislation for sharing the costs of hospital services with the provinces. This legislation was extended to physicians' services in 1962, and all provinces and territories had physician insurance plans by 1968.

THE *CANADA HEALTH ACT*

The *Canada Health Act* of 1984 is an amalgamation of previous federal legislation. It sets out the national

health insurance plan as well as federal, provincial, and territorial roles in the health care system. Health care is administered and delivered by the provinces and territories; the Canadian "system" is 13 interlinked provincial and territorial systems. The responsibilities of the federal government include the following:

- Setting and administering national principles for the health care system through the *Canada Health Act*
- Collaborating with provinces and territories on national health policies
- Contributing to the funding of health care services through transfer payments to the provinces and territories

The transfer of funds for health care from the federal government to provincial governments is contingent on adherence to the principles of the *Canada Health Act* (Box 22.1). The federal government's responsibilities are limited in regard to the provision of health care services for specific groups (e.g., First Nations, Inuit, and veterans). Aside from this limited health care delivery by the federal government, the management, financing, and delivery of publicly insured health services is the responsibility of the provinces and territories, each with its own health care insurance plan. Under the *Canada Health Act*, "medically necessary" services are publicly insured, including primary health care, care in hospitals, and dental surgery in hospitals. However, the term "medically necessary" is not explicitly defined and is thus somewhat open to interpretation. Hence, there is variability across the country in the provision of some services such as home care, long-term care (LTC), medications outside of hospital, physiotherapy, optometry services, and others. The level of funding provided for these services varies from province to province. For example, provincial variations in LTC mean differences in the amount that residents pay (McDonald, 2015), the hours of care provided per day (see Chapter 26), and the requirements for length of residency in the province to determine eligibility for government-funded LTC. Furthermore, services have been added and deleted from provincial health insurance plans at various times.

HEALTH CARE FINANCING

According to a report from the Canadian Institute for Health Information (Canadian Institute for Health

BOX 22.1	Principles of the *Canada Health Act*
Public administration	The provincial and territorial plans must be administered and operated on a nonprofit basis by a public authority accountable to the provincial or territorial government.
Comprehensiveness	The provincial and territorial plans must insure all medically necessary services provided by hospitals, medical practitioners, and dentists working within a hospital setting.
Universality	The provincial and territorial plans must entitle all insured persons to health insurance coverage on uniform terms and conditions.
Portability	The provincial and territorial plans must cover all insured persons when they move to another province or territory within Canada and when they travel abroad. The provinces and territories have some limits on coverage for services provided outside Canada and may require prior approval for non-emergency services delivered outside their jurisdiction.
Accessibility	The provincial and territorial plans must provide all insured persons reasonable access to medically necessary hospital and physician services without financial or other barriers.

Source: Health Canada. (2012). *Canada's health care system.* Retrieved from http://www.hc-sc.gc.ca/hcs-sss/pubs/system-regime/2011-hcs-sss/index-eng.php.

Information [CIHI], 2016), total health care spending in Canada in 2016 was about $228.1 billion. Government spending consistently accounts for about 70% of total health care spending, while private-sector spending (i.e., private insurance and out-of-pocket expenses) accounts for 30% of spending. Per capita spending varies by province; the highest per-person expenditure ($14,065) is in the Northwest Territories, and the lowest ($5,822) is in Quebec. At 29.5%, spending on hospitals accounts for the largest proportion of health expenditures, followed by expenditures on medications (16.0%) and physicians' services (15.3%). Health care spending on LTC homes and residential care facilities accounts for 10.6% of health expenditures.

According to Canadian Institute for Health Information, health care spending for older persons is stable (CIHI, 2016). The proportion of government health care expenditures for older persons has been about 46% since 1998. Per capita expenditures for older persons are higher than those for younger adults—$6,424 for people aged 65 to 69 years and $21,150 for people older than 80 years. (Overall expenditure is $6,299 per Canadian.) Health care funding has not increased in proportion to inflation and to the growth of the Canadian population.

The myth that population aging will overwhelm the Canadian health care system has repeatedly been shown to be false, but the myth still persists (Canadian Health Services Research Foundation [CHSRF], 2011;

CIHI, 2016; Sheets & Gallagher, 2013). Historically, the increased use of services by older persons in poor health accounted for small portions of the increased health care expenditures for the entire population of older persons (CHSRF, 2011; Canadian Institute for Health Information [CIHI], 2011). Increased costs of services and increased use of expensive technologies (such as diagnostic imaging) in the general population have had a much bigger impact on government health care spending and may continue to do so (CIHI, 2011).

The Canadian Institute for Health Information predicts a gradual increase of about 1% in health care costs attributable to population aging (CIHI, 2016). Government health care spending as a proportion of **gross domestic product** is not significantly affected by expenditures on older Canadians. Over the years, the biggest cost increase in the health care system has been spending on prescription medication. However, most of this expense is paid out of pocket and by private insurance. The extent to which provincial governments pay for prescription medications for older persons varies considerably from province to province. For example, Albertans aged 65 years and older pay 30% of each prescription, to a maximum of $25 per prescription (Alberta Health, 2017). In Ontario, those aged 65 years and older pay the first $100 of prescription costs and then up to $6.11 for each prescription filled or renewed (Government of Ontario, 2017). The rising costs of prescription medications will have an effect on both government expenditures and individual Canadians. The way in which health services are provided to older Canadians will continue to be monitored; there will be continued pressure to use research evidence about the best models of health care and health promotion.

SOCIAL SECURITY RETIREMENT INCOME PROGRAMS

Social security retirement income programs are designed to minimize the chances that retirees and older people will live in poverty. The first publicly funded income support program for older Canadians came with the establishment of the Old Age Security program in 1952 at about the same time as the establishment of the first publicly funded health insurance programs. The Canada Pension Plan and the parallel Quebec Pension Plan were established in 1966.

OLD AGE SECURITY PROGRAM

The Old Age Security (OAS) program is an income support program for older Canadians. It includes the OAS pension, the Guaranteed Income Supplement, the Allowance, and the Allowance for the Survivor. It is federally financed through general tax revenues.

Old Age Security Pension

The OAS pension is a monthly payment available to Canadian citizens and legal residents, aged 65 years and older, who have lived in Canada for at least 10 years after the age of 18 years. Citizens and legal residents who do not reside in Canada may receive the OAS pension if they have lived in Canada for at least 20 years after the age of 18 years. Older persons must apply to receive OAS, and they can apply 6 months before their sixty-fifth birthday. Whether the older person receives a full or partial OAS pension depends on his or her length of residency in Canada after the age of 18 years. The full OAS pension is provided to (1) people who have lived in Canada for at least 40 years after turning 18 years of age, and (2) people who lived in Canada for 10 years immediately before approval of their OAS application and who meet additional residency or immigration status requirements. This means that some people who immigrated to Canada as older persons are not eligible for OAS for the first

10 years of residence. In 2017, the maximum monthly OAS pension benefit was $578.53. The amount is "indexed" to the cost of living; every four months the amount is adjusted if the cost of living increases. The OAS is taxable income. Persons with an annual **net income** over $119,615 do not receive OAS. Pensioners with individual net incomes over $73,756 must repay part of the OAS. Updated rates for all benefits are available at the Service Canada website (https://www.canada.ca/en/services/benefits/publicpensions/cpp/old-age-security/payments.html#tbl1).

Guaranteed Income Supplement

The Guaranteed Income Supplement (GIS), sometimes referred to as "the supplement," is a monthly benefit for OAS recipients who have little or no other income. Recipients apply at the same time they apply for the OAS and must reapply annually. Sponsored immigrants are not eligible for the GIS or the Allowance during the period of their sponsorship (up to 10 years) except under limited conditions. The amount of the benefit depends on the amount of other income, marital status, and whether or not the spouse is receiving OAS or the GIS; the rate for single persons is higher than that for persons who are married or living as common-law partners. In 2017, the maximum monthly benefit was $864.09 for a single person and $520.17 for the spouse of someone who receives OAS. Like OAS, the GIS is indexed to the cost of living.

Allowance and Allowance for the Survivor

The Allowance is paid to the spouse or common-law partner of an OAS pensioner. The Allowance for the Survivor is paid to the survivor (widow or widower) of an OAS pensioner. It is an income-tested benefit based on the combined yearly income of a couple or the survivor. Persons between the ages of 60 and 64 years who meet Canadian citizenship and residency requirements are eligible to apply and must reapply annually. The benefits are not taxable income and stop at age 65 years, when the person becomes eligible for the OAS. The maximum monthly benefit for the Allowance was $1,098.70 in 2017, and the maximum monthly benefit for the Allowance for the Survivor was $1,309.67. The Allowance and the Allowance for the Survivor are indexed to the cost of living.

CANADA PENSION PLAN AND QUEBEC PENSION PLAN

The Canada Pension Plan (CPP) and the Quebec Pension Plan (QPP) provide retirement pensions and disability benefits for persons who have made contributions to the plans. When a contributor to the plan dies, the CPP and QPP also provide survivor benefits for eligible spouses, common-law partners (including same-sex partners), and dependent children. The CPP and the QPP were established after years of provincial–federal negotiations. Provinces may opt out of the CPP (the federal pension plan). Quebec is the only province with its own plan, the QPP. The CPP and the QPP are similar; neither is funded from tax revenues but rather from mandatory contributions from all employers, employees, and self-employed persons.

Older persons are eligible to receive the CPP or the QPP retirement pension if they have contributed to one of the plans and they are either 65 years old or more or if they are between 60 and 64 years of age and meet additional requirements. To receive the CPP or QPP between 60 and 64 years of age, the person either must stop working and have no earnings for 1 month before the pension begins or must earn less than the current monthly CPP retirement pension amount. The person must apply to receive the CPP or QPP retirement pension. The amount received depends on how much and how long the person contributed to the CPP or QPP and on their age when they start receiving the pension. The maximum monthly benefit was $1,114.15 in 2017; this amount is indexed to the cost of living and is adjusted annually. The maximum amount is less for persons who start receiving the pension before age 65 years. The average monthly CPP benefit for new beneficiaries in 2016 was $644.34 (Service Canada, 2017).

Survivor benefits include the CPP death benefit, the CPP survivor's pension, and the CPP children's benefit. The CPP death benefit is a maximum $2,500 payment to the deceased contributor's estate. The CPP survivor's pension is a monthly payment to the spouse or common-law partner of a person who received or was eligible to receive the CPP. The amount of the survivor pension benefit depends on contributions the spouse made to the CPP and on the surviving spouse's age and income. If the surviving spouse is 65 or more years of age and is not receiving other CPP benefits, he or she receives 60% of the contributor's CPP pension. The benefit amount for surviving spouses who are aged 64 years or less depends on a number of other conditions.

Workers between the ages of 65 and 70 years can continue to contribute to CPP and QPP funds. It may be possible for people who made contributions to a social security system in a country with which Canada has a social security agreement to use those contributions to meet minimum qualifying conditions. For further information about the QPP, see http://www.retraitequebec.gouv.qc.ca. For information about the CPP, see https://www.canada.ca/en/services.

FINANCING OAS, CPP, AND QPP

Old age security (OAS) is financed through federal tax revenues. The CPP and QPP are financed through mandatory contributions from employers, employees, and self-employed workers and from revenue from investments of funds in the CPP and QPP. Funds in the CPP and QPP are independently managed by the Canada Pension Plan Investment Board and by La caisse de dépôt et placement du Québec (referred to as the "Caisse"), respectively. Both fund-management bodies operate at arm's length from the government, are accountable to the public, and are responsible for maximizing returns on investment without undue risk.

The amount that employers, employees, and self-employed workers contribute to the CPP and QPP is set to ensure the long-term viability of the CPP and QPP. The current contribution rates are 9.9% of earnings (under the CPP) and 10.8% of earnings (under the QPP) up to $55,300 per year; the first $3,500 of earnings are exempt. Self-employed workers contribute the full amount. In the case of employees, the employee and the employer each contribute half of the maximum amount. The plan is designed to replace about 25% of earnings up to $42,620 per year. Pensions to current pensioners are paid from contributions of current workers and employers; the surplus is added to the CPP and QPP fund and invested.

Public opinion surveys indicate that Canadians are not well informed about the CPP and have doubts about the future viability of the CPP (Press, 2017). However, since reforms to the contribution system were made in 1996, actuarial reports and audits of the fund have consistently shown that the CPP and QPP are financially sound. As of December 2016, the CPP fund was $298.1 billion (CPP Investment Board, 2016a). Currently, the fund is not used to pay pension benefits; this will not occur until 2020, when a small portion of investment earnings will be used to pay benefits. It is projected that additional contributions to the CPP fund will be higher than additional payouts and costs to run the fund until 2058. By that time, the fund will have grown considerably, producing more investment income to continue to finance pensions (Office of the Chief Actuary, 2016; CPP Investment Board, 2016b). The Chief Actuary of Canada asserts that the CPP is sustainable over a very long term (Office of the Chief Actuary, 2016). As with Medicare, the growing number of older Canadians will not "bankrupt" the current CPP and QPP pensions.

 ## IMPLICATIONS FOR GERONTOLOGICAL NURSING AND HEALTHY AGING

Medicare and the social security income programs that are part of the social safety net in Canada directly affect the health of older Canadians. Medicare is designed to ensure that Canadians receive required health care regardless of their financial means. The OAS programs and the CPP and QPP are designed to ensure that older Canadians do not live in poverty.

Gerontological nurses will nonetheless find that, despite the principles of universality and accessibility enshrined in the *Canada Health Act*, the health care services that older persons need are not always equally available across the country. Many services that support older people's health are not deemed "medically necessary" as defined by the *Canada Health Act* and may fall outside provincial health plans. This does not mean that these services are unavailable; rather, access may depend on the older person's income or on where he or she lives. For example, the amount that residents pay for accommodation in LTC homes varies across provinces (see Chapter 26); access to respite services is limited in rural and remote areas (see Chapter 26); access to end-of-life care is uneven, especially for those living in rural and remote areas (see Chapter 25); and culturally and ethnically specific

services for older persons are limited (see Chapter 23). Gerontological nurses have a role in individually and collectively advocating policies that improve access to health care services for older Canadians.

The OAS program and the CPP and QPP are two parts of financial security in retirement. The third "pillar" of financial security is private savings, including Registered Retirement Savings Plans (RRSPs). Not everyone has adequate retirement savings; many older women are not eligible for CPP or QPP, and some immigrants may not be eligible for OAS or for CPP or QPP. Consequently, 12.5% of Canadians aged 65 years and older live under low-income circumstances (Statistics Canada, 2013).

The two commonly used measures of poverty in Canada are the low income cut-off (LICO) and the low income measure (LIM). (The latter is now favoured by Statistics Canada.) The LICO is the point at which a family is spending 70% or more of their income on necessities (i.e., food, clothing, and shelter). The LICO depends on family size and community size. In 2014, the LICO for one person living alone ranged from $13,188 for a person living in a rural area to $20,160 for a person living in an area with a population of 500,000. For two-person families, the corresponding LICOs were $16,051 to $24,536 (Statistics Canada, 2015). A single older Canadian with no other income would receive $17,311.44 per year from a combination of the OAS program and the GIS.

Thanks to the growth in the numbers of people receiving full CPP and QPP benefits, the percentage of older Canadians living in poverty has declined over the years, from 21% in 1980 to a low of 3.9% in the mid-1990s (Schirle, 2013). According to Statistics Canada, 5.2% of males and 3.8% of females 65 years of age were living below the LICO in 2011 (Statistics Canada, 2013). Statistics Canada (2013) reported an increase in the proportion of older Canadians living below the LICO in recent years.

Recent use of the LIM, a more contemporary and valid estimate of low income than the LICO, reveals higher levels of poverty among Canadians, including older Canadians—13.4% among older Canadians in 2011 and 12.5% in 2014 (Statistics Canada, 2016). These findings cannot be compared to previously reported rates because of different ways of defining low income. There is considerable variation in poverty rates among specific groups of older persons. Rates are higher for women (14.4%) than for men (10.3%) and for people who live alone (28.8%) (Statistics Canada, 2016). Poverty rates are also high for Indigenous and immigrant older persons (Preston et al., 2012/2013).

The process of applying for the GIS, the Allowance, and the Allowance for the Survivor can be challenging. A significant number of older Canadians miss out on benefits they are entitled to and need because of late applications or missed renewal application deadlines. Nurses' assessments should include information about total income, all sources of income, and the person's knowledge about the process of applying for OAS and CPP or QPP benefits. Because some older people may be reluctant to reveal the extent of their financial need, assessment in the context of the therapeutic relationship is important. Nurses can provide the person with information about income supports and the process of applying. Detailed information is available on the Service Canada website (https://www.canada.ca/en.html).

Receiving the GIS may entitle the recipient to additional benefits from their province or territory. Gerontological nurses should be aware of additional benefits that older persons with low income can apply for in their province or territory and be familiar with the process of applying for these benefits. Recipients must reapply for the GIS and the Allowance every spring. They can reapply by completing an income tax return. If a tax return is not filed by April 30, a renewal form is mailed to the recipient. Completing a tax return may also be tied to other entitlements, such as provincial tax rebates. In many communities, nurses can provide older persons with information about charitable organizations that help people with a low income complete and file tax returns.

Gerontological nurses can promote age-friendly attitudes and combat ageism by being knowledgeable about the financing of both the health care system and the pension system. Statements that older persons will overwhelm either system are unfounded.

HEALTH CARE AND SERVICES FOR VETERANS

The Canadian health care system includes services for veterans that are provided or funded directly by the federal government. As of March 2014, there were approximately 685,300 veterans in Canada. (A "veteran" is a person who served in the Canadian Forces.)

"Traditional" veterans are those who served in the First World War (of which there are no living survivors), the Second World War, and the Korean War. The average age of the 75,900 WWII veterans is 91 years; the average age of the 9,100 Korean War veterans is 83 years. "Nontraditional" veterans are those who served in the Regular Forces or Primary Reserves after 1947 (except those who served in the Korean War). The average age of the 600,300 Canadian Forces Veterans (Regular Forces and Primary Reserves) is 57 years (Veterans Affairs Canada, 2016).

The federal government, through Veterans Affairs Canada, provides treatment and other health-related benefits and services to veterans and to civilians who served in wartime. It also provides services to retired members of the Royal Canadian Mounted Police. Services and benefits include disability pensions; war veterans allowance; home care services; financial support for LTC; counselling; personalized case planning; medical needs assessment, advice, information, and referral; legal help with pension or allowance matters; and help with the cost of funerals and burials. Health care services are provided directly or through community or contract facilities. There are some differences in eligibility for and types of services provided for traditional and nontraditional veterans.

WAR VETERANS ALLOWANCE AND DISABILITY PENSION

The War Veterans Allowance (WVA) provides monthly financial assistance to meet basic needs and is provided in recognition of the war service of veterans and qualified civilians. The following veterans and civilians meet war service requirements:

1. Canadian Armed Forces veterans and Merchant Navy veterans who served in the First or Second World War or in the Korean War
2. Veterans of allied countries who served in the First or Second World War or in the Korean War and lived in Canada either before or after the war
3. Civilians who served in close support of the Canadian Armed Forces during wartime

Eligibility is based on age or health, income, and residency in Canada at the time of application.

The WVA is an income-tested benefit that supplements income up to a maximum ceiling. Surviving spouses, common-law partners, or orphans may also qualify.

Disability pensions are provided to eligible veterans who have a medical disability related to their service. Eligibility for the disability pension and eligibility for the WVA are based on the same three criteria. Disability pensions are monthly payments; additional payments to disability pensioners, depending on the pensioner's eligibility, may include the exceptional incapacity allowance, the attendance allowance, and the clothing allowance. Veterans who served after 1947 and were disabled as a result of their service are eligible for a lump-sum disability payment rather than a monthly disability pension.

Veterans Health Care Program

Persons who receive the WVA and some recipients of disability pensions are also eligible for other programs and benefits, including health care benefits. The Veterans Health Care Program promotes independence and assists in keeping veterans at home and in their communities. This program includes the Veterans Independence Program, treatment benefits, and long-term care.

Veterans Independence Program. The Veterans Independence Program complements other federal, provincial, and municipal programs that help veterans remain in their homes and communities. Services depend on the individual's circumstances and health needs and may include the following: grounds maintenance; housekeeping; personal care services; nutrition services (such as Meals on Wheels); health and support services; outpatient health care, including the provision of adult day programs; payment of transportation costs for adult day programs, social activities, and activities of daily living; and home adaptation. Disabled and low-income survivors of certain categories of veterans are eligible for the housekeeping and grounds maintenance services.

Health Care Benefits. Recipients of the WVA or the disability pension are eligible for treatment benefits. For disability pensioners, eligibility is limited to services that are directly related to the condition for which the disability pension was granted. Treatment benefit programs are listed in Box 22.2.

BOX 22.2 Veterans Health Care Benefit Programs

- Aids for daily living (e.g., walking, bedroom, and bathroom assistive devices)
- Ambulance and medical travel
- Hearing services
- Dental services
- Acute care, chronic care, and rehabilitative care hospital services
- Physician services not covered by provincial health plans
- Medical and surgical equipment
- Nursing services for assessments, foot care, and visits
- Oxygen therapy and supplies
- Prescription medications
- Prosthetics and orthotics
- Health services including chiropractic, massage therapy, physiotherapy, acupuncture, occupational therapy, speech therapy, and psychological counselling
- Vision care
- Special equipment (e.g., hospital beds, lifts, home adaptations, wheelchairs, driving aids)

Source: Adapted from Veterans Affairs Canada. (2014). *Programs of choice (POC)*. Retrieved from http://www.veterans.gc.ca/eng/services/health/treatment-benefits/poc#poc8.

Long-Term Care. For eligible veterans, Veterans Affairs Canada shares with provincial and territorial LTC programs the cost of care at an LTC home. Veterans pay the cost of accommodations and meals (see Chapter 26). The cost of LTC is subsidized according to the person's military service, the person's income, and whether the person's admission to an LTC home is due to the condition for which he or she is receiving the disability pension. Veterans Affairs Canada works with veterans, their families, LTC homes, and provincial and municipal governments to ensure that veterans' needs are met. An outreach and visitation program operated by the Royal Canadian Legion provides volunteer visitors to veterans who receive financial assistance and live in LTC homes.

 IMPLICATIONS FOR GERONTOLOGICAL NURSING AND HEALTHY AGING

Gerontological nurses need to be aware of the services and support that are available for veterans. Currently, people are provided with information about programs and eligibility when they retire. However, this was not the case at the end of the Second World War or the Korean War, and nurses will encounter veterans and family caregivers who may not be aware of the benefits and assistance to which they are entitled. Assessments of older persons should include questions about military service or civilian service during wartime. Those persons who may be eligible for veterans' benefits can be assisted in obtaining additional information. Veterans and civilians who served during wartime can get information about programs and services by contacting Veterans Affairs Canada. Details regarding eligibility and application procedures for each program are available on the Veterans Affairs Canada website at http://www.veterans.gc.ca/eng.

LEGAL ISSUES IN GERONTOLOGICAL NURSING

Knowledge of the most common legal issues that may arise when working with older persons is as important as knowledge of the financial issues just discussed. The lack of knowledge about health care laws and the misapplication of laws have been cited as a cause of ageist practices (Spencer, 2009). Legal concerns are most often related to an individual's ability to make financial, personal, or health care decisions and to consent to treatment.

MENTAL CAPACITY

Mental capacity is the ability to make decisions. It is a legal construct, not a clinical condition. The exact legal definition of capacity varies from province to province and from country to country. In general, to be deemed capable of making a decision, a person must understand information that is relevant to making a decision, evaluate the data, and appreciate the consequences of the decision (or the consequences of not making a decision) (Law Commission of Ontario, 2015). People are presumed to have capacity unless there is clear evidence to the contrary and the person has been legally deemed incapable.

The concept of capacity applies to different kinds of decisions, including financial decisions; decisions about daily activities, housing, and personal care; and medical and health-related decisions, including consent to treatments and procedures.

Capacity exists on a continuum and is issue or task specific; there is no such thing as global incapacity. A person may have capacity for a particular decision or kind of decision but not for another decision or kind of decision. For example, a person may not be able to adequately take care of day-to-day personal business such as paying bills but may still be able to make personal health care decisions. Capacity can improve, decrease, or fluctuate.

Mental capacity is assessed by different caregivers, depending on the kind of decision being made (e.g., health care consent, admission to an LTC home, or a financial contract) and relevant provincial laws, including health care consent laws, guardianship laws, substitute decision maker and personal directives laws, privacy and personal information laws, and mental health laws. For example, capacity to provide health care consent is assessed by the nurse or another health care provider offering the health care. Under mental health laws, whenever a person is admitted to a psychiatric facility, a physician assesses the person's capacity to provide health care consent and capacity (sometimes referred to as *competency*) to manage his or her property. The mechanisms by which a person can dispute a finding of incapacity vary from province to province and within provinces according to the type of decision.

For persons who are unable to speak for themselves or are not able to understand the consequences of their decisions, legal protection may be needed. However, every attempt should be made to match the level of protection to the person's need, taking actions that provide the needed protection with the minimum restriction of personal autonomy.

Legal protection of the person with impaired capacity ranges from power of attorney for finances, to power of attorney for personal care, to guardianship (a mechanism by which the person becomes a "ward" under the protection of a guardian).

Power of Attorney

A power of attorney (POA) is a legal document in which one person designates another person (e.g., a family member or a friend) to act on his or her behalf. The appointed person is called the *attorney* and may or may not be a lawyer. The two types of POA for financial affairs are *continuing* or *enduring* POA, and *noncontinuing* POA (appointed for a limited time, such as when the person is out of the country). An attorney for financial affairs does not have the authority to make decisions about the person's health or personal care. (Information about relevant provincial laws are available on the websites of provincial Public Guardians and Trustees.)

An individual may appoint an attorney with a POA for personal care (who is also referred to as the personal guardian, agent, or delegate for personal care). The attorney has the authority to make health-related decisions for the individual when that individual is unable to do so themself. The attorney with POA is expected to use "substituted judgement" in making decisions; that is, the decision is expected to be the decision the person would make were the person able to do so and not the decision the attorney would make for herself or himself in the same situation. Therefore, it is always advisable that the person selected as attorney be someone who knows and is willing to uphold the wishes and preferences of the individual.

A POA for finances comes into effect as soon as it is signed, unless the document clearly indicates that it takes effect only after the individual becomes mentally incapable of managing finances. A POA for personal care comes into effect when the individual becomes mentally incapable of making decisions about personal care. An important aspect of POA is that the person who is given decision-making rights is chosen by the older individual rather than by a court. This type of advance planning is generally recommended because it is the least restrictive and is most likely to ensure that the wishes of the older person are followed. It does not, however, ensure that the POA will not be misused.

Guardians

When a person becomes mentally incapable of managing personal or financial affairs and does not have a POA in place, a guardian may be appointed. Guardians may have responsibility for finances and property, personal care, or both. The appointment is made at a court hearing in which someone provides evidence of the incapacity of the person, who often is not present. Such a person is declared *incapacitated* (sometimes called *incompetent*) in a process that differs by province. The guardian continues in the role until the court rescinds the order. When there is no suitable person to be appointed guardian, a provincial Public Guardian or Trustee may be appointed.

 IMPLICATIONS FOR GERONTOLOGICAL NURSING AND HEALTHY AGING

Nurses are responsible for assessing the person's capacity to consent to health care and for obtaining consent from the appropriate legal designate when a person is not capable of providing consent. There is no specific test for capacity, such as a score on an assessment of cognitive functioning. Nurses must be fully informed about the laws in their province or territory that are related to consent, capacity, and substitute consent, and they must also be aware that the laws are changing. Instances of nurses and other health care providers acting against the older person's rights because they do not fully understand the law include inappropriate decisions about moving to LTC homes (Meadus, 2014), inappropriate use of advance directives (Wahl, 2013), and inappropriate documents and policies (see Chapter 25).

Nurses who are consulted by older persons and their families about legal issues should not attempt to provide legal advice. Instead, nurses should refer them to legal resources, legal clinics, or specialized lawyers. The provincial bar association is a resource for nurses and for older people and their advocates (http://www.cba.org). A number of organizations dedicated to legal issues and advocacy for older persons are listed in the Resources section at the end of the chapter.

ABUSE, MISTREATMENT, AND NEGLECT OF OLDER PERSONS

"Elder abuse is any action by someone in a relationship of trust that results in harm or distress to an older person. Neglect is a lack of action by that person in a relationship of trust with the same result" (Public Health Agency of Canada, 2012, ¶ 3). Abuses of older persons include physical abuse, sexual abuse and exploitation, neglect, psychological or emotional

TABLE 22.1   Types of Abuse of Older Persons

DEFINITION	EXAMPLES	INDICATORS
Emotional (Psychological) Abuse Using words or actions to control, frighten, isolate, or erode a person's self-respect.	• Threatening • Blaming, insulting, lying • Deciding what the person can do or not do • Not keeping promises • Humiliation • Alienating others from the older person • Making fun of the person's heritage, traditions, or religious or spiritual beliefs • Constant yelling	• Fear, anxiety, withdrawal • Depression • Cowering • Reluctance to talk openly • Fearful interaction with caregiver • Family or caregiver talking on behalf of the person and not allowing privacy
Financial Abuse Acting without the older person's consent in a way that benefits the abuser at the expense of the older person through threats, intimidation, or deceit. Most forms of financial abuse are crimes.	• Misuse of power of attorney • Theft • Misusing control over a person's funds by not providing them for the person's benefit • Pressuring the person to provide financial support • Making the person sign a legal document • Overcharging for services • Failing to repay loans • Pressuring the person to sign over house or property	• Standard of living inconsistent with income or assets • Theft or missing property noted • Unusual or inappropriate activity in bank accounts • Forged signatures on cheques • Overdue bills • Missing mail
Physical Abuse Using physical force against a person without the person's consent. It can cause pain, injury, or impairment.	• Hitting, punching, slapping, pushing, biting, or throwing the older person • Burning the person • Confining the older person, including unnecessary use of restraints • Throwing objects at the older person	• Unexplained injuries (bruises, burns, bites, fractures) • Untreated medical problems • History of "accidents" • Signs of over- or underuse of medication • Wasting • Dehydration
Neglect Failing to adequately provide necessities or care for a dependent older person.	• Failing to provide adequate nutrition, personal care, or a clean, warm, safe environment • Withholding medical services or treatments • Failing to provide proper needed supervision • Failing to prevent physical harm	• Unkempt appearance • Inappropriate or dirty clothing • Signs of infrequent bathing • Unhealthy living conditions • Dangers or disrepair in home environment • Hoarding • Lack of social contact • No regular health care appointments

Source: Adapted from Department of Justice Canada. (2015). *Elder abuse is wrong*. Retrieved from http://www.justice.gc.ca/eng/rp-pr/cj-jp/fv-vf/eaw-mai/index.html; National Initiative for Care of the Elderly. (n.d.). *Elder abuse: Assessment and intervention reference guide*. Retrieved from http://www.nicenet.ca/tools-elder-abuse-assessment-and-intervention-reference-guide.

abuse, economic or financial abuse, and spiritual abuse (Table 22.1). A person may experience more than one form of abuse. The abuse may occur in private homes, in places where the older person lives alone or with other persons, or in residential care homes and health care facilities. The abuse of persons living in LTC homes and residential care facilities is called *institutional abuse*. It "involves inadequate care and nutrition, low standards of nursing care, inappropriate and aggressive staff–client interactions, or substandard, overcrowded or unsanitary living environments" (Department of Justice Canada, 2015).

The most common forms of the abuse of older persons are emotional abuse and financial abuse (National Initiative for Care of the Elderly [NICE], 2016). The abuse may be intentional or unintentional. Neglect may occur because the perpetrator does not know how to provide medical care or does not realize that what she or he is doing could be harmful.

Accurate prevalence is difficult to ascertain because of underreporting and differences in the ways this abuse is defined and measured. About 5 to 10% of older Canadians are abused (Wang et al., 2015). A 2015 national survey found that 8.2% of community-dwelling older Canadians had experienced abuse or neglect in the previous year (NICE, 2016). A 2014 survey found that 16% of older persons attending primary health clinics in one region of Quebec had experienced abuse from a family member in the past year (Préville et al., 2014). The rate of family violence was lower for persons aged 75 years and older than for those aged between 65 and 74 years. Persons who have cognitive impairment are more likely than those who are not cognitively impaired to experience abuse (Pillimer et al., 2016). Experts on the abuse of older persons caution that prevalence estimates are probably low because older persons are reluctant to report and disclose abuse and because people who are more vulnerable are less likely to participate in surveys of the abuse of older persons (Pillimer et al., 2016).

The abuse of older persons is a complex problem. Psychological, social, and economic factors, along with the mental and physical conditions of the victim and the perpetrator, contribute to the occurrence of the abuse of the older person (Registered Nurses' Association of Ontario [RNAO], 2014). Most abuse of older persons is committed by family members (NICE, 2016). Older women are most likely to be abused by their spouse or adult children, and older men are most likely to be abused by adult children or close friends (Centre for Addiction and Mental Health [CAMH], 2008). Intimate partner violence in older age is most likely to be a continuation of domestic violence that began earlier in the relationship (CAMH, 2008).

Older women are more likely than older men to experience abuse (Burnes et al., 2015; NICE, 2016). (Other risk factors for the abuse and neglect of older

TABLE 22.2	Risk Factors for Abuse and Neglect

- Isolation
- Lack of support
- Cognitive impairment (i.e., dementia)
- Responsive behaviours
- Living with a person who has a mental illness
- Living with people who engage in excessive consumption of alcohol or illegal drugs
- Dependency on others to complete activities of daily living (including banking)
- Recent worsening of health
- Arguing frequently with relatives

Source: Extracted from Registered Nurses' Association of Ontario [RNAO]. (2014). *Preventing and addressing abuse and neglect of older adults: Person-centred, collaborative, system-wide approaches* (p. 26, Table 2). Toronto, ON: Author.

persons are listed in Table 22.2.) Some risk factors may be more relevant to a particular type of abuse or neglect. For example, functional impairment appears to be a risk factor for physical and emotional abuse but not for neglect (Burnes et al., 2015; NICE, 2016). A recent national survey of more than 8,000 older Canadians indicated that the following factors are independently associated with abuse: being depressed, having been abused at another age (i.e., childhood, youth, or middle age), feeling unsafe with the people who are closest, having unmet needs in regard to activities of daily living and instrumental activities of daily living, being unmarried, and being female (NICE, 2016).

Abusers are often dependent on victims for financial assistance or shelter. Personal problems or stressors may increase a person's likelihood of abusing an older person. "It is important to avoid characterizing abuse as 'caregiver stress.' Caregiving situations should never be used to excuse or downplay an abusive person's criminal conduct" (CAMH, 2008, p. 100).

Most often, older victims are unwilling or afraid to report the problem because of shame, embarrassment, intimidation, or fear of retaliation. The abuser may be the only caregiver available; reporting or complaining could leave the victim without any care at all. The abuse may be part of a lifelong pattern in which the victim has always felt somewhat at fault; thus, he or she will remain in the abusive situation.

INSTITUTIONAL ABUSE

Older persons who live in LTC homes, hospitals, or retirement homes are vulnerable to abuse because of their isolation and dependence and because of the characteristics of some facilities. There are two types of institutional abuse: *resident-to-resident abuse* and *staff-to-resident abuse.*

Resident-to-resident abuse (also known as resident-to-resident aggression, violence, or mistreatment) differs from the typical abuse of older persons because of its potential harm to both residents and because abuse is typically defined as occurring in the context of a relationship of trust (which does not apply to resident-to-resident relationships) (McDonald et al., 2015). Resident-to-resident abuse is a relatively new area of research. A recent review indicated that 1 to 41% of residents experienced resident-to-resident abuse (McDonald et al., 2015). According to the review, resident-to-resident abuse is less frequently reported than staff-to-resident abuse but makes up the majority of cases that are reported to the police.

Sexual abuse that is reported is more likely to be from another resident than from a staff member. Residents with one or more of the following characteristics are at higher risk of resident-to-resident abuse: female gender, cognitive impairment, wandering behaviour, and limited mobility. Less is known about perpetrators' characteristics. Frequently, residents are unlikely or unable to report abuse. In a survey of relatives of LTC home residents in Michigan, 24.3% reported that their relative in the home had experienced physical abuse—including physical mistreatment, sexual abuse, or the forced use of restraint—from staff members (Schiamberg et al., 2012).

Surveys confirm that institutional abuse is a problem, but their research methods make it difficult to conclusively quantify the problem. Much of the research asks how many staff members have observed resident abuse (36 to 80% have witnessed resident abuse), not how many incidents of abuse occur (Castle et al., 2015). Most research asks staff members or families about their perspectives. Box 22.3 describes

---

BOX 22.3   Research for Evidence-Informed Practice: Residents May Minimize Their Experiences of Abuse to Avoid Retaliation and Other Negative Consequences

Problem: Most literature about the potential for abuse in residential care homes approaches the problem from the perspective of how policies and practices can be changed to prevent abuse. Residents "are seen as passive victims with no say in the reflection process" (p. 341), and their perspective is missing. The research objective was to understand residents' perception of abuse and the strategies they develop to exercise their rights.

Methods: In depth, semistructured interviews were conducted with 20 residents in diverse residential care homes in Quebec. Over two interviews, participants were asked about their personal history, their lives in the residential home, and their views of the rights of residents and what constitutes abuse. The average age of the participants was 83 years, and most were women. Thematic analyses were conducted.

Findings: Views of what constitutes abuse were influenced by sensationalistic media stories. Many participants' ideas of abuse were limited to physical abuse; they felt safe from the tragic abuses reported in the media. This narrow focus on extreme instances of physical abuse caused them to "trivialize the disrespectful and sometimes

even violent acts committed against or witnessed by seniors living in institutional settings" (p. 346). Participants recounted experiences that fit the definitions of psychological abuse (such as infantilization, negligence, passive retaliation, and psychological violence) and physical abuse (physical "roughness") but did not view them as abuse.

Participants reported that positive relationships with staff members "seem to counterbalance what they consider to be unfortunate but inevitable incidents" (p. 348). Some residents had given up hope of defending their rights, some reported that they would report abuse, and most had found ways to maintain control over some aspects of their lives.

Application to Nursing Practice: Nurses can acknowledge the loss of power and control that accompanies moving to a residential care home. The authors suggest that although it is important to increase residents', families', and staff members' awareness of abuse and residents' rights, it is also important to address issues that result in residents' failure to report abuse, such as "poor knowledge or recourse mechanisms, fear of getting someone fired, and above all, fear of retaliation and of being labeled as a disruptive elderly person or family" (p. 352).

Source: Charpentier, M., & Soulières, M. (2013). Elder abuse and neglect in institutional settings: The resident's perspective. *Journal of Elder Abuse & Neglect, 25*(4), 339–354. doi:10.1080/08946566.2012.751838.

a study of the abuse of older persons in residential homes from the perspective of the residents.

Risk factors for institutional abuse include the environment and organizational culture, staff characteristics, and resident characteristics (Hutchison & Kroese, 2015). These factors interact. For example, important organization-level risk factors (such as how work is organized, inadequate staffing levels, inadequate or ineffective supervision, intimidation, and a low proportion of qualified staff) influence staff-level risk factors, such as staff burnout. Staff characteristics associated with abuse include workplace stress, dissatisfaction with management or the workplace, emotional exhaustion, job pressures, inexperience, lack of knowledge about older persons, negative attitudes such as ageism, personal problems, a personal history of abuse, alcohol or substance misuse, and deficiencies in communication skills or problem-solving ability (Hutchison & Kroese, 2015; RNAO, 2014). Resident characteristics that are associated with higher risk include aggressive, hyperactive, or responsive behaviours (see Chapter 21); dependency in regard to activities of daily living; a history of previous abuse; social isolation; and impaired communication (Hutchison & Kroese, 2015; RNAO, 2014).

IMPLICATIONS FOR GERONTOLOGICAL NURSING AND HEALTHY AGING

ASSESSMENT

The importance of skillful communication (see Chapter 3), the therapeutic relationship, and the establishment and maintenance of trust cannot be understated in the context of the abuse of older persons. Nurses must be vigilant and sensitive to the potential for abuse and neglect, watching for signs and symptoms in all their interactions with older people (see Table 22.1). In addition to signs of physical abuse, look for more subtle signals. Is there an unusual delay between the beginning of a health problem and when help is sought? Are appointments often missed without reasonable explanations? Are there inconsistencies between the history given by a dependent older person and by his or her caregiver?

Certain behaviours may be suggestive of an abusive situation. Does the family member or caregiver do all of the talking in a situation, even though the older person is capable? Does the family member or caregiver appear angry, frustrated, or indifferent, while the older person appears hesitant or frightened? Is either the family member or the older person aggressive toward the other or the nurse? The nurse should pay particular attention to a caregiver who is alone and has no support from others and no opportunities for respite.

The accuracy of screening tools is questionable and controversial. Nurses and other health care providers who use screening tools for older-person abuse should be trained in their use. If abuse is suspected, a full assessment should be done, including a determination of the immediate safety of the victim; the desires of the victim, if capable; and supports available to reduce the person's risk of abuse (RNAO, 2014). Assessment will typically involve the interprofessional health care team and possibly police and legal experts. It should include diagnostic tests and referrals and consultations (RNAO, 2014). Privacy in regard to the person's family and care providers should be ensured. It is important to be nonjudgemental and accepting of the person and the suspected abuser (RNAO, 2014). In addition to the RNAO (2014) practice guideline on the abuse of older persons, a practice guideline on the abuse of women is relevant to assessing older women (Registered Nurses' Association of Ontario [RNAO], 2005/2012). Instructions for a detailed assessment are provided as part of a practice protocol at *ConsultGeri.org* (Fulmer & Caceres, 2012). The questions to ask in the assessment depend on the type of suspected abuse. The questions "Are you afraid of anyone?" "Do you live in a household where there is stress or frustration?" "Do you live with anyone who abuses alcohol or drugs?" and "Do you live with anyone who was abused as a child?" can be asked in most types of assessments (Caceres & Fulmer, 2016). Box 22.4 provides some other questions.

INTERVENTION

The goals of intervention are to prevent, detect, and stop mistreatment and neglect of older people; provide care and treatment of the consequences of abuse; protect the victim and society from inappropriate and illegal acts; hold abusers accountable; rehabilitate the offender; and order restitution of property

BOX 22.4	Questions to Ask When Assessing Suspected Abuse

Physical Abuse
Has anyone ever tried to hurt you in any way?
Have you had any recent injuries?
Has anyone ever touched you or tried to touch you without permission?
Have you ever been tied down?

Emotional Abuse
Has anyone ever yelled at you or threatened you?
Has anyone been insulting you and using degrading language?
Are you cared for by anyone who abuses drugs or alcohol?

Financial Abuse
Who pays your bills? Do you ever go to the bank with him or her? Does this person have access to your accounts? Does this person have power of attorney?
Have you ever signed documents you did not understand?
Are any of your family members exhibiting a great interest in your assets?
Has anyone ever taken anything that was yours without asking?

Neglect
Are you alone a lot?
Has anyone ever failed you when you needed help?
Does anyone care for you or provide regular assistance to you?
Are you cared for by anyone who abuses drugs or alcohol?

Source: Extracted from Caceres, B. A., & Fulmer, T. (2016). Mistreatment detection (p. 184, Table 13.2). In M. Boltz, E. Capezuti, T. T. Fulmer, et al. (Eds.). *Evidence-based Geriatric Nursing Protocols for Best Practice* (5th ed.). New York, NY: Springer Publishing Co.

BOX 22.5	Developing a Safety Plan With Potential Victims of Older-Person Abuse

Encourage the older persons to do the following:
- Tell someone they trust about what is happening to them.
- Ask others for help, and be specific about the type of help needed.
- Think ahead about what to do if someone is hurting them or if they do not feel safe.
- Do the following for their protection if they are facing possible abuse:
  - Have emergency phone numbers written in a safe place.
  - Have a safe place to go, both inside and outside the house.
- Create an emergency kit containing money, copies of important documents, a list of all medications, and a 3-day supply of medications, extra clothing, and assistive devices.
  - Dial 911.

Source: Adapted from Ontario Seniors' Secretariat. (n.d.). *Safety planning for older persons.* Retrieved from http://www.seniors.gov.on.ca/en/elderabuse/docs/safetyplanning.pdf.

and payment for expenses incurred as a result of exploitation. Many interventions are done in the justice system and are beyond the nurse's usual scope of practice. Most important, nurses must know how to participate in the prevention and early recognition of abuse; how to refer victims and perpetrators to social, health, and legal services in their community; and how to report the abuse of older persons.

Prevention

Prevention of older-person abuse is a priority of the World Health Organization and the Canadian government, and there are international, national, provincial, and local initiatives to increase awareness and prevent the abuse of older persons. Two such initiatives are the International Network for the Prevention of Elder Abuse and the Canadian Network for the Prevention of Elder Abuse. Prevention requires **intersectoral collaboration** between health, social service, and justice (law enforcement and legal) sectors. Canadian prevention networks include representatives from all sectors as well as members of the public, including older persons.

Gerontological nurses need to be alert to situations that entail risk for the mistreatment of vulnerable older people and need to take steps to prevent abuse or neglect. In some situations, the abuse may be preventable. Nurses can develop a safety plan with potential victims to ensure that they know how to get help if needed and know what resources are available to them (Box 22.5). Nurses can also provide support, encouragement, and assurance that it is possible to leave the situation. Unfortunately, few shelters will accept a frail older person. If the abusive behaviour is learned behaviour or a response to stress, the situation may allow for change.

Addressing Abuse and Preventing Recurrence

Multiple strategies are likely required to effectively address abuse and prevent recurrence. Older persons who are victims of abuse are often unaware of services that are available to them. Nurses should provide information about local services, such as crisis hotlines, victim support groups, and victim volunteer companions, as well as information about how to access them and about the kinds of support they provide. Some communities, through their elder abuse prevention networks, have created intersectoral, interdisciplinary, and interprofessional networks for responding to the abuse of older persons (for example, the BC Community Response Networks [http://www.bccrns.ca]).

If the abuse is associated with caregiving, nurses can be proactive and provide support to all involved in order to reduce caregiver stress. This may include finding respite services, changing the situation entirely (e.g., giving the caregiver permission to give up the role), providing referrals to support groups, teaching about the care recipient's illness, teaching how to use crisis hotlines, and teaching anger management strategies.

Culturally and ethnically appropriate services related to the abuse of older persons need to be developed (Haukioja, 2016). Older persons who are members of minority ethnic groups or are immigrants may be more isolated, more dependent on family members, and less aware of their rights and the resources available to them (Matsuoka et al., 2012/2013; Ploeg et al., 2013). Education and support materials for health care providers working with Indigenous persons have been developed by the Vancouver Coastal Health Authority (http://www.vchreact.ca/aboriginal_manual.htm).

Older people who have experienced abuse decline to use offered services 33% of the time (CAMH, 2008). Failure on the part of the nurse to develop a therapeutic relationship with the older person can contribute to the person's decision to decline services. Some other reasons for declining to use offered services are that the person thinks that she or he does not need help; the person does not think that the services offered will help; the financial and emotional costs of accepting services are too high; the person feels under pressure to maintain the family's reputation; the services are culturally and linguistically inappropriate; the person holds culturally based beliefs that are inconsistent with accepting services; and the cost of legal services is too great.

Criminal Code and Reporting

Many police officers and some lawyers have additional training in how to respond to the abuse of older persons. Canada has legislation and legal tools that protect the rights of older persons. There are at least 19 *Criminal Code* offences that may apply to the abuse of older persons (see http://www.advocacycentreelderly.org/elder_abuse_-_faq.php). However, lack of awareness of legislation and legal tools is a problem among front-line health care providers and law enforcement professionals who encounter abuse of older persons. Provincial laws may require that police be notified when there is evidence of abuse of a person who is incapable of seeking assistance. However, a person with mental capacity has the right to make all personal decisions and can refuse assessment and intervention. In most provinces and territories, the reporting of suspected abuse or neglect of residents in LTC homes and assisted-living facilities is mandatory.

Preventing Institutional Abuse

Much of the responsibility for preventing the abuse of older people in health care facilities rests with the organizations that run the facilities. Management practices can address risk factors, such organization of work, staffing levels, staff qualifications, quality of supervision, staff well-being, and job pressures, all of which are thought to be underlying causes of institutional abuse (Hutchison & Kroese, 2015). Approaches to culture change are consistent with recommendations to adopt person-centred approaches (see Chapter 26).

Employers should ensure that all staff are educated about ageism; residents' rights; abuse, neglect, and the factors that contribute to them; and staff members' responsibilities to report abuse (RNAO, 2014). Health care providers within LTC homes should be educated about assessing and responding to abuse; their roles and responsibilities; relevant laws; positive care approaches; managing responsive behaviours; and fostering a safe and healthy work environment. Collaborative teams, including experts from outside the

BOX 22.6	Institutional Approaches to Preventing Abuse of Older Persons

Adopt a combination of approaches, including the following:
- Screening potential employees, hiring the most qualified employees, and providing proper supervision and monitoring in the workplace
- Securing appropriate staffing
- Providing mandatory training to all employees
- Supporting the needs of individuals with cognitive impairment, including those with responsive behaviours
- Upholding resident rights
- Establishing and maintaining person-centred care and a healthy work environment
- Educating older adults and families on abuse and neglect and their rights, and establishing routes for complaints and quality improvement

Source: Extracted from Registered Nurses' Association of Ontario (RNAO). (2014). *Preventing and addressing abuse and neglect of older adults: Person-centred, collaborative, system-wide approaches* (p. 52, Recommendation 6.3). Toronto, ON: Author.

facility, should be in place to work on prevention and response to abuse. Policies and procedures about recognizing and responding to abuse should be explicit. A no-blame process for reporting abuse and neglect is important. A combination of approaches is required, as outlined in Box 22.6.

SUMMARY

Nurses are expected to provide safety and security for the persons under their care to the extent possible, regardless of the capacity of the person. This responsibility increases as the limitations of the older person increase. The nurse is often the one who provides much of the information that older persons and their significant others need in order to make informed decisions; it is essential that this exchange be documented in the health care record (see Chapter 5). The nurse often deals with difficult and problematic legal and ethical issues when providing care to older persons and when interacting with the families of these persons. Nurses must be knowledgeable about the rights of older persons with respect to access to health care and social security programs. Nurses are responsible for acting in accordance with laws pertaining to capacity and consent. Recognition that the

abuse of older persons is a problem in our society is growing. Interprofessional and intersectoral collaboration is required to prevent older-person abuse and neglect and to effectively intervene in cases of such abuse. Providing appropriate care within the context of a person's changing cognitive capacity and judgement is at the core of many ethical and legal dilemmas in gerontological nursing.

KEY CONCEPTS

- The Canadian health care system is made up of 13 interlinked provincial and territorial systems. The extent to which health services other than hospital-based care, primary care, and some dental surgery are part of provincial health insurance plans varies from province to province.
- The Old Age Security program provides eligible persons with a regular income after the age of 65 years. Benefits from the Canada Pension Plan are available only to people who contributed to the plan when they worked; the amount of benefits depends on the number of years a person contributed to the plan.
- Through power of attorney and guardians, protective measures are available for persons with limited or absent capacity.
- The nurse has a responsibility to ensure the safety and security of those persons to whom care is provided. This responsibility does not alter with changes in the person's legal status or capacity.
- At least 5 to 10% of older Canadians experience abuse or neglect, most often perpetrated by family members.
- Abuse of older persons occurs in institutions. One in four relatives of residents of LTC homes report that their relative experienced physical abuse.
- In most jurisdictions, the nurse is required to report suspicions of abuse of older persons who live in care homes.

ACTIVITIES AND DISCUSSION QUESTIONS

1. Interview an older person who receives benefits from the Old Age Security (OAS) program and the Canada Pension Plan or Quebec Pension Plan

about what difference these programs make in his or her daily life. Compare your findings with those of a classmate.

2. Explain the fundamentals of the OAS program sufficiently to assist older persons in applying for benefits.

3. Learn about the laws regarding capacity, consent, and guardianship in your province or territory. Compare these laws to practices you have experienced in clinical settings. Discuss with your classmates.

4. Learn about the laws pertaining to reporting the abuse of older persons in your province or territory.

5. Find legal resources for older people in your community, and obtain information about the costs of these services to the older person and about the process of accessing them.

6. Interview a member of your local elder abuse prevention network. Find out what motivates him or her to do this work, what initiatives are in place in your community, what challenges are being faced by the network, and what priorities for future work have been decided upon.

7. Review instructions for assessing the abuse of older persons. Take turns with classmates in conducting role-play interviews in which you are screening for older-person abuse, alternately taking the role of the victim and the role of the perpetrator. Discuss what it was like to participate in the role-playing.

RESOURCES

Advocacy Centre for the Elderly
http://www.advocacycentreelderly.org

Canadian Association of Retired Persons (CARP)
http://www.carp.ca

Canadian Centre for Elder Law
http://www.bcli.org/ccel

Canadian Network for the Prevention of Elder Abuse (CNPEA)
http://cnpea.ca/en/

Centre for Public Legal Education Alberta. Legal resources by province and territory
http://www.oaknet.ca/abuse/more-information/organizations-and-resources-re-elder-abuse-in-canada/

Centre for Public Legal Education Alberta. OakNet: Canadian law for older adults
https://www.oaknet.ca/

College of Registered Nurses of Nova Scotia. Guidelines to assist registered nurses with the *Personal Directives Act*
http://cotns.ca/assets/documents/GuidelinestoAssistRNswiththePersonalDirectivesAct.pdf

Employment and Social Development Canada. Provincial and territorial resources on the abuse of older persons
https://www.canada.ca/en/employment-social-development/corporate/seniors/forum.html

Public Health Agency of Canada. Elder abuse: It's time to face the reality
https://www.canada.ca/en/public-health/services/health-promotion/stop-family-violence/prevention-resource-centre/prevention-resources-older-adults/elder-abuses-time-face-reality.html

For additional resources, please visit *http://evolve.elsevier.com/Canada/Ebersole/gerontological/*

REFERENCES

Alberta Health. (2017). *Coverage for seniors benefit*. Retrieved from http://www.health.alberta.ca/services/drugs-seniors.html.

Black, J., Hashimzade, N., & Myles, G. (2009). *Gross domestic product*. From *A dictionary of economics. Oxford reference online*. Oxford University Press. Retrieved from http://www.oxfordreference.com/views/ENTRY.html?entry=t19.e1403&srn=1&ssid=525632653#FIRSTHIT.

Burnes, D., Pillemer, K., Caccamise, P. L., et al. (2015). Prevalence and risk factors for elder abuse and neglect in the community: A population-based study. *Journal of the American Geriatrics Society, 63*(9), 1906–1912. doi:10.1111/jgs.13601.

Canada Pension Plan (CPP) Investment Board. (2016a). *Our performance*. Retrieved from http://www.cppib.com/en/our-performance/.

Canada Pension Plan (CPP) Investment Board. (2016b). *Sustainability of the CPP*. Retrieved from http://www.cppib.com/en/our-performance/cpp-sustainability/.

Canadian Gerontological Nursing Association (CGNA). (2010). *Gerontological nursing competencies and standards of practice*. Vancouver, BC: Author.

Canadian Health Service Research Foundation (CHSRF). (2011). *Research synthesis on cost drivers in the health sector and proposed policy options*. Ottawa, ON: Author. Retrieved from http://www.cfhi-fcass.ca/SearchResultsNews/11-02-18/029025cd-350f-4f7f-87cf-b207f8514aa6.aspx.

Canadian Institute for Health Information (CIHI). (2011). *Health care in Canada 2011: A focus on seniors and aging*. Ottawa, ON: Author. Retrieved from https://secure.cihi.ca/estore/productFamily.htm?locale=en&pf=PFC1677.

Canadian Institute for Health Information (CIHI). (2016). *National health expenditure trends, 1975 to 2016*. Ottawa, ON: Author. Retrieved from https://www.cihi.ca/en/national-health-expenditure-trends.

Caceres, B. A., & Fulmer, T. (2016). Mistreatment detection. In M. Boltz, E. Capezuti, T. T. Fulmer, et al. (Eds.), *Evidence-based geriatric nursing protocols for best practice* (5th ed., pp. 179–194). New York, NY: Springer Publishing Co.

Castle, N., Ferguson-Rome, J., & Teresi, J. A. (2015). Elder abuse in residential long-term care: An update to the 2003 National Research Council report. *Journal of Applied Gerontology, 34*(4), 407–443. doi:10.1177/0733464813492583.

Centre for Addiction and Mental Health (CAMH). (2008). *Improving our response to older adults with substance use, mental health and gambling problems: A guide for supervisors, managers and clinical staff*. Toronto, ON: Author.

Department of Justice Canada. (2015). *Elder abuse is wrong: Institutional abuse*. Retrieved from http://www.justice.gc.ca/eng/rp-pr/cj-jp/fv-vf/eaw-mai/p9.html.

Fulmer, T., & Caceres, B. A. (2012). *Elder mistreatment and abuse*. Retrieved from https://consultgeri.org/geriatric-topics/elder-mistreatment-and-abuse.

Government of Ontario. (2017). *What you pay*. Retrieved from https://www.ontario.ca/page/get-coverage-prescription-drugs#section-4.

Haukioja, H. (2016). Exploring the nature of elder abuse in ethno-cultural minority groups: A community-based participatory research study. *The Arbutus Review, 7*(1), 51–67. doi:10.18357/tar71201615681.

Hutchison, A., & Kroese, B. S. (2015). A review of the literature exploring the possible causes of abuse and neglect in adult residential care. *The Journal of Adult Protection, 17*(4), 216–233. doi:10.1108/JAP-11-2014-0034.

Law Commission of Ontario. (2015). *Legal capacity, decision-making and guardianship: Interim report*. Toronto, ON: Author. Retrieved from http://www.lco-cdo.org/en/our-current-projects/legal-capacity-decision-making-and-guardianship/legal-capacity-decision-making-and-guardianship-interim-report/.

Matsuoka, A., Guruge, S., Koehn, S., et al. (2012/2013). Moving forward: Prevention of abuse of older women in the postmigration context in Canada. *Canadian Review of Social Policy, 68*(69), 108–120. Retrieved from http://crsp.journals.yorku.ca/index.php/crsp/article/view/34745.

McDonald, L., Sheppard, C., Hitzig, S. L., et al. (2015). Resident-to-resident abuse: A scoping review. *Canadian Journal on Aging, 34*(2), 215–236. doi:10.1017/S0714980815000094.

McDonald, M. (2015). Regulating individual charges for long-term residential care in Canada. *Studies in Political Economy a Socialist Review, 95*(1), 83–114. doi:10.1080/19187033.2014.11674947.

Meadus, J. (2014). *Admission to long-term care homes: Are evaluations of capacity being conducted in accordance with the law?*

Toronto, ON: Advocacy Centre for the Elderly. Retrieved from http://www.advocacycentreelderly.org/ace_library.php.

National Initiative for Care of the Elderly (NICE). (2016). *Into the light: National survey on the mistreatment of older Canadians*. Toronto, ON: Author. Retrieved from http://cnpea.ca/en/publications/studies/68-the-national-survey-on-the-mistreatment-of-older-canadians-a-prevalence-study.

Office of the Chief Actuary. (2016). *27th Actuarial report on the Canada Pension Plan as at 31 December 2015*. Ottawa, ON: Author. Retrieved from http://www.osfi-bsif.gc.ca/Eng/Docs/cpp27.pdf.

Pillimer, K., Burnes, D., Riffin, C., et al. (2016). Elder abuse: Global situation, risk factors and prevention strategies. *The Gerontologist, 56*(S2), S194–S205. doi:10.1093/geront/gnw004.

Ploeg, J., Lohfeld, L., & Walsh, C. A. (2013). What is "elder abuse"? Voices from the margin: The views of underrepresented Canadian older adults. *Journal of Elder Abuse & Neglect, 25*(5), 396–424. doi:10.1080/08946566.2013.780956.

Press, J. (2017). Most Canadians have a poor understanding of CPP, reports show. *Toronto Star*. Retrieved from https://www.thestar.com/news/canada/2017/01/25/most-canadians-have-a-poor-understanding-of-cpp-reports-reveal.html.

Preston, V., Kim, A., Hudyma, S., et al. (2012/2013). Gender, race, and immigration: Aging and economic security in Canada. *Canadian Review of Social Policy, 68*(69), 90–106. Retrieved from http://crsp.journals.yorku.ca/index.php/crsp/article/view/34386.

Préville, M., Mechakra-Tahiri, S. D., Vasiliadis, H., et al. (2014). Family violence among older patients consulting family care clinics: Results from the ESA (Enquête sure las santé des aînés) services study on mental health and aging. *Canadian Journal of Psychiatry, 59*(8), 426–433. Retrieved from http://journals.sagepub.com/home/cpa.

Public Health Agency of Canada [PHAC]. (2012). *Elder abuse: It's time to face the reality*. Retrieved from https://www.canada.ca/en/public-health/services/health-promotion/stop-family-violence/prevention-resource-centre/prevention-resources-older-adults/elder-abuses-time-face-reality.html.

Registered Nurses' Association of Ontario [RNAO]. (2014). *Preventing and addressing abuse and neglect of older adults: Person-centred, collaborative, system-wide approaches*. Toronto, ON: Author. Retrieved from http://rnao.ca/bpg/guidelines/abuse-and-neglect-older-adults.

Registered Nurses' Association of Ontario [RNAO]. (2005/2012). *Woman abuse: Screening, identification and initial response*. Toronto, ON: Author. Retrieved from http://rnao.ca/bpg/guidelines/woman-abuse-screening-identification-and-initial-response.

Schiamberg, L. B., Oehmke, J., Zhang, Z., et al. (2012). Physical abuse of older adults in nursing homes: A random sample survey of adults with an elderly family member in a nursing home. *Journal of Elder Abuse & Neglect, 24*(1), 65–83. doi:10.1080/08946566.2011.608056.

Schirle, T. (2013). Seniors in poverty in Canada: A decomposition analysis. *Canadian Public Policy, 39*(4), 517–540. doi:10.3138/CPP.39.4.517.

Service Canada. (2017). *Canada Pension Plan – How much you could receive.* Retrieved from https://www.canada.ca/en/services/benefits/publicpensions/cpp/cpp-benefit/amount.html.

Sheets, D. J., & Gallager, E. M. (2013). Aging in Canada: State of the art and science. *The Gerontologist, 53*(1), 1–8. doi:10.1093/geront/gns150.

Spencer, C. (2009). *Ageism and the law: Emerging concepts and practices in housing and health.* Toronto, ON: Law Commission of Ontario. Retrieved from http://www.lco-cdo.org/en/older-adults-lco-funded-papers-charmaine-spencer.

Statistics Canada. (2013). *Persons in low income after tax (In percent, - 2007 to 2011).* Retrieved from http://www.statcan.gc.ca/tables-tableaux/sum-som/l01/cst01/famil19a-eng.htm.

Statistics Canada. (2015). *Table 1: Low income cut-offs (1992 base) after tax.* Retrieved from http://www.statcan.gc.ca/pub/75f0002m/2015001/tbl/tbl01-eng.htm.

Statistics Canada. (2016). *Table 206-0041: Low income statistics by age, sex and economic family type, Canada, provinces and selected census metropolitan areas (CMAs).* Retrieved from http://www5.statcan.gc.ca/cansim/a26?lang=eng&id=2060041.

Veterans Affairs Canada. (2016). *General statistics.* Retrieved from http://www.veterans.gc.ca/eng/news/general-statistics.

Wahl, J. (2013). *Advance care planning and end of life decision-making: More than just documents.* Toronto, ON: Advocacy Centre for the Elderly. Retrieved from http://www.advocacycentreelderly.org/advance_care_planning_-_publications.php.

Wang, X. M., Brisbin, S., Loo, T., et al. (2015). Elder abuse: An approach to identification, assessment and intervention. *Canadian Medical Association Journal (CMAJ), 187*(8), 575–581. doi:10.1503/cmaj.141329.

LEARNING OBJECTIVES

Upon completion of this chapter, the reader will be able to:

- Identify the various relationships that people identify as constituting "family."
- Examine family relationships in later life.
- Describe the various roles of grandparents.
- Explain the issues involved in adapting to a major transition such as retirement or widowhood.
- Identify the range of caregiving situations and associated potential challenges and opportunities.
- Discuss nursing responses with older persons and with their families who are assuming caregiver roles or experiencing other transitions.
- Discuss intimacy and sexuality in later life and the appropriate nursing responses.

GLOSSARY

Capacity The ability to understand and appreciate the reasonably foreseeable consequences of decisions or lack of decisions.

Caregiving The act of providing assistance to those who are unable to care entirely for themselves. Caregivers, also referred to as carers, may be informal (family, friends, and others who volunteer this service) or formal (persons hired to provide the care).

Filial piety Respecting parents and feeling gratitude toward them, placing family needs above individual needs, and caring for parents. Filial piety is a fundamental value in Confucian ethics and is part of other cultures as well.

Familism A "strong identification and solidarity of individuals with their family as well as strong normative feelings of allegiance, dedication, reciprocity, and attachment to their family members, both nuclear and extended" (Sayegh & Knight, 2010, p. 3).

Respite Relief in caregiving, providing benefit to both the caregiver and the care recipient.

THE LIVED EXPERIENCE

It is so irritating when Madge tries to help me do things. After all, I have lived 85 years and have done very well. I think she wants to put me away somewhere. I wish she would just leave me alone. I'm sure I could manage if she just wouldn't interfere.

    John, the father

I just can't stand watching as my father becomes weaker and is unable to do the things he always did so naturally and well. Yesterday he got lost on his way to the market. He was always my guide and protector. I knew I could count on him no matter what. It makes me feel sort of alone in the world.

    Madge, the daughter

RELATIONSHIPS, ROLES, AND TRANSITIONS

This chapter focuses on the various relationships, roles, and transitions that characteristically play a part in later life. Concepts of family structure and function; intimacy and sexuality; and the transitions of retirement, widowhood, and **caregiving** are examined. Nursing responses to supporting older persons in maintaining fulfilling roles and relationships are discussed.

FAMILIES

The idea of family evokes strong impressions of whatever an individual believes the typical family should be. Because everyone comes from a family, these impressions have powerful symbolic meaning. However, in today's world, the definition of a family is in a state of flux. As recently as 100 years ago, the norm was the extended family, made up of parents, grown children, and the children's children—often living together and sharing resources, strengths, and challenges. As cities grew and adult children moved to them in pursuit of work, parents did not always come along, and the primacy of the nuclear family evolved. The norm in North America became two parents with two children. This pattern has not been as common in many Indigenous families or immigrant families.

Other variations on the idea of family have developed, and today there is no typical Canadian family. Approximately 38% of today's families are couples without children. The high divorce and remarriage rate result in households of blended families, with children from both previous and new marriages. Lone-parent families, blended families, and childless couples are common. Multigenerational families are becoming more common; the number of three-generation households has increased, in part because of a higher proportion of three-generation households among recent Canadian immigrants (Milan et al., 2015). Still other families are composed of couples of the same gender and may or may not include children. Others without biological families (either by choice or by circumstance) have created their own "families" through communal living with siblings, friends, or others.

Family members, however they are defined, form the nucleus of relationships for the majority of older persons and, if they become dependent, their support systems. A longstanding myth in society is that families are alienated from their older members and abandon them to institutions. Nothing could be further from the truth; family relationships remain strong in a family member's old age. Most older people have frequent contact with their families and possess a large intergenerational web of significant people, including sons, daughters, stepchildren, in-laws, former in-laws, nieces, nephews, grandchildren, and great-grandchildren, as well as partners and former partners of their offspring. All of these people may play an important part in maintaining a person's satisfaction in later life.

As families change, the roles of the family members or their expectations of one another may change as well. Grandparents may assume parental roles for their grandchildren if their children are unable to care for them, or grandparents and older aunts and uncles may assume temporary caregiving roles while the children, nieces, and nephews work. Adult children of any age may provide limited or extensive caregiving to their own parents or aging relatives when needed. A spouse or sometimes a sibling may become a temporary or long-term caregiver when needed. Close-knit families are more aware of the needs of their members, work to resolve problems, and find ways to meet the needs of other family members, even if they are not always successful. Emotionally distant families are less available in times of need and have greater potential for conflict. If the family has never been close and supportive, it will not magically become so when members have unmet needs. Resentments long buried may crop up and produce friction or psychological pain. Long-submerged conflicts and feelings may return if the needs of any one family member exceed those of the others.

In coming to know the older person, the gerontological nurse comes to know the family as well, learning of their special gifts and life challenges. Knowledge about families and family relationships, the ability to establish and maintain therapeutic relationships with older persons and their family members, and the ability to work collaboratively with older persons and their family members are required to meet Standard

IV of the Canadian *Gerontological Nursing Competencies and Standards of Practice* (Canadian Gerontological Nursing Association, 2010). The nurse works with the older person within the culture of the person's family of origin, present family, and support networks, including friends.

TRADITIONAL COUPLES

The marital or partnered relationship is a critical source of support for older people. About 76% of Canadians aged 65 years and older are married and living with a spouse (Milan et al., 2014). Although this relationship is often the most binding if it extends into later life, the chance of a couple going through old age together is exceedingly slim. Among those over 65 years of age, about 75% of men and 50% of women live with spouses or common-law partners (Milan et al., 2014). Older women are more likely to be widows; about 80% of widowed Canadians are women (Statistics Canada, 2016). A man who survives his spouse into old age ordinarily has more than one opportunity to remarry if he wishes; a woman is less likely to have an opportunity for remarriage in later life. Often, older couples live together but do not marry owing to economic and inheritance reasons.

The needs, tasks, and expectations of couples in late life differ from those in their earlier years. Some couples have been married more than 60 years. These years together may have been filled with love and companionship, abuse and resentment, or anything in between. However, in general, being married (or the presence of a long-time partner) is positively related to health, life satisfaction, and well-being. For all couples, the normal physical and sociological circumstances in late life present challenges. Some of the issues that strain many of these relationships are (1) the deteriorating health of one or both partners, (2) limitations in income, (3) conflicts with children or other relatives, (4) incompatible sexual needs, and (5) mismatched needs for activity and social activities.

Divorce

In the past, divorce was considered a stigmatizing event. However, it is so common today that nurses may forget the ostracizing effects of divorce 50 years ago. In 2016, divorced and separated persons represented 10% of older Canadians (Statistics Canada,

2016). While there are generational and individual differences in people's expectations of marriage, older couples are becoming less likely to stay in unsatisfactory marriages. Nurses need to avoid making assumptions and be alert to the possibility of marital dissatisfaction in old age. Nurses should ask, "How would you describe your marriage?"

Long-term relationships are varied and complex, and many factors form the glue that holds them together. Marital breakdown may be more devastating in old age because it is often unanticipated and may occur concurrently with other significant losses. Nurses should support clients' decisions to divorce and assist them in seeking counselling in the transition. The person should be informed that divorce will bring on a grieving process similar to that brought on by the death of a spouse, and that a severe disruption in coping **capacity** may occur as the person adjusts to a new life. The grief may be more difficult to cope with because socially sanctioned patterns of grief have not been established, as is the case with widowhood. In addition, tax and fiscal policies favour married couples, and many divorced older women are at a serious economic disadvantage.

NONTRADITIONAL COUPLES

As the variations in families grow, so too do the types of couple relationships. Among the types of couples we see today are lesbian, gay, bisexual, transgender, and queer (LGBTQ) couples. Although the accurate number of LGBTQ people of any age remains difficult to determine, in the 2014 Canadian Community Health Survey, 1.9% of adult Canadians between the ages of 18 and 59 years self-identified as gay or lesbian, and 1.3% self-identified as bisexual (Statistics Canada, 2015). This is likely an underestimate because of the hesitancy of some persons to publicly identify as being LGBTQ. Less than 1% of Canadians aged 65 years and older are in same-sex partnerships. These partnerships will become more common in coming generations of older Canadians (Milan et al., 2014).

Although these couples are less often seen in the aging population, they are still there. They may not be obvious, owing to longstanding discrimination and fear. The experiences of younger LGBTQ individuals are considerably different from those of older persons. Older LGBTQ individuals did not have the benefit

TABLE 23.1 Timeline of LGBTQ Rights Events for a 77-Year-Old Canadian

YEARS	LGBTQ RIGHTS EVENT	YEARS OF AGE
1969	Decriminalization of same-sex acts between consenting adults	29
1973	Homosexuality removed from list of mental illnesses	33
1974	LGBTQ people allowed to immigrate to Canada	34
1977–1998	Provinces and territories prohibit discrimination on basis of sexual orientation	37–58
2003	Ontario legalizes same-sex marriage	63
2005	Ontario opens door to same-sex marriage and immigration	64
2012	Ontario includes protection of gender expression under the *Human Rights Code*	72

LBGTQ, Lesbian, gay, bisexual, transgender, and queer.
Source: Extracted from Moore, D. (February, 2017). *Older adults: Considerations for Care* (PowerPoint Slide Presentation). Presented at Brock University, St. Catharines, ON.

of antidiscrimination laws and support for same-sex partners. They were also more likely to keep their sexual orientation, gender identity, and relationships "hidden." A timeline of rights events in the life of a 77-year-old Canadian is presented in Table 23.1.

Many older LGBTQ persons have been part of a live-in couple at some time during their life. However, they are more likely to live alone in older age. Some may have social networks consisting of friends, members of their family of origin, and the larger community, but many lack social support. In some cases, they may be estranged from their families of origin and come to later life with a network of close friends who make up their "family." These nonrelatives become a surrogate family and take on the instrumental and affective attributes of a family. Because these family members are not relatives in the traditional sense, they may not be recognized by the health care system, leading to considerable stress for all involved.

Some research indicates the possibility that older lesbian women and gay men may adapt more successfully to old age because of having coped with discrimination and prejudice over a lifetime. However, other research appears to indicate that a life of managing stigma can have significant negative health effects.

Older gay and lesbian adults describe their experience of invisibility in senior organizations, health care, and society (Daley et al., 2017). Experiences of discrimination and prejudice from health care agencies and the resultant, realistic fears of disclosing LGBTQ identity are barriers to accessing health care services, including mental health, long-term care (LTC) and assisted living, palliative care, services for persons infected with human immunodeficiency virus (HIV), and caregiver support (Daley et al., 2017; Grigorovich, 2015). Gerontological nurses and the health care organizations for which they work can improve accessibility and create a welcoming, safe environment for older LGBTQ persons by engaging older LGBTQ community members; advocating openness and acceptance; using inclusive language, positive messages, and images of LGBTQ older persons in documents and brochures and on websites; enacting inclusive policies; hiring LGBTQ staff; and providing education and training for staff and volunteers (Daley et al., 2017; Grigorovich, 2015).

Older lesbian women and gay men have identified other concerns, such as pension benefits, health insurance, and access to appropriate housing and services. Most research has involved gay and lesbian couples; much less is known about partnerships of bisexual or transgendered older persons. More knowledge of cohort, cultural, and generational differences among age groups is needed to understand the recent, dramatic changes in family configurations among LGBTQ individuals. Few organizations are designed for LGBTQ older persons. Aînés et Retraités de la Communauté, in Montreal, is one such group. Some organizations, such as The 519 (an LGBTQ agency in Toronto), have programs for older persons.

OLDER PEOPLE AND THEIR ADULT CHILDREN

In adulthood, relationships between the generations become increasingly important for most people. Older parents enjoy being told about the various activities and successes of their offspring, and these adult children begin to see aspects of themselves that have developed from their parents. At times, the relationships may become strained because the younger adults are more concerned with their own spouses, partners, and children. The parents are no longer central to the younger adults' lives, although they may be central to their parents' lives. The most difficult situations occur when the older parents are openly critical or judgemental about the lives of their offspring. In the best of situations, adult children shift to the roles of friend, companion, and confidante to the older person, a concept known as *filial maturity*.

Most older people see their children on a regular basis. Even children who do not live close to their older parents can maintain their close connections, and "intimacy at a distance" can occur (Hooyman & Kiyak, 2011). Approximately 50% of older people have daily contact with their adult children; nearly 80% see an adult child at least once a week; and more than 75% talk on the phone at least weekly with an adult child (Hooyman & Kiyak, 2011).

OLDER PERSONS WHO HAVE NEVER MARRIED

Approximately 6% of older persons today have never married (Statistics Canada, 2015). Older people who have lived alone most of their lives often develop supportive networks with siblings, friends, and neighbors. As a result of their independence, older persons who have never married may be resilient to the challenges of aging and may not feel lonely or isolated. Furthermore, they may have longer lifetime employment and enjoy greater financial security as they age. The number of single older persons will increase in the future, because being single is increasingly common in younger years (Hooyman & Kiyak, 2011).

GRANDPARENTING

Grandparenthood and, increasingly, great-grandparenthood are experienced by most older persons. There are over 7.1 million grandparents in Canada (Milan et al., 2015). The average age at which Canadians become grandparents is increasing because of the older ages at which people have had children over the past several decades. For example, in 1985, 80% of women aged 60 to 64 years were grandmothers, whereas in 2011, 66% of women in this age group were grandmothers (Margolis, 2016). About 80% of Canadians aged 65 years and older are currently grandparents (Margolis, 2016).

As the term implies, "grands" are a step ahead of parents in their concerns, exposure, and responsibility. Most grandparents derive great emotional satisfaction from their grandchildren. Historically, the emphasis has been on the aging of the grandparent as it affects the relationship with the grandchild, but little has been said about the effects of the growth and maturation of the grandchild on the relationship. Many young adults who have had close contact with their grandparents report that this relationship was very meaningful in their lives. Growing numbers of adult grandchildren are assisting in caregiving for frail grandparents.

The age, vitality, and proximity of both the child and grandparent produce a kaleidoscope of possible activities and interactions as both progress through the aging process. Approximately 80% of grandparents see a grandchild at least monthly, and nearly 50% do so weekly. Geographic distance does not significantly affect the quality of the relationships between grandparents and their grandchildren. The Internet is increasingly being used by distant grandparents as a way of staying involved in their grandchildren's lives and forging close bonds (Hooyman & Kiyak, 2011).

Younger grandparents and grandparents who live near their grandchildren are more likely to be involved in child care and recreational activities (Margolis & Wright, 2016). About 75% of grandparents provide financial assistance to their adult children or grandchildren (Margolis & Wright, 2016). About 11% of grandparents live in the same household as a grandchild, most often with an adult child. Among ethno-culturally diverse families and families from visible minority groups, there may be greater interaction and more grandparent responsibility for child-rearing. Living with grandchildren is more common among the Inuit (22.3%), First Nations (14.4%), and immigrants (21%) (Milan et al., 2015). More and more grandparents are assuming the role of primary caregiver to their grandchildren, a phenomenon discussed later in this chapter.

SIBLINGS

Sibling relationships in late life are poorly understood and have been neglected by researchers. As individuals age, they often have more contact with siblings than they did in the years when family and work demands were more pressing. About 80% of older people have at least one sibling, and siblings are often strong sources of support in the lives of never-married older persons, widowed persons, and those without children. For many older persons, these relationships become increasingly important because siblings have a long history of memories, are of the same generation, and have similar backgrounds. Sibling relationships become particularly important when siblings are part of the support system, especially for single or widowed older women living alone. The strongest sibling bond is thought to be the relationship between sisters. Sibling relationships remain important into late old age. Nurses should ask about sibling relationships of past and present significance.

The death of a sibling has a profound effect on a person's awareness of his or her own mortality, particularly when the sibling is of the same gender. When an older person reaches the age of the sibling who died, the reaction can be quite disruptive. Grieving is activated, and a rehearsal of a person's own death may occur. In some cases when an older sibling survives younger ones, there may be not only deep grief but also pangs of guilt—"Why them and not me?" (see Chapter 25).

OTHER KIN

Interaction with collateral kin (cousins, aunts, uncles, nieces, and nephews) generally depends on proximity, preference, and the availability of primary kin. The quality of relationships varies but is still a potential source of joy, support, assistance, or conflict. As compared to paternal kin (related through male bloodlines), maternal kin may be emotionally closer. These relatives may provide a reservoir of kin from which to find replacements for missing or lost intimate relationships for single or childless people as they grow older.

FICTIVE KIN

Fictive kin relationships are family-like reciprocal relationships between persons who are not related by blood or marriage. Such relationships cope with change, hardship, and marginalization (Allen, 2016, p. 3). Fictive kin become surrogate family and take on some of the instrumental and affectional attributes of families. They are important in the lives of many older persons, especially those who have no close or satisfying family relationships and those who live alone. Older persons who have been marginalized throughout their lives—for example, LGBTQ persons—may have long-established fictive kin networks. Nurses who work with older people need to recognize the instrumental and emotional support provided by these networks and the mutually satisfying relationships that develop between friends, neighbors, and others who are fictive kin of older persons.

Relationships between older persons and paid caregivers must be acknowledged as important to the older person. They are not, however, reciprocal in the ways that family relationships and fictive kin relationships are.

LATE-LIFE TRANSITIONS

Transition is "a process of convoluted passage during which people redefine their sense of self and develop self-agency in response to disruptive life events" (Kralik et al., 2006, p. 321). Transitions are classified as developmental (e.g., retirement, grandparenthood), situational (e.g., widowhood, becoming a caregiver, moving to seniors' housing, moving to receive care), or health–illness (e.g., experiencing persistent illness, transition between hospital and home, transition from home to an LTC home) (Schumacher & Meleis, 1994). Often, transitions are not discrete; people experience one or more related transitions at the same time.

Transitions may occur predictably or may be imposed by unanticipated events. Retirement is a predictable event that can and should be planned long in advance; for some persons, however, it can occur unexpectedly as a result of illness, disability, or being terminated from a job. To the degree that an event is perceived as expected and occurring at the "right" time, a transition may be comfortable and even welcomed. Persons who must retire "too early" or are widowed "too soon" will have more difficulty adapting than those who are at an age when these events are expected.

The speed and intensity of a major change may make the difference between a transitional crisis and a gradual, comfortable adaptation. The most difficult transitions are those that incorporate losses rather than gains in status, influence, and opportunity. The move from independence to dependence and becoming a care recipient is particularly difficult.

Conditions that influence the process and outcome of transitions include personal meanings, expectations, knowledge, planning, socioeconomic status, and emotional and physical reserves, as well as community and societal conditions. Cohort, cultural, and gender differences are inherent in all of life's major transitions. Transitions that make use of past skills and adaptations may be less stressful. The ideal outcome occurs when gains in satisfaction and new roles offset losses.

RETIREMENT

Historically, retirement was compulsory at the age of 65 years. However, Canada does not have a mandatory retirement age. "Retirement" no longer means simply a few years of rest from the rigours of work before death. It is a developmental stage that may occupy 30 or more years of a person's life and may involve many stages. The transitions are blurring, and the numerous patterns and styles of retiring have produced more varied experiences of retirement. Over the past decade, there has been a trend for retirement at a later age; 13.0% of Canadians aged 65 years and older are employed (Statistics Canada, 2016). Many retirees work for pay at some point after retirement. Some do so because of economic need, whereas others want to remain involved and productive.

Obviously, health and financial status affect people's abilities and decisions to work or to engage in new work opportunities. The "baby boomers" increasingly face the prospect of working longer, and many are concerned about the possibility of outliving their retirement savings. The Canadian government estimates that 24% of persons approaching retirement will not have sufficient income to maintain their standard of living (Department of Finance, 2016).

Older people who did not expect retirement at the time they left the workforce may experience detrimental effects and need counselling or assistance. Some may experience job separation as a crisis and a traumatic role transition triggered by an unplanned job termination—for example, as a result of illness or company downsizing. Others, given the opportunity

---

| BOX 23.1 | Predictors of Retirement Satisfaction |

Good health
Functional abilities
Adequate income
Suitable living environment
Strong social support system characterized by reciprocal relationships
Decision to retire that involved choice, autonomy, adequate preparation, higher-status job prior to retirement
Retirement activities that offer an opportunity to feel useful, learn, grow, and enjoy oneself
Positive outlook, sense of mastery, resilience, resourcefulness
Good marital relationship
Interests similar to interests of spouse or significant other

Source: Data from Hooyman, N., & Kiyak, H. (2011). *Social gerontology: A multidisciplinary perspective.* Boston, MA: Allyn and Bacon.

to work past retirement age, must weigh the benefits of doing so. Part-time work during retirement may be an option. Employers value older workers because they are experienced and dependable. Canadians older than 65 years can earn any amount without endangering their Canada Pension Plan benefits. A portion of Old Age Security benefits is repaid if income is over $73,756.

Retirement Planning

Current research indicates that retirement may have positive effects on life satisfaction and health, although this may vary depending on the individual's circumstances. Predictors of satisfaction in retirement are presented in Box 23.1. Decisions to retire are often based on financial resources, age, health, attitude toward work, and self-perceptions of the ability to adjust to retirement. Retirement planning is advisable during early adulthood and is essential in middle age. However, people differ in their focus on the past, present, and future and in their realistic ability to "put away something" for future needs.

Retirement preparation programs are usually aimed at employees with high levels of education and occupational status, those with private pension coverage, and government employees. Thus, the people with the fewest resources for retirement, who are most in need of planning assistance, may be least likely to have access to such assistance. People who are retiring in poor health, people who live at lower socioeconomic levels, and ethnoculturally diverse persons may have greater financial concerns in retirement and may need specialized counselling. These groups are often neglected in retirement planning programs.

Working couples must plan together for retirement. Decisions will depend on their career goals, their shared future interests, and the quality of their interpersonal relationship. The following are some questions a person must weigh when deciding to retire or continue working:

- What do I want to do?
- Who needs me, and what are my best opportunities?
- What am I best able to do?
- What is the meaning of my life?
- What should my life accomplish or contribute?
- Am I financially secure for the rest of my life if I live 30 or more years?
- Can I afford to completely retire from paid work?

Information about retirement planning is supplied through group lectures, individual counselling, booklets, and online resources. However, in light of the current economy and the many financial hazards experienced before retirement, planning for retirement is often insufficient. Many individuals have very high expectations for the final third of their lives. Federal tax laws encourage contributions to private savings plans such as Registered Retirement Savings Plans (RRSPs); in any given year, however, less than 25% of Canadians who file a tax return make RRSP contributions (Statistics Canada, 2017a). Less than 40% of employed Canadians have a pension plan sponsored by an employer or union (Statistics Canada, 2017b). When considering retirement, people need to take into account the adequacy of (1) employer-provided retirement benefits, (2) government pension benefits, (3) employer-provided postretirement health care, and (4) personal savings.

The adequacy of retirement income depends not only on a person's work history but also on marital history and marital status. The poverty rates of women are excessively high. Couples who had previous marriages and divorces may have significantly fewer economic resources available than couples in first marriages have. Child support, divorce settlements, and pension apportionment to ex-spouses may result in diminished retirement income. This problem is an ever-increasing impediment to retirement, because less than half of couples presently approaching retirement age are in a first marriage. Policies based on the traditional lifelong marriage are no longer appropriate.

Special Considerations in Retirement

Retirement security depends on the following "three pillars" or "three-legged stool" of income protection: (1) the federal Old Age Security (OAS) and Guaranteed Income Supplement (GIS) programs; (2) income from the Canada Pension Plan (CPP) or Quebec Pension Plan (QPP); and (3) income from private retirement savings, including investments and savings, RRSPs, and employer-sponsored pension plans (Moussaly, 2010).

People with higher incomes are most likely to participate in retirement savings plans. Less than 10% of Canadians in the lowest income quintile contribute to RRSPs, compared to 60% of those in the highest income quintile (Statistics Canada, 2017b). Canadians are eligible to receive CPP or QPP payments if they have worked and made contributions to the plan and are at least 60 years old. The amount received depends on the amount contributed, how long the person has been making contributions, and the person's age at retirement. Old age security (i.e., OAS pension, GIS, and the Allowance) is provided to Canadian residents who are citizens or legal residents who have lived in Canada for at least 10 years. Eligibility does not depend on work history. Persons with very low income or no sources of income are eligible for an income supplement benefit (see Chapter 22).

Older people with disabilities, persons who lacked access to education or held low-paying jobs that provided no benefits, and persons who are not eligible for CPP or QPP benefits are at economic risk during their retirement years. In addition, older persons who are members of an ethnocultural minority group, women (especially widows and divorced or never–married women), immigrants, and LGBTQ persons often face greater difficulties in obtaining adequate income and benefits in retirement than others face.

Inadequate coverage for women in retirement is common, because their work histories are sporadic and diverse. Women often retire earlier than anticipated because of family needs. Whereas most men have always worked outside the home, only within the past 30 years has this has been expected of women. When today's retired women were working, they earned significantly less than men; therefore, large cohort differences exist. Traditionally, the variability of women's work histories, interrupted careers, the residuals of sexist pension policies, pension inequities, and low-paying jobs created hazards for adequate income in retirement. Older women are likely to have several years of no earnings included in the averages that determine the amount of their CPP or QPP benefits.

Barriers to equal treatment for LGBTQ couples include job discrimination and historical unequal treatment under government pension plans. To help rectify this situation, Canadian legislation introduced in 2000 extended benefits to persons in same-sex common-law relationships, giving them access to CPP and OAS survivor benefits (McLaren & Manery, 2001).

IMPLICATIONS FOR GERONTOLOGICAL NURSING AND HEALTHY AGING

Successful retirement adjustment depends on socialization needs, energy levels, health, adequate income, a variety of interests, the amount of self-esteem derived from work, the presence of intimate relationships, social support, and general adaptability. Nurses may have the opportunity to work with older persons in different phases of retirement or participate in retirement education and counselling programs (Box 23.2). Talking with people older than 50 years about

---

BOX 23.2   Phases of Retirement

Remote: Future anticipation with little real planning
Near: Preparation and fantasizing regarding retirement
Honeymoon: Euphoria and testing of the fantasies
Disenchantment: Letdown, boredom, depression sometimes
Reorientation: Development of a realistic and satisfactory lifestyle
Stability: Personal investment in meaningful activities
Termination: Loss of retirement role as a result of illness or return to work

---

retirement plans, providing proactive guidance in the transition to retirement, identifying those who may be at risk for lowered income and health concerns, and referring individuals to appropriate resources for retirement planning and support are important nursing interventions.

It is important to build on the strengths of older persons' life experiences and coping skills and to provide appropriate counselling and support to help older people continue to grow and develop in meaningful ways during the various transitions. In ideal situations, retirement offers older persons the opportunity to pursue interests that may have been neglected while fulfilling other obligations. However, for too many older people, retirement presents challenges that affect both health and well-being, and nurses must be advocates for policies and conditions that allow all older people to maintain their quality of life in retirement.

WIDOWS AND WIDOWERS

Widowhood is common; 37% of all women and 11% of all men aged 65 years and older are widowed (Statistics Canada, 2016). The rate is lower for men because men are more likely to remarry after a spouse dies. Losing a partner after a long, close, and satisfying relationship is one of the most difficult transitions a person can face. It "shatters persons' familiar and taken-for-granted world" (Naef et al., 2013, p. 1109). The transition involves grief, the psychological and physical reactions to the loss, as well as the process of grieving, coping with the loss, and reconstructing meaning. Over time, most people come to terms with bereavement. However, even widows and widowers who reorganize their lives and invest in family, friends, and activities often find that many years later they still profoundly miss their "other half."

The core features of grief are depression, anxiety, and loneliness. Table 23.2 presents four dimensions—affective, cognitive, behavioural, and physiological-somatic—of the many symptoms of normal, uncomplicated grief. A fifth dimension of grief (an existential dimension) involves the search for meaning in death and the questioning of spiritual beliefs (Love, 2007). It is important to note that not every grieving person experiences all of these reactions. Furthermore, the intensity, duration, and

TABLE 23.2	Four Dimensions of Grief Reactions

REACTION	SYMPTOMS
Affective	Depression, despair, dejection, distress Anxiety, fears, dreads Guilt, self-blame, self-accusation Anger, hostility, irritability Anhedonia (loss of pleasure) Loneliness Yearning, longing, pining Shock, numbness
Cognitive	Preoccupation with thoughts of the deceased, intrusive ruminations Sense of presence of the deceased Suppression, denial Lowered self-esteem Self-reproach Helplessness, hopelessness Sense of unreality Memory, concentration problems
Behavioural	Agitation, tenseness, restlessness Fatigue Overactivity Searching Weeping, sobbing, crying Social withdrawal
Physiological-somatic	Loss of appetite Sleep disturbances Energy loss, exhaustion Somatic complaints Physical complaints similar to those of the deceased Immunological and endocrine changes Susceptibility to illness, disease

Source: Extracted from Hansson, R. O. & Stroebe, M. S. (2007). *Bereavement in late life: Coping, adaptation, and developmental influences* (p. 14, Table 1.3). Washington, DC: American Psychological Association.

impact of these reactions vary from person to person and across cultures.

The bereaved partner experiences stress from the loss of the loved person and their companionship, as well as stress that is a secondary consequence of the loss (Stroebe & Schut, 2010). Thus, grieving involves two kinds of coping: (1) dealing with the loss of the partner and (2) adjusting to secondary losses, such as changes in living arrangements; loss of income; no longer having a partner who does certain tasks (e.g., cooking, doing chores, or managing finances); and changes in identity, from being a spouse or partner to being a widow or widower and from being part of a couple to being single. Grieving involves moving back and forth between these two kinds of coping; the person copes with loss, adjusts to secondary losses, and establishes new activities and relationships.

A person's bereavement is influenced by the circumstances of the spouse's death, by other stressors (such as financial stress or social isolation), and by the supports that are available to the person. There are gender differences in regard to bereavement. Bereaved husbands may be more socially and emotionally vulnerable. Suicide risk is highest among men over 80 years of age who have experienced the death of a spouse. Widowers adapt more slowly than widows to the loss of a spouse and often remarry quickly. Loneliness and the need to be cared for are factors influencing widowers to seek out new partners. Associating with family and friends, being members of a church community, and continuing to work or engage in activities can all be helpful for men in the adjustment period following the death of a spouse. Widows are more likely to experience financial hardship and poverty. Adjusting to social life as a single person is difficult for both men and women (Naef et al., 2013).

 IMPLICATIONS FOR GERONTOLOGICAL NURSING AND HEALTHY AGING

ASSESSMENT

Nurses interact with bereaved older people in many settings. When working with widows and widowers, nurses need to understand the complexity and variability of normal grief reactions, as well as the resilience of older persons. It is important to avoid judging coping as being adaptive or maladaptive. Rather, the nurse should focus on understanding the meaning of the loss, the resources available to the person, and the strategies the person is using to cope (Naef et al., 2013).

Assessment should include the person's grief and response to the loss of the spouse, as well as how the person is adjusting to secondary losses and role changes. Grief reactions must be accepted as personally valid and useful evidence of healing. Intense emotions in the weeks after the death of the spouse are common. Emotions commonly experienced over a longer period include loneliness, shock, pain, sadness, anger, and regret. Sleep difficulties are common and may persist for up to 2 years. Loss of appetite and weight loss are also common, especially in the first few months of bereavement (Naef et al., 2013). Many widows and widowers are comforted by ongoing bonds and connections with their spouse (e.g., dreaming of them, conversing with them, taking up an activity their spouse engaged in, or keeping objects that belonged to their spouse) long after the spouse's death (Naef et al., 2013). Several tools can be used to assess the following aspects of the bereavement process: coping, grief symptoms, personal growth, continuing bonds, and health risk (Minton & Barron, 2008; Sealey et al., 2015).

Grief is not a linear process; each person has a unique grief and adjustment experience. However, there are patterns of adjustment (Box 23.3). Re-integration can usually be expected in 2 to 4 years.

INTERVENTIONS

People respond to losses in ways that reflect the nature and meaning of the lost relationships, as well as the unique characteristics of the bereaved. To support grieving persons, nurses need to extend themselves with warmth and caring in order to connect with the person.

With the support of friends and family, most people cope and grieve without complication and without professional help. Some may find that grief counselling or bereavement support groups facilitate normal, uncomplicated grieving. However, grief counselling may not be necessary or beneficial (Naef et al., 2013). Information in Box 23.3 can be used to plan interventions to support widows and widowers.

People with little family or social support may need professional help to get through the early months of grief. Widows and widowers may need more support with the secondary stressors of grief—finding new ways to manage at home, seeking social support, or managing financial hardship. Some widows and widowers (10 to 20%) experience *complicated grief* (an unusual duration and intensity of grief symptoms)

BOX 23.3   Patterns of Adjustment to Widowhood

Stage One: Reactionary (First Few Weeks)
Disbelief, anger, indecision, detachment, and inability to communicate in a logical, sustained manner are common. Searching for the partner, visions, hallucinations, and depersonalization may be experienced.
    Interventions: Support, validate, be available, listen to talk about the partner, and reduce the person's expectations.

Stage Two: Withdrawal (First Few Months)
Depression, apathy, physiological vulnerability occur; movement and cognition are slowed; insomnia, unpredictable waves of grief, sighing, and anorexia occur.
    Interventions: Protect against suicide, and involve the person in support groups.

Stage Three: Recuperation (Second 6 Months)
Periods of depression are interspersed with characteristic capability. Feelings of personal control begin to return.
    Intervention: Support accustomed lifestyle patterns that sustain and assist the person in exploring new possibilities.

Stage Four: Exploration (Second Year)
The person begins new ventures, testing the suitability of new roles. Wedding anniversary, holidays, birthdays, and the anniversary of the death may be especially difficult.
    Intervention: Prepare the individual for unexpected reactions during anniversaries. Encourage and support new trial roles.

Stage Five: Integration (Fifth Year)
The person will feel fully integrated into new and satisfying roles if grief has been resolved in a healthy manner.
    Intervention: Help the person recognize and share his or her own pattern of growth through the trauma of loss.

---

for at least 6 months, causing functional impairment (Lobb et al., 2010). Grief therapy, a specialized therapy for persons experiencing or at high risk for complicated grief, can be effective (Hansson & Stroebe, 2007). (See Chapter 25 for additional information about dying, death, and grief.)

CAREGIVING

Former US First Lady Rosalyn Carter said, "There are only four kinds of people in the world: those who have been caregivers, those who currently are caregivers, those who will be caregivers, and those who will need caregivers" (Alzheimer's Association, 2017, ¶ 1).

Family caregiving has become a normative experience (similar to marriage, work, or retirement) for many families and cuts across racial, ethnic, and social class distinctions. Gerontological nurses are most likely to encounter older persons and their family and friends in situations relating to caregiving of some kind. In any given year, 13 million Canadians (28% of the population) provide care for a chronically ill, disabled, or older family member or friend (Sinha, 2013). Most of these caregivers provide care for at least a year; periods longer than 4 years are common. Informal caregivers include friends, unpaid workers, and volunteers in the home.

Family caregiving activities vary. They can include assistance with activities of daily living and instrumental activities of daily living; illness-related care such as carrying out treatments, managing symptoms, and managing equipment; and case management, including care coordination, communication with health professionals, and advocacy. Most caregivers spend fewer than 10 hours per week giving care, but 1 in 10 caregivers spends 30 or more hours per week providing care. Those who are caring for a spouse spend the most time (Sinha, 2013). Our health care system relies heavily on family caregiving. The value of caregiving is estimated to be at least $24 billion per year (National Seniors Strategy, 2017). The cost of replacing family caregiving with formal care within the health care system would be devastating for society.

Just over half (54%) of family caregivers are women. Women are more likely than men to spend 20 or more hours per week giving care. They are also more likely to provide personal care, assist with medical treatments, and complete household tasks. More than a quarter of caregivers (28%) have at least one child under 18 years of age living at home. Caregiving can also be a financial burden, and women who are family caregivers are more likely to live in poverty than those who are not caregivers. Even though caregiving is generally considered a women's issue, more and more men, including those who are not spouses (e.g., brothers, nephews, and sons), are assuming the full range of caregiving roles. Forty-six percent of caregivers are men, and more research is needed to identify their special needs and challenges. In addition, a

substantial number of children and youths provide care for an adult relative. The number of children providing care in Canada is not known, but just under a half-million youths aged 15 to 17 years provide care for an adult relative, and 40% of them provide care to an older person (Stamatopoulos, 2015).

Caregiving is considered a major public health issue, and the physical and mental health of caregivers is receiving increased attention. The aging of the population, medical advances, shorter hospital stays, and the expansion of home care technology will increase the demand for family caregivers. At the same time, however, the number of family members who are available to provide care will decrease.

IMPACT OF CAREGIVING

Although caregiving is a way to "give back" to a loved one and joy can be found in the giving, it is also stressful and can be physically and emotionally demanding, leading to greater risks for illness and mortality. The caregiver is considered to be "the hidden patient" (Schulz & Beach, 1999, p. 2216). Family caregiving is associated with increased depression and anxiety, poorer self-reported physical health, compromised immune function, and increased mortality (Sinha, 2013; Turcotte, 2013). "Caregiving is a very complex issue, and assuming a caregiving role is a time of transition that requires a restructuring of one's goals, behaviors, and responsibilities. It requires taking on something new but it is also about loss—of what was and what could have been" (Lund, 2005, p. 152).

The financial consequences of caregiving can be significant. A national survey found that 41% of Canadians caring for a parent and 61% of those caring for a spouse spent at least $500 per year on out-of-pocket expenses. One in five spousal caregivers and 7% of those caring for a parent experienced financial hardship due to caregiving (Turcotte, 2013). Expenses include those of transportation, travel, accommodation, and the purchasing of medications for the care recipient. Financial problems also result from lost wages due to work absences, early retirement, or job resignation. One in ten Canadians who provide care for a parent says that caregiving prevents him or her from working (Turcotte, 2013).

Most caregivers report that they can cope with the demands of caregiving, and caregiving does not

BOX 23.4	Nursing Suggestions for Reducing Caregiver Stress

Restore a sense of control and effectiveness in the situation.

Reinforce any social supports that are available to the caregiver.

Find opportunities for group participation with other caregivers.

Advise routine times of respite, and assist the caregiver in finding respite sources.

Tailor programs and services to the unique situation of the caregiver and care recipient.

Urge the caregiver to take care of himself or herself.

Encourage the caregiver to maintain activities that are important to his or her well-being.

Allow the caregiver to express negative and angry feelings they may have about the care recipient and the caregiving experience.

Encourage the caregiver's efforts to use all available resources and assistance.

Include all directly involved parties in decisions about care.

Praise whatever is being done well, and encourage the letting go of things that have not gone well.

Source: From Schmall, V. L., & Stiehl, R. (2003). *Coping with caregiving: How to manage stress when caring for older relatives.* Corvallis, OR: Pacific Northwest Extension. Retrieved from http://extension.oregonstate.edu/catalog/PDF/PNW/PNW315.pdf.

BOX 23.5	Research for Evidence-Informed Practice: Immigrant Women Caregivers Experience Barriers to Services

Problem: Cultural diversity is often not considered in programs and policies about caregiving.

Methods: In this descriptive qualitative study, individual and group interviews were conducted with 29 women who provided care to an older relative and who were immigrants from China or South Asia and with 15 service providers and policy-makers in Edmonton, Alberta.

Findings: More than half of the women did not access any services. One barrier to access was immigration policy; because of sponsorship rules, immigrants under family reunification policy have limited access to community resources for 10 years. Other barriers were an inability to speak English, time demands related to employment, a lack of access to transportation, and waiting lists and inconvenient hours of services. Participants' recommended strategies to improve services included linguistically and culturally relevant support services, peer support, outreach, and the use of the language of the caregivers when information about services is being distributed.

Application to Nursing Practice: Linguistically and ethnoculturally sensitive services for family carers are needed. To increase accessibility, services should be advertised in the family carers' languages, possibly through cultural brokers. Flexible hours would improve access for caregivers whose working hours are not flexible.

Source: Stewart, M. J., Neufeld, A., Harrison, M. J. et al. (2006). Immigrant women family caregivers in Canada: Implications for policies and programmes in health and social sectors. *Health and Social Care in the Community, 14*(4), 329–340.

necessarily result in negative outcomes. However, the circumstances that are more likely to cause problems with caregiving include competing role responsibilities (e.g., work, home, parenting), advanced age of the caregiver, high-intensity caregiving needs, insufficient resources, a care recipient with dementia, and prior relational conflicts between the caregiver and care recipient. Caregivers of persons with dementia may experience even greater emotional and physical stress than other caregivers experience. Suggestions for reducing caregiver stress are presented in Box 23.4.

Some research, particularly in the United States, indicates that the burden of caregiving may be lower among African Americans and that family caregivers who are members of an ethnocultural minority rely less on formal support than ethnic-majority family caregivers do. However, it has been suggested that this is not because of differences in value systems (Pinquart & Sörensen, 2005). Rather, the lack of access

to culturally competent support services and the lack of knowledge about available resources may influence caregiving more than ethnicity or culture influences it (Koehn et al., 2016; Pinquart & Sörensen, 2005). **Filial piety** and **familism**—prevalent values in Asian, Indigenous, and other minority ethnic cultures in Canada—play an important role in family caregiving (Liu & McDaniel, 2015; McCleary & Blain, 2013). Further research into ethnicity, culture, and caregiving is needed in light of the increasing ethnocultural diversity of older Canadians. Box 23.5 describes a Canadian study of immigrant women caregivers.

Some of the benefits of caregiving are enhanced self-esteem, well-being, and ability to empathize with others; personal growth, satisfaction, and pride in caregiving; finding meaning or making meaning through caregiving; and the development of an interest in activism (Giesbrecht et al., 2016; Meisner & Binnington, 2016). Further research is needed to understand that factors that influence how family caregivers perceive the experience. Most attention in caregiving research has been given to the caregiver. Less attention has been given to the care recipient or to the relationship between caregiver and care recipient.

Archbold et al. (1990) studied caregiving as a role, examining how the relationships between the family caregiver and care recipient (*mutuality*) and the preparation of the family caregiver (preparedness) influence reactions to caregiving. Mutuality is "an enduring quality of a relationship with four components: shared values, love, shared activities, and reciprocity" (Sebern, 2005, p. 175). Family caregivers who have a positive relationship with the care recipient experience less stress and find caregiving more meaningful. Nursing interventions to assist in preparing a person for the caregiving role, particularly at the time of the patient's discharge from hospital, also seem to prevent or reduce role strain. Further research is needed to understand the complexities of these roles. Box 23.6 describes the needs of caregivers. Box 23.7 gives suggestions for family caregivers.

SPOUSAL CAREGIVING

Of family caregivers over 60 years of age, spouses provide the most care, and 80% of persons who live with spouses with disabilities provide care for them. Many have health problems that are neglected in deference to the needs of the spouse. Although spousal caregivers provide more intensive, time-consuming care than other family caregivers provide, the spouse may need care that is beyond the capabilities of the caregiver.

A comparison of needs of spouses and adult children who were primary caregivers for persons with dementia found that for both groups of caregivers, the burden of caregiving was associated with needing more support from family, feeling lonely, and feeling underappreciated. For spouses, having a poor relationship with the person before the person became ill was associated with a greater burden, as was caring

| BOX 23.6 | Caregiver Needs |

- Finding time for one's self
- Keeping the person being cared for safe
- Balancing work and family responsibilities
- Managing emotional and physical stress
- Finding easy and satisfying activities to do with the care recipient
- Learning how to talk to physicians
- Making end-of-life decisions
- Moving or lifting the care recipient (bathing and dressing)
- Managing the challenging behaviours of the care recipient
- Negotiating health care and home- and community-based services
- Managing complex medication schedules or high-tech medical equipment
- Choosing a home health agency or assisted living or long-term care home
- Managing incontinence or toileting problems
- Finding non-English educational material

Sources: Adapted from Curry, L., Walker, C., & Hogstel, M. O. (2006). Educational needs of employed family caregivers of older adults: Evaluation of a workplace project. *Geriatric Nursing, 27*(3), 166–173; Family Caregiver Alliance. (2006). *Caregiver assessment: Principles, guidelines and strategies for change.* Report from a National Consensus Development Conference (Vol. 1). San Francisco, CA: Author.

for a person experiencing agitation or sleep problems (Chappell, et al. 2014).

Older family caregivers are at greater risk for negative consequences. The nurse should be alert for situations in which health care providers may be able to provide supports and resources that make it possible for a family caregiver to assume new responsibilities without being totally overwhelmed. When a spouse is ill and the partner needs to take over functions for both of them, someone must be available to provide reinforcement, encouragement, and relief. An adult day program, **respite** care services, routine visits from a community health nurse, or periodic assistance from a home health aide or a housekeeper may make it possible for the couple to continue to live together. It is important to pay attention to the physical and mental health needs of the caregiver as well as those of the care recipient.

BOX 23.7   Self-Care Suggestions for Family Caregivers

- Check in; make time to think about how you are feeling physically, emotionally, and mentally.
- Seek information about the disease or medical condition(s) and about community resources that might help you as a caregiver.
- Set realistic goals, recognize what you can or cannot do, and set priorities accordingly.
- Ask for help from health professionals, family, friends, or neighbours.
- Practise good communication; try to listen carefully, be aware of your feelings, be clear in your requests or inquiries, and be assertive about your needs without imposing on the rights of others.
- Keep lines of communication with family and friends open. Consider joining a caregiver support group.
- Take care of your physical health, including diet, exercise, sleep, and rest.
- Take care of your spiritual health, whatever your spiritual or religious belief system; investigate opportunities for support and rejuvenation in your community.
- Plan for and seek opportunities for respite and breaks from caregiving (either with the help of your social network or through formal respite services).

Source: Extracted from VON Canada. (2008). *Caregiver connect guide: Caregiver health information*. Retrieved from http://www.caregiver-con-nect.ca/en-us/caregiverconnectguide/CaregiverHealthInformation/Pages/Whatdoesitmeantobeafamilycaregiver.aspx.

AGING PARENTS CARING FOR DEVELOPMENTALLY DISABLED CHILDREN

Although we tend to think of caregivers as middle-aged adults caring for older persons, an unknown number of older people are caring for their middle-aged children who are physically and mentally disabled. Earlier in the past century, developmentally disabled children usually died before reaching adulthood. Now, with improved care, they are surviving.

With increased survival, these adults with developmental disabilities are also at risk for developing chronic illness, thus needing more care and services. For example, people with Down syndrome are much more likely to develop dementia, and they develop it at a younger age. Often, the responsibility for managing or providing care is carried by parents for their entire adult life, ending only with the death of the

parent or the adult child. The most stressful issues for parents are long-term planning for care of the adult child after the parent dies, planning for emotional and social support, handling financial concerns, and creating opportunities for their child to socialize. Families also report lack of access to sufficient respite care (Lunsky et al., 2014). The phenomenon of an aging parent caring for an aging child is beginning to receive more attention both from organizations for aging and from organizations for developmentally disabled persons.

GRANDPARENTS RAISING GRANDCHILDREN

In recent years, more grandparents have become primary caregivers for their grandchildren when the parents are unable to provide needed care. The reasons include child abuse, teen pregnancy, imprisonment, joblessness, military deployment, drug and alcohol addictions, illness, death, and other social problems. In Canada in 2011, 58,500 children lived solely with their grandparents (Statistics Canada, 2015).

Caregiving by grandparents is more common among Indigenous peoples (Fuller-Thomson, 2005). This is partly a reflection of Indigenous cultures in which grandmothers and the community are traditionally involved in child-rearing but is also a result of historic and current government policies and a legacy of the residential schools (Hsieh et al., 2017) (see Chapter 4). Two consequences of the residential schools policy (which was in place until the last quarter of the twentieth century) were the destruction of family relationships and the loss of traditional child-rearing practices (Fontaine et al., 2015). A qualitative study found that grandmother caregivers in Manitoba Indigenous communities took pride in preserving their culture (Eni et al., 2009). Grandmothers talked about dangers in their communities and about their role in monitoring and protecting their grandchildren. Problems for grandmothers included overcrowded housing, low community and personal income levels, balance of work and family responsibilities, lack of employment opportunities, and difficulty in accessing health care services. Grandmothers received support from friends and relatives, as well as nurses and community services.

For many grandparents, economic, health, and social challenges associated with caregiving include limited income and financial support through the welfare system, lack of informal support systems, loss of leisure and social activities in retirement, and shame or guilt related to their children's inability to parent. Research on the physical and mental health consequences of grandparents' raising grandchildren is limited, but some of the research suggests that custodial grandparents are at risk for psychological distress and depression, especially in a context of poverty (Hadfield, 2014). Many custodial grandparents are happy and satisfied with their roles (Hsieh et al., 2017), but they also experience caregiver stress, particularly when resources are inadequate, there is conflict with the child's parents, or the grandchild has emotional or health problems (Hsieh et al., 2017). Too often, both the children and their grandparents are in need of help. Children in the care of a custodial grandparent are more likely to have emotional or behavioural problems than are children in two-parent families.

Routine screening for psychological distress in custodial grandparents is important, as is offering support and referrals to reduce stressors. Custodial grandparents may need information about financial resources, subsidies, and tax benefits (National Initiative for Care of the Elderly [NICE], n.d.). Box 23.8 provides research-informed suggestions for nursing interventions with older persons who are providing primary care to their grandchildren. Grassroots non-profit organizations of grandparents, such as Grand Parenting Again Canada and CANGRANDS, have developed resources and support groups in many communities. Nurses can be instrumental in collaborating with community organizations to provide needed support. Resources and online information are available for custodial grandparents (see the Resources section at the end of this chapter).

LONG-DISTANCE CAREGIVING

Because of the increasing mobility of today's society, more children move away from home for education or employment. Help for a parent must, then, be provided "long distance." One in five Canadians who provide care to a parent or parent-in-law live more than an hour away (Vézina & Turcotte, 2010). Caregivers at a distance provide similar types of assistance and care although less frequently than those living closer to the older person. Distance caregivers incur more expenses for caregiving and have higher incomes. This is perhaps one of the most difficult situations, and it presents unique challenges. See Chapter 26 for a discussion of residential care options for older people, including moving in with an adult child.

A caregiving industry is emerging in Canada, following a trend in the United States, to assist the geographically distant family member to ensure that an older relative will be cared for; this industry is made up of geriatric care managers, some of whom are nurses or social workers. The services are provided on a fee-for-service basis.

IMPLICATIONS FOR GERONTOLOGICAL NURSING AND HEALTHY AGING

Nurses are often care providers and case managers for older people and their families, both in the home and in retirement homes, assisted living, and LTC home settings. Support for families in the caregiving role is an important nursing intervention.

ASSESSMENT

Family Assessment

A comprehensive assessment of the older person includes an assessment of the family—its members; family history; usual roles; family members' strengths and contributions; and deterrents to the functioning of the family unit. In order to know the family

---

BOX 23.8	Suggested Nursing Interventions With Grandparent Caregivers

- Early identification of at-risk grandparents
- Comprehensive assessment of physical, psychosocial, and environmental factors affecting grandparents who are caring for grandchildren
- Anticipatory guidance and counselling about child growth and development and other child-raising issues
- Referral to resources for support and counselling
- Advocate for policies supportive of grandparents who have assumed a caregiving role for grandchildren

Source: Butler, F., & Zakari, N. (2005). Grandparents parenting grandchildren: Assessing health status. *Journal of Gerontological Nursing, 31*(3), 43–54.

and design responses that may strengthen the family unit, the nurse must assess the family's needs and strengths and the meaning family members assign to caregiving, as well as their sources of stress, particular methods of coping, cultural values, support system, and family dynamics.

Often, nurses see families in times of crisis, when an older family member needs care. It is important that nurses encourage the expression of feelings from all involved family members as well as from the older person and maintain a nonjudgemental attitude. The nurse must also be aware of his or her vision of what a family should be and do. The nurse's values should not enter into assessment and intervention, and nurses should not label families as "dysfunctional." As Meiner (2011, p. 113) stated, "It is necessary to identify the strengths within each family and to build on those strengths while recognizing the family's limitations in providing support and caregiving." Thus, the nurse's role is to teach, monitor, and strengthen the family system so as to maintain the health and wellness of the entire family.

Caregiver Assessment

The stresses, expectations of future needs and problems, and positive aspects of the caregiving situation should be explored with family caregivers. Assessing a caregiver includes determining how the caregiver can help the care recipient and how the health care team can help the caregiver. In light of the physical and emotional stressors often associated with the caregiving role, nurses need to monitor the physical and emotional health of both the caregiver and the care recipient and provide support as necessary. A partnership model "blending the nurse's knowledge and expertise in health care with the caregiver's knowledge of the family members and the caregiving situation" is necessary (Messecar, 2016, p. 152).

The assessment should focus on identifying the caregiver's priorities and include (1) the caregiving context (i.e., relationship of caregiver to care recipient, roles and responsibilities, home and physical environments, financial status, potential caregiving resources, and cultural background); (2) the caregiver's perception of the health and functional status of the care recipient; (3) the caregiver's preparedness for caregiving; (4) the quality of family relationships;

BOX 23.9   Nursing Actions to Create and Sustain a Partnership With Caregivers

- Monitoring: conducting ongoing surveillance
- Coaching: helping caregivers apply knowledge and develop skills
- Teaching: providing information and instruction
- Fostering partnerships: fostering communication and collaboration between the caregiver and the care recipient and between them and the nurse
- Providing psychosocial support: attending to psychosocial well-being
- Rescuing: providing a safety net by stepping in to provide direct care and by making clinical decisions
- Coordinating: orchestrating the work of other health care team members and the activities of the caregiver

Sources: Data from Eilers, J., Heermann, J., Wilson, M., et al. (2005). Independent nursing actions in cooperative care. *Oncology Nursing Forum, 32*(4), 849–855; Schumacher, K., Beck, C., & Marren, J. (2006). Family caregivers: caring for older adults working with their families. *American Journal of Nursing, 106*(8), 40–49.

(5) indications of problems with quality of care; (6) the caregiver's physical and mental health; and (7) the caregiver's strengths (Messecar, 2016). Several validated caregiver assessment instruments are available in the Try This series section of the *ConsultGeri* website, which includes the Modified Caregiver Strain Index, Let's PREPARE, and the Elder Assessment Instrument. Box 23.9 presents a research-based model to guide nursing interventions with caregivers.

INTERVENTIONS

Caregiver interventions have the goal of either reducing the amount of caregiving provided by a caregiver or improving the caregiver's well-being and coping. Some interventions aim to achieve both outcomes. The six types of caregiver interventions are psychoeducational interventions, supportive interventions, respite interventions, psychotherapy interventions, interventions to improve care receiver competence, and multicomponent interventions. These interventions have all been tested for their effects in regard to caregiver burden, depression, and well-being; the care provider's satisfaction with caregiving; the caregiver's knowledge and caregiving ability; and the care

TABLE 23.3	Influence of Caregiver Interventions on Caregiver Outcomes	
CAREGIVER INTERVENTION	**CHARACTERISTICS OF INTERVENTION**	**CAREGIVER OUTCOME**
Psychoeducational interventions	Structured program providing: • Information about care recipient's disease process • Information about resources and services • Training to caregivers in responding effectively to disease-related problems	• Burden • Depression • Well-being • Satisfaction • Knowledge and ability
Supportive interventions	Professional or peer-led unstructured support groups Reliance on group members to provide mutual support, information, and advice	• Burden • Knowledge and ability
Respite and adult day program interventions	In-home or site-specific (e.g., adult day program or temporary stay in an LTC home) supervision and assistance for the care recipient, designed to give the caregiver time off	• Burden • Depression • Well-being
Psychotherapy and counselling interventions	Most use a cognitive–behavioural approach involving self-monitoring, challenging of negative thoughts and assumptions, development of problem-solving skills and emotional reactivity management, and re-engagement in pleasurable activities	• Burden • Depression • Well-being • Satisfaction • Knowledge and ability
Interventions to improve care-receiver competence	For example, memory clinics for people with dementia and activity programs	• Well-being
Multicomponent interventions	Combinations of education, support, psychotherapy, and respite	• Burden • Well-being • Knowledge and ability

Source: Adapted from Sörensen, S., Pinquart, M., & Duberstein, P. (2002). How effective are interventions with caregivers? An updated meta-analysis. *The Gerontologist, 42*(3), 356–372.

receiver's functioning. Caregiver interventions are not equally effective, and their effectiveness varies according to the characteristics of the caregiver and the care recipient (Messecar, 2016). Table 23.3 outlines the characteristics of the six caregiver interventions and the outcomes they influence. In general, caregiver interventions have a bigger effect on caregiver knowledge than on other outcomes. Group interventions are less effective than individual interventions. Psychoeducation, counselling, and interventions with multiple components show the strongest evidence of effectiveness. The effectiveness is less when care receivers have dementia or other illness conditions that worsen over time (Messecar, 2016).

Interventions with caregivers must always be made with consideration of the great variability in family structures, resources, traditions, and history. The range of adaptations is enormous, and the goal is always to restore the balance of the system to the greatest extent possible and to support caregivers in their caring. The family can be visualized as a mobile with many parts; when the mobile is touched, each part shifts to regain the balance. The intrusion of health care providers into a family system will temporarily unbalance the system but may provide an opportunity to restore the balance in a healthier manner, sometimes by adding an element or by increasing the weight of one or decreasing the weight of another.

When the nurse works with a family from a culture different from his or her own culture—for instance, a culture whose rituals and routines are unfamiliar to the nurse—the nurse must be particularly careful to respect the differences. The nurse can work with the family to make the best use of their strengths; each family member can be valued for what he or she brings to the situation.

INTIMACY AND SEXUALITY

INTIMACY

Although intimacy is often thought of in the context of sexual performance, it encompasses more than sexuality and includes the following major components: commitment, affective intimacy, cognitive intimacy, physical intimacy, and interdependence (Youngkin, 2004). "Intimacy is from a Greek work meaning 'closest to; inner lining of blood vessels'" (Steinke, 2005, p. 40). It is a warm, meaningful feeling of joy. Intimacy involves the need for close friendships; relationships with family, friends, and formal caregivers; spiritual connections; and knowing that one matters in another person's life (Steinke, 2005).

Youngkin (2004) pointed out that older people may be concerned about changes in sexual intimacy, but "social relationships with people important in their lives, the ability to interact intellectually with people who share similar interests, the supportive love that grows between human beings (whether romantic or platonic), and physical nonsexual intimacy are equally—and in many instances more—important than physical intimacy of direct sexual relations. All of these facets of intimate life are integrally woven into the fabric of aging, along with other influences that can make life rewarding" (Youngkin, 2004, p. 46). Intimacy needs with others change over time, but intimacy and satisfying social relationships are important components of successful aging.

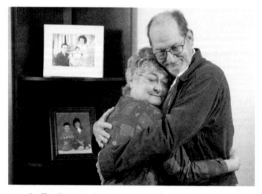

Love and affection are important to older persons. From Sorrentino, S. A., & Gorek, B. (2007). *Mosby's textbook for long-term care assistants* (5th ed.). St. Louis: Mosby.

SEXUALITY

Sexuality is a central aspect of being human throughout life and encompasses sex, gender identities and roles, sexual orientation, eroticism, pleasure, intimacy, and reproduction (World Health Organization, 2004). As a major aspect of intimacy, sexuality includes the physical act of intercourse, as well as many other intimate activities. Sexuality provides the opportunity to express passion, affection, admiration, and loyalty; it can also enhance personal growth and communication. Sexuality also allows a general affirmation of life and a continuing opportunity to search for new growth and experience.

Sexuality, like food and water, is a basic human need, yet it goes beyond the biological realm and has psychological, social, and moral dimensions (Fig. 23.1). The constant interactions among these spheres of sexuality produce harmony. The linkage of the four dimensions makes up the holistic quality of an individual's sexuality.

The social sphere of sexuality is the sum of cultural factors that influence the individual's thoughts and actions with respect to interpersonal relationships and the individual's ideas and learned behaviour related to sexuality. Television, radio, literature, and the more traditional sources of family, school, and religious teachings combine to influence social sexuality. A person's belief of what constitutes masculine and feminine is deeply rooted in cultural factors.

The psychological domain of sexuality reflects a person's attitudes, feelings toward self and others, and learning from experiences. From birth, people are bombarded with cues and signals of how a person should act and think about the use of "dirty words" or body parts. Conversation is self-censored in the presence of or in discussion with certain people. The moral aspect of sexuality (the "I should" or "I shouldn't") is based in religious beliefs or in a pragmatic or humanistic outlook.

The final dimension, biological sexuality, is reflected in physiological responses to sexual stimulation, reproduction, puberty, and growth and development.

Because of their interrelatedness, these dimensions affect each other directly or indirectly whenever an aspect of sexuality is out of harmony. Sexuality is a vital aspect to consider in the care of the older person,

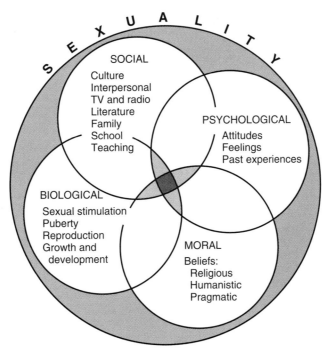

FIGURE 23.1 Interrelationship of dimensions of sexuality. *Source:* Ebersole, P., Touhy, T., Hess, P., et al. (2008). *Toward healthy aging: Human needs and nursing response* (7th ed.) (p. 464, Fig. 19-2). St. Louis, MO: Mosby.

regardless of the setting. Sexuality exists throughout life in one form or another in everyone. All older people have a need to express sexual feelings, whether the individuals are healthy and active or frail. Sexuality in the older person shifts from a focus on procreation to a focus on companionship, physical nearness, intimate communication, and a pleasure-seeking physical relationship. Some researchers have coined the phrase, "from procreation to recreation," to refer to this change in sexual emphasis.

Sexual Health

The World Health Organization defines sexual health as a state of physical, emotional, mental, and social well-being related to sexuality (World Health Organization, 2004). This definition illustrates the multifaceted nature of the biological, psychosocial, cultural, and spiritual components of sexuality and implies that sexual behaviour has the capacity to enhance the self and others. Sexual health is individually defined and wholesome if it leads to intimacy (not necessarily coitus) and enriches the involved parties.

Factors Influencing Sexual Health

Expectations. A large number of cultural, biological, psychosocial, and environmental factors influence older persons' sexual expression and sexual behaviour. Factors affecting a person's attitudes toward intimacy and sexuality include family dynamics and upbringing and cultural and religious beliefs. Older people often internalize the broad cultural proscriptions of sexual behaviour in late life that hinder the continuance of sexual expression. Much sexual behaviour stems from the incorporation of other people's reactions. Older people may be influenced to feel asexual when faced with others around them who consider them to be old and asexual.

Normal sexual interest and activity in the older population are sometimes regarded as deviant behaviour. The same activity engaged in by a younger person would be viewed as appropriate. The following often-quoted statement by Alex Comfort (1974) sums it up nicely: "In our experiences, old folks stop having sex for the same reasons they stop riding a bicycle—general infirmity, thinking it looks ridiculous, no

BOX 23.10   Sexuality and Aging: Common Myths

- Masturbation is an immature activity of youngsters and adolescents, not older people.
- Sexual prowess and desire wane during the climacteric, and menopause is the death of a woman's sexuality.
- Hysterectomy creates a physical disability that results in the inability to function sexually.
- Sex has no role in the lives of older people, except as perversion or remembrance of times past.
- Sexual expression in old age is taboo.
- Older persons are too old and frail to engage in sex.
- The young are considered lusty and virile; older people are considered lecherous.
- Sex is unimportant or over when a person is older.
- Older people do not wish to discuss their sexuality with health care providers.

bicycle." Box 23.10 presents some of the myths about sexuality in older people that may be held by older people themselves and by society in general.

Activity Levels. While sexual desire may change as people age, older men and women remain sexually active and interested and find their sexual lives satisfying. The results of a large national probability survey of sexual attitudes, behaviours, and problems among 57- to 85-year-old community residents in the United States revealed that about 75% were married or living with a partner and that three-quarters of those persons were sexually active. Sexual activity was defined as "any mutually voluntary activity with another person that involves sexual contact, whether or not intercourse or orgasm occurs" (Lindau & Gavrilova, 2010, p. 2). The prevalence of sexual activity declined with age; 73% of people between 57 and 64 years of age, 53% of those between 65 and 74 years of age, and 26% of those between 75 and 85 years of age reported being sexually active. A large Quebec survey indicated that genital sex becomes less frequent and important in older age in favour of other intimate activities and demonstrations of sexuality, such as caressing and hugging (Trudel et al., 2014). About two-thirds of men and half of women over the age of 50 years reported having masturbated during the previous year (Schwartz et al., 2014).

Sexual activity and satisfaction with sexual activity are associated with physical and mental health, the quality of the relationship, the availability of a partner, past history of sexual activity, attitudes towards sex and marriage, and self-esteem (Lindau & Gavrilova, 2010; Schwartz et al., 2014; Trudel et al., 2014). Sexual activity and sexual satisfaction differ between genders, partly due to the lesser availability of sexual partners for older women, who are less likely to be in a relationship, owing to their longer lifespan. Older women are less likely than men to report decreased sexual pleasure or satisfaction and are more likely to have consistent sexual preferences. Over time, women consistently prefer kissing, loving, and caring to other sexual activities, whereas men's preferences for these other activities increase as they age (Schwartz et al., 2014).

Cohort and Cultural Influences. The era in which a person was born influences his or her attitudes about sexuality. Women in their eighties today may have been influenced by the conservative atmosphere of their youth, when sexuality was not openly discussed. The next generation of older people (the "baby boomers") experienced the women's movement, increasing numbers of gay and lesbian couples, more divorced adults, more-liberal attitudes toward sexuality, and the human immunodeficiency virus (HIV) epidemic, all of which affect their views and attitudes as they age. The boomers and people of future generations, as they find themselves experiencing sexuality, may alter society's perceptions of aging and sexuality.

Most of what is known about sexuality in aging has been gained through research with well-educated, healthy, White older persons. More research on culturally, socially, and ethnically diverse older people; those with persistent illness; and LGBTQ persons needs to be done. It is important to know and understand older persons within their social and cultural backgrounds and not to make judgements based on one's own belief system.

Lesbian, Gay, Bisexual, Transgender, and Queer Older Persons. Older LGBTQ people are as diverse as the heterosexual older population. Most age successfully, are healthy and active, and have satisfying lives. Some live as couples, have children, and are open about their sexual orientation. Some of these individuals have only recently "come out"; others have been "out" most of their lives; and some find themselves isolated in the larger society. Older gay persons and lesbians are more likely to have kept their relationships hidden than are those who grew up in the modern-day gay liberation movement (Daley et al., 2017). For older lesbian and gay couples, as for heterosexual couples, relationship satisfaction is linked to sexual activity and satisfaction (Schwartz et al., 2014). Little research has been conducted on sexual activity and sexual satisfaction among older LGBTQ persons, and more research is needed in this area.

Older LGBTQ persons are much less likely than their heterosexual peers to access needed health and social services or to identify themselves as gay, lesbian, bisexual, transgendered, or queer to health care providers (LGBT Movement Advancement Project [MAP] & Services and Advocacy for Gay, Lesbian, Bisexual and Transgender Elders [SAGE], 2010). Health care providers may assume that their LGBTQ patients are heterosexual and neglect to obtain a sexual history, discuss sexuality, or be aware of their particular health needs.

Health care providers receive little education and training in the needs of this population and may lack sensitivity when caring for older LGBTQ individuals. Sensitivity is of utmost importance when obtaining a health history. Asking open-ended questions such as "Who is most important to you?" or "Do you have a significant other?" is much better than asking "Are you married?" This form of questioning allows the nurse to be open to diverse responses. Euphemisms (e.g., roommate or close friend) are frequently used to describe a life partner. Asking individuals if they consider themselves primarily heterosexual, bisexual, or gay (or lesbian) persons conveys the questioner's recognition and acceptance of sexual variety. An older lesbian woman in a health care situation may refer to herself indirectly by saying "people like us." Nurses must be aware of these nuances and try to understand the fear of discovery that is felt by older LGBTQ individuals, who may still be "closeted" because of the homophobic experiences they had in their younger years.

Better support and care services for LGBTQ persons by care providers should include the care providers working through any personal homophobic attitudes and discomfort when discussing sexuality, learning about special issues facing older gay men and lesbians, and becoming aware of resources for them in the community. Programs to increase awareness of the needs of LGBTQ older persons and to reduce discrimination are necessary.

Biological Changes With Age. Acknowledgement and understanding of age-related changes that influence coitus may partially explain alterations in sexual behaviour that accommodate these changes and facilitate the continuation of pleasurable sex (see Chapter 6). Characteristic physiological changes during the sexual response cycle do occur with aging, but these changes vary from person to person, depending on general health factors. The more sexually active a person is, the fewer changes he or she is likely to experience in their patterns of sexual response. Illness and medication also affect sexual response. Changes in the appearance of the body (e.g., wrinkles and sagging skin) may affect the older persons' security about their sexual attractiveness, especially in North American culture, which equates youth and beauty (Schwartz et al., 2014).

Older people who do not understand the physical changes that affect sexual activity become concerned that their sex life is approaching its natural conclusion. Some women make this assumption with the onset of menopause. Men may assume so when they discover a reduced firmness of their erection, less need for ejaculation with each orgasm, or a lengthier refractory period between episodes of intercourse. A major nursing role is to provide information about these changes, as well as appropriate assessment and counselling in the context of the individual's needs.

Sexual Dysfunction

"Sexual dysfunction" is defined as the impairment of normal sexual functioning and can have both physical and psychological causes. Sexual disorders have not been well studied among older people, but the following four categories are generally described: hypoactive sexual desire disorder, sexual arousal disorder, orgasmic disorder, and sexual pain disorders (Steinke, 2016).

Male Sexual Dysfunction. Erectile dysfunction is the inability to achieve and sustain an erection sufficient for satisfactory sexual intercourse in at least 50% of attempts. It is the most prevalent sexual problem in men. Erectile dysfunction (ED) occurs transiently to men of all ages at some point in their life. However, the prevalence of ED increases with age and is reported by 31% of men aged 57 to 65 years and by about 44% of those over 65 years of age (Waite et al., 2009).

For most older men, ED is caused by an underlying medical condition. The interaction among the hormonal, vascular, and nervous systems governs an erection; a problem in any of these systems can cause ED. In nearly one-third of cases, ED is a complication of diabetes. Alcoholism, depression, medications, and prostate disease and treatment are also causes of ED in older men. Various medications that affect the sympathetic and parasympathetic nervous systems interfere with the capacity to have an erection or to ejaculate. Erectile dysfunction is associated with the prescription of vasodilators, selective serotonin reuptake inhibitor (SSRI) antidepressants, and cardiac, antihypertensive, and antihyperglycemic medications (Buttaro et al., 2014; Lochlainn & Kenny, 2013).

Because of health care providers' discomfort with discussing sexuality or because of a lack of knowledge about the sexuality of older people, medications are often prescribed to older persons without consideration of sexual side effects. If medications that affect sexual function are necessary, adjustments of doses, the use of alternative drugs, and the prescription of antidotes to reverse sexual side effects are important.

The use of phosphodiesterase type 5 inhibitors such as sildenafil (Viagra), vardenafil (Levitra), and tadalafil (Cialis) has revolutionized the treatment of ED regardless of cause. Contraindications to the use of these medications include nitrate therapy, heart failure with low blood pressure, certain antihypertensive regimens, and other medications and cardiovascular conditions. (See Chapter 14 for a discussion of contraindications and side effects.) Penile implants of the semi-rigid, adjustable-malleable, or hinged and inflatable types are available when impotence does not respond to other treatments or is irreversible.

Female Dysfunction. Female dysfunction is considered a "persistent impediment to a women's normal pattern of sexual interest, response, or both" (Kaiser, 2003, p. 1174). Female sexual function can be influenced by culture, ethnicity, emotional state, age, and previous sexual experiences, as well as by changes in sexual response with normal aging. For women, the

frequency of intercourse depends more on the age, health, and sexual function of the partner or on the availability of a partner than it depends on their own sexual capacity.

Pain resulting from vaginal atrophy and dryness can result in painful intercourse (dyspareunia) and the avoidance of sexual activity. The use of water-soluble lubricants such as K-Y Jelly, Astroglide, and HR lubricating jellies can help with vaginal dryness. Topical low-dose estrogen creams, rings, or pills that are introduced into the vagina may also help to plump tissues and restore lubrication, with less absorption than with oral hormones (Buttaro et al., 2014).

Women can experience arousal disorders that result from the use of medications such as anticholinergics, antidepressants, and chemotherapeutic agents and from a lack of lubrication, resulting from radiation, surgery, or stress. Orgasmic disorders also may result from medications used to treat depression. Prolapse of the uterus, rectoceles, and cystoceles can be surgically repaired to facilitate continued sexual activity. Urinary incontinence (UI) is another condition that may affect sexual activity for both men and women. Appropriate assessment and treatment are important because many causes of UI are treatable (see Chapter 9).

INTIMACY AND PERSISTENT ILLNESS

Persistent chronic illnesses and their related treatments may bring many challenges to intimacy and sexual activity. Some research has been done on the effects of myocardial infarction on sexual function. Less information is available for people who have heart failure, implantable cardioverter-defibrillators, hypertension, arthritis, persistent pain, or chronic obstructive pulmonary disease (Steinke, 2005).

Often, older people and their partners are given little or no information about the effect of illnesses on sexual activity or about strategies for continuing sexual activity within functional limitations. The timing of intercourse (e.g., mornings or when energy level is highest); oral or anal sex; masturbation; appropriate pain relief; different sexual positions; and the use of sex toys may all help persons continue sexual activity. If pain due to arthritis is a concern, taking pain medications or a warm bath prior to lovemaking may be helpful. Alternate sexual positions such as the side-by-side, back-to-belly (spoon), and crosswise (i.e., one partner supine and the other on his or her side) positions require less flexion of the hip and knee and may reduce the body weight pressure associated with the "missionary" position (Kennedy et al., 2010). Table 23.4 presents other suggestions for individuals with chronic illness.

INTIMACY AND SEXUALITY IN LONG-TERM CARE HOMES

Surveys indicate that a significant number of older people residing in LTC settings might choose to express themselves sexually and, if they had privacy and an available partner, would be sexually active (Mahieu & Gastmans, 2015). Intimacy and sexuality among residents encompasses not only coitus but also other forms of intimate expressions, such as hugging, kissing, handholding, and masturbation. Wallace (2003) commented that the sexual needs of older persons in LTC homes should have the same priority as nutrition, hydration, and other well-accepted needs. A person who lives in an LTC home or assisted-living facility has the same right to engage in or abstain from sexual activity as a person living in the community has.

Depending on the province or territory, LTC homes may be required by law to allow residents to share a room with their spouse or same-sex partner. Residents also have the right to meet privately with their spouse or partner. Participants of studies on older gays and lesbians and their families reported being terrified of going into care homes and having to hide their relationships or losing their partners and friends. One lesbian couple who had been living together for several decades were separated by health care providers and family members who were not aware of

TABLE 23.4	Chronic Illness and Sexual Function: Effects and Interventions	
ILLNESS	**EFFECTS AND PROBLEMS**	**INTERVENTIONS**
Arthritis	Pain, fatigue, limited motion. Steroid therapy may decrease sexual interest or desire.	Advise the person to perform sexual activity at a time of day when they are less fatigued and most relaxed. Suggest use of analgesics and other pain-relief methods before sexual activity. Encourage use of relaxation techniques before sexual activity, such as a warm bath or shower or the application of hot packs to affected joints. Advise the person to maintain optimum health through a balance of good nutrition, proper rest, and activity. Suggest the person experiment with different positions or use pillows for comfort and support. Recommend use of a vibrator if massage ability is limited. Suggest use of water-soluble jelly for vaginal lubrication.
Cancers Breast cancer	No direct physical effect. Psychological effects: • Loss of sexual desire • Body-image change • Depression • Reaction of partner	Encourage individual or group counselling.

Continued

TABLE 23.4   Chronic Illness and Sexual Function: Effects and Interventions—cont'd

ILLNESS	EFFECTS AND PROBLEMS	INTERVENTIONS
Most other cancers	Temporary loss of sexual desire. In men, potential erectile dysfunction; dry ejaculation; retrograde ejaculation. In women, potential vaginal dryness or dyspareunia. Anxiety, depression, pain, or nausea from chemotherapy, radiation, pelvic surgery, or hormone therapy, or nerve damage from pelvic surgery.	
Cardiovascular disease	Most men have no change in physical effects on sexual function. One-fourth may not return to pre–heart attack function; one-fourth may not resume sexual activity. Women do not experience sexual dysfunction after a heart attack. Fear of another heart attack (or death) during sex. Shortness of breath.	Encourage counselling about realistic restrictions that may be necessary. Teach the person alternative positions that avoid strain. Suggest the person avoid large meals for several hours before sex. Advise the person to relax. Plan medications for effectiveness during sex.
Cerebrovascular accident (stroke)	Depression. May or may not have sexual activity changes. Often, erectile disorders; decrease in frequency of intercourse and sexual relations. Change in role and function of partners. Fatigue, decreased physical endurance. Mobility and sensory deficits. Perceptual and visual deficits. Communication deficit. Cognitive and behavioural deficits. Fear of relapse or sudden death.	Encourage counselling. Instruct the person to use alternative positions. Suggest use of a vibrator if massage ability is limited. Suggest use of pillows for positioning and support. Suggest use of water-soluble jelly for lubrication. Instruct the person to use alternative forms of sexual expression.
Chronic obstructive pulmonary disease	No direct impairment of sexual activity, although coughing, exertional dyspnea, positions, and activity intolerance can have an effect. Medications may lead to erectile difficulties.	Encourage the person to plan sexual activity when energy is highest. Instruct the person to use alternative positions. Advise the person to plan sexual activity at a time when medications are most effective. Suggest the person use oxygen before, during, or after sex, depending on when it provides the most benefit.
Diabetes	Sexual desire and interest unaffected. Erectile function interference from neuropathy, vascular damage, or both. (About 50 to 75% of men have erectile disorders; a small portion have retrograde ejaculation. Some men regain function if diagnosis of diabetes is well accepted, if diabetes is well controlled, or both. Women have less sexual desire and vaginal lubrication.) Potential decrease in orgasms, or absence of orgasm. Less-frequent sexual activity. Local genital infections.	Recommend possible candidates for penile prosthesis. Instruct the person to use alternative forms of sexual expression. Recommend immediate treatment of genital infections.

the nature of their partnership. Another partner in a lesbian relationship changed her last name to her partner's so that they would be taken for sisters and put in the same room (Brotman et al., 2003).

Lack of privacy is a major issue in LTC homes and assisted living facilities and can prevent the fulfillment of intimacy and sexual needs. Suggested actions for providing privacy and an atmosphere accepting of sexual activity include making available a private room, not interrupting when doors are closed and sexual activity is taking place, allowing residents to have sexually explicit materials in their rooms, and providing adaptive equipment such as side rails and double beds.

Attitudes about intimacy and sexuality among LTC home staff and, often, family members may reflect general societal attitudes that older people do not have sexual needs or that their engaging in sexual activity is inappropriate. Family members may have difficulty understanding that their older relative may want to have a new relationship. Health care providers often view residents' sexual acts as problems rather than expressions of the need for love and intimacy. Reactions may include disapproval, discomfort, and embarrassment, and health care providers may explicitly or implicitly discourage or deny intimacy needs.

Staff, family, and resident programs to promote awareness, provide education on sexuality and intimacy in late life, involve residents in discussions of sexuality, and discuss interventions that respond to residents' needs are important in LTC settings. Staff education should include the opportunity to discuss personal feelings about sexuality, normal changes of aging, and the impact of diseases and medications on sexual function, as well as skill training in sexual assessment and intervention through simulation or role play.

INTIMACY, SEXUALITY, AND DEMENTIA

Intimacy and sexuality remain important in the lives of persons with dementia and their partners throughout the illness. Intimacy and sexuality may "serve as a nonverbal form of communication and intimacy when other cognitive skills and functions have declined" (Agronin, 2004, p. 13). As dementia progresses, particularly in persons living in LTC homes, intimacy and sexuality issues may present challenges, especially in regard to the impaired person's ability to consent to sexual activity, which requires accurate assessment and documentation. Issues of intimacy and sexuality of persons with dementia in LTC homes are complex. Practice standards and applicable laws must guide nursing practice (Christie et al., n.d.; Wahl, 2009a).

Determination of a cognitively impaired person's ability to consent to participation in a sexual activity involves consideration of (1) the person's mental **capacity,** (2) the risks and benefits of such activity for the person, and (3) what constitutes voluntary participation. Assessing the person's capacity to consent to sexual activity involves assessing the resident's awareness of the relationship, ability to avoid exploitation, and awareness of potential risks (Lichtenberg, 2014). If the person does not have the capacity to consent to sexual activity, the LTC home has a duty to protect that person from abuse and harm (Wahl, 2009b). An interprofessional working group in Hamilton, Ontario, has created a toolkit for developing policies about intimacy, sexuality, and sexual behaviour in dementia in LTC homes (http://www.rgpc.ca/resources/).

Persons with dementia in LTC homes may also express sexuality, including by holding hands, cuddling, having sexual intercourse, and using sexual language, as well as by engaging in behaviour that may be labelled inappropriate (e.g., exposing themselves, masturbating in public, or making inappropriate sexual advances or comments). These behaviours can be distressing to staff, residents, and families. The extent to which sexual expression and sexual behaviour of residents who have dementia are accepted varies between settings (Makimoto et al., 2015). When sexually inappropriate behaviour occurs, it should be assessed (as is any other behaviour) for cause, precipitating factors, and response to interventions. Encouraging family and friends to touch, hug, kiss, and hold hands when visiting may help to meet touch and intimacy needs and reduce inappropriate sexual behaviour. Also, allowing the person with dementia to stroke a pet or hold a stuffed animal may be helpful. Providing an environment that allows for the expression of sexuality in private may also be a solution (Steinke, 2016). It is important to provide staff with opportunities for discussion, assistance with interventions, and education about written policies on sexuality and capacity assessment (Lichtenberg, 2014).

SEXUALLY TRANSMITTED INFECTIONS

The prevalence of sexually transmitted infections (STIs) such as chlamydia, gonorrhea, syphilis, HIV infection, and genital herpes is increasing in Canada. Although younger Canadians have the highest incidence of STIs, older Canadians are also at risk. Among Canadians aged 60 years and older, the rates for chlamydia are 6.3 and 3.2 per 100,000 for men and women, respectively; for gonorrhea, 3.7 and 0.7 per 100,000 for men and women, respectively; and for syphilis, 2.8 and 0.1 per 100,000 for men and women, respectively (Public Health Agency of Canada [PHAC], 2015). Among older persons, widows and widowers who date and have new sexual partners are at highest risk (Canadian Public Health Association, 2015/2016).

In the context of reporting HIV infection statistics, the Public Health Agency of Canada (PHAC), as do international reporting bodies, considers an older person to be a person older than 50 years. In 2014, persons aged 50 years and older accounted for 21.3% of acquired immunodeficiency syndrome (AIDS) cases in Canada, an increase from 12.2% in 2006 (Government of Canada, 2015; PHAC, 2007). This increase is caused by the following two factors: (1) people diagnosed at a younger age are now more likely to survive into older age because of the availability of antiretroviral therapy and other treatments, and (2) there has been an increase in the incidence of new cases of HIV infection among older persons. In 2014, persons over the age of 50 years accounted for 21.9% of annual positive HIV test reports, compared to 13.8% in 2006 (Government of Canada, 2015; PHAC, 2007). As these trends continue, the prevalence of HIV infection and AIDS in older people will continue to increase. There are more positive HIV test results among those aged 50 years and older than there are among persons in the 20- to 29-year-old age group (Government of Canada, 2015).

The compromised immune system of older persons, associated with normal age-related changes, makes them more susceptible than younger adults to HIV or AIDS. AIDS is not exclusively a young person's disease, but it is frequently underreported in the older population because the symptoms of fatigue, weakness, weight loss, and anorexia are common to other disease conditions or may be falsely attributed to "normal aging." Older persons are often diagnosed in the later stages of HIV infection, often with AIDS illnesses (PHAC, 2013). Lack of knowledge about HIV and AIDS and a belief that it "just does not happen in my generation" contribute to underreporting and late diagnosis. In addition, the idea that older people are not sexually active limits health care providers' objectivity and thus their ability to recognize HIV infection and AIDS as possible diagnoses.

Older persons who are sexually active are at risk for HIV infection and AIDS and other sexually transmitted diseases. Heterosexual contact and sex between men are the most common modes of transmission among older Canadians (35% of cases each), followed by injection drug use (Canadian AIDS Society, 2013). Older women who are sexually active are at high risk for HIV infection and for AIDS and other STIs from an infected partner, resulting in part from the normal age-related changes of the vaginal tissue (such as a thinner, drier, and more friable vaginal lining). They are also less likely than younger women to use condoms.

Testing for HIV is less common among older persons. However, assessment and screening for other STIs should be part of primary care for sexually active older persons. If symptoms of another STI arise, HIV testing should be done as well. The Public Health Agency of Canada (2014) recommends that HIV testing be part of routine care, regardless of a person's age.

Nurses and other health care providers must become comfortable with taking a complete sexual history, talking about sex and STIs with older patients, and providing education about condom use and safer sex practices. (Websites with specific information about HIV, AIDS, and older people for prevention and education are listed in the Resources section at the end of this chapter.)

IMPLICATIONS FOR GERONTOLOGICAL NURSING AND HEALTHY AGING

Nurses have many roles in the area of sexuality and older people. The nurse is a facilitator of a milieu that is conducive to the older person asking questions and expressing sexuality. The nurse has the responsibility to help maintain the sexuality of older people by offering an opportunity for discussion. Some older people remain or want to remain sexually active, whereas others do not see this as an important part of their lives. Nurses should open the door to discussions of sexual concerns in a nonjudgemental manner, helping those who want to continue to be sexually active and making it clear to others that stopping sex is an acceptable option (Lindau et al., 2007). The nurse should be an educator and provide information and guidance to older people who need it.

ASSESSMENT

To assist and support older persons' sexual needs, nurses should be aware of their own feelings about sexuality and their attitudes toward intimacy and sexuality in older people, whether those persons are single, married, or LGBTQ. Only after nurses confront their own attitudes, values, and beliefs can they provide support without being judgemental. Sex histories are rarely elicited from older persons, and physical examinations often do not include the reproductive system unless it is directly involved in a current illness. However, when questions about sexual issues are asked or when an older person is assessed, the nurse needs to be particularly cognizant of the era the person has lived through and the person's culture in order to understand the factors affecting the person's conduct.

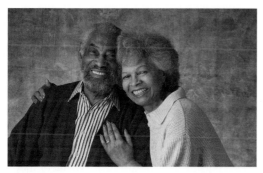

Sexuality is an important need in late life; it affects pleasure, adaptation, and a person's general feeling of well-being. Copyright Getty Images.

Older persons should be asked about their sexual satisfaction because they may not mention it voluntarily. Anticipating problems in older individuals'

sexual experiences can ward off anxiety, misconceptions, and an arbitrary cessation of pleasurable sexual activity. The normalcy of sexual activity may need validation. Also needed may be a discussion of the physiological changes that occur with age or of the effects of illness and treatment that may interfere with sexual activity by altering its routine or interfering with physical performance. Counselling may also be needed for the older person to adapt to natural physiological changes and image-altering surgical procedures. Assessment of any medical conditions or medications that are associated with poor sexual health and functioning, screening for HIV infection and for AIDS and other STIs, and education about safer sex are also important.

Discussion of sexuality and sexuality problems may be uncomfortable for the nurse or the older person. Nonetheless, it is important that the nurse learn the significance that sexual function has for the older person and the person's perception of sexual function, without bringing the nurse's own biases into the interaction.

The PLISSIT model (Annon, 1976) is a helpful guide for the discussion of sexuality (Box 23.11). Also, *Nursing Standard of Practice Protocol: Sexuality in Older Adults* (Wallace, 2012) is available at https://consultgeri.org/geriatric-topics/sexuality-issues-aging.

Youngkin (2004) provides the following suggestions for using the PLISSIT model with older people:

- **Permission.** Obtain permission from the person to initiate sexual discussion. Allow the person to

---

BOX 23.11 The PLISSIT Model

P	Having **P**ermission from the person to initiate sexual discussion.
LI	Providing the **L**imited **I**nformation needed to function sexually.
SS	Giving **S**pecific **S**uggestions to the individual for proceeding with sexual relations.
IT	Providing **I**ntensive **T**herapy around the issues of sexuality for the person. (This may mean referral to specialist.)

Sources: Adapted from Annon, J. (1976). The PLISSIT model: A proposed conceptual theme for behavioral treatment of sexual problems. *Journal of Sexual Education & Therapy, 2*(2), 1–15; Kazer, M. W. (2007). *Sexuality assessment for older adults.* Try This Series (Issue 10). Retrieved from https://consultgeri.org/try-this/general-assessment/issue-10.

discuss concerns related to sexual issues, and gather information about what might have changed in the person's life to affect sexual needs and response. Ask questions such as "What concerns or questions do you have about fulfilling your sexual needs?" or "In this era of HIV and other sexually transmitted infections, I ask all my patients about sexual practices and concerns. Are there any questions I can answer for you?"

- **Limited Information.** Limit the information provided to that needed for sexual function. Offer teaching about the normal age-associated changes that affect sexual performance or how illness may affect sexuality. Encourage the person to learn more about their concerns from books and other sources.
- **Specific Suggestions.** Offer suggestions for dealing with the following: lubricants for atrophic vaginitis; the use of condoms to prevent STIs; the proper use of medications for erectile dysfunction; how to communicate sexual and other needs; and ways to increase the comfortability of coitus or ways to be intimate without coital relations.
- **Intensive Therapy.** Refer as appropriate for complex problems that call for specialist intervention.

The *Seniors A GOGO (Growing Older, Getting it On)* project in Calgary is an example of an innovative enactment of intersectoral collaboration, public participation, and the promotion of sexual health for older persons. The Calgary Sexual Health Centre, the Seniors Action Group, and the Foundation Lab (an art, research, and human development organization) collaborated to explore sexuality issues among older persons and used theatre to discuss sexuality and ageism (Arts Health Network Canada, n.d.). Three short video documentaries are available on YouTube (http://www.youtube.com/watch?v=L6e0BXxhGHI).

INTERVENTIONS

Interventions will vary depending on the needs identified by the assessment. Following a comprehensive assessment, interventions may centre on the following categories: (1) education regarding age-associated change in sexual function, (2) ways of compensating for normal aging changes, (3) effective management of acute and chronic illness affecting sexual function, (4) removal of barriers associated with difficulty in fulfilling sexual needs, and (5) special interventions to promote sexual health in cognitively impaired older persons (Steinke, 2016).

Education about the prevention of HIV infection and STIs is also important for sexually active older persons.

KEY CONCEPTS

- The ability to successfully negotiate transitions and develop new and gratifying roles depends on personal and environmental supports, timing, clarity of expectations, personality, and the degree of change required.
- Older people and their family members carry a long history. Current family dynamics must be understood within the context of family history.
- Sibling relationships may increase in importance during old age as individuals cope with various losses.
- Grandparenting is a significant role among older persons. In an increasing number of families, grandparents are the primary providers for young children and function as parents.
- Caregiving is one of the major social issues of our times. Most spouses will spend some time caring for one another, and most adult children will spend some time caring for aged parents.
- Sexuality comprises love, sharing, trust, and warmth, as well as physical acts. Sexuality provides a person with self-identity and affirms life.
- Sexuality continues in late life, although older persons need to adapt to age-related changes and the effects of chronic illness.
- Further research is needed to promote knowledge and understanding of the sexual health of older persons who live alternative lifestyles, such as LGBTQ persons.
- Awareness of HIV and AIDS and the practice of safer sex among older persons are still lacking. Older persons and health care providers may not consider the risk for HIV infection and AIDS, even though the incidence of both in the older population is increasing.
- To optimize the sexuality of older persons in the community or in an LTC setting, the nurse provides education and counselling about sexual function,

adaptations for age-related changes and chronic conditions, the prevention of HIV infection and AIDS and other STIs in sexually active older persons, and the maintenance of intimacy and sexuality for the older person who desires them.

ACTIVITIES AND DISCUSSION QUESTIONS

1. Discuss your position in the family and how that has affected your relationship with siblings and parents.
2. What do you suppose your role will be when your parent or parents need help?
3. What would you find most difficult in regard to assisting your older parent?
4. With a classmate, role-play how you would conduct a review of systems in the area of sexual health with an older person. What would be the most important factors to consider when teaching about sexuality and sexual health?
5. What resources are available for older LGBTQ persons in your community?

RESOURCES

BC Centre for Disease Control. Sexually transmitted infections
http://www.bccdc.ca/health-info/disease-types/sexually-transmitted-infections

CANGRANDS National Kinship Support
http://www.cangrands.com/

Hartford Institute for Geriatric Nursing. Sexuality assessment for older adults (streaming video)
https://consultgeri.org/try-this/general-assessment/issue-10

Health Canada. Seniors and aging—Sexual activity
http://publications.gc.ca/collections/collection_2007/hc-sc/H13-7-15-2006E.pdf

Helpguide.org. Grandparents raising grandchildren
https://www.helpguide.org/articles/grandparenting/grandparents-as-parents.htm

National Initiative for the Care of the Elderly (NICE). Financial resources for Ontario grandparents raising their grandchildren

http://www.nicenet.ca/tools-financial-resources-for-ontario-grandparents-raising-their-grandchildren

Parent Support Services Society of BC. Resources for grandparents raising grandchildren
http://www.parentsupportbc.ca/for-grandparents/

Rainbow Health Ontario
http://www.rainbowhealthontario.ca/

Realize. HIV and aging fact sheets
http://www.realizecanada.org/en/doc-category/hiv-and-aging/

Senior Pride Network
http://www.seniorpridenetwork.com/home.htm

Seniors A GOGO (Growing Older, Getting it On) theatre project with the Calgary Sexual Health Centre
https://www.calgarysexualhealth.ca/programs-workshops/older-adults-seniors/

Services & Advocacy for LGBT Elders (SAGE). Resources for LGBT older people and those interested in LGBT aging issues
http://www.sageusa.org/index.cfm

For additional resources, please visit *http://evolve.elsevier.com/Canada/Ebersole/gerontological/*

REFERENCES

Agronin, M. (2004). Sexuality and aging: An introduction. *CNS Long-Term Care, Summer,* 12–13.

Allen, K. R. (2016). Fictive kin. *The Encyclopedia of Adulthood and Aging,* 1–4. doi:10.1002/9781118528921.wbeaa292\.

Alzheimer's Association. (2017). *Caregiver resources.* Retrieved from http://www.alz.org/cacentral/in_my_community_21690.asp.

Annon, J. (1976). The PLISSIT model: A proposed conceptual theme for behavioral treatment of sexual problems. *Journal of Sexual Education & Therapy, 2*(2), 1–15. doi:10.1016/B978-0-08-020373-7.50019-X.

Archbold, P. G., Stewart, B. J., Greenlick, M. R., et al. (1990). Mutuality and preparedness as predictors of caregiver role strain. *Research in Nursing & Health, 13*(6), 375–384. doi:10.1002/nur.4770130605.

Arts Health Network Canada. (n.d.). *Seniors A GOGO.* Retrieved from https://artshealthnetwork.ca/initiatives/seniors-gogo.

Brotman, S., Ryan, B., & Cormier, R. (2003). The health and social service needs of gay and lesbian elders and their families in Canada. *The Gerontologist, 43*(2), 172–202. doi:10.1093/geront/43.2.192.

Buttaro, T. M., Koeniger-Donohue, R., & Hawkins, J. (2014). Sexuality and quality of life in aging: Implications for practice. *The*

Journal for Nurses Practitioners, 10(7), 480–485. doi:10.1016/j.nurpra.2014.04.008.

Canadian AIDS Society. (2013). *HIV and aging*. Retrieved from http://www.realizecanada.org/en/our-work/hiv-and-aging/.

Canadian Gerontological Nursing Association (CGNA). (2010). *Gerontological nursing competencies and standards of practice.* Retrieved from http://cgna.net/uploads/CGNAStandardsOfPractice_English.pdf.

Canadian Public Health Association. (2015/2016). *Sex and seniors: A perspective.* Retrieved from http://www.cpha.ca/en/about/digest/39-4/15.aspx.

Chappell, N. L., Dujela, C., & Smith, A. (2014). Spouse and adult child differences in caregiver burden. *Canadian Journal on Aging, 33*(4), 462–472. doi:10.1017/S0714980814000336.

Christie, D., Botham, L., Gilbert, S., et al. (n.d.). *Intimacy, sexuality and sexual behaviour in dementia: How to develop practice guidelines and policy for long term care facilities.* Retrieved from http://brainxchange.ca/Public/Files/Sexuality/Intimacy-Sexuality-and-Sexual-Behaviour-in-Dementi.aspx.

Comfort, A. (1974). Sexuality in old age. *Journal of the American Geriatrics Society, 22*(10), 440–442. doi:10.1111/j.1532-5415.1974.tb04811.x.

Daley, A., MacDonnell, J. A., Brotman, S., et al. (2017). Providing health and social services to older LGBT adults. *Annual Review of Gerontology and Geriatrics, 37*(1), 143–160. doi:10.1891/0198-8794.37.143.

Department of Finance, Government of Canada. (2016). *Backgrounder: Canada Pension Plan (CPP) enhancement.* Retrieved from http://www.fin.gc.ca/n16/data/16-113_3-eng.asp.

Eni, R., Harvey, C. D. H., & Phillips-Beck, W. (2009). In consideration of the needs of caregivers: Grandparenting experiences in Manitoba First Nation Communities. *First Peoples Child & Family Review, 4*, 85–98. Retrieved from http://journals.sfu.ca/fpcfr/index.php/FPCFR/index.

Fontaine, P., Craft, A., & The Truth and Reconciliation Commission of Canada (2015). *A knock on the door: The essential history of residential schools from the Truth and Reconciliation Commission of Canada.* Winnipeg, MB: University of Manitoba Press.

Fuller-Thomson, E. (2005). *Grandparents raising grandchildren in Canada: A profile of skipped generation families.* SEDAP Research Paper No. 132. Hamilton, ON: SEDAP Research Program. Retrieved from http://socserv.mcmaster.ca/sedap/p/sedap132.pdf.

Giesbrecht, M., William, A., Duggleby, W., et al. (2016). Exploring the daily geographies of diverse men caregiving for family members with multiple chronic conditions. *Gender, Place and Culture, 23*(11), 1586–1598. doi:10.1080/0966369X.2016.1219329.

Government of Canada. (2015). *Page 8: HIV and AIDS in Canada: Surveillance report to December 31, 2014—Results: At a glance.* Retrieved from https://www.canada.ca/en/public-health/services/publications/diseases-conditions/hiv-aids-canada-surveillance-report-december-31-2014/page-8-results-glance.html#s7a2_2.

Grigorovich, A. (2015). The meaning of quality of care in home care settings: Older lesbian and bisexual women's perspectives.

Scandinavian Journal of Caring Sciences, 30(1), 108–1160. doi:10.1111/scs.12228.

Hadfield, J. C. (2014). The health of grandparents raising grandchildren: A literature review. *Journal of Gerontological Nursing, 40*(4), 32–42. doi:10.3928/00989134-20140219-01.

Hansson, R. O., & Stroebe, M. S. (2007). *Bereavement in late life: Coping, adaptation, and developmental influences.* Washington, DC: American Psychological Association.

Hooyman, N., & Kiyak, H. (2011). *Social gerontology a multidisciplinary perspective* (9th ed.). Boston, MA: Allyn & Bacon.

Hsieh, J. Y., Mercer, K. J., & Costa, S. A. (2017). Parenting a second time around: The strengths and challenges of Indigenous grandparent caregivers. *GrandFamilies: The Contemporary Journal of Research, Practice and Policy, 4*(1), 76–114. Retrieved from http://scholarworks.wmich.edu/grandfamilies/.

Kaiser, F. (2003). Sexual function and the older woman. *Clinics in Geriatric Medicine, 19*(3), 463–472. doi:10.1016/S0749-0690(02)00144-1.

Kennedy, G. J., Martinez, M. M., & Garo, N. (2010). Sex and mental health in old age. *Primary Psychiatry, 17*(1), 22–30. Retrieved from http://primarypsychiatry.com/sex-and-mental-health-in-old-age/.

Koehn, S., Badger, M., Cohen, C., et al. (2016). Negotiating access to diagnosis of dementia: Implications for policies in health and social care. *Dementia (Basel, Switzerland), 15*(6), 1436–1456. doi:10.1177/1471301214563551.

Kralik, D., Visentin, K., & van Loon, A. (2006). Transition: A literature review. *Journal of Advanced Nursing, 55*(3), 320–329. doi:10.1111/j.1365-2648.2006.03899.x/full.

LGBT Movement Advancement Project (MAP) and Services and Advocacy for Gay, Lesbian, Bisexual and Transgender Elders (SAGE). (2010). *Improving the lives of LGBT older adults.* Retrieved from http://www.lgbtmap.org/file/improving-the-lives-of-lgbt-older-adults.pdf.

Lichtenberg, P. A. (2014). Sexuality and physical intimacy in long term care: Sexuality, long term care, capacity assessment. *Occupational Therapy in Health Care, 28*(1), 42–50. doi:10.3109/07380577.2013.865858.

Lindau, S. T., Schumm, L. P., Laumann, E. O., et al. (2007). A study of sexuality and health among older adults in the United States. *The New England Journal of Medicine, 357*, 762–774. doi:10.1056/NEJMoa067423.

Lindau, S. T., & Gavrilova, N. (2010). Sex, health, and years of sexually active life gained due to good health: Evidence from two US population based cross sectional surveys of ageing. *British Medical Journal, 340*, c810. doi:10.1136/bmj.c810.

Liu, L. W., & McDaniel, S. A. (2015). Family caregivers for immigrant seniors living with heart disease and stroke: Chinese Canadian perspective. *Health Care for Women International, 36*(12), 1327–1345. doi:10.1080/07399332.2015.1038346.

Lobb, E. A., Kristjanson, L. J., Aoun, S. M., et al. (2010). Predictors of complicated grief: A systematic review of empirical studies. *Death Studies, 34*(8), 673–698. doi:10.1080/07481187.2010.496686.

Lochlainn, M. N., & Kenny, R. A. (2013). Sexual activity and aging. *The Journal of Post-Acute and Long-Term Care Medicine, 14*(8), 565–572. doi:10.1016/j.jamda.2013.01.022.

Love, A. W. (2007). Progress in understanding grief, complicated grief, and caring for the bereaved. *Contemporary Nurse, 27*(1), 73–83. doi:10.5172/conu.2007.27.1.73.

Lund, M. (2005). Caregiver, take care. *Geriatric Nursing, 26*(3), 152–153. doi:10.1016/j.gerinurse.2005.03.009.

Lunsky, Y., Tint, A., Robinson, S., et al. (2014). System-wide information about family carers of adults with intellectual/developmental disabilities: A systemic review of the literature. *Journal of Policy and Practice in Intellectual Disabilities, 11*(1), 8–18. doi:10.1111/jppi.12068.

Mahieu, L., & Gastmans, C. (2015). Older residents' perspectives on aged sexuality in institutionalized elderly care: A systematic literature review. *International Journal of Nursing Studies, 52*(12), 1891–1905. doi:10.1016/j.ijnurstu.2015.07.007.

Makimoto, K., Kang, H. S., Yamakawa, M., et al. (2015). An integrated literature review on sexuality of elderly nursing home residents with dementia. *International Journal of Nursing Practice, 21*(52), 80–90. doi:10.1111/ijn.12317.

Margolis, R. (2016). The changing demography of grandparenthood. *Journal of Marriage and Family, 78*(3), 610–622. doi:10.1111/jomf.12286.

Margolis, R., & Wright, L. (2016). Older adults with three generations of kin: Prevalence, correlates, and transfers. *The Journals of Gerontology. Series B, Psychological Sciences and Social Sciences, gbv158*, 1–6. doi:10.1093/geronb/gbv158.

McCleary, L., & Blain, J. (2013). Cultural values and family caregiving for persons with dementia. *Indian Journal of Gerontology, 27*(1), 178–201.

McLaren, A. T., & Manery, M. M. (2001). *Factors affecting the economic status of older women in Canada: Implications for mandatory retirement.* Victoria, BC: British Columbia Human Rights Commission. Retrieved from https://books.google.ca/books/about/Factors_Affecting_the_Economic_Status_of.html?id=evqDvgAACAAJ&redir_esc=y.

Meiner, S. E. (2011). *Gerontological nursing* (4th ed.). St. Louis, MO: Mosby.

Meisner, B. A., & Binnington, L. E. (2016). I'm so glad you're here: Positive aspects of informal caregiving. *Journal of the American Geriatrics Society, 65*(1), e25–e26. doi:10.1111/jgs.14655.

Messecar, D. C. (2016). Family caregiving. In M. Boltz, E. Capezuti, T. T. Fulmer, et al. (Eds.), *Evidence-based geriatric nursing protocols for best practice* (5th ed., pp. 137–163). New York, NY: Springer Publishing Company.

Milan, A., Laflamme, N., & Wong, I. (2015). *Diversity of grandparents living with their grandchildren.* Catalogue no. 75-006-X. Ottawa, ON: Statistics Canada. Retrieved from http://www.statcan.gc.ca/pub/75-006-x/2015001/article/14154-eng.htm.

Milan, A., Wong, I., & Vézina, M. (2014). *Emerging trend in living arrangements and conjugal unions for current and future seniors.* Retrieved from http://www.statcan.gc.ca/pub/75-006-x/2014001/article/11904-eng.htm.

Minton, M., & Barron, C. (2008). Spousal bereavement assessment: A review of bereavement specific measures. *Journal of Gerontological Nursing, 34*, 34–48. doi:10.3928/00989134-20080801-08.

Moussaly, K. (2010). *Participation in private retirement savings plans, 1997–2008.* Catalogue no. 13F0026M, no 1. Ottawa, ON: Statistics Canada. Retrieved from http://www.statcan.gc.ca/pub/13f0026m/13f0026m2010001-eng.htm.

Naef, R., Ward, R., Mahrer-Imhof, R., et al. (2013). Characteristics of the bereavement experience of older adults after spousal loss: An integrative review. *International Journal of Nursing Studies, 50*(8), 1108–1121. doi:10.1016/j.ijnurstu.2012.11.026.

National Initiative for the Care of the Elderly (NICE). (n.d.). *Financial resources for Ontario grandparents raising their grandchildren.* Retrieved from http://www.nicenet.ca/tools-financial-resources-for-ontario-grandparents-raising-their-grandchildren.

National Seniors Strategy. (2017). *Ensuring caregivers are not unnecessarily financially penalized for taking on caregiving roles.* Retrieved from http://nationalseniorsstrategy.ca/pillar-4-old/financial-support-caregivers/.

Pinquart, M., & Sörensen, S. (2005). Ethnic differences in stressors, resources, and psychological outcomes of family caregiving: A meta-analysis. *The Gerontologist, 45*(1), 90–106. doi:10.1093/geront/45.1.90.

Public Health Agency of Canada (PHAC). (2007). *HIV/AIDS Epi Updates 2007.* Catalogue no. HP37-7/2007E. Ottawa, ON: Author. Retrieved from http://www.phac-aspc.gc.ca/aids-sida/publication/epi/pdf/epi2007_e.pdf.

Public Health Agency of Canada (PHAC). (2013). *HIV and AIDS in Canada: Surveillance report to December 31st, 2012.* Retrieved from http://www.phac-aspc.gc.ca/aids-sida/publication/survreport/2013/dec/index-eng.php.

Public Health Agency of Canada (PHAC). (2014). *Human immunodeficiency virus—HIV screening and testing guide.* Retrieved from https://www.canada.ca/en/public-health/services/hiv-aids/hiv-screening-testing-guide.html#c1.

Public Health Agency of Canada (PHAC). (2015). *Table equivalents: Report on sexually transmitted infections in Canada: 2012.* Retrieved from http://www.phac-aspc.gc.ca/sti-its-surv-epi/rep-rap-2012/assets/longdesc/longdesc-eng.php#figure-2.

Sayegh, P., & Knight, B. G. (2010). The effects of familism and cultural justification on the mental and physical health of family caregivers. *The Journals of Gerontology. Series B, Psychological Science and Social Sciences, 66B*(1), 3–14. doi:10.1093/geronb/gbq061.

Schulz, R., & Beach, S. R. (1999). Caregiving as a risk factor for mortality: The Caregiver Health Effects Study. *Journal of the American Medical Association, 282*(23), 2215–2219. doi:10.1001/jama.282.23.2215.

Schumacher, K. L., & Meleis, A. I. (1994). Transitions: A central concept in nursing. *IMAGE-The Journal of Nursing Scholarship, 26*(2), 119–127. doi:10.1111/j.1547-5069.1994.tb00929.x/pdf.

Schwartz, P., Diefendorf, S., & McGlynn-Wright, A. (2014). Sexuality in aging. *APA Handbook of Sexuality and Psychology, 1*, 523–551. doi:10.1037/14193-017.

Sealey, M., Breen, L. J., O'Connor, M., et al. (2015). A scoping review of bereavement risk assessment measures:

Implications for palliative care. *Palliative Medicine, 29*(7), 577–589. doi:10.1177/0269216315576262.

Sebern, M. (2005). Shared care, elder and family member skills used to manage burden. *Journal of Advanced Nursing, 52*(2), 170–179. doi:10.1111/j.1365-2648.2005.03580.x.

Sinha, M. (2013). *Portrait of caregivers, 2012.* Catalogue no. 89-652-X. Ottawa, ON: Statistics Canada. Retrieved from http://www.statcan.gc.ca/pub/89-652-x/89-652-x2013001-eng.htm.

Stamatopoulos, V. (2015). One million and counting: The hidden army of young carers in Canada. *Journal of Youth Studies, 18*(6), 809–822. doi:10.1080/13676261.2014.992329.

Statistics Canada. (2015). *Marital Status: Overview 2011.* Proportion of population aged 15 and over that was never married by age group and sex, Canada, 1981 and 2011. Retrieved from http://www.statcan.gc.ca/pub/91-209-x/2013001/article/11788/fig/desc/desc02-eng.htm.

Statistics Canada. (2016). *Table 051-0042: Populations by marital status and sex.* Retrieved from http://www.statcan.gc.ca/tables-tableaux/sum-som/l01/cst01/famil01-eng.htm.

Statistics Canada. (2017a). *Table 111-0039: Registered Retirement Savings Plan (RRSP) contributions, by contributor characteristics.* Retrieved from http://www5.statcan.gc.ca/cansim/a26?lang=eng&id=1110039.

Statistics Canada. (2017b). *Table 111-0039: Pensions: The ups and downs of pension coverage in Canada.* Retrieved from http://www5.statcan.gc.ca/cansim/pick-choisir?lang=eng&p2=33&id=1110039.

Steinke, E. (2005). Intimacy needs and chronic illness. *Journal of Gerontological Nursing, 31*(5), 40–50.

Steinke, E. (2016). Issues regarding sexuality. In M. Boltz, E. Capezuti, T. T. Fulmer, et al. (Eds.), *Evidence-based geriatric nursing protocols for best practice* (5th ed., pp. 165–188). New York, NY: Springer Publishing Company.

Stroebe, M., & Schut, H. (2010). The dual process model of coping with bereavement: A decade on. *Omega, 61*(4), 273–289. doi:10.2190/OM.61.4.b.

Trudel, G., Dargis, L., Villeneuve, L., et al. (2014). Marital, sexual and psychological functioning of older couples living at home: The results of a national survey using longitudinal methodology (Part II). *Sexologies, 23*(2), e35–e48. doi:10.1016/j.sexol.2013.03.007.

Turcotte, M. (2013). *Family caregiving: What are the consequences?* Catalogue no. 75-006-X. Ottawa, ON: Statistics Canada. Retrieved from http://www.statcan.gc.ca/pub/75-006-x/2013001/article/11858-eng.htm.

Vézina, M., & Turcotte, M. (2010). Caring for a parent who lives far away: The consequences. *Canadian Social Trends, 89,* 3–13. Retrieved from http://dsp-psd.pwgsc.gc.ca/collections/collection_2010/statcan/11-008-X/11-008-x2010001-eng.pdf.

Wahl, J. (2009a). *Sexuality in long term care.* Retrieved from http://www.advocacycentreelderly.org/appimages/file/Sexuality%20in%20LTC.pdf.

Wahl, J. (2009b). *Sexuality in long term care—the legal issues.* Retrieved from http://www.advocacycentreelderly.org/appimages/file/Sexuality%20in%20LTC.pdf.

Waite, L. J., Laumann, E. O., Das, A., et al. (2009). Sexuality: Measures of partnerships, practices, attitudes, and problems in the national social life, health and aging study. *The Journal of Gerontology. Series B, Psychological Sciences and Social Sciences, 64B*(Suppl. 1), 56–66. doi:10.1093/geronb/gbp038.

Wallace, M. (2003). Sexuality and aging in long-term care. *The Annals of Long-Term Care, 11,* 53–59. Retrieved from http://www.managedhealthcareconnect.com/home/altc.

Wallace, M. (2012). *Nursing standard of practice protocol: Sexuality in the older adult.* Retrieved from https://consultgeri.org/geriatric-topics/sexuality-issues-aging.

World Health Organization. (2004). *Sexual health: A new focus for WHO.* Progress in Reproductive Health Research. Retrieved from http://www.who.int/en/.

Youngkin, E. (2004). The myths and truths of mature intimacy. *Advance for Nurse Practitioners, 12*(8), 45–48.

Mental Health and Wellness in Later Life

 LEARNING OBJECTIVES

Upon completion of this chapter, the reader will be able to:

- Discuss factors contributing to mental health and wellness in later life.
- List symptoms of late-life anxiety and depression, and discuss assessment, treatment, and nursing interventions.
- Recognize older persons who are at risk for suicide, and use appropriate techniques for suicide prevention, assessment, and intervention.
- Specify several indications of substance abuse in older persons, and discuss appropriate nursing responses.
- Recognize signs of problem gambling and use appropriate techniques to screen for problem gambling.
- Evaluate interventions aimed at promoting mental health and wellness in older persons.

GLOSSARY

Affect   A person's prevailing emotion as observed by an interviewer or assessor.

Attention   The ability to attend to and concentrate on stimuli and to follow directions.

Delusion   A fixed, false belief.

Dysthymia   At least 2 years of depressed mood for more days than not, accompanied by additional depressive symptoms that do not meet the criteria for a major depressive episode.

Hallucination   The perception of a sensory experience with no external stimulus (e.g., hearing voices that no one else can hear).

Illusion   Misinterpretation of a real experience (e.g., thinking a curled rope is a snake).

Insight   Recognition that one has a health problem or illness.

Judgement   Ability to evaluate alternate courses of action in difficult situations.

Mental disorder   Mental illness diagnosed on the basis of criteria from the American Psychiatric Association *Diagnostic and Statistical Manual of Mental Disorders*.

Mood   A person's internal, self-reported emotional state.

Paranoia   An intense and strongly defended irrational suspicion.

Suicidal behaviour   Potentially self-injurious behaviour with a nonfatal outcome but for which there is evidence of the person's intention to die.

THE LIVED EXPERIENCE

During those bad times, I didn't get along with my family at all. I didn't know if they felt I [was] not doing a good job, like maybe they weren't sympathetic enough, but I think they just didn't know how people can feel when things like this [not working, being sick] happen.... I didn't get along with them for a long time. I had to, but I didn't. Just like that. That was tough.

   A 68-year-old man

I feel down, or depressed.... I thank God for every year of life that he gives me, but I still think that the older one gets the fewer the things one can do, right? ... I am sick right now, sometimes I fall and I can't get up on my own.... They [older men] do need to be understood, not for others to argue with them, to contradict them.

A 67-year-old man

From Apesoa-Varano, E. C., Barker, J. C., & Hinton, L. (2015). Shards of sorrow: Older men's accounts of their depression experience. *Social Science & Medicine, 124:* 1-8. doi:10.1016/j.socscimed.2014.10.054, pages 4 and 5.

Mental health in later life is not different than mental health earlier in life, but the challenges of maintaining mental health may be different in later life. Developmental transitions, life events, physical illness, cognitive impairment, and situations calling for psychic energy may interfere with mental health in older persons. These factors, although not unique to older persons, often influence adaptation. However, anyone who has survived for 80 or so years has been exposed to many stressors and crises and has developed resilience. Most older people face life's challenges with equanimity, good humour, and courage. The nurse's task is to discover the strengths and adaptive mechanisms that will help the person cope with the challenges.

The focus of this chapter is on the differing presentations of mental disorders that may occur in older persons and the appropriate assessments and interventions. Readers should refer to a comprehensive psychiatric–mental health text for more in-depth discussion of mental disorders.

MENTAL HEALTH AND MENTAL DISORDER IN LATER LIFE

The meaning of mental health is subject to many interpretations and many familial and cultural influences. According to the World Health Organization (WHO), mental health is "a state of well-being in which every individual realizes his or her own potential, can cope with the normal stresses of life, can work productively and fruitfully, and is able to make a contribution to her or his community" (World Health Organization [WHO], 2007, ¶ 2). Qualls (2002) defines a mentally healthy person as "one who accepts the aging self as an active being, engaging available strengths to compensate for weaknesses in order to create personal meaning, maintain maximum autonomy by mastering

the environment, and sustain positive relationships with others" (p. 12). Erikson et al. (1986) proposed that autonomy, intimacy, integrity, and generativity are all aspects of mentally healthy adult adaptation (see Chapter 7).

These definitions of mental health do not mention psychiatric symptoms or symptoms of mental disorder. Mental health is conceptually distinct from **mental disorder.** A mental disorder, or diagnosable mental illness, is a health condition "characterized by alterations in a variety of factors that include mood and affect, behaviour, and thinking and cognition. The disorders are associated with various degrees of distress and impaired functioning" (Austin & Boyd, 2010, p. 23). There are many causes of mental disorders, including genetic and biological factors and their interaction with social, psychological, and economic factors.

Four populations of people live with mental illness in older age (Mental Health Commission of Canada [MHCC], 2012). The first consists of people who have had a recurrent or persistent mental illness for many years. Because most mental illnesses have their initial onset in young adulthood, the most common experience of mental illness in older age is this recurrent or persistent illness. The second population consists of people who have a mental illness with onset in older age. The third group of older persons with mental illness is made up of those with dementia (see Chapter 21). The fourth population consists of older persons who experience mental illness in conjunction with a medical condition that has mental health symptoms, such as Parkinson's disease or cerebro-vascular disease (see Chapter 21).

People can achieve mental health, as defined by the WHO and Qualls (2002), despite the presence of a mental disorder or symptoms of a mental illness. Likewise, the absence of symptoms of mental illness does not guarantee mental health. The Canadian framework for a national mental health strategy builds on the WHO definition of mental health and explains the interaction between mental health and mental disorder as follows: "People can have varying degrees of mental health, regardless of whether or not they have a mental illness. For example, some people, whether they have a mental illness or not, have tremendous resilience, strength, healthy relationships, and a positive outlook. Others, whether they have a mental illness or not, may feel that day-to-day life is a struggle, that they have limited prospects, few friends, and are more easily set back by life's challenges" (Mental Health Commission of Canada [MHCC], 2009, p. 11).

It is important for nurses working with older persons to create relationships and environments that contribute to mental health and wellness, happiness, and meaning throughout life, even at the end of life, regardless of whether the older person experiences a mental disorder.

MENTAL HEALTH CARE

One in five Canadians experiences mental illness at some time in their lives (Health Canada, 2002). The prevalence of mental illness is the same in older persons as in the general population, except for a higher prevalence of dementia and delirium (Canadian Mental Health Association [CMHA], n.d.). Mental disorders are associated with increased use of health care resources and overall costs of care for older Canadians (Adams et al., 2015). Like younger Canadians, in a given year about 10% of older Canadians will experience a mental illness other than dementia or delirium (Pearson et al., 2015). The most prevalent mental disorders in late life are anxiety, dementia, and mood disorders such as depression. Addictions and substance use disorders among older persons are also concerning.

The stigma of having a mental illness discourages many people from seeking treatment. For example, up to two-thirds of older persons experiencing depression do not seek health care for the depression (Mackenzie et al., 2012). The rate of utilization of mental health services for older persons, even when such services are available, is less than that of any other age group. Some of the reasons for this are a stoic acceptance of difficulty, an unawareness of resources, a reluctance to seek help because of pride of independence, and the fear of being "put away." Ageism also affects the identification and treatment of mental health disorders in older people.

Symptoms of mental health problems may be overlooked, mistakenly seen as normal consequences of aging, or blamed on dementia by both older people and health care providers. In older people, the presence of comorbid medical conditions complicates the recognition and diagnosis of mental disorders. Also, the myth that older people do not respond well to treatment is still prevalent. Other factors—including health care providers' knowledge deficits; inadequate numbers of mental health care providers; and limited availability of specialized seniors' mental health services—are barriers (Adams et al., 2015; Mental Health Commission of Canada, 2011).

Older people receive psychiatric services across a wide range of settings, including acute and long-term inpatient psychiatric units, primary care, home care, and long-term care homes. Nurses will encounter older persons with mental disorders in all of these settings. Acute care admissions for medical problems are often exacerbated by depression, anxiety, cognitive impairment, substance abuse, or chronic mental illness. Length of stay, re-admission rate, and resource use are higher for older persons admitted to acute care with a comorbid mental illness (Adams et al., 2015).

Cultural and Ethnic Disparities

Lack of knowledge and awareness of cultural differences in regard to the meaning of mental health, differences in the way concerns may become apparent, limited access to culturally competent mental health treatment, and insufficient research in this area must be addressed in light of increasing ethnocultural diversity among older persons in Canada. These persons have less access to mental health services and are at risk of receiving poorer quality mental health care. Some identified barriers to the use of services are cultural beliefs, lack of culturally appropriate services, lack of services in the older person's language, lack of awareness of services, and ageism (Guruge et al., 2015).

In all assessment situations, it is important to include a cultural assessment and a discussion of what culturally and ethnically diverse older persons

BOX 24.1   Research for Evidence-Informed Practice: Help Seeking for Mental Health Problems Among Older Chinese Canadian Immigrants

Problem: Older persons are less likely than younger adults to seek help for mental disorders and mental health problems. Older persons who are members of minority ethnic groups are even less likely to seek help, even though their rates of mental disorder are higher. This study examined whether seeking help for mental health problems was associated with demographic and health factors, social support, and cultural values.

Method: Data were collected through a survey and semistructured interviews of Chinese Canadians aged 55 years and older who lived in the community or in assisted-living residences. A convenience sample of 149 participants completed questionnaires about social support, health-related quality of life, mental health care use, help-seeking attitudes, intentions to seek help, and Chinese cultural beliefs and values.

Findings: Sixteen percent of the participants sought help for mental problems in the previous year, more often from other types of practitioners than from health care providers. Positive help-seeking attitudes were associated with higher social support, better physical health, and lower levels of the influence of Chinese cultural beliefs and values.

Application to Nursing Practice: Attitudes toward seeking help were less positive than those in the general population. Older individuals from cultures that stigmatize mental illness, distress, and help seeking may be less likely to seek help. Outreach to immigrant communities may increase awareness of resources and reduce stigmatization. When discussing mental health, nurses should consider the person's cultural values and beliefs about mental illness.

Source: Tieu, U., & Konnert, C. A. (2014). Mental health help-seeking attitudes, utilization and intentions among older Chinese immigrants in Canada. *Aging & Mental Health, 18*(2), 140–147. doi:10.1080/1360786 3.2013.814104.

believe about their mental health problems. Box 24.1 describes a study about older Chinese Canadian immigrants seeking mental health help. Culturally appropriate education about mental health concerns is also important. Research on all aspects of culture and mental health is needed. (See Chapter 4 for an in-depth discussion of culture and aging.)

ASSESSMENT AND MENTAL ILLNESS

Accurate and appropriate assessment is critical. See Chapter 13 for a discussion about assessment tools for gerontological nursing. Specific information on instruments for assessment of depression, suicide, and substance abuse are described in this chapter. Assessment includes the mental status examination (MSE) and a holistic assessment. The components of the MSE are appearance and behaviour, **affect** and **mood,** speech and language, thought processes, thought content, perceptual disturbances (e.g., hallucinations), memory, level of consciousness, concentration and **attention,** and **insight** and **judgement**. Thought processes are the way a person's thoughts are organized (e.g., coherence and logical connections). Thought content is what a person is thinking about, including delusions, obsessions, phobias, suicide, and homicide. Mental status is assessed through careful observation and interviewing and also by standardized assessments. Psychosocial functioning and biological factors, such as medical conditions and medication side effects that may result in symptoms of mental disorders, must be considered. Mental health assessment is best done during short sessions after rapport has been established. Performing repeated assessments at various times of the day and in different situations will lead to a more complete and accurate assessment. The assessment should focus on the person's resilience, strengths, and skills, as well as his or her deficiencies. Assessment should include past experiences of mental illness and treatment.

ANXIETY DISORDERS

Anxiety is defined as unpleasant and unwarranted feelings of apprehension, which may be accompanied by physical symptoms. Anxiety itself is a normal human reaction and part of a fear response; it is rational, within reason. When a person experiences problematic anxiety, called *anxiety disorder*, the anxiety is prolonged and exaggerated and interferes with function. Anxiety disorders are not considered part of the normal aging process, but the changes and challenges that older persons often face may contribute to the development of anxiety symptoms and disorders. Many older people with anxiety disorders had an anxiety disorder earlier in their lives; however, late-onset anxiety is common. Anxiety disorders that may occur in older people include generalized anxiety disorder, phobic disorder, obsessive-compulsive disorder, panic disorder, and post-traumatic stress disorder (PTSD). Anxiety disorders are frequently comorbid with depression.

Prevalence

Epidemiological studies indicate that anxiety disorders are common in older persons; about 11% of older persons experience an anxiety disorder in any given year (Bower & Wetherell, 2015). However, relatively few people are diagnosed with these disorders in clinical practice. Anxiety disorders are more common among women and younger old persons (Katzman et al., 2014).

Generalized anxiety disorder (GAD) and specific phobias are the most common anxiety disorders in older people (Bower & Wetherell, 2015). In addition to unwarranted worries and feelings of apprehension that interfere with functioning, the symptoms of GAD include unrealistic and excessive worries; restlessness or a feeling of being keyed up or on edge; fatigue that develops readily; difficulty concentrating, or the mind's going blank; irritability; muscle tension; and sleep disturbance (American Psychiatric Association [APA], 2013). About 2% of older persons experience GAD in a given year (Volkert et al., 2013).

Phobia is an unrealistic or irrational fear that interferes with a person's life. Between 2% and 10% of older persons experience phobias. This may be an underestimate, because older persons tend to have less insight into the extent to which phobias and associated avoidance affect their lives (Bower & Wetherell, 2015). Fear of falling is likely the most common phobia among older persons.

Some of the risk factors for anxiety disorders in older people are female gender, a history of worry or rumination, poor physical health or physical illness, low socioeconomic status, high-stress life events, early childhood abuse, depression, cognitive impairment, a family history of anxiety disorder, and alcohol or drug misuse. Protective factors that decrease the risk for anxiety disorders include receiving social support from family, having a spouse or living with someone, and being physically active (Bower & Wetherell, 2015).

Anxiety in older persons is associated with more visits to primary care providers and an increase in the average length of visits. Some of the negative consequences of anxiety symptoms and disorders are decreased physical activity, decreased functional status, decreased satisfaction with life, and an increased risk of mortality (Bower & Wetherell, 2015; Katzman et al., 2014). Unidentified or untreated anxiety disorders in older people adversely affect well-being and quality of life.

IMPLICATIONS FOR GERONTOLOGICAL NURSING AND HEALTHY AGING

ASSESSMENT

Approximately 70% of primary care visits are driven by psychological factors (e.g., panic, generalized anxiety, and somatization) (American Psychological Association, 2014). This means that nurses often encounter anxious older people and can identify anxiety-related symptoms and initiate assessments that will lead to appropriate treatment and management. When assessing older patients, nurses should be aware of factors that can reduce the chance of recognizing anxiety (Box 24.2).

Older people are less likely to report psychiatric symptoms or acknowledge anxiety, often attribute their symptoms to physical health problems, and are likely to have coexistent medical conditions that mimic symptoms of anxiety. Some of the medical disorders that cause anxiety symptoms are cardiac arrhythmias, delirium, dementia, chronic obstructive pulmonary disease, heart failure, hyperthyroidism, hypoglycemia, postural hypotension, pulmonary edema, and pulmonary embolism. Distinguishing a medical condition from the physical symptoms of an anxiety disorder may be difficult.

Anxiety is also a common adverse effect of many drugs, including anticholinergics, digitalis, theophylline, antihypertensives, beta-blockers, beta-adrenergic stimulators, corticosteroids, and over-the-counter (OTC) medications such as appetite suppressants and cough and cold preparations. Caffeine; nicotine; and withdrawal from alcohol, sedatives, and hypnotics cause symptoms of anxiety.

BOX 24.2	Factors That Reduce the Chances of Seeking Help for and Recognizing Anxiety

1. Stigmatization of mental illness; discomfort when talking to health care providers about anxiety
2. Attribution of psychological symptoms to physical causes
3. Nonrecognition of the impact of symptoms on daily life and functioning
4. Labels and words that are used to describe anxiety (e.g., "worry," as opposed to "concerns" or "issues")
5. Ageist attitudes and beliefs
6. Pessimism about treatment effectiveness
7. Diagnostic difficulties
8. Time constraints in primary care settings

Source: Adapted from Bower, E. S., & Wetherell, J. L. (2015). Late-life anxiety disorders. In P. A. Lichtenberg, B. T. Mast, B. D. Carpenter, et al. (Eds.), *APA handbook of clinical geropsychology. Vol. 2, Assessment, treatment, and issues in later life.* Washington, DC: American Psychological Association.

BOX 24.3	Suggested Questions for Identifying Anxiety in Older People

1. Can you say what triggers your feeling anxious?
2. Have you been concerned about or fretted over a number of things?
3. Is there anything going on in your life that is causing you concern?
4. Do you find that you have a hard time putting things out of your mind?

The following questions are useful in identifying how and when physical symptoms began:

1. What were you doing when you noticed the chest pain?
2. What were you thinking about when you felt your heart start to race?
3. When you can't sleep, what is usually going through your head?

Source: The Anxiety Disorder Association of America. (2010-2016). *Symptoms.* Retrieved from http://www.adaa.org/living-with-anxiety/older-adults/symptoms

Assessment of anxiety in older people focuses on physical, social, and environmental factors, as well as past life history and recent events. Older people more often report somatic complaints such as gastrointestinal symptoms, headaches, dizziness, pain, dyspnea, and palpitations, rather than cognitive symptoms such as excessive worrying. It is important to remember that expressed fears and worries may be realistic or unrealistic, so the nurse must investigate and obtain collateral information from family or caregivers. For example, fear of leaving the home may be related to frequent falling or to crime in the neighbourhood. Worries about financial stability may be related to the economy or financial abuse by others.

It is important to investigate other possible causes of anxiety, such as medical conditions and depression. Diagnostic and laboratory tests may be ordered as indicated to rule out medical conditions. Cognitive assessment, brain imaging, and neuro-psychological evaluation are included if cognitive impairment is suspected (see Chapter 21). When comorbid conditions are present, they must be treated. A review of medications, including OTC medications and herbal or home remedies, is essential, as is the elimination of those that cause anxiety symptoms.

Scales may be used to supplement the clinical assessment. Numerous self-report rating scales are available, but few have been adequately tested with older persons (Bower & Wetherell, 2015). Rating scales developed for use with older persons include the Geriatric Anxiety Inventory (Pachana et al., 2007), the Worry Scale (Wisocki et al., 1986), and the Geriatric Anxiety Scale (Segal et al., 2010). Box 24.3 lists suggested questions to identify anxiety disorders in older people.

INTERVENTIONS

Anxiety disorders in older people can be treated effectively. Treatment choices depend on the symptoms, the specific anxiety diagnosis, comorbid medical conditions, and any current medication regimen. Pharmacological and nonpharmacological interventions are effective and may be used conjointly (Katzman et al., 2014). Many older people prefer nonpharmacological treatments.

Nonpharmacological Interventions

The therapeutic relationship is the foundation for any intervention. Family support, community resources and therapists, support groups, and the provision of information are all important.

Cognitive behavioural therapy, relaxation training, mindfulness meditation, acceptance and commitment therapy, supportive therapy, and psychoeducation are used to treat older persons' anxiety disorders. Many of these approaches can be provided individually or in groups, and some may also be provided via the Internet. Cognitive behavioural therapy (CBT) is a widely used approach for the treatment of both anxiety and depression. It is designed to modify thought patterns, improve skills, and alter the environmental states that contribute to anxiety. This therapy may involve relaxation training, cognitive restructuring (i.e., replacing anxiety-producing thoughts with more realistic, less catastrophic ones), and education about signs and symptoms of anxiety. It is moderately effective for older people but less effective than it is for younger people (Ayers et al., 2015). Cognitive behavioural therapy is time consuming and requires a commitment to daily homework and practice. Given that other approaches such as mindfulness and supportive therapy may be equally as effective for older persons, CBT may not be the first-line nonpharmacological approach (Ayers et al., 2015).

Mindfulness approaches encourage the person to have a focused nonjudgemental awareness of the present instead of worrying. The training involves practising mindfulness, meditation, yoga, and awareness of breathing (Lenze et al., 2014). Some studies show positive results for older persons with anxiety symptoms or disorders (Geiger et al., 2016).

Pharmacological Interventions

Issues of polypharmacy and age-related changes in pharmaco-dynamics make prescribing and monitoring medications in older people a complex undertaking (see Chapter 14). Antidepressants in the form of selective serotonin reuptake inhibitors and serotonin-norepinephrine reuptake inhibitors have been found to be effective for the treatment of GAD and panic disorder. Within these classes of medications, those with sedating rather than stimulating properties are preferred (e.g., citalopram, paroxetine, and sertraline). When selective serotonin reuptake inhibitors (SSRIs) are prescribed, it is important to educate the patient about (and to watch for) potential side effects, such as initial increased nervousness, insomnia, nausea, and sexual dysfunction. A discontinuation syndrome of dizziness, insomnia, and flu-like symptoms is common when SSRIs are stopped.

Second-line treatment may include short-acting benzodiazepines, such as alprazolam (Xanax) and lorazepam (Ativan). Treatment with benzodiazepines should be used only for short-term therapy (less than 6 months) and for relief of immediate symptoms; these medications must be used carefully in older persons. Older medications, such as diazepam (Valium), should be avoided because of their long half-lives and the increased risk of accumulation and toxicity in older people. All of these medications can have problematic side effects such as sedation, falls, cognitive impairment, and dependence (see Chapter 14). Non-benzodiazepine anxiolytic agents, such as buspirone, may also be used. Buspirone has fewer side effects but requires a longer period of administration (up to 4 weeks) for effectiveness.

OBSESSIVE-COMPULSIVE DISORDERS

Obsessive-compulsive disorder is characterized by recurrent and persistent thoughts, impulses, or images (obsessions) that are repetitive and purposeful and by intentional ritualistic behaviours (compulsions) that improve the person's comfort level. The person cannot control compulsions even when recognizing that they are excessive and unreasonable. Obsessive-compulsive disorder (OCD) significantly impairs function for more than an hour each day (American Psychiatric Association, 2013). Symptoms in older persons are often not sufficient to disrupt function seriously and thus may not be considered symptoms of a true disorder but rather a coping strategy. If symptoms progress to the point at which they disrupt function, the older person will need clinical attention. Recommended treatments include exercise and CBT combined with pharmacological treatment (i.e., SSRIs) if indicated.

POST-TRAUMATIC STRESS DISORDER

Post-traumatic stress disorder (PTSD) is a syndrome characterized by the development of symptoms after a traumatic event that involved (1) the person's witnessing or unexpectedly hearing about an actual or threatened death or (2) serious injury to the person or someone close to the person. Most older people have experienced a potentially traumatic event at some time, and some of them develop PTSD as a consequence (Bower & Wetherell, 2015). The *Diagnostic and Statistical Manual of Mental Disorders, 5th ed.* (DSM-5) changed the classification of PTSD from an anxiety disorder to a new disorder called *trauma and stress-related disorder* (American Psychiatric Association, 2013).

Individuals with PTSD often re-experience the traumatic event in episodes of fear, and they experience symptoms such as helplessness, flashbacks, intrusive thoughts, memories, images, emotional numbing, loss of interest, avoidance of any place that reminds the person of the traumatic event, poor concentration, irritability, startle reactions, jumpiness, and hypervigilance. They may experience ongoing sleep problems, somatic disturbances, anxiety, depression, and restlessness. The severity of the symptoms tends to decline over time. Older persons with a history of PTSD have high rates of several physical health conditions, as well as worse physical functioning and cognitive performance (Bower & Wetherell, 2015). Compared to other older persons, older American veterans with PTSD have a higher risk for dementia and cognitive impairment (Cook & Dinnen, 2015).

The lifetime prevalence of PTSD among Canadian adults is 9.2% (Katzman et al., 2014). According to epidemiological studies, in a given year about 1% to 2% of older persons experience PTSD (Volkert et al., 2013), but its prevalence may be higher in clinical populations. A study of older persons attending primary care clinics in Quebec found that 11% had significant post-traumatic stress symptoms in the previous 6 months (Lamoureux-Lamarche et al., 2016). The disorder is more common in women. Sexual assault is the most common cause of PTSD in women, followed by being abused as a child, being threatened with a weapon, being molested, being neglected as a child, and being subject to physical violence. For men, the most common cause is also sexual assault, followed by abuse as a child, combat (war), and molestation.

In older persons, PTSD may develop as a new disorder in response to a recent trauma, or it may be related to trauma long past. Compared to younger adults, older people are more likely to experience PTSD after natural disasters and human-induced disasters such as war and terrorist attacks (Parker et al., 2016; Siskind et al., 2016). Older persons who are at greatest risk for PTSD after a disaster are those with lower socioeconomic status; poor subjective health and functioning; a mental illness; chronic medical conditions; or low levels of social support (Heid et al., 2016).

Although trauma has long been associated with PTSD symptoms (e.g., First World War soldiers with these symptoms were labelled as having "shell shock"), it was first recognized as a psychiatric diagnosis in 1980. At that time, attention to PTSD symptoms was an outcome of overwhelmingly stressful experiences of individuals who took part in the American war in Vietnam. Many Second World War veterans have lived most of their lives under the shadow of PTSD without its being recognized. Older persons under care now also experienced the Great Depression, the Holocaust and other genocides, racism, and the Korean conflict—events that also may have precipitated PTSD.

 IMPLICATIONS FOR GERONTOLOGICAL NURSING AND HEALTHY AGING

ASSESSMENT

The care of the individual with PTSD involves an awareness that certain events may trigger PTSD reactions; the pattern of these reactions should be identified when possible. Provision of intimate bodily care can trigger a traumatic response among older persons with a history of sexual assault or abuse as a child. Knowing the person's past history and life experiences is essential to understanding the person's behaviour and implementing appropriate interventions. However, the person's history of trauma may be unknown, and if the person has dementia, the history may be difficult to ascertain. Self-protective behaviours of individuals who have dementia may be linked to their past experiences of trauma (see Chapter 21). Nurses who work in hospitals and long-term care (LTC) homes should be aware of potential environmental triggers of traumatic memories for older persons with dementia who have a history of trauma. The *ConsultGeri.org* website describes a tool for assessing the impact of trauma on older persons (Weiss & Marmar, 1997).

INTERVENTIONS

Effectively coping with traumatic events seems to be associated with the following: secure and supportive relationships; the ability to freely express or fully suppress the experience; favourable circumstances immediately following the trauma; a productive and active lifestyle; strong faith, religion, and hope; a sense of humour; and biological integrity. CBT with prolonged exposure involves psychoeduction, breathing retraining, imagining the past traumatic event, and exposure to situations that have been avoided since the traumatic event. CBT is effective for PTSD, and there is some evidence of its effectiveness with older persons (Cook & Dinnen, 2015). Pharmacological treatment with antidepressant SSRIs and serotonin-norepinephrine reuptake inhibitors (SNRIs) may be helpful. Paroxetine (Paxil) and venflafaxine (Effexor) are recommended as first-line treatments of PTSD in adults (Katzman et al., 2014). However, older persons have not been included in most clinical trials of medications for PTSD.

PSYCHOSIS AND PSYCHOTIC SYMPTOMS IN LATE LIFE

Psychosis is a syndrome or constellation of psychiatric symptoms that occurs in a number of physical and mental disorders. The predominating symptoms are hallucinations and delusions. Older persons may experience psychosis from a persistent, recurrent mental illness such as schizophrenia, delusional disorder, depression, or bipolar affective disorder. In older persons, a new onset of psychosis may occur as a secondary syndrome in a variety of disorders, the most common being dementia and Parkinson's disease. Temporal lobe epilepsy, untreated endocrine disorders, tumours, and the use of some medications and illicit drugs also may result in psychosis (Varcarolis & Clements, 2013). Risk factors for psychosis in older persons are social isolation, sensory deficits, physical illness, cognitive impairment, and polypharmacy (Ceglowski et al., 2015).

Paranoia

Symptoms of **paranoia** can signify an acute change in mental status as a result of a medical illness or delirium (see Chapter 21), or they can be caused by an underlying mental disorder such as depression, PTSD, or substance use disorder. Paranoia is also an early symptom of Alzheimer's disease. Medications, vision and hearing loss, social isolation, negative life events, financial strain, and PTSD can also precipitate symptoms of paranoia. The dynamics of paranoia seem to be loss of control, the inability to evaluate the social milieu appropriately, and the feeling that external forces are controlling life (which in many instances may be true).

Delusions

A **delusion** is a fixed, false belief that guides a person's interpretation of events but is not shared by others. Delusions may be comforting or threatening, but they always form a structure for understanding situations that otherwise might seem unmanageable. A delusional disorder is one in which conceivable ideas that are without factual foundation persist for more than 1 month.

More-common delusions of older persons are of being poisoned, their children taking their assets, being held prisoner, or being deceived by a spouse or lover. The delusions of older persons often incorporate significant persons. Fear and a lack of trust originating from a basis in reality may become magnified, especially when the person is isolated from others and does not receive reality feedback. Delusions related to family members and their actions or intentions may occur among older people. Some delusions may aid in coping, but most are troubling to the person. One study found that 21% of new LTC–home residents had delusions (Canadian Coalition for Seniors' Mental Health [CCSMH], 2006). It is always important to determine whether what "appears" to be a delusion is in fact based in reality.

Hallucinations

A **hallucination** is the sensory perception of a non-existent object. Any of the five senses can be subject to hallucinations. Although not attributable to environmental stimuli, hallucinations may occur as the result of a combination of environmental factors. Among older persons, hallucinations that arise from psychotic disorders (e.g., schizophrenia) are less common than hallucinations that arise from other causes.

The character and stages of hallucinatory experiences in late life have not been adequately defined. Many hallucinations are associated with medications, neurological disorders such as dementia and Parkinson's disease, and physiological and sensory disorders. The hallucinations of older persons most often appear along with disorientation, **illusion,** intense grief, or immersion in retrospection, the origins being difficult to separate. Older people with hearing and vision deficits may also hear voices or see people and objects that are not actually present (illusions). Some researchers have explained these illusions as the brain's attempt to create stimulation in the absence of adequate sensory input. Illusions and hallucinations that are not disturbing to the person may not necessitate treatment.

IMPLICATIONS FOR GERONTOLOGICAL NURSING AND HEALTHY AGING

ASSESSMENT

Determining whether a person's psychotic symptoms (paranoia, delusions, and hallucinations) are the result of medical illnesses, medications, dementia, psychoses, deprivations, or overload is challenging, because the treatment will vary accordingly. Treatment must be based on a comprehensive assessment and a determination of the nature of the psychotic behaviour (primary or secondary psychosis) and the time of onset of first symptoms (early or late). Treating the underlying cause of a secondary psychosis brought on by medical illnesses, head trauma, dementia, illicit substances, medication misuse, or delirium is a priority (Ceglowski et al., 2015).

An assessment of vision and hearing is important, since impairments of vision and hearing may predispose the person to paranoia and suspiciousness. Screening for depression should be conducted. Assessment of suicide potential is also indicated, because individuals experiencing paranoid symptoms are at significant risk for self-harm.

It is never safe to conclude that someone is delusional or paranoid or experiencing hallucinations unless the claims have been thoroughly investigated, physical and cognitive status evaluated, and the environment assessed for contributing factors to the behaviours.

INTERVENTIONS

Frightening hallucinations or delusions (e.g., of being poisoned) usually arise in response to anxiety-provoking situations, and caregivers may best manage these symptoms by reducing the situational stress, being available to the person, providing a safe and nonjudgemental environment, and attending to the person's fears more than to the content of the delusion or hallucination. Direct confrontation is likely to increase person's anxiety and agitation and sense of vulnerability; it also may disrupt the relationship with the care provider. A more useful approach is to establish a trusting relationship that is not demanding and not too intense.

It is important to identify the person's strengths and build on them. Demonstrating respect and a willingness to listen to complaints and fears is important. The nurse must be trustworthy, give clear information, and present clear choices. The nurse should not pretend to agree with paranoid beliefs or delusions but rather should ask what is troubling to the person and provide reassurance of safety. It is important to try to understand what the experience is like for the person and how distressing it is. Other suggestions are to avoid television, which can be confusing, especially if the person has a hearing or vision impairment and awakens with the television on. In addition, clutter in the person's room should be reduced, large mirrors should be removed, and shadows that can appear threatening should be eliminated. Eyeglasses and hearing aids need to be provided to maximize sensory input and reduce misinterpretations.

If symptoms are interfering with function and environmental strategies and if nonpharmacological approaches are not effective, antipsychotic medications may be used. The newer atypical antipsychotics such as risperidone (Risperdal) and olanzapine (Zyprexa) are preferred but must be used judiciously, with careful attention to side effects and monitoring response. Antipsychotic medications are not recommended as a first-line treatment of psychotic symptoms associated with dementia, except in cases of severe agitation or psychosis (see Chapter 21).

SCHIZOPHRENIA

Schizophrenia is a severe mental disorder characterized by two or more of the following symptoms: delusions, hallucinations, disorganized thinking, disorganized or catatonic behaviour (called "positive" symptoms), and affective flattening, poverty of speech, or apathy (called "negative" symptoms). These symptoms cause significant social or occupational dysfunction and are not accompanied by prominent mood symptoms or substance misuse or attributed to medical causes (American Psychiatric Association, 2013).

The prevalence of schizophrenia in older people is approximately 0.5%, about half of its prevalence in younger adults (Ceglowski et al., 2015). The onset of schizophrenia usually occurs between adolescence and the midthirties. It can first appear in later life, but this is rare. Late-onset schizophrenia is more common among women, and the symptoms are more likely to include persecutory delusions and hallucinations.

Cognitive impairment is common in schizophrenia. It affects memory, verbal and language functioning, attention, concentration, and executive functioning. These impairments persist even with effective treatment. Cognitive impairment is worse for persons whose schizophrenia began when they were young adults (Ceglowski et al., 2015; Mausbach & Ho, 2015). Social skills impairment is also common and persistent. Older people with schizophrenia are more likely to live in LTC homes or receive residential care (Dixon, 2009).

Metabolic syndrome, common in schizophrenia, is a constellation of clinical and metabolic risk factors for cardiovascular disease, including elevated blood pressure and cholesterol, insulin resistance and diabetes, and abdominal obesity. Metabolic syndrome is partly attributed to the effects of antipsychotic medications. The prevalence of metabolic syndrome associated with schizophrenia is about 40%, and the condition is more common among older people with a longer history of schizophrenia (Ceglowski et al., 2015). Individuals with schizophrenia have a 20% lower life expectancy and have a higher prevalence of many physical illnesses, especially diabetes. These health disparities are a result of limited access to adequate preventative and primary health care as well as

health risks associated with antipsychotic medications (Kredenster et al., 2014).

 IMPLICATIONS FOR GERONTOLOGICAL NURSING AND HEALTHY AGING

ASSESSMENT

Holistic assessment should include assessment of social skills, social functioning, and social support. Monitoring for metabolic syndrome is important. Relatives of older people with schizophrenia may have been providing care for years and into very old age. Caregiver needs and resources should be assessed. Trauma history should be considered, since people with schizophrenia are vulnerable to housing insecurity, assault, and mistreatment.

TREATMENT

Nursing interventions with persons with schizophrenia focus on recovery and well-being. This means supporting the persons in living a meaningful life, contributing to their community, and achieving their potential regardless of their age or the effects of their schizophrenia (Mental Health Commission of Canada [MHCC], 2011). Hope, choice, self-care, and self-determination are important within a recovery approach. The nurse supports both pharmacological and nonpharmacological treatment. Conventional neuroleptic medications such as haloperidol (Haldol) have been effective in managing the positive symptoms but are problematic with older people and carry a high risk of disabling and persistent adverse effects such as tardive dyskinesia (TD) (see Chapter 14). When given in low doses, the newer atypical antipsychotic medications—such as risperidone (Risperdal), olanzapine (Zyprexa), and quetiapine (Seroquel)—are associated with a lower risk for extrapyramidal symptoms and TD. Psychosocial treatments include CBT, family psychoeducation, social skills therapy, cognitive remediation therapy, and a combination of these approaches. Some of these treatments have been modified and tested with older persons, and the results for social skills training and cognitive behaviour social skills training are promising (Mausbach & Ho, 2015). Other important interventions include case management, weight management, and support for the self-care of chronic physical illnesses.

BIPOLAR DISORDER AND MANIA

Although bipolar disorder is not common in later life, more cases will be seen as the number of older persons grows. Ten percent of inpatient psychiatric admissions of older persons are for bipolar disorder. Bipolar disorders, characterized by periods of mania and depression, often level out in later life, and bipolar individuals tend to have longer periods of depression. Mania is a more frequent cause of hospitalization than depression is, but depression may account for more disability. New episodes of mania in older age are often due to underlying medical conditions that must be identified and treated (Carlino et al., 2013). Metabolic syndrome is common among older persons with bipolar disorder (Dols et al., 2014).

IMPLICATIONS FOR GERONTOLOGICAL NURSING AND HEALTHY AGING

Recommended treatment consists of a combination of one or more mood stabilizers and intensive psycho-social intervention. Lithium is a mood stabilizer and the first-line pharmacological treatment for bipolar disorder. Lithium's side effects of fine hand tremor, polyuria, mild thirst, mild nausea, and weight gain make it difficult for older people to tolerate the medication. However, most older people who use lithium are positive about it, despite the side effects (Rej et al., 2016). Lithium has a long half-life (more than 36 hours) and a narrow therapeutic window, meaning that there is a small difference between a therapeutic level and a toxic level. Serum lithium levels must be monitored regularly. Lithium is excreted by the kidneys, so adequate kidney function and salt and fluid intake are necessary to maintain a therapeutic level. Signs of toxicity include nausea, vomiting, diarrhea, thirst, polyuria, lethargy, slurred speech, muscle weakness, and coarse hand tremors. Confusion and other neurological changes are signs of severe toxicity. Antidepressants (i.e., SSRIs) may be used for individuals who have little or no history of mania.

Patient and family education and support are essential, and the family must understand that the individual is unable to control mania and irritating behaviours. Education about lithium therapy should include information about the importance of a maintaining a normal diet, maintaining hydration, taking lithium with meals to avoid nausea, and knowing what to do if signs of toxicity develop. Other resources for bipolar disorder can be found in the Resources section at the end of the chapter.

DEPRESSION

Depression is not a normal part of aging, and studies show that most older people are satisfied with their lives, despite physical problems. To understand depression, nurses must comprehend the influence of late-life stressors, culture, and the beliefs that older people, society, and health care providers may have about depression and its treatment.

Prevalence and Consequences

Depression is the most common mental health problem in later life. The estimated prevalence of major depressive disorder in later life is between 1.5% and 3.3% (Statistics Canada, 2016; Volkert et al., 2013). Estimates of prevalence vary, depending on how depression is measured and the clinical setting. Major depression is more prevalent in hospitalized older persons (13% to 22%) and those in LTC homes (6% to 16%) (DiNapoli & Scogin, 2015).

The prevalence of milder forms of depression is much higher, between 4% and 18% (DiNapoli & Scogin, 2015). Like major depression, milder forms of depression are more common in clinical populations. Depression symptoms are present in 25 to 33% of hospitalized older persons, 22 to 44% of home care clients, and 44% of LTC home residents (Canadian Institute for Health Information [CIHI], 2010; DiNapoli & Scogin, 2015; Markle-Reid et al., 2014). More than 15% of older persons with persistent physical conditions are depressed, and depression has been called "the unwanted co-traveler" accompanying many medical illnesses (Byrd, 2005, p. 132). Many medications that older people take can also cause depression.

Depression and depressive symptoms are associated with negative consequences, such as increased disability and functional decline, delayed recovery from illness and surgery, increased use of health services, cognitive impairment, malnutrition, decreased quality of life, substance misuse, and an elevated risk of suicide and non-suicide-related death (DiNapoli & Scogin, 2015; McKenzie & Harvath, 2016).

Depression remains underdiagnosed and under-treated, which may be explained by the attitudes and beliefs of older persons and health care providers and by how difficult it is to differentiate the symptoms of depression from those of other illnesses. Although public attitudes about mental illness and depression are improving, the stigma associated with depression may be more prevalent for older people, and older persons may not acknowledge depressive symptoms or seek treatment. Some older persons, particularly those who have survived wars and other tragedies, may see depression as shameful, evidence of flawed character, being self-centred, a spiritual weakness, sin, or retribution.

Health care providers may mistakenly believe that depression is normal in aging and may not take appropriate action to assess and treat depression in older persons. The differing presentation of depression in older people, as well as the high prevalence of medical problems that may cause depressive symptoms, also contributes to inadequate recognition and treatment.

Older persons of various ethnic and cultural groups have different risk factors for depression. For example, older visible minority Canadian immigrants have a higher prevalence of depression symptoms, owing to their experiences of discrimination (Kim & Noh, 2014). They also face additional barriers to accessing depression treatment. Culturally based beliefs may contribute to a reluctance to seek help for depression (Tieu & Konnert, 2014). However, there is considerable variability between and among ethnic and cultural groups (Jiminez et al., 2013; Kim et al., 2015), and the lack of accessible services is problematic (Guruge et al., 2015).

Failure to treat depression increases morbidity and mortality. Yet, treatments for depression are as effective for older individuals as they are for the general population. It is highly likely that nurses in all settings will encounter a large number of older people with depressive symptoms. The nurse's recognition of depression and the nurse's role in enhancing the access to appropriate mental health care are important for improving outcomes for older people.

Etiology and Risk Factors

The causes of depression in older persons are complex and must be examined within a biopsychosocial framework. It is thought that an interaction of biological and psychosocial vulnerabilities and stressful life events explain risk for depression in older age (Edelstein, Bamonti, Gregg, & Gerolimatos, 2015).

Genetic risk is linked with depression onset in younger adulthood and is thus more relevant to older persons with recurrent depression (Edelstein et al., 2015). Medical illnesses are commonly comorbid. Some of the medical conditions that contribute to depression are cardiovascular disorders, chronic lung diseases, end-stage renal disease, arthritis, endocrine disorders (such as thyroid problems and diabetes mellitus), and insomnia (McKenzie & Harvath, 2016; Edelstein et al., 2015). Medications used to treat medical disorders can also results in depressive symptoms. Psychosocial and environmental risk factors for depression in older age include low levels of social support; financial strain; neurotic personality; low self-efficacy; stressful life events and losses; and family caregiving (DiNapoli & Scogin, 2015; McKenzie & Harvath, 2016). Depression in older persons is commonly comorbid with other mental illnesses, particularly anxiety disorder, personality disorder, dementia, and alcohol use disorder (DiNapoli & Scogin, 2015). Some common risk factors for depression are presented in Box 24.4.

Factors that protect older persons who have these risks for depression include socioeconomic and health resources, coping, and engagement in meaningful activities. Through life experience, older persons learn coping strategies that work for them. Many stressful events in older age can be anticipated and may thus be viewed as manageable. Lastly, older persons who remain engaged in activities and relationships despite their physical limitations are less likely to experience depression (DiNapoli & Scogin, 2015).

Differing Presentation of Depression in Older Persons

The *DSM-5* provides criteria for the diagnosis of major depression and **dysthymia** (American Psychiatric

BOX 24.4   Common Risk Factors for Depression in Older Persons

Predisposing Factors
- Female
- Widowed or divorced
- History of depression
- Vascular brain changes
- Neurotic personality characteristics
- Major physical and chronic illnesses
- Medications—antihypertensives, narcotic analgesics, indomethacin, steroids, L-dopa, antimicrobials, benzodiazepines, digoxin, cimetidine, cancer chemotherapeutics
- Excessive alcohol consumption
- Social disadvantages and low social support
- Family caregiving

Precipitating Factors
- Recent bereavement
- Moving to an LTC home (within first year)
- Adverse life events
- Long-term stress
- Persistent sleep difficulties

Source: Adapted from Canadian Coalition for Seniors' Mental Health (CCSMH). (2006). *National guidelines for seniors' mental health: The assessment and treatment of depression.* Toronto, ON: Author (p. 23); McKenzie, G. L., & Harvath, T. A. (2016). Late-life depression. In M. Boltz, E. Capezuti, T. Fulmer, et al. (Eds.), *Evidenced-based geriatric nursing protocols for best practice* (5th ed.) (pp. 211–232). New York, NY: Springer Publishing Company.

Association, 2013). Depression is a syndrome consisting of an array of affective, cognitive, and somatic or physiological symptoms. Affective symptoms include depressed, sad, or irritable mood; loss of pleasure in usual activities; and feelings of worthlessness or guilt. Two cognitive symptoms are decreased concentration and suicidal thoughts or behaviour. Some of the somatic and physiological symptoms are fatigue and decreased energy, increased or decreased appetite or weight, sleep disturbance, and psychomotor agitation or retardation (American Psychiatric Association, 2013). Depression may result in dependency, poor grooming, difficulty completing activities of daily living, decreased motivation, and decreased sexual interest. Depression may range in severity from mild symptoms to more severe forms, both of which can persist over long periods. Suicidal ideation and

psychotic features (e.g., delusional thinking) accompany more severe depression (McKenzie & Harvath, 2016).

The symptoms of depression in older people are different from those in people in other age groups. Older people who are depressed report more somatic complaints, such as physical symptoms, insomnia, loss of appetite and weight loss, memory problems, and persistent pain. They are less likely to have the feelings of guilt and worthlessness seen in younger depressed individuals. The somatic complaints "are often difficult to distinguish from the somatic or physical symptoms associated with acute or chronic physical illness… or the somatic symptoms that are part of common aging processes" (McKenzie & Harvath, 2016, p. 212). Compared to younger adults with depression, persons with late-life depression are also less likely to have a family history of depression (Edelstein et al., 2015).

Hypochondriasis, complaining, and criticism may actually be expressions of depression. Depression may be an early symptom of dementia, but it is unclear whether it is a prodrome for the onset of dementia, a risk factor for dementia, or an independent event (Edelstein et al., 2015). Symptoms such as agitation and repetitive verbalizations in persons with dementia may be symptoms of depression. It is important that older people with memory impairment be evaluated for depression (see Chapters 7 and 21).

 IMPLICATIONS FOR GERONTOLOGICAL NURSING AND HEALTHY AGING

ASSESSMENT

Assessment involves a systematic and thorough evaluation with a depression screening instrument, interview, history and physical assessment, functional assessment, cognitive assessment, laboratory tests, medication review, determination of iatrogenic or medical causes, and family interview, as indicated. Assessment for depressogenic medications and for related comorbid conditions that may contribute to or complicate treatment of depression must also be included. A comprehensive guide to the assessment and treatment of depression in older persons, *Nursing*

Standard of Practice Protocol (Harvath & McKenzie, 2012), is available at http://consultgeri.org.

Screening of all older persons for depression should be incorporated into routine health assessments across the continuum of care—in hospitals, primary care, LTC, home care, and community-based settings (McKenzie & Harvath, 2016). The Geriatric Depression Scale Short Form (GDS-SF) has been validated and used extensively with older persons (see Chapter 13). The GDS-SF takes approximately 5 minutes to administer, and although it is not a substitute for individualized assessment, it is an effective screening tool for older persons. A video demonstrating use of the GDS-SF is available at http://consultgeri .org. The Cornell Scale for Depression in Dementia, a caregiver report tool, is used to screen for depression in older persons with dementia (Alexopoulos et al., 1988).

INTERVENTIONS

When depression is diagnosed, treatment should begin as soon as possible, and appropriate follow-up should be provided. Depressed people are often unable to follow through on their own; without appropriate treatment and monitoring, they may develop deeper depression or die by suicide. Persons with severe depression or high suicide risk are often initially treated as inpatients.

The major treatment options for depression are pharmacotherapy and electroconvulsive therapy (ECT), psychotherapy, and psychosocial interventions. The most effective treatment is a combination of pharmacological therapy and psychosocial interventions or psychotherapy. Older patients tend to prefer psychosocial interventions. Interventions are individualized and are based on history, severity of symptoms, concomitant illnesses, and level of disability.

Effective psychosocial treatments include behavioural therapy, CBT, problem-solving therapy, cognitive bibliotherapy, reminiscence therapy, and brief dynamic psychotherapy (Edelstein et al., 2015). Behavioural therapy addresses the link between mood and behaviour. The depressed person learns to monitor mood and activity, increase engagement in activities that improve mood, decrease involvement in unpleasant activities, and develop problem-solving skills to overcome barriers to engaging in activities

(Edelstein et al., 2015). Problem-solving therapy teaches people to manage and cope with stressors; it is effective in primary care settings and for medially ill persons at home (DiNapoli & Scogin, 2015). Cognitive bibliotherapy is structured, self-administered CBT in which a person follows written directions with minimal input from a therapist (Edelstein et al., 2015). Reminiscence and life review therapy (see Chapter 3) is an effective treatment for depression in older persons and improves depression symptoms of persons with dementia (Edelstein et al., 2015). Although there is less research about the effects of exercise on depression, some studies have found that exercise is an effective treatment for major depression and dysthymia (Edelstein et al., 2015). In addition, family and social support, education, grief management, and reminiscence and life-review therapy (see Chapter 3) have been helpful for depression. Box 24.5 lists suggestions for families and providers who are caring for older persons with depression.

A collaborative-care approach in primary care, home care, and LTC is recommended. This model involves an interprofessional approach in which team members, including nurses, are trained in geropsychiatry. Nurses often function as case managers. Nurse-led collaborative care for persons with persistent illness results in improved depression symptoms (McKenzie & Harvath, 2016; Markle-Reid et al., 2014). (See Chapter 15 for an in-depth discussion of care models.)

Nursing care of a person with depression should take into account the person's comorbid medical conditions and abilities. Priorities for nursing care are outlined in Box 24.6.

Somatic Therapies and Medications

Electroconvulsive therapy (ECT) is considered a somatic therapy. It is more often used for older people with psychotic depression, those who do not respond to antidepressant medications, and those who have a high suicide risk. People who have received no treatment, treatment of short duration, or treatment with inadequate doses of medication may respond quite well to ECT. The advantage of ECT as compared to medications is its rapid treatment response with minimal side effects (McKenzie & Harvath, 2016; Edelstein et al., 2015).

BOX 24.5   Suggestions for Family and Providers of Interpersonal Support

- Provide relief from the discomfort of physical illness.
- Enhance physical function (i.e., regular exercise or activity; physical, occupational, and recreational therapies).
- Develop a daily activity schedule that includes pleasant activities.
- Increase opportunities for socialization and enhance social support.
- Provide opportunities for decision making and exercising control.
- Focus on spiritual renewal and rediscovery of meaning.
- Reactivate latent interests, or help develop new ones.
- Validate depressed feelings as a means of aiding recovery (i.e., do not try to bolster the person's mood or deny his or her despair).
- Help the person become aware of the presence of depression, the nature of the symptoms, and the time-limited nature of depression.
- Provide an accepting atmosphere and an empathic response.
- Share yourself with the person.
- Demonstrate faith in the person's strengths.
- Praise any and all efforts at recovery, no matter how small.
- Assist the person in expressing and dealing with anger.
- Avoid stifling the grief process; grief cannot be hurried.
- Create a hopeful environment where self-esteem is fostered and life is meaningful.
- Assist the person in dealing with guilt.
- Foster the development of connections with others.

BOX 24.6   Nursing Interventions for Persons With Depression

- Provide a therapeutic relationship with the person.
- Ensure a suicidal person's safety.
- Promote adequate nutrition, elimination, and sleep and rest.
- Provide adequate pain control, including the use of adjunctive relaxation strategies.
- Encourage daily exercise.
- Facilitate support from family and friends.
- Facilitate engagement in pleasant activities.
- Maximize patient control and autonomy.
- Acknowledge and support strengths, capabilities, and hope.

Source: Adapted from McKenzie, G. L., & Harvath, T. A. (2016). Late-life depression. In M. Boltz, E. Capezuti, T. T. Fulmer, et al. (Eds.), *Evidenced-based geriatric nursing protocols for best practice* (5th ed.) (pp. 211–232). New York, NY: Springer Publishing Company.

---

is similar to that in younger adults, and about half of the people who are prescribed a given antidepressant respond to it. Even with therapeutic doses, many people do not experience complete symptom resolution and may have to try several different antidepressants before finding one that is effective (McKenzie & Harvath, 2016). Therapy is continued for 4 to 6 months. For those with more severe or recurring depression, it is recommended that medication be continued for up to 3 years (Edelstein et al., 2015).

SUICIDE

In 2013, 623 Canadians aged 65 years and older (488 men and 135 women) were known to have died by suicide (Statistics Canada, 2017a). The rate of suicide among men aged 85 years and older is the highest in the population, over twice the national rate (34 per 100,000 for men aged 85–89 years and 24.7 per 100,000 for men aged 90 years and older) (Statistics Canada, 2017b). Reported suicide rates are believed to underestimate the true number of suicides, because suicide is often mistaken for accidental death, and stigmatization leads to a reluctance to label a death suicide. Rates of **suicidal behaviour** are thought to be lower for older persons than for younger adults. However, older persons who have suicidal behaviour

Medication therapies are effective in managing depression. The most commonly prescribed are selective serotonin reuptake inhibitors (SSRIs) and serotonin-norepinephrine reuptake inhibitors (SNRIs). Tricyclic antidepressants are rarely used for older persons because of significant side effects and risks. The SSRIs are generally well tolerated in older people; common side effects include nausea, vomiting, dizziness, drowsiness, and hyponatremia (see Chapter 14).

Medications must be closely monitored for side effects and therapeutic response. Doses should be lower at first and titrated as indicated (McKenzie & Harvath, 2016). Most antidepressants take about 6 weeks to have a therapeutic effect. The response rate

are more likely to use lethal methods such as hanging, poisoning, and firearms.

One of the most significant risk factors for suicide is depressive disorder. Other mental disorders (including anxiety, schizophrenia, and substance use disorders) are also important risk factors for suicide in older persons (Vasiliadis et al., 2017). As many as 97% of older persons who die of suicide have a mental illness (Fiske et al., 2015). Hopelessness, a symptom of depression, is also an indicator of suicide risk. Physical health problems such as disability, pain, or multiple serious illnesses—particularly when they are accompanied by depression—confer risk for suicide (McKenzie & Harvath, 2016). Social isolation, loneliness, family discord, and the perception of oneself as a burden are associated with suicidal thoughts (Fiske et al., 2015). Suicide risk is higher for persons who have access to lethal means.

As many as half of older persons who die by suicide have visited a physician within 1 month before death, but their depression symptoms and suicidal ideation are not recognized (McKenzie & Harvath, 2016). Older persons who are depressed or suicidal often present to their primary care providers with somatic rather than psychological symptoms, which suggests that opportunities for assessing suicidal risk may be missed.

Risk factors and resiliency or protective factors are presented in Boxes 24.7 and 24.8. Having a purpose in life and feeling that life is meaningful are important resiliency factors for older persons (Heisel & Flett, 2016). Of importance, risk factors interact with one another.

 IMPLICATIONS FOR GERONTOLOGICAL NURSING AND HEALTHY AGING

ASSESSMENT

Older people with suicidal ideas and intent are encountered in many settings. It is the nurse's obligation to prevent suicide whenever possible. Nurses should be vigilant in recognizing suicide risk factors and assessing suicide potential, not only among persons who experience mood disorders but also among those with no apparent mental disorder. The

---

BOX 24.7 Suicide Risk Factors Among Older Persons

- Older age
- Previous suicidal behaviour
- Thoughts of suicide or wanting to die
- Mental illness (major depressive disorder, mood disorder, psychotic disorder, or any mental disorder)
- Substance misuse
- Medical illness (visual impairment, seizure disorder, neurological disorder, cancer, chronic obstructive pulmonary disease, arthritis, pain)
- Functional impairment
- Personality disorders, rigid personality
- Social, physical, or financial loss
- Negative life events and transitions (including changes in housing)
- Lack of a confidante, or being lonely
- Being unmarried, living alone, or having limited social interaction

Source: Adapted from Canadian Coalition for Seniors' Mental Health (CCSMH). (2006). *National guidelines for seniors' mental health: Assessment of suicide risk and prevention of suicide.* Toronto, ON: Author. Retrieved from http://www.ccsmh.ca.

BOX 24.8 Suicide Resiliency Factors Among Older Persons

Positive Health Care Practices and Adaptive Coping
- Contact with family and friends
- Moderate alcohol consumption
- Active interests
- Religious practice and spirituality
- Extroversion, openness to experience, and conscientiousness
- Perceived meaning in life
- Future orientation

Source: Adapted from Canadian Coalition for Seniors' Mental Health (CCSMH). (2006). *National guidelines for seniors' mental health: Assessment of suicide risk and prevention of suicide.* Toronto, ON: Author. Retrieved from http://www.ccsmh.ca.

---

major risk factors for suicide are detectable and any direct, indirect, or enigmatic references to the ending of life must be taken seriously and discussed with the person. Putting affairs in order in preparation for death (e.g., giving away possessions and making wills and funeral plans) is a warning sign of suicide. However, this behaviour may be difficult to interpret among older persons, as such behaviours are typically indications of maturity.

The most important task for the nurse is to establish a trusting and respectful relationship with the person. Since many older people grew up in an era when suicide bore stigma and even criminal implications, they may not bring up their suicidal thoughts. It is important to accept and validate the person's suicidal symptoms. Self-awareness on the part of the nurse is important. Nurses should be careful to avoid statements that normalize thoughts of suicide and should avoid statements that could be perceived as judgemental.

Nurses may be reluctant to ask questions about suicide because of a myth that talking about suicide will incite suicidal ideation. This is not true. Talking about suicide does not increase suicide risk. Rather, in the context of assessment and discussion about the meaning of stressors in life, the person experiences being asked about suicide as validation of the person's experience and as, therefore, relieving. By talking about suicide, nurses demonstrate interest in the individual and open the door to honest interaction and connection at deep levels of psychological need. Superficial interest and mechanical questioning will not be meaningful. What will make a difference is the nature of the nurse's concern and nurse's ability to connect with the alienation and desperation of the individual.

If there is suspicion that the older person is suicidal, the use of direct and straightforward questions, such as the following, is most helpful:

- How often have you thought about dying or killing yourself?
- How often do you feel like life isn't worth living?
- How would you kill yourself if you decided to do it?

In addition to examining risk factors and suicide intent, the assessment should also include lethality, access to means, and the presence of protective factors. It is important to obtain collateral information from family, friends, and other care providers who know the older person. Detailed interview questions for assessing suicidal ideation and plans are available in the Registered Nurses' Association of Ontario's Best Practice Guideline, *Assessment and Care of Adults at Risk for Suicidal Ideation and Behaviour*. When

a person is intoxicated, it is difficult to complete an accurate assessment. In such cases, immediate risk should be assessed and the person's safety ensured until the person is sober and the assessment can be completed (Registered Nurses' Association of Ontario [RNAO], 2009).

INTERVENTIONS

It is important to have in place a suicide protocol that clearly defines how the nurse will intervene if a positive response is obtained from the suicide assessment. The person should not be left alone until help arrives to assist and care for them. If a person is at risk of suicide, access to lethal means of suicide should be limited. People at high risk should be hospitalized, especially if they have current psychological stressors, access to lethal means of suicide, or both. People at moderate risk may be treated as outpatients, provided they have adequate social support and no access to lethal means. Persons at lower risk should have a full psychiatric evaluation and be followed up carefully (Das et al., 2007). Box 24.9 presents interventions to perform if suicidal intent has been established. Interventions should address underlying mental disorders and risk factors such as isolation, hopelessness, pain, and loss.

SUBSTANCE USE DISORDERS

Substance use disorders in older people can be a continuation of long-term problems, or they can arise in older age, often in the context of stressful life events or other stressors. One-third of older persons who are seen by addiction specialists experience the onset of their problems in older age (Centre for Addiction and Mental Health [CAMH], 2008).

This section discusses substance use disorders and substance misuse and focuses on alcohol, prescription medication, and illicit drugs. See Chapter 6 for information about smoking cessation. Risk factors for substance use disorders in older persons are presented in Box 24.10. Terms used to describe substance use disorder are defined in Table 24.1.

ALCOHOL

The most common type of substance use disorder is problem drinking (Naegle & McCabe, 2016).

BOX 24.9	Interventions for the Older Adult With Suicidal Intent

If suicidal intent has been established, the following interventions, arranged in order of immediacy, are necessary:

1. Reduce immediate danger by removing hazardous articles.
2. Do not leave the person alone; evaluate the need for constant attendance; and arrange for a family member, a friend, or a health care provider to be present during the period of immediate danger.
3. Provide an honest expression of concern, such as "I do not want you to take your life. I will help you with this troubling situation."
4. Consult with a mental health professional and evaluate the person for possible hospitalization.
5. Find out whether a "no-suicide contract" can be drawn up with the person; however, there is no evidence that such an agreement is effective in preventing suicide.
6. Evaluate the need for medication.
7. Focus on the hazard or crisis that is currently causing the most stress on the person.
8. Mobilize internal and external resources by getting the person reinvolved with external supports and reconnected with his or her internal capabilities. The health care provider, family, or caregiver may have to take the initiative to find activities, support systems, transportation, and other resources for the individual.
9. Implement a specific plan of action with an ongoing structured program. Develop a lifeline of individuals who can be called on at any hour of distress, and plan regular calls and follow-up for the individual.

BOX 24.10	Risk Factors for Substance Use Disorders

1. Family history of dependence on alcohol, tobacco, or prescription or illicit drugs
2. Co-occurrence of addiction with dependency or abuse of another substance dependence (e.g., alcohol and tobacco)
3. Lifelong pattern of substance use, including heavy drinking
4. Male gender
5. Social isolation
6. Recent and multiple losses
7. Persistent pain
8. Co-occurrence with depression
9. Unmarried, living alone, or both

Source: Extracted from Naegle, M. (2012). *Nursing standard of practice protocol: Substance abuse in older adults.* Retrieved from https://consultgeri.org/geriatric-topics/substance-abuse.

TABLE 24.1	Definitions of Substance Misuse Terms

TERM	DEFINITION
Substance use disorder	A broad category of disorders that include a continuum of use or misuse of alcohol, tobacco, prescription or illicit drugs, and the abuse or dependence on these drugs.
Substance abuse	A maladaptive pattern of substance use evidenced by recurrent and significant adverse consequences related to the repeated use of substances.
Substance dependence	A pattern of self-administration of a drug that is maladaptive and results in the development of tolerance, withdrawal, and compulsive drug-taking behaviour. Dependence is both physiological and psychological.
Medication misuse	Use of a medication for purposes other than that for which it was intended.

Source: Extracted from Naegle, M. (2012). *Nursing standard of practice protocol: Substance abuse in older adults.* Retrieved from https://consultgeri.org/geriatric-topics/substance-abuse.

Alcohol-related problems in the older population often go unrecognized, although the long-term effects of alcohol misuse complicate the presentation and treatment of many persistent disorders of older people. About three-quarters of older men and two-thirds of older women drink alcohol occasionally or regularly; for the majority of them, this is not a problem. However, 10 to 13% of older persons have a problem with alcohol use, and the prevalence of unhealthy drinking among men is higher than that among women (Satre & Wolf, 2015). Alcohol use disorders are more likely to emerge in adulthood than in older age, and many people reduce their drinking as they age. For some people, however, the problem emerges or recurs in older age. Late-onset problem drinking may be related to situational events such as illness, retirement, or the death of a spouse, and is more common among women than among men (Satre & Wolf, 2015).

Gender Issues

Men (particularly older widowers) are four times more likely than women to misuse alcohol, but the prevalence of alcohol misuse in women may be underestimated. The number and impact of older female drinkers are expected to increase in the coming years as the disparity between men's and women's drinking decreases (Epstein et al., 2007). Women of all ages are significantly more vulnerable to the effects of alcohol misuse, including drug interactions, physical injury from alcohol-related falls and accidents, cognitive impairment, and liver and heart disease. Health care providers may assume that older women do not drink problematically and not screen for alcohol misuse. Often, alcohol misuse among women is undetected until the consequences are severe.

Medication Effects

Many medications that older persons use for persistent illnesses have adverse effects when combined with alcohol. Alcohol interacts with at least 50% of prescription medications (Naegle & McCabe, 2016). Medications that interact with alcohol include analgesics, antibiotics, antidepressants, benzodiazepines, H_2 receptor antagonists, nonsteroidal anti-inflammatory drugs, and herbal medications (e.g., echinacea and valerian). When combined with alcohol, acetaminophen taken on a regular basis may lead to liver failure. Alcohol diminishes the effects of oral hypoglycemics, anticoagulants, and anticonvulsants. All older people should be given precise information about the interaction of alcohol with their medications.

Other effects of alcohol use disorder in older people include urinary incontinence, which results from rapid bladder filling and diminished neuromuscular control of the bladder; gait disturbances from alcohol-induced cerebellar degeneration and peripheral neuropathy; depression and suicide; sleep disturbances and insomnia; dementia; and delirium. Older

persons with alcohol use disorder are also susceptible to cognitive, physical, and functional decline and have increased risk for injury.

Physiology

Normal physiological changes of aging may make older persons more susceptible to problems when they drink alcohol. Increased body fat, decreased lean body mass, and decreased total body water content can result in a higher blood alcohol level for a given dose of alcohol and alter the absorption and distribution of alcohol (Satre & Wolf, 2015). Reduced liver and kidney functioning result in slower alcohol metabolism and elimination. A decrease in the gastric enzyme alcohol dehydrogenase results in slower metabolism of alcohol and higher blood levels for a longer time. Risks of gastro-intestinal ulceration and bleeding may be higher in older people because of the decrease in gastric pH that occurs in aging (Letizia & Reinboltz, 2005).

Because of the high risk of adverse effects from alcohol use, the US National Institute on Alcohol Abuse and Alcoholism recommends that individuals over the age of 65 years limit alcohol consumption to no more than one standard drink per day (that is, 12 ounces of beer, 5 ounces of wine, or 1.5 ounces of liquor) (Barry & Blow, 2015).

OTHER SUBSTANCES

Illicit Drugs

Historically, the use of illicit drugs was rare among older persons. However, this is changing as the "baby boomers" age. Marijuana is the most frequently used illicit drug. A survey conducted by the Centre for Addiction and Mental Health (Ialomiteaunu et al., 2015) indicated that 7.2% of individuals aged 50 years and older had used cannabis in the previous year, an increase from 2.6% in 2005. The same survey found that 3.5% of those aged 50 years and older reported nonmedical use of an opioid. The prevalence of substance misuse among older persons is expected to increase as the last of the baby boomers (who are more likely than their older counterparts to use illicit drugs) enter older age. A person's use of an illicit substance does not necessarily mean that the person has a substance use disorder; the use of illicit drugs is problematic when it interferes with the person's health, functioning, relationships, responsibilities, or safety.

Prescription and Over-the-Counter Medications

Among older persons, the misuse of prescription and OTC medications is more common than illicit drug use. Medication misuse is defined as use of a medication for reasons other than those for which it was prescribed. More than 33% of all prescriptions for medications are to older people, and the nonmedical use of prescription medications is increasing in people over 60 years of age. The inappropriate use of benzodiazepines and barbiturates is especially problematic for older women, who are more likely than men to receive prescriptions for these medications (Epstein et al., 2007). One-quarter of older persons are prescribed a medication that potentially can be misused, such as benzodiazepines and opioid analgesics (Naegle & McCabe, 2016). Higher rates of illness and mortality are associated with misusing prescription and nonprescription medications.

Most older persons who misuse medications do so unintentionally in the following ways: not taking the medication as directed; using a medication for reasons other than those for which it was intended (e.g., taking dimenhydrinate [Gravol] for sleep); using old medications to treat new or recurring symptoms; taking herbal remedies without consulting a pharmacist; sharing medications with other people; obtaining prescriptions from multiple physicians; drinking alcohol while taking prescription medication; and taking prescription and OTC medications that interact (CAMH, 2008). Some of the reasons for the misuse of psychoactive prescription medications may be inappropriate prescribing, inadequate health teaching about medication, ineffective monitoring of response, and ineffective follow-up. In many instances, older people are given prescriptions for benzodiazepines or sedatives because of complaints of insomnia or nervousness, without adequate assessment for depression, anxiety, or other conditions that may be causing the symptoms. Misuse of benzodiazepines and barbiturates increases the risk for sedation, balance problems, falls, and delirium (see Chapter 21). These risks increase with concurrent use of alcohol. Withdrawal from benzodiazepines in older persons is risky and complex and requires careful monitoring.

IMPLICATIONS FOR GERONTOLOGICAL NURSING AND HEALTHY AGING

ASSESSMENT

Routine screening for misuse of alcohol, prescription drugs, and illicit drugs is recommended. It is important to establish rapport and explain the reasons for the questions. The questions should be easy to understand and be presented in a manner similar to that of questions in a routine assessment. Screening may include short self-report questionnaires or may be part of an assessment interview (Barry & Blow, 2015). A caring and supportive approach that provides a safe and open atmosphere is the foundation of the therapeutic relationship. It may also be helpful to discuss the issue factually. For example, the nurse might explain that "Many older people find that the stresses, loneliness, and losses of aging are very hard to bear. Some retreat into alcohol or medication use as a way of coping. There are treatments and groups that help people make these difficult adjustments. If this is a problem for you, or if it becomes a problem, please let us know so we may provide resources or referrals for you." It is always important to search for the pain beneath the behaviour. Box 24.11 lists pre-screening questions whose answers may alert the nurse to a need for more complete screening and assessment.

Positive responses to screening questions or suspected substance misuse indicates the need for a more comprehensive assessment, including medical history, physical examination, cognitive assessment, functional assessment, and review of medications. Screening for alcohol use, drug use, and depression is important. Diagnostic tests should include a complete blood count, liver function tests, chemistries, and an electro-cardiogram.

Similar to previously described mental disorders, many health care providers do not routinely screen for alcohol misuse or other substance misuse in older persons. This lack of screening may be related to poor symptom recognition, inadequate knowledge about screening instruments, lack of age-appropriate diagnostic criteria for misuse by older people, and ageism. The signs of substance use disorders and misuse among older people may be mistaken for dementia or depression. Furthermore, health care providers

BOX 24.11	Pre-Screening Questions for Alcohol and Prescription Drug Misuse

Pre-screening question: "Do you drink beer, wine, or other alcoholic beverages?"

Follow-up (if yes): "How many times in the [past year; past three months; past six months] have you had five or more drinks in a day (for men)/four or more drinks in a day (for women)?"

"On average, how many days per week do you drink alcoholic beverages?" *If weekly or more,* "On a day when you drink alcohol, how many drinks do you have?"

Pre-screening questions: "Do you use prescription medicines for pain? Anxiety? Sleep? Do you use any of these prescription drugs in a way that is different from how they were prescribed?"

Follow-up: If yes, follow up with additional questions regarding which substances, frequency, and quantity of use.

Source: Extracted from Barry, K. L., & Blow, F. C. (2015). Substance use, misuse, and abuse: Special issues for older adults. In N. A. Pachana & K. Laidlaw (Eds.), *The Oxford Handbook of Clinical Geropsychology* (p. 10). Oxford: Oxford University Press. By permission of Oxford University Press. doi:10.1093/oxfordhb/9780199663170.013.015.

BOX 24.12	Signs and Symptoms of Potential Alcohol Problems in Older Adults

Mental
- Memory difficulties after having a drink
- Trouble finishing sentences
- Being unsure of oneself
- Irritability, sadness, depression, trouble concentrating
- Not remembering to pay bills; spending money on alcohol rather than paying bills

Physical
- Intoxication
- Loss of coordination (walking unsteadily, frequent falls)
- Broad-based gait (lurching quality; difficulty turning; difficulty walking in a straight line)
- Digestion problems such as gastric reflux, irritation in the stomach lining
- Significant weight gain in abdominal area or weight loss
- Poor nutrition
- Flu-like symptoms
- Problems swallowing
- Changes in sleeping or eating habits
- Unexplained bruises (especially at furniture level)
- Unexplained persistent pain
- Jaundice or anemia
- Swollen abdomen
- Not bathing or keeping clean
- Urinary incontinence

Social
- Difficulty staying in touch with family or friends
- Lack of interest in usual activities
- Desire to remain alone much of the time
- Socializes only with drinking buddies
- Gives up activities that the person used to enjoy

Environmental
- Furniture, carpet burns
- Difficulty keeping housing

Source: Extracted from Centre for Addiction and Mental Health [CAMH]. (2008). *Improving our response to older adults with substance use, mental health and gambling problems: A guide for supervisors, managers and clinical staff.* Toronto, ON: Author (pp. 40–41).

may be pessimistic about the ability of older people to change longstanding problems (Naegle & McCabe, 2016).

Alcohol

People with alcohol use disorders often reject or deny the diagnosis, or they may take offense at the suggestion of it. Feelings of shame or disgrace may make older persons reluctant to disclose a drinking problem. This may be especially true among older women from cultural backgrounds in which alcohol use is highly discouraged (Finfgeld-Connett, 2004). Members of the families of older people with substance misuse disorders (particularly adult children) may be ashamed of the problem and may choose not to address it. Box 24.12 lists signs and symptoms that may indicate alcohol problems in older persons.

Positive responses to pre-screening questions about alcohol use may be followed by the use of a screening instrument such as the Michigan Alcoholism Screening Test, Geriatric Version (MAST-G) (available at https://consultgeri.org) or the Alcohol Use Disorders Identification Test (AUDIT) to identify problem drinking or dependence. The AUDIT has good validity for ethnically mixed groups and for older persons (Naegle & McCabe, 2016).

Because of the high risk for depression among heavy drinkers, assessment and screening for depression is also important when alcohol misuse is

BOX 24.13 Questions to Ask the Person About Potential Medication Misuse

- Do you take your medication regularly?
- How often do you skip or forget to take your medication?
- Do you ever have difficulty remembering when to take your medication?
- Do you ever take medication that belongs to someone else?
- Which doctor knows all the medications you are taking?
- Do you ever drink alcohol while you are also taking medication, without checking with a doctor or pharmacist?
- What do you do with old unused medications that are no long prescribed?

Source: Extracted from Centre for Addiction and Mental Health [CAMH]. (2008). *Improving our response to older adults with substance use, mental health and gambling problems: A guide for supervisors, managers and clinical staff.* Toronto, ON: Author (pp. 72–73).

BOX 24.14 Adapting Alcohol Treatment Interventions for Older Persons

- Take into account vision, hearing, and other functional impairments.
- Provide easy access and transportation if needed.
- Address issues such as loss, grief, and health problems.
- Include relevant topics such as worries about the future, including worries about independent living, grandparenting, being retired, and having a fixed income.
- Consider using life review and reminiscence techniques.
- Use a respectful rather than confrontational approach.
- Slow the pace of treatment.
- Use case management and interprofessional approaches.
- Address spiritual needs.
- Tailor treatment to the level of cognitive function.
- Provide opportunities for interesting activities and socialization opportunities that do not involve drinking.
- Focus on strengths and past coping skills used during difficult times.
- Demonstrate faith in the person's ability to change, and avoid ageist attitudes.
- Consider groups designed for women only, as their needs are different.

Sources: Adapted from Epstein, E., Fischer-Elber, K., & Al-Otaiba, Z. (2007). Women, aging, and alcohol use disorders. *Journal of Women & Aging, 19*(1/2), 31–48; Malatesta, V. (Ed.). (2007). *Mental health issues of older women: A comprehensive review for health care professionals.* Florence, KY: Routledge.

suspected. Screening should also be done before the prescription of any new medications that may interact with alcohol and should be done as needed after life-changing events.

Other Substances

The signs and symptoms of illicit drug use disorder or prescription medication misuse are similar to the signs and symptoms of alcohol use disorder. Additional signs include the presence of the odour of the drug (e.g., as with marijuana) or of drug paraphernalia, problems with memory and concentration, sexual dysfunction, drug-seeking behaviour, headaches, nausea, and constipation (CAMH, 2008). For information about signs of problems specific to particular drugs, see http://www.camh.ca.

When assessing potential misuse of prescription and OTC medications, assessment should include obtaining a comprehensive list of all medications and determining whether they are being used as directed. Some questions to ask as part of this assessment are listed in Box 24.13.

INTERVENTIONS

Nurses should share information with older people about safe drinking and the deleterious effects of alcohol. Alcohol and substance use problems affect physical, mental, spiritual, and emotional health. Nurses should use nonjudgmental approaches. Interventions must address quality of life in all of these spheres and be adapted to meet the unique needs of the older adult (Box 24.14).

Abstinence or reduced harm are the goals of interventions. Older persons may refuse addiction treatment that requires abstinence, and a harm-reduction approach may be more appropriate. "Programs with a harm reduction approach focus on reducing the health, social, financial and other harms of substance use....Clients choose their own goals for making change" (CAMH, 2008, p. 92). Increasing the awareness of older persons about the risks and benefits of consuming alcohol and other substances in the context of their own situation is an important goal

(Merrick et al., 2008). Treatment and intervention strategies include cognitive behavioural approaches, individual and group counselling, medical and psychiatric approaches, referral to Alcoholics Anonymous, family therapy, case management and community and home care services, and formalized substance abuse treatment. Treatment outcomes for older people are similar to or better than outcomes for younger people (Naegle & McCabe, 2016).

Unless the person is in immediate danger, a stepped-care approach should be used, beginning with brief interventions followed by more intensive therapies if necessary. Brief intervention is a time-limited (one meeting to four or five short sessions) patient-centred strategy focused on changing behaviour and assessing the person's readiness to change. Sessions can range from one meeting of 10 to 30 minutes to four or five short sessions. The goals of brief intervention are to (1) reduce or stop consumption of the substance and (2) facilitate entry into formalized treatment if needed. Research results indicate that this type of intervention has positive outcomes for older persons with alcohol use disorders (Barry & Blow, 2015). Older people may be more likely to accept treatment given by their primary care provider (Naegle & McCabe, 2016).

Long-term self-help treatment programs for older persons show high rates of success, especially when social outlets are emphasized and cohort supports are available. A significant concern is the lack of programs designed specifically for older people, particularly older women, whose concerns are very different from those of younger people who misuse drugs or alcohol. Health status, availability of transportation, or impaired mobility may further limit access to treatment. Accessibility can be improved by locating treatment in more accessible settings, such as community health centres, senior centres, and assisted-living residences.

Acute Alcohol Withdrawal

When there is significant physical dependence, withdrawal from alcohol can become a life-threatening emergency. Detoxification should be done in an inpatient setting because of the potential medical complications and because withdrawal symptoms in older persons can be prolonged.

Older people who drink heavily are at risk of experiencing acute alcohol withdrawal if they are admitted to the hospital for treatment of acute illnesses or emergencies. All older persons admitted to acute care settings should be screened for alcohol use and assessed for signs and symptoms of alcohol-related problems. Older persons with a long history of consuming excess alcohol, previous episodes of acute withdrawal, or a history of prior detoxification are at increased risk of acute alcohol withdrawal (Naegle & McCabe, 2016). Symptoms of acute alcohol withdrawal vary. They may be more severe and last longer in older people. Minor withdrawal (withdrawal tremulousness) begins 6 to 12 hours after a person has consumed the last drink. Symptoms include tremor, anxiety, nausea, insomnia, tachycardia, and increased blood pressure, and withdrawal may frequently be mistaken for common problems in older persons. Major withdrawal is seen 10 to 72 hours after cessation of alcohol intake, and the symptoms include vomiting, diaphoresis, hallucinations, tremors, and seizures (Naegle & McCabe, 2016).

Delirium tremens (DT) is alcohol withdrawal delirium; it usually occurs 24 to 72 hours after the last drink but may occur up to 10 days later. Delirium tremens occurs in 5% of persons in acute alcohol withdrawal and is considered a medical emergency; the mortality rate is as high as 15% from respiratory failure and cardiac arrhythmia. Other signs and symptoms include confusion, disorientation, hallucinations, hyperthermia, and hypertension. The Clinical Institute Withdrawal Assessment (CIWA) scale a valid and reliable screening instrument (Larose & Renner, 2016).

Recommended treatment is the use of short-acting benzodiazepines at one-half to one-third the normal dose around the clock or as needed during withdrawal. Disulfiram (Antabuse) use in older persons to promote abstinence is not recommended, because of the potential for serious cardio-vascular complications. The use of oral or intravenous alcohol to prevent or treat withdrawal is not established.

The CIWA scale aids the adjustment of medication. Other interventions are assessing mental status, monitoring vital signs, and maintaining fluid balance without overhydrating the patient. Calm and quiet surroundings, no unnecessary stimuli, consistent caregivers, frequent reorientation, prevention of injury, and support and caring are additional suggested interventions. Nutritional assessment is indicated, as well as the addition of a thiamine and multivitamins (Naegle & McCabe, 2016).

PROBLEM GAMBLING

About three-quarters of Canadians participate in some form of gambling, whether it be through lotteries or bingo; at casinos or race tracks; or, in some provinces, at video lottery terminals (Cox et al., 2005). An Ontario survey indicated that older persons are less likely than middle-aged adults to gamble (77% and 85%, respectively) (Williams & Volberg, 2013). On average, Canadians spend about $536 per person per year on gambling, and the total revenue from government-operated gambling in 2013 was $13.7 billion (Canadian Partnership for Responsible Gambling, 2015). When asked why they gamble, older persons most commonly answer that they gamble for entertainment or fun, to socialize, to support charitable causes, to relieve boredom or loneliness, to make money, and to take advantage of promotions offered to older persons at casinos and race tracks (Community Links, 2010).

Problem gambling is gambling that (1) interferes with work, school, or other activities; (2) harms the person's mental or physical health; (3) hurts the person financially; (4) damages the person's reputation; or (5) causes problems with family or social relationships (CAMH, 2008). Between 1% and 2% of older persons report problem gambling (Subramaniam et al., 2015). Problem gambling can cause anxiety and depression and is a risk factor for suicide. It is more common among those with a history of mental illness or substance abuse. When problem gambling emerges in older persons, it is often related to emotional distress (Tira et al., 2014). The negative effects of problem gambling include financial loss for the person and his or her family, strained family relationships, a higher risk of experiencing physical and emotional abuse, and a higher risk for physical and mental illnesses, both for the person and for family members (Subramaniam et al., 2015).

 IMPLICATIONS FOR GERONTOLOGICAL NURSING AND HEALTHY AGING

ASSESSMENT

That persons affected by problem gambling may hide or deny the problem (possibly owing to shame, embarrassment, fear of the consequences of disclosure, or hopelessness) complicates assessment. A direct question about problem gambling is not likely to be effective (CAMH, 2009). A nonjudgemental approach is important. Screening for problem gambling can be integrated into the assessment of recreation and leisure activities and the assessment of financial well-being. Nurses should be aware of the signs of problem gambling (Box 24.15). A detailed list of behavioural, emotional, financial, and health signs of problem gambling, as well as screening tools for problem gambling, are available from the Centre for Addiction and Mental Health (CAMH) (https://www.problemgambling.ca). The CAMH gambling screen is a short self-assessment and screening tool (Box 24.16). A score of 0 indicates that the person does not have a gambling problem; a score of 3 or higher is highly indicative of a gambling problem. If the score is 3 or higher but the person responded "once" to the last question, the person probably does not have a gambling problem. A score of 2 indicates that the person may be developing a problem. If problem gambling is suspected, the Problem Gambling Severity Index can be used (available at https://www.problemgambling.ca).

BOX 24.15 Signs of Problem Gambling

- Spending more on gambling than intended
- Feeling bad, sad, or guilty about gambling
- Not having enough money for food, rent, or bills
- Being unable to account for blocks of time
- Experiencing social withdrawal
- Experiencing anxiety or depression

Source: Extracted from Centre for Addiction and Mental Health. (2006). *Responding to older adults with substance use, mental health and gambling challenges: A guide for workers and volunteers.* Toronto, ON: Author (p. 31). Retrieved from http://www.camh.net/Publications/Resources_for_Professionals/Older_Adults/responding_older_adults.pdf.

BOX 24.16   Centre for Addiction and Mental Health Gambling Screen

1. In the past 12 months, have you gambled more than you intended to?
2. In the past 12 months, have you claimed to be winning money when you were not?
3. In the past 12 months, have you felt guilty about the way you gamble or about what happens when you gamble?
4. In the past 12 months, have people criticized you for your gambling?
5. In the past 12 months, have you had money arguments centred on gambling?
6. In the past 12 months, did you feel you had to persist until you won?
7. If you answered "yes" to two or more of these questions, how often has it happened? Once, only sometimes, or often?

Source: Centre for Addition and Mental Health. (2011). *CAMH Gambling Screen.* Retrieved from http://www.problemgambling.ca/EN/Resources-ForProfessionals/Pages/CAMHGamblingScreen.aspx.

INTERVENTIONS

Public education and increased public awareness of problem gambling contributes to prevention, early identification, and earlier treatment of gambling. A good educational tool is *Betting on Older Adults: A Problem Gambling Awareness Kit,* which includes a video, interactive games, and a facilitator's guide (https://www.problemgambling.ca). All provinces have gambling help lines and websites with information about accessing services. When problem gambling is identified, the person should be referred to a mental health provider. Specialized gambling counselling is available through addiction treatment services. Peer support may be especially important for reaching and helping older persons who are at risk for or are experiencing problem gambling (Community Links, 2010). Therapeutic approaches include CBT, motivational interviewing (MI), psychotherapy, aversion therapy, the 12-step program, and self-exclusion. The evidence of effectiveness is greatest for CBT and MI; evidence for other approaches is weaker (Merkouris et al., 2016). Although older people may be more likely to drop out of treatment, older age is associated with better treatment outcomes (Merkouris et al., 2016). It is important to address the comorbid medical and mental health conditions of persons who have problem gambling. Self-help tools and resources for families are available in 22 languages at https://www.problemgambling.ca.

IMPLICATIONS FOR GERONTOLOGICAL NURSING AND HEALTHY AGING

The development of holistic and humanistic models of care for older people experiencing mental health disturbances is critically important in gerontological nursing. Much of the distress associated with mental disorders in late life can be relieved through competent, caring, and compassionate gerontological nursing care. An awareness of appropriate assessment and treatment of the mental illnesses that can occur in late life is a very important component of best practice care.

Knowing and appreciating each older person's uniqueness, his or her past and present experiences, and how these experiences colour the present are important to promoting mental health and wellness. Believing in and supporting the strength and wisdom of older people supports their self-confidence and feelings of worth, important components of mental health and wellness. To appreciate the nature of loss and grief in old age, gerontological nurses need to really listen and offer support. Nurses' work must focus on the development of environments of care that enhance physical and mental health and wellness, create conditions of hope, and support older persons.

KEY CONCEPTS

- Mental health in later life is difficult to determine, because the accrual of life experiences results in great variability in the mental health of older persons.
- Mental health is a fluctuating situation for most individuals, with peaks and valleys of happiness and pain.

- The prevalence of mental disorders is expected to increase significantly with the aging of the baby boomers.
- Mental disorders are underreported and underdiagnosed among older persons. Somatic complaints are often the presenting symptoms of mental disorders, making diagnosis difficult.
- The incidence of psychotic disorders with late-life onset is low among older people, but psychotic manifestations can occur as secondary symptoms in a variety of disorders, the most common of which is Alzheimer's disease. The psychotic symptoms of Alzheimer's disease necessitate different assessment and treatment from those of long-standing psychotic disorders.
- Anxiety disorders are common in later life and can be successfully treated.
- Post-traumatic stress disorder is finally being recognized in older persons who have been subjected to extremely traumatic events.
- Depression is the most common mental disorder of aging and is the most treatable. Unfortunately, it is often neglected or assumed to be a condition of aging that one must "learn to live with." An important nursing intervention is assessment of depression.
- Suicide is a significant problem among older men. Assessment of suicidal intent is important, especially in the light of loss. Many older persons who die of suicide are seen by a health care provider and present with physical complaints shortly before they die.
- Substance misuse (particularly that of alcohol) and the misuse of prescription medications are often underrecognized and undertreated problems of older persons, especially for women. Screening and appropriate assessment and intervention are important in all settings.
- Problem gambling can have significant consequences for older persons and their families. Public education and increased awareness of problem gambling are needed for prevention, early identification, and effective treatment.
- Further research is needed to fully understand the cultural and ethnic differences in peoples' mental health concerns and to appropriately assess and treat older people of various cultures and ethnicities.

ACTIVITIES AND DISCUSSION QUESTIONS

1. List the various stressors you have encountered with the older people you have cared for and discuss what was done about them.
2. Discuss the three most common mental disorders that older persons are likely to experience, and describe appropriate assessment and treatment.
3. Explain what is likely to be different in the appearance of depression in a person who is 70 years old from that in a person who is 20 years old.
4. Describe the behaviours that are indicative of suicidal intent in an older person. Discuss the methods of assessment and your reactions to them.
5. Discuss the various situations that may result in an older person's substance abuse and ways to effectively intervene.
6. Describe the type of teaching on the use of alcohol and medications you would use to provide this information to an older person.
7. Formulate strategies that may be used to promote mental health and wellness in late life.

RESOURCES

AUDIT alcohol screening
https://patient.info/doctor/alcohol-use-disorders -identification-test-audit

Betting on Older Adults: A Problem Gambling Prevention Clinical Manual for Service Providers
https://www.problemgambling.ca/EN/Documents/ Betting%20on%20Older%20Adults%20Manual.pdf

Canadian Academy of Geriatric Psychiatry (CAGP)
http://www.cagp.ca

Canadian Coalition for Seniors' Mental Health (CCSMH)
https://www.ccsmh.ca

Canadian Mental Health Association (CMHA)
https://www.cmha.ca

Centre for Addiction and Mental Health (CAMH)
http://www.camh.ca

Mental Health Commission of Canada
https://www.mentalhealthcommission.ca

Mood Disorders Society of Canada
https://mdsc.ca/

National Coalition on Mental Health and Aging (NCMHA)
http://www.ncmha.org

Schizophrenia Society of Canada
http://www.schizophrenia.ca

For additional resources, please visit *http://evolve .elsevier.com/Canada/Ebersole/gerontological/*

REFERENCES

Adams, L. Y., Koop, P., Quan, H., et al. (2015). A population-based comparison of the use of acute healthcare services by older adults with and without mental illness diagnoses. *Journal of Psychiatric and Mental Health Nursing*, 22(1), 39–46. doi:10.1111/jpm.12169.

Alexopoulos, G., Young, J., & Shamoian, C. (1988). Cornell Scale for Depression in Dementia. *Biological Psychiatry*, 23, 271–284. doi:10.1016/0006-3223(88)90038-8.

American Psychiatric Association (APA). (2013). *Diagnostic and statistical manual for mental disorders* (5th ed.). Washington, DC: American Psychiatric Association.

American Psychological Association (APA). (2014). *Primary care.* Retrieved from https://www.apa.org/health/briefs/primary-care .pdf.

Austin, W., & Boyd, M. A. (2010). *Psychiatric and mental health nursing for Canadian practice* (2nd ed.). New York, NY: Lippincott Williams & Wilkins.

Ayers, C., Strickland, K., & Wetherell, J. L. (2015). Evidence-based treatment for late-life generalized anxiety disorder. In P. A. Areán (Ed.), *Treatment of late-life depression, anxiety, trauma, and substance abuse* (pp. 111–139). Washington, DC: American Psychological Association.

Barry, K. L., & Blow, F. C. (2015). Substance use, misuse, and abuse: Special issues for older adults. In N. A. Pachana & K. Laidlaw (Eds.), *The Oxford handbook of clinical geropsychology.* Oxford, UK: Oxford University Press. doi:10.1093/oxfordhb/9780199663170.013.015.

Bower, E. S., & Wetherell, J. L. (2015). Late-life anxiety disorders. In P. A. Lichtenberg, B. T. Mast, B. D. Carpenter, et al. (Eds.), *APA handbook of clinical geropsychology* (Vol. 2). Assessment, treatment, and issues in later life. Washington, DC: American Psychological Association.

Byrd, E. (2005). Nursing assessment and treatment of depressive disorders of late life. In K. Mellilo & S. Houde (Eds.), *Geropsychiatric and mental health nursing.* Sudbury, MA: Jones and Bartlett.

Canadian Coalition for Seniors' Mental Health (CCSMH). (2006). *National guidelines for seniors' mental health: The assessment and treatment of mental health issues in long term care homes.* Toronto, ON: Author. Retrieved from http://www.ccsmh.ca.

Canadian Institute for Health Information (CIHI). (2010). *Analysis in brief: Depression among seniors in residential care: Highlights of study findings.* Retrieved from https://secure.cihi.ca/free_products/ccrs_depression_among_seniors_e.pdf.

Canadian Mental Health Association (CMHA). (n.d.). *Demographic and prevalence statistics.* Retrieved from www.ontario.cmha.ca/seniors.asp?cID=5801.

Canadian Partnership for Responsible Gambling. (2015). *Canadian gambling digest 2013-2014.* Retrieved from http://www .responsiblegambling.org/docs/default-source/default-document -library/cprg_canadian-gambling-digest_2013-14.pdf.

Carlino, A. R., Stinnett, J. L., & Kim, D. R. (2013). New onset of bipolar disorder in late life. *Psychosomatics*, 54(1), 94–97. doi:10.1016/j.psym.2012.01.006.

Ceglowski, J., de Dios, L. V., & Depp, C. A. (2015). Psychosis in older adults. In N. A. Pachana & K. Laidlaw (Eds.), *The Oxford handbook of clinical geropsychology.* Oxford, UK: Oxford University Press. doi:10.1093/oxfordhb/9780199663170.013 .041.

Centre for Addiction and Mental Health (CAMH). (2008). *Improving our response to older adults with substance use, mental health and gambling problems: A guide for supervisors, managers and clinical staff.* Toronto, ON: Author.

Centre for Addiction and Mental Health (CAMH). (2009). *Info on problem gambling.* Retrieved from http://www.camh.net/About _Addiction_Mental_Health/AMH101/top_searched_prob _gambling.html#effectsofpg.

Community Links. (2010). *Seniors and gambling: A hidden problem? A report of the Seniors and Gambling Project.* Retrieved from http://www.nscommunitylinks.ca/publications/Seniorsand Gambling.pdf.

Cook, J. M., & Dinnen, S. (2015). Exposure therapy for late-life trauma. In P. A. Areán (Ed.), *Treatment of late-life depression, anxiety, trauma, and substance abuse* (pp. 133–161). Washington, DC: American Psychological Association.

Cox, B. J., Yu, N., Afifi, T., et al. (2005). A national survey of gambling problems in Canada. *Canadian Journal of Psychiatry*, 50(4), 213–217.

Das, B., Greenspan, M., Muralee, S., et al. (2007). Late-life depression: A review. *Clinical Geriatrics*, 15(10), 35–44.

DiNapoli, E. A., & Scogin, F. R. (2015). Late-life depression. In N. A. Pachana & K. Laidlaw (Eds.), *The Oxford handbook of clinical geropsychology.* Oxford, UK: Oxford University Press. doi:10.1093/oxfordhb/9780199663170.001.0001.

Dixon, C. M. (2009). The unmet needs of those aging with schizophrenia. *Occupational Therapy Now*, 11(1), 4–5. Retrieved from http://www.caot.ca/site/fm/archivesotnow?nav=sidebar.

Dols, A., Rhebergen, D., Beekman, A., et al. (2014). Psychiatric and medical comorbidities: Results from a bipolar elderly cohort study. *The American Journal of Geriatric Psychiatry*, 22(11), 1066–1074. doi:10.1016/j.jagp.2013.12.176.

Edelstein, B. A., Bamonti, P. M., Gregg, J. J., et al. (2015). Depression in later life. In P. A. Lichtenberg, B. T. Mast, B. D. Carpenter, et al. (Eds.), *APA handbook of clinical geropsychology*: Vol. 2, Assessment, treatment, and issues in later life (pp. 15–59). Washington, DC: American Psychological Association.

Epstein, E., Fischer-Elber, K., & Al-Otaiba, Z. (2007). Women, aging, and alcohol use disorders. *Journal of Women & Aging*, 19(1–2), 31–48. doi:10.1300/J074v19n01_03.

Erikson, E. H., Erikson, J. M., & Kivnick, H. Q. (1986). *Vital involvement in old age: The experience of old age in our time*. New York, NY: W.W. Norton.

Finfgeld-Connett, D. L. (2004). Treatment of substance misuse in older women: Using a brief intervention model. *Journal of Gerontological Nursing*, 30(8), 31–37. Retrieved from https://www.healio.com/nursing/journals/jgn.

Fiske, A., Smith, M. D., & Price, E. C. (2015). Suicidal behavior in older adults. In P. A. Lichtenberg, B. T. Mast, B. D. Carpenter, et al. (Eds.), *APA handbook of clinical geropsychology*: Vol. 2, Assessment, treatment, and issues in later life (pp. 154–181). Washington, DC: American Psychological Association.

Geiger, P. J., Boggero, I. A., Brake, C. A., et al. (2016). Mindfulness-based interventions for older adults: A review of the effects on physical and emotional well-being. *Mindfulness*, 7(2), 296–307. doi:10.1007/s12671-015-0444-1.

Guruge, S., Thomson, M. S., & Seifi, S. G. (2015). Mental health and service issues faced by older immigrants in Canada: A scoping review. *Canadian Journal on Aging/La Revue Canadienne du Vieillissement*, 34(04), 431–444. doi:10.1017/S0714980815000379.

Harvath, T. A., & McKenzie, G. L. (2012). *Nursing standard of practice protocol: Depression in older adults*. Retrieved from https://consultgeri.org/geriatric-topics/depression.

Health Canada (2002). *A report on mental illnesses in Canada*. Ottawa, ON: Author. Retrieved from http://www.phac-aspc.gc.ca/publicat/miic-mmac/pdf/men_ill_e.pdf.

Heid, A. R., Christman, Z., Pruchno, R., et al. (2016). Vulnerable, but why? Post-traumatic stress symptoms in older adults exposed to Hurricane Sandy. *Disaster Medicine and Public Health Preparedness*, 10(03), 362–370. doi:10.1017/dmp.2016.15.

Heisel, M. J., & Flett, G. L. (2016). Investigating the psychometric properties of the Geriatric Suicide Ideation Scale (GSIS) among community-residing older adults. *Aging & Mental Health*, 20(2), 208–221. doi:10.1080/13607863.2015.1072798.

Ialomiteanu, A. R., Hamilton, H. A., Adlaf, E. M., et al. (2015). *CAMH monitor ereport 2015: Substance use, mental health and well-being among Ontario adults* (CAMH research document series no. 45). Toronto, ON: CAMH. Retrieved from http://www.camh.ca/en/research/news_and_publications/CAMH%20Monitor/CAMH-Monitor-2015-eReport-Final-Web.pdf.

Jiminez, D. E., Bartels, S. J., Carenas, V., et al. (2013). Stigmatizing attitudes toward mental illness among ethnic older adults in primary care. *International Journal of Geriatric Psychiatry*, 28(10), 1061–1068. doi:10.1002/gps.3928.

Katzman, M. A., Bleau, P., Blier, P., et al. (2014). Canadian clinical practice guidelines for the management of anxiety, posttraumatic stress and obsessive-compulsive disorders. *BMC Psychiatry*, 14(1), S1. doi:10.1186/1471-244X-14-S1-S1.

Kim, W., Kang, S. Y., & Kim, I. (2015). Depression among Korean immigrant elders living in Canada and the United States: A comparative study. *Journal of Gerontological Social Work*, 58(1), 86–103. doi:10.1080/01634372.2014.919977.

Kim, I. H., & Noh, S. (2014). Ethnic and gender differences in the association between discrimination and depressive symptoms among five immigrant groups. *Journal of Immigrant and Minority Health*, 16(6), 1167–1175. doi:10.1007/s10903-013-9969-3.

Kredenster, M. S., Martens, P. J., Chochinov, H. M., et al. (2014). Cause and rate of death in people with schizophrenia across the lifespan: A population-based study in Manitoba, Canada. *The Journal of Clinical Psychiatry*, 75(2), 154–161. doi:10.1016/j.apnu.2015.11.005.

Lamoureux-Lamarche, C., Vasiliadis, H. M., Préville, M., et al. (2016). Post-traumatic stress syndrome in a large sample of older adults: Determinants and quality of life. *Aging & Mental Health*, 20(4), 401–406. doi:10.1080/13607863.2015.1018864.

Larose, A. T., & Renner, J. (2016). Alcohol and older adults. In M. A. Sullivan & F. R. Levin (Eds.), *Addiction in the older patient* (pp. 69–104). Oxford, UK: Oxford University Press.

Lenze, E. J., Hickman, S., Hershey, T., et al. (2014). Mindfulness-based stress reduction for older adults with worry symptoms and co-occurring cognitive dysfunction. *International Journal of Geriatric Psychiatry*, 29(10), 991–1000. doi:10.1002/gps.4086.

Letizia, M., & Reinboltz, M. (2005). Identifying and managing acute alcohol withdrawal in the elderly. *Geriatric Nursing*, 26(3), 176–183. doi:10.1016/j.gerinurse.2005.03.018.

Mackenzie, C. S., Reynolds, K., Cairney, J., et al. (2012). Disorder-specific mental health service use for mood and anxiety disorders: Associations with age, sex, and psychiatric comorbidity. *Depression and Anxiety*, 29(3), 234–242. doi:10.1002/da.20911.

Markle-Reid, M., McAiney, C., Forbes, D., et al. (2014). An interprofessional nurse-led mental health promotion intervention for older home care clients with depressive symptoms. *BMC Geriatrics*, 14(1), 62. doi:10.1186/1471-2318-14-62.

Mausbach, B. T., & Ho, J. (2015). Schizophrenia in late-life. In P. A. Lichtenberg, B. T. Mast, B. D. Carpenter, et al. (Eds.), *APA handbook of clinical geropsychology*: Vol. 2, Assessment, treatment, and issues in later life (pp. 105–129). Washington, DC: American Psychological Association.

McKenzie, G. L., & Harvath, T. A. (2016). Late-life depression. In M. Boltz, L. Capezuti, T. T. Fulmer, et al. (Eds.), *Evidence-based geriatric nursing protocols for best practice* (5th ed., pp. 211–232). New York, NY: Springer Publishing Company.

Mental Health Commission of Canada [MHCC] (2009). *Towards recovery and well-being: A framework for a mental health strategy for Canada*. Ottawa, ON: Author. Retrieved from www.mentalhealthcommission.ca/SiteCollectionDocuments/boarddocs/15507_MHCC_EN_final.pdf.

Mental Health Commission of Canada [MHCC]. (2011). *Guidelines for comprehensive mental health services for older adults in Canada*. Retrieved from http://www.mentalhealthcommission.ca/sites/default/files/mhcc_seniors_guidelines_1.pdf.

Mental Health Commission of Canada [MHCC]. (2012). *Changing directions, changing lives: The mental health strategy for Canada*. Retrieved from http://strategy.mentalhealthcommission.ca/pdf/strategy-images-en.pdf.

Merkouris, S. S., Thomas, S. A., Browning, C. J., et al. (2016). Predictors of outcomes of psychological treatments for disordered gambling: A systematic review. *Clinical Psychology Review, 48*, 7–31. doi:10.1016/j.cpr.2016.06.004.

Merrick, E. L., Horgan, C. M., Hodgkin, D., et al. (2008). Unhealthy drinking patterns in older adults: Prevalence and associated characteristics. *Journal of the American Geriatrics Society, 56*(2), 214–223. doi:10.1111/j.1532-5415.2007.10539.x.

Naegle, M. A., & McCabe, D. (2016). Substance misuse and alcohol use disorders. In M. Boltz, L. Capezuti, T. T. Fulmer, et al. (Eds.), *Evidence-based geriatric nursing protocols for best practice* (5th ed., pp. 457–477). New York, NY: Springer Publishing Company.

Pachana, N. A., Byrne, G. J., Siddle, H., et al. (2007). Development and validation of the Geriatric Anxiety Inventory. *International Psychogeriatrics, 19*(1), 103–114. doi:10.1017/S1041610206003504.

Parker, G., Lie, D., Siskind, D. J., et al. (2016). Mental health implications for older adults after natural disasters – A systematic review and meta-analysis. *International Psychogeriatrics, 28*(1), 11–20. doi:10.1017/S1041610215001210.

Pearson, C., Janz, T., & Ali, J. (2015). *Mental and substance use disorders in Canada: Health at a glance.* (Catalogue no. 82-624-X.) Retrieved from http://www.statcan.gc.ca/pub/82-624-x/2013001/article/11855-eng.htm.

Qualls, S. (2002). Defining mental health in later life. *Generations (San Francisco, Calif.), 26*(7), 9–13.

Registered Nurses' Association of Ontario (RNAO) (2009). *Nursing Best Practice Guideline: Assessment and care of adults at risk for suicidal ideation and behaviour.* Toronto, ON: Author.

Rej, S., Schuurmans, J., Elie, D., et al. (2016). Attitudes towards pharmacotherapy in late-life bipolar disorder. *International Psychogeriatrics, 28*(6), 945–950. doi:10.1017/S1041610215002380.

Satre, D. D., & Wolf, J. P. (2015). Alcohol abuse and substance misuse in later life. In P. A. Lichtenberg, B. T. Mast, B. D. Carpenter, et al. (Eds.), *APA handbook of clinical geropsychology* (Vol. 2, pp. 130–153). assessment, treatment, and issues of later life. Washington, DC: American Psychological Association.

Segal, D. L., June, A., Payne, M., et al. (2010). Development and initial validation of a self-report assessment tool for anxiety among older adults: The Geriatric Anxiety Scale. *Journal of Anxiety Disorders, 24*(7), 709–714. doi:10.1016/j.janxdis.2010.05.002.

Siskind, D. J., Sawyer, E., Lee, I., et al. (2016). The mental health of older persons after human-induced disasters: A systematic review and meta-analysis of epidemiological data. *The American Journal of Geriatric Psychiatry, 24*(5), 379–388. doi:10.1016/j.jagp.2015.12.010.

Statistics Canada. (2016). *Rates of depression, 12 month, by age and sex, Canada, household population 15 and older, 2012.* (Catalogue no. 82-624-X). Retrieved from http://www.statcan.gc.ca/pub/82-624-x/2013001/article/c-g/11855-c-g-01-eng.htm.

Statistics Canada. (2017a). *Suicides and suicide rate, by sex and by age group (both sexes no.).* Retrieved from http://www.statcan.gc.ca/tables-tableaux/sum-som/l01/cst01/hlth66a-eng.htm.

Statistics Canada. (2017b). *Suicides and suicide rate, by sex and by age group (both sexes rate).* Retrieved from http://www.statcan.gc.ca/tables-tableaux/sum-som/l01/cst01/hlth66d-eng.htm.

Subramaniam, M., Wang, P., Soh, P., et al. (2015). Prevalence and determinants of gambling disorder among older adults: A systematic review. *Addictive Behaviors, 41*, 199–209. doi:10.1016/j.addbeh.2014.10.007.

Tieu, U., & Konnert, C. A. (2014). Mental health help-seeking attitudes, utilization and intentions among older Chinese immigrants in Canada. *Aging & Mental Health, 18*(2), 140–147. doi:10.1080/13607863.2013.814104.

Tira, C., Jackson, A. C., & Tomnay, J. E. (2014). Pathways to late-life problematic gambling in seniors: A grounded theory approach. *The Gerontologist, 54*(6), 1035–1048. doi:10.1093/geront/gnt107.

Varcarolis, E. M., & Clements, K. (2013). The nursing process and standards of care for psychiatric mental health clients. In M. J. Halter, C. L. Pollard, S. L. Ray, et al. (Eds.), *Varcarolis's Canadian psychiatric mental health nursing* (1st ed., pp. 132–146). Toronto, ON: Elsevier.

Vasiliadis, H. M., Lamoureux-Lamarche, C., & Guerra, S. G. (2017). Gender and age group differences in suicide risk associated with co-morbid physical and psychiatric disorders in older adults. *International Psychogeriatrics, 29*(2), 249–257. doi:10.1017/S1041610216001290.

Volkert, J., Schulz, H., Härter, M., et al. (2013). The prevalence of mental disorders in older people in Western countries – A meta-analysis. *Ageing Research Reviews, 12*(1), 339–353. doi:10.1016/j.arr.2012.09.004.

Weiss, D. S., & Marmar, C. R. (1997). The impact of event scale-revised. In J. P. Wilson & T. M. Keane (Eds.), *Assessing psychological trauma and PTSD: A practitioner's handbook* (pp. 399–411). New York, NY: Guilford Press.

Williams, R. J., & Volberg, R. A. (2013). *Gambling and problem gambling in Ontario.* Report prepared for the Ontario Problem Gambling Research Centre and the Ontario Ministry of Health and Long Term Care. Retrieved from https://www.uleth.ca/dspace/bitstream/handle/10133/3378/2013-GPG%20ONT-OPGRC.pdf?sequence=3&isAllowed=y.

Wisocki, P. A., Handen, B., & Morse, C. (1986). The Worry Scale as a measure of anxiety among home bound and community active elderly. *The Behavior Therapist, 5*, 91–95.

World Health Organization. (2007). *What is mental health?* Retrieved from http://www.who.int/features/qa/62/en/index.html.

Loss, Death, and Palliative Care

 LEARNING OBJECTIVES

Upon completion of this chapter, the reader will be able to:

- Differentiate between loss and grief.
- Explain the different types of grief and the dynamics of the grieving process.
- Explain the nursing competencies required to effectively intervene in the older person's grief and bereavement.
- Identify and discuss the needs of people who are in the process of dying, as well as appropriate interventions.
- Explain the role and responsibility of the nurse in advance directives.
- Explain the role of the nurse in medically assisted dying.

 GLOSSARY

Bereavement overload   Multiple losses occurring in a short period of time.

End-of-life care   Care provided when death is imminent.

Grief   An emotional response to loss.

Mourning   The process by which grief is experienced.

Palliative care   Care which is directed toward maximizing comfort rather than achieving a cure.

THE LIVED EXPERIENCE

When we were in our sixties, my friends and I met over cards, went on trips, and experienced all of the joys of retirement. We didn't have much time to worry about aches and pains. In our seventies, we had less time to play, because we were busy visiting one another in hospital or in nursing homes. In our eighties, we met frequently again, but it was usually at our friends' funerals, leaving little time for cards or travel. Now that I am in my nineties, hardly any of my friends are still alive; you know, it gets kind of lonely, so you just have to make new younger friends!

Theresa, aged 93 years

Loss, dying, and death are universal, incontestable events of the human experience. Some loss is associated with the normal changes of aging, such as the loss of flexibility in the joints. Loss is also related to normal changes in everyday life and to life transitions such as moving and retirement. Still other losses are those of loved ones through death. Some deaths, such as those of parents and friends, are considered

normative and are expected. Other deaths, such as the deaths of adult children or grandchildren, are considered non-normative and are unexpected.

Regardless of the type of loss, each one has the potential to trigger **grief** and a process called bereavement or **mourning**. "Grief" and "mourning" are usually used synonymously. However, grief is an individual's response to a loss, and mourning is an active and evolving process that includes behaviours through which the experience of loss is incorporated into one's life. Mourning behaviours are strongly influenced by social and cultural norms that prescribe the appropriate ways of both reacting to the loss and coping with it (Thompson et al., 2016; Williams et al., 2015). There is no single way to grieve or respond to loss; each person grieves in his or her own way.

Although there are cultural expectations of grief behaviours for loss through death, there are no guidelines for behaviour when the loss is of another type. For example, an individual who is seriously ill, or who moves to a long-term care (LTC) home (thereby experiencing the loss of his or her home), or who retires (willingly or unwillingly) may be sad, irritable, and forgetful. The person may be suspected of developing dementia, when he or she is actually grieving. When the losses accumulate in quick succession, **bereavement overload** may result. The griever may become incapacitated and require skilled support and guidance.

Gerontological nurses should be knowledgeable about the grieving process and how to comfort and care for grievers. This includes being able to self-care in their own experiences of grief. Knowledge about the dying process is also needed, as are skills related to care of the dying person and the bereaved. This chapter provides the basic information necessary to promote effective grieving, peaceful dying, and good and appropriate deaths.

THE GRIEVING PROCESS

Researchers have tried for years to understand the grieving process, and their efforts have resulted in a number of proposed models to explain and predict the experience. Most of the models, developed in the 1970s and 1980s, influence how grief is understood by care providers and society in general. Although intended to describe death-related grief, these same models can be applied to other significant and meaningful losses experienced by older persons.

All models recognize similar physical and psychological manifestations of acute grief (i.e., when it is first felt), a middle period when the manifestations of grief (e.g., despair or depression) affect the person's day-to-day functioning, and an ending phase during which the person learns to adjust to life in a new way without that which has been lost. At the same time, it is also recognized that the grieving process is not rigidly structured and that a predictable pattern of responses does not always occur.

WORDEN'S MODEL OF BEREAVEMENT

The model of bereavement developed by Worden (2008) has been frequently cited and adapted. The model represents the grieving process as a series of evolving tasks that are repeated for all losses or parts of losses. The four tasks are to (1) accept the reality of the loss, (2) work through the physical and emotional pain associated with the loss, (3) adjust to life without the lost person, and (4) find an enduring connection with the deceased person and move on with life.

If this model is applied to someone (such as Helen) who has lost a loved one (such as her life partner, Chris), the nurse may look for signs that the person is accepting the reality of the loved one's death (e.g., the deceased person is referred to in the past tense rather than the present tense). For example, Helen may speak of Chris as someone who "just loved to garden," not as someone who "just loves to garden." Although her working through the pain is an individual process, Helen does have a support network of family, friends, and church members. They encourage her to "tell her story" of not only Chris's life but also their life together and gently move her to thinking of her life without Chris. In working through acute grief, the grieving person may try to avoid grief pain by using medications such as anxiolytics (e.g., benzodiazepines). Although these medications may be necessary in some cases to enable the griever to accomplish some needed tasks, they are not recommended for everyday use. They interfere with resolution and with dealing with the pain caused by grief and are generally not recommended for older persons (see Chapters 14 and 24).

Adjusting to loss may take a considerable period of time, especially if the relationship with the deceased was a long and close one. Changes in the environment—such as a re-arrangement of furniture or a different seating pattern at the dinner table—may be physical, emotional, or spiritual.

As Helen proceeds through the grieving process, her memories of life with Chris will be those of the past, and she will be able to develop new memories of her life without Chris. Although there may be a lot of pain associated with the first birthday, anniversary, and holiday without Chris, the pain will lessen with subsequent years as the loss is relocated from the present to the past.

LOSS RESPONSE MODEL

Jett's Loss Response Model (Jett, 2004) is a modification of a model proposed by Giacquinta for families facing cancer (Giacquinta, 1977). This adapted model incorporates a systems approach that provides a framework for the design of nursing interventions. When loss occurs within a system, such as a family, the experience is one of acute grief. The system's equilibrium is thrown off and undergoes a functional disruption; that is, the system cannot perform its usual activities. Family members are in a state of disequilibrium. The loss seems unreal. The grieving family searches for meaning. Why did this happen? How will they survive the loss? Older persons who are reacting to the loss of a child or a grandchild commonly ask themselves, "Why wasn't it me?"

The family may then become active in informing others. Each time the story is repeated, the loss becomes more real, and the system moves toward a new steady state. The story is also different each time it is told, because it is told from a new perspective. Informing others involves engaging emotions that may have been previously withheld or subdued because of the shock of the loss. The expression of emotions can release energy that can be used to reorganize the family structure. As roles change, adaptation and accommodation are necessary. Someone else steps in to perform the roles of the person who is now absent or to complete the tasks of that person. For example, when the older patriarch dies, the eldest child may step up and assume some of the parent's roles and responsibilities.

Finally, if the system is to survive, it needs to redefine itself. One way this is done is through the reframing of memories—that is, families understand that portraits and reunions are still possible, just different from what they were before the loss; or they realize that a person can still be vital, active, and important even after the loss of the ability to drive a car, walk unassisted, or live alone (Fig. 25.1).

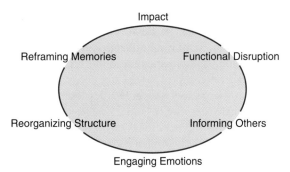

FIGURE 25.1 The Loss Response Model. *Source:* Jett, K. F. (2004). *The Loss Response Model.* Unpublished manuscript. Adapted from Giacquinta, B. (1977). Helping families face the crisis of cancer. *American Journal of Nursing, 77*(10), 1585–1588.

TYPES OF GRIEF

Grieving takes enormous amounts of physical and emotional energy. It is the hardest thing that anyone does and may be especially hard for older persons. Emotions can be intense, and this intensity may manifest as confusion, depression, or a preoccupation with thoughts of the deceased or the loss. This reaction may be mistaken for other conditions, such as dementia. The gerontological nurse will likely work with older people who are experiencing anticipatory grief, acute grief, or persistent grief. A fourth type, disenfranchised grief, may be hidden but is significant when it does occur.

Anticipatory Grief

Anticipatory grief is the response to a real or perceived loss before that loss occurs. This grief can be in anticipation of a loss, such as loss of belongings (e.g., through the selling of a home), loss of home (e.g., through moving into an LTC home), loss of a body part or function (e.g., through mastectomy), or loss of a spouse or oneself (through dementia or death). Behaviours that may signal anticipatory grief include preoccupation with the expected loss, unusually detailed planning, or a sudden change in attitude toward the thing, body part, or person to be lost (Lewis & McBride, 2004). End-of-life communication is associated with anticipatory grief and improved bereavement-related outcomes (Metzger & Gray, 2008).

The grieving process described by the various models may occur in the context of anticipatory grief, with one significant difference: the loss has not yet occurred. If the loss is certain but no one can say when it will occur, or if it does not occur when or as expected, the person who is awaiting the actual loss or death may become irritable, hostile, or impatient in response to the emotional ups and downs of the waiting. Glaser and Strauss (1968) described what they call an interruption in the sentimental order of a nursing unit when this occurs—no one quite knows how to behave.

Anticipatory grief can result in the premature detachment from an individual who is dying or the detachment of the dying person from the environment. Pattison (1977) called the premature withdrawal of others "sociological death" and the premature withdrawal of the person "psychological death." In either case, the person who is dying is no longer involved in day-to-day activities of living and essentially suffers a premature death.

Acute Grief

Acute grief is a crisis. It has a definite syndrome of somatic and psychological symptoms of distress that occur in waves lasting for varying periods of time. These symptoms may occur every time the loss is acknowledged, others are informed, or another person offers condolences. This preoccupation with the loss is similar to daydreaming and is accompanied by a sense of unreality. Depending on the situation, feelings of self-blame or guilt may be present and manifest themselves as hostility or anger toward friends, as depression, or as withdrawal.

It is often difficult for persons who are acutely grieving to accomplish their usual activities of daily living or to meet other responsibilities (a condition called functional disruption). Even if the tasks are accomplished, the person may complain of feeling distracted, restless, and "at loose ends." Deciding what to wear may seem too complex a task. Fortunately, the signs and symptoms of acute grief eventually diminish. Acute grief is most intense in the months immediately following the loss, especially the first 6 months; the intensity lessens over time (Zisook et al., 2014).

Helen, in the first months after Chris died, cried any time he was mentioned. Later, she was still grieving, but her tears were replaced with a surging sense of loss and sadness and still later by more-fleeting reactions.

Persistent or Complicated Grief

Although grief may temporarily inhibit some activity, it is considered a normal response to loss. The intermittent pain of grief is often exacerbated on birthdays, holidays, and wedding anniversaries. For the survivors of tragedies such as war, terrorist attacks, or natural disasters, the grief may never completely go away. This type of lingering grief has been described as "shadow grief," grief that resurfaces from time to time but does not persist. It produces a temporary grief, usually triggered by a sight, smell, or sound (Coryell, 2007).

Some persistent grief is more than shadow grief and evolves into *complicated grief*. Complicated grief is thought to begin as a normal grief response, but the evolution toward adjustment and the re-establishment of equilibrium is blocked. The memories resist being reframed. Reactions are exaggerated, and memories are experienced as recurrent acute grief, over and over again, months and years later. The signs of complicated grief include preoccupation with the loss, avoidance of reminders of the loss, the feeling that others are not trustworthy or do not understand the loss, bitterness and anger, numbness or anhedonia, a feeling of shock, and a grief episode that triggers a major depressive episode (Neimeyer & Holland, 2015). Those with a relative who died from suicide have a greater risk for complicated grief (Tal et al., 2016). Complicated grief occurs in up to 7% of bereaved persons (Zisook et al., 2014). This type of grief requires the intervention of a professional grief counsellor, a psychiatric nurse practitioner, or a psychologist who is skilled in helping grieving persons.

Disenfranchised Grief

Disenfranchised grief is an experience of the person whose loss cannot be openly acknowledged or publicly mourned. The grief is socially disallowed or unsupported and is incongruent with norms of grief in the person's culture (Doka, 2002). The person does not have a socially recognized right to be perceived as a bereaved person or to function as one. The relationship is not recognized, the loss is not sanctioned, or the grieved one is not recognized or cannot be made public. A common theme with disenfranchised grief is that persons close to the grieving person do not know about the loss or do not understand the full meaning of the loss to that person.

Situations that are associated with disenfranchised grief include hidden or secret relationships (e.g., some lesbian, gay, bisexual, transgender, or queer [LGBTQ] relationships and relationships that are part of extramarital affairs). Disenfranchised grief can also occur when the cause of death is stigmatized (e.g., suicide, HIV and AIDS) or when the loss is not seen as worthy of sympathy (e.g., the death of a pet, retirement). Families grieving the loss of a person who had dementia may also experience disenfranchised grief, particularly when others perceive the death of the older person as a blessing and fail to support the grieving family members, who have struggled for years with losses and anticipatory grief and now must cope with the acute grief of the actual death (Doka, 2002).

FACTORS AFFECTING COPING WITH LOSS

Coping, as it relates to loss and grief, is the ability of the individual or family to find ways to deal with the stress. In the language of the Loss Response Model (Jett, 2004), it is the ability to move from a state of chaos and disequilibrium to one of renewed order, equilibrium, and peace. Many factors affect the ability to cope with loss and grief (Box 25.1).

Older spouses and life partners are at higher risk for the effects of grief than are younger spouses and life partners. Intense grief may cause a temporary decrease in cognitive function that can be misinterpreted as dementia, isolating the grieving person (Ward et al., 2007).

The psychiatrist Avery Weisman, a classic authority on death and dying, described people who are more likely to effectively deal with grief as "good copers" (Weisman, 1979, p. 42). These are individuals or families who have experience with the successful management of crisis. They are resourceful and are able to draw on coping strategies that have worked in the past. Weisman (1979; 1984) found that persons who cope effectively with cancer do the following:

- Avoid avoidance
- Confront realities and take appropriate action
- Focus on solutions
- Redefine problems

BOX 25.1	Factors Influencing the Grieving Process

- Number of losses caused by the illness
- Recognition of each loss
- Importance of the loss to the person
- Appropriateness of the use of psychotropic medications
- Level of health and fitness before the loss (e.g., nutritional status, sleep, and exercise)
- Coping skills and the types of coping responses available to the person
- Past experience with loss or death
- Immediate circumstances surrounding the loss
- Timing of the loss
- Number, type, and quality of secondary losses occurring at the same time

Additional Factors Specific to Dying and Death
- Role that the deceased occupied in the family or social system
- Amount of unfinished business
- Perception of the deceased's fulfillment in life
- Immediate circumstances surrounding the death
- Length of illness before death
- Anticipatory grief and involvement with the dying person

Source: Adapted from Hess, P. A. (1994). Loss, grief, and dying. In P. G. Beare & J. L. Myers (Eds.), *Principles and practice of adult health nursing* (2nd ed.). St. Louis. MO: Mosby.

- Consider alternatives
- Have good communication with loved ones
- Seek and use constructive help
- Accept support when offered
- Keep up their morale

In other words, effective copers are people who can acknowledge their loss and try to make sense of it. They are able to maintain composure, use generally good judgement, and remain optimistic without denying their loss. Good copers seek guidance when they need it. By contrast, people who cope less effectively have few if any of these abilities. They tend to be more rigid and pessimistic, are demanding, and are given to emotional extremes. They may be dogmatic and expect perfection from themselves and others. Ineffective copers are also more likely to be people who live alone, socialize little, and have few close friends or an ineffective support network. They may have a history of mental illness, or they may have guilt, anger, and ambivalence toward the person who has died or toward that which has been lost. People at risk for pathological grief will more likely have unresolved past conflicts or be simultaneously facing the loss and facing other, secondary stressors. Older people with these qualities are most in need of expert interventions by grief counsellors and skilled gerontological nurses.

 ## IMPLICATIONS FOR GERONTOLOGICAL NURSING AND HEALTHY AGING

The nursing goal is not to prevent grief but to support those who are grieving. Although the loss will never change, its potential long-term detrimental effects can be lessened. Working with grieving older people is part of what gerontological nurses do on a daily basis. Even small actions taken by the nurse can make a large difference in the grieving person's quality of life.

ASSESSMENT

In grief assessment, the nurse aims to understand the person's grieving experience so that the person can be appropriately supported. It is also important for the nurse to try to differentiate persons who are likely to cope effectively from those who are at risk of coping ineffectively so that appropriate interventions can be planned. A grief assessment is based on a knowledge of the grieving process and subsequent mourning. Data are obtained through observation of the person's behaviour, and the assessment is conducted while considering the cultural context (Neimeyer & Holland, 2015).

A thorough grief assessment includes questions about recent significant life events, life or religious values, and the person's relationship to who or what has been lost. It is important to take time to hear the person's account of the death and attend to cues about the meaning of the loss. The bereaved person should be asked about his or her concerns about grieving and loss (Neimeyer & Holland, 2015). Knowing more about the loss and the effect of the loss on the older person's life enables the nurse to identify persons who are at risk for complicated grief and to construct and implement appropriate and caring responses. Box 25.2 lists the components of the bereavement assessment.

BOX 25.2 Components of a Bereavement Assessment of an Older Person

- Physical and cognitive functions, including a full record of medications and medical interventions prescribed now and prior to the loss.
- Reactions and behaviours of the bereaved person since the death.
- Quality of relationship with the deceased person, as described by the bereaved person.
- Changes and losses in role investment and in daily life since the loss.
- Reactions and expectations of family members and other significant people in the bereaved individual's life.
- Past experiences of loss, traumatic experiences, circumstances of the loss (e.g., prolonged illness or sudden death), and the history of adaptive or maladaptive functioning.
- Contextual and economic realities (i.e., location and neighbourhood, financial status).
- Social networks and social support from friends and professional health care providers and especially from relationships and from family caregivers who can provide support and enhance therapeutic involvement.
- Cohort and personal beliefs; generational issues and attitudes; spiritual and religious beliefs; cultural context; and values regarding old age, psychological interventions, widowhood, and illnesses.
- Sociocultural and religious context within which bereavement is experienced by the older person.

Source: Malkinson, R., & Bar-Tur, L. (2014). Cognitive grief therapy: Coping with the inevitability of loss and grief in later life. In N. A. Pachana & K. Laidlaw (Eds.). *The Oxford Handbook of Clinical Geropsychology* (p. 8). Oxford, UK: Oxford University Press. doi:10.1093/oxfordhb/9780199663170.013.024.

INTERVENTIONS

A goal of intervention is to assist the individual or family in attaining a healthy adjustment to the loss experience and in re-establishing equilibrium. Actions that can meet this goal are basic and simple; however, the emotional overlay can make these interventions difficult. For the new nurse who is confronted with a person's grief for the first time, there may be discomfort, fear, and insecurity. The tendency is to be sympathetic rather than empathetic. Questions such as following arise in one's mind: What do I say? Should I be cheerful or serious? Should I talk about or even mention the dead person's name?

Nursing interventions, especially when older people are in crisis, begin with the gentle establishment of rapport. Nurses need to introduce themselves and explain the nature of their roles (e.g., charge nurse, staff nurse) and their availability. If it is the time of impact (e.g., just after a serious diagnosis, at the death of a family member, or upon becoming a resident of an LTC home), nurses can provide support and a safe environment and ensure that basic needs are met. The nurse can soften the despair by saying things that foster reasonable hope, such as "You will make it through this time, one moment at a time, and I will be here to help."

Nurses need to be observant for *functional disruption* and offer support and direction. They may have to help the family figure out what has to be done immediately and find ways to do it. The nurse can offer to either complete the task or find a friend or family member who can step in so the disruption does not have any deleterious effects.

As grieving persons search for meaning, they may require help to find what they are looking for. Sometimes it is information about a disease, a situation, or a person. Sometimes it is a spiritual search. Sometimes they need help in finding a resource or a place of peace. Often, what is needed most is someone to listen to the "whys" and "hows"—questions that cannot be answered.

Sometimes nurses offer to contact others on behalf of those who are grieving, assuming that this is something that will help. However, it is far more therapeutic for the grieving person to be the one who informs others, because doing so helps the loss to become real. The nurse can offer to find a phone number, old the grieving person's hand during the conversation, or just "be there" when the news is being shared. In this way, the nurse can be available to provide support when the grieving person's emotions are difficult.

As the grieving person moves forward in adjusting to the loss (e.g., moving from his or her home to an LTC home), the nurse can help the person reorganize the structure of life. For example, the nurse can talk with the person about what was most valued about living at home and what habits were comforting; the nurse can then help the person find ways to incorporate these into the new environment. If, for instance, the older person always had a cup of tea before bed but does not have access to a kitchen, addressing this circumstance can be a part of the individualized plan of care.

According to the Loss Response Model, memories are reframed as part of the completion of the cycle of grieving. The grandmother who lives in an LTC home who always hosted her granddaughter's birthday party can still host it. The nurse who knows about this important ritual can help the resident reserve a private space, send out invitations, and have the birthday party as always, just reframed in that it is catered by the grandmother's new "home."

Countercoping

Weisman (1979) described the grief-related work of health care providers as "countercoping." Although he was speaking of working with people with cancer, the concept is equally applicable to working with people who are grieving for any loss. "Countercoping is like counterpoint in music, which blends melodies together into a basic harmony. The patient copes; the therapist [nurse] countercopes; together they work out a better fit" (Weisman, 1979, p. 109). Weisman suggests four very specific types of interventions or countercoping strategies: (1) clarification and control, (2) collaboration, (3) directed relief, and (4) cooling off.

Clarification and Control

The nurse can help the person cope with loss by helping him or her confront the loss, assisting the person with getting or receiving information, considering alternative ideas and actions, and finding a way to make the grief manageable. The nurse can help the person resume control by encouraging him or her to avoid acting on impulse.

Collaboration

The nurse can act collaboratively by encouraging the grieving person to share stories with others and to repeat the stories as often as is necessary to "talk it out." In this situation, the nurse is more directive than usual; it may be acceptable for the nurse to say, "No, this is not a good time to make any major decisions."

Directed Relief

Some temporary directed relief may be necessary, especially during a period of acute grief. Catharsis may be helpful. In many instances, it is the nurse who encourages the grieving person to cry or otherwise express feelings such as hurt or anger. The nurse may have to say something such as "Expressing your feelings might help." Activity may also be recommended as a natural extension of feelings. Intense physical activity provides emotional relief. In some cultures, people may tear their clothes or cut their hair. There are numerous ways of acting out feelings—for example, by throwing things, taking a walk, busying oneself with tasks, and expressing feelings through creative work.

Cooling Off

From time to time, the grieving person might be encouraged to temporarily avoid active mourning by way of diversions that worked in the past during times of stress, especially when things have to be done or decisions have to be made. The nurse may need to suggest new tactics that may prove helpful. Although there is considerable cultural variation, "cooling off" is also facilitated by encouraging the person to modulate emotional extremes and to think about ways to make sense of the loss, build a new sense of self-esteem after the loss, and re-establish life patterns.

In all interventions related to grief, the nurse must have therapeutic communication skills. Active listening is greatly preferable to giving advice. When listening, the nurse soon discovers that the actual loss is not of utmost concern; rather, the fear associated with the loss is. If the nurse listens carefully to both what is stated and what is implied, the nurse may hear expressions such as the following: "How will I go on?", "What will I do now?", "What will become of me?", "I don't know what to do," and "How could he (she) do this to me?" Because the nurse knows that there will be a resolution of some kind, such comments may seem exaggerated. To the one who is grieving, however, there seems to be no resolution. The person who is actively grieving cannot yet look ahead and know that the despair and other feelings will resolve. The nurse must be flexible, practical, resourceful, and abundantly optimistic.

DYING, DEATH, AND PALLIATIVE CARE

Many people have said that death is not the problem; it is dying that takes the work. This is true for all

involved—the person who is dying; the dying person's loved ones; and the professional caregivers, such as nurses and health care aides.

Dying is both a challenging and a private life experience. How a person deals with dying is a reflection of the person's culture and the way the person has handled earlier losses and stressors. Although not all older persons have had fulfilling lives or have a sense of completion, transcendence, or self-actualization, death at or after the age of their parents when they died is considered normative. If the dying process is particularly long or if the death occurs after a painful illness, some people may rationalize the death or view it as a relief, at least in part. Death at a younger age or as the result of trauma or catastrophe is viewed as tragic and sometimes incomprehensible. Death as a result of natural disaster, war, or violence is seldom rationalized; even the deaths of older victims are considered an unacceptable loss of human potential.

CONCEPTUAL MODELS

Just as models have been proposed to explain the grieving process, so too have models been proposed to explain the process of dying. One of the most well-known models is by Kübler-Ross. In her book *On Death and Dying*, she reported on observations of inpatients on the psychiatric ward where she completed her psychiatry residency. She defined the stages of dying as denial, anger, bargaining, depression, and acceptance. Nurses and many others have tried to help dying persons work past their denial and accept their death. However, professional caregivers have come to realize that the "stages" are actually types of emotional reactions to dying and not parts of a model at all. An alternative concept that has been very useful to nursing practice is presented next.

The Living–Dying Interval

Whereas dying physically begins early in life (see Chapter 6), in personal terms, dying begins at a moment called the "crisis knowledge of death" (Pattison, 1977, p. 44) and ends at the moment of physiological death. Pattison (1977) calls the time between these two points the "living–dying interval," made up of the acute, chronic, and terminal phases. The chronological time of the living–dying interval is accordion-like because of remissions and exacerbations in the

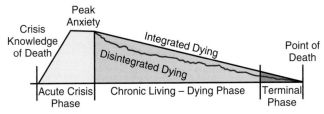

FIGURE 25.2 The living–dying interval. *Source:* Pattison, E. M. (1977). *The experience of dying.* Englewood Cliffs, NJ: Prentice-Hall.

terminal illness; it may last days, weeks, months, or years. The manner in which a person faces dying is an expression of personality, circumstances, illness, and culture.

The "crisis knowledge of death" occurs when someone receives the information that he or she will not live as long as previously anticipated. Certainly it would appear that the greater the discrepancy between the previously assumed length of life and the newly projected length of life, the greater the required adjustment and, perhaps, the intensity of the grief.

The point of crisis is a moment in time that is followed by the acute phase of the living–dying interval. The point of crisis is usually the peak time of stress and anxiety, because it is the time when the life and future of the individual and the family are thrown into disequilibrium. Crisis intervention is most effective at this time because the individual, the family, and the caregivers are struggling to come to terms with the knowledge. A significant amount of anticipatory grieving may be observed.

Since no one can withstand a crisis indefinitely, most of the dying time is spent in the chronic phase. During this time, the dying and those around them are forced to resume some sense of normalcy. Bills still need to be paid, dishes still need to be washed, and life can still be lived. The challenge for persons with terminal illnesses and for their families is to work toward living while dying and not toward dying while still living. Entertainment, work, and relationships can be maintained as the individual's condition permits. Life goes on despite the anticipation of its end.

The terminal phase is reached when the speed of the physical dying is accelerated and the person no longer has the energy to maintain the activities of everyday life. The person may withdraw or turn away from the outside world, or the person may engage in coded communication (such as saying "good-bye" instead of the usual "good night," giving away cherished possessions as gifts, or urgently contacting friends and relatives with whom he or she has not communicated for a long time). The focus then turns to preserving energy and completing life's journey. In some cultures, this period of time is called the "death watch" and is associated with prescribed rituals.

The living–dying interval can reflect an integrated or disintegrated trajectory (Fig. 25.2) (Pattison, 1977). The interval is integrated when each new crisis is dealt with effectively and the quality of life while dying is preserved. The interval is disintegrated if one crisis tumbles on to the next one without any effective resolution and if the quality of life while dying is compromised.

IMPLICATIONS FOR GERONTOLOGICAL NURSING AND HEALTHY AGING

Most often, death is not sudden or unexpected. For most people, the dying process lasts from a few weeks to many months. Persons with progressive persistent illnesses experience three distinct illness and death trajectories (Murray et al., 2005). Nurses who are aware of these trajectories can anticipate the needs of those who are dying and help them and their families to cope and plan. The first trajectory (typical of cancer) is a short period of decline over weeks, months, and occasionally years. The second trajectory (more typical of conditions such as heart failure and chronic obstructive pulmonary disease) consists of long-term functional limitations and gradual deterioration in health and functioning, with intermittent exacerbations. Death may occur as part of one of these exacerbations, but the timing of death is unpredictable

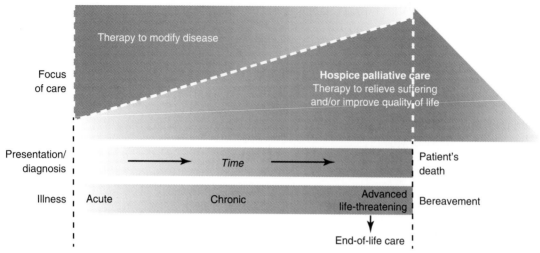

FIGURE 25.3 The role of hospice palliative care during illness. *Source:* Canadian Hospice Palliative Care Association. (2013). *A model to guide hospice palliative care* (p. 7). Ottawa, ON: Author. Retrieved from http://www.chpca.net/media/319547/norms-of-practice-eng-web.pdf.

and uncertain. The third trajectory (more typical of dementia or frailty) is called *prolonged dwindling* and lasts for years. Death may occur as a result of an acute condition such as pneumonia, or it may result from a combination of minor physical events that the person does not have the reserve to surmount. The role of **palliative care** in the illness trajectory is illustrated in Fig. 25.3.

The responsibility of the nurse is to work within the interprofessional team to provide safe conduct as the dying and their families navigate through unknown waters to a good and appropriate death. A good and appropriate death is one that a person would choose (if choosing were possible) and one in which the person's needs are met to the greatest extent possible. There are several ways to approach an understanding of the dying and to meet their needs. The approach discussed here is called the "six C's approach."

THE SIX C'S APPROACH

Weisman (1984) identified six needs of the dying: care, control, composure, communication, continuity, and closure.

Care

Persons who are dying should receive the best care possible; this includes expert management of symptoms and support at all times. Care includes the adequate treatment of physical pain (see Chapter 16). Care also addresses the psychological pain—induced by depression, anxiety, fear, and other unresolved emotional concerns—that can be just as strong and just as real as physical pain. When emotional needs are not met, the total pain experience is intensified. Medications alone cannot relieve pain. Instead, empathic listening and allowing the person to express his or her thoughts is an important intervention (see Chapter 4). If tears and sadness are present, gentle touch, closeness, and sitting near the person are helpful when culturally appropriate. As an advocate, the gerontological nurse should also make sure that the person receives the care that is needed.

Caring for a dying person also means helping the person conserve energy. Dying calls for great amounts of energy to cope with the emotional and physical assault of illness on the body. How much can the individual do without becoming physically and emotionally taxed? What activities of daily living are most important for the person to do independently? How much energy is needed for the person to be able to talk with visitors or staff without becoming exhausted? Only the person can answer these questions, and the nurse can advocate for the person to be given the opportunity to do so. The person will thus be able to remain more in control and to maintain composure.

Control

As a person proceeds along the living–dying interval, he or she often feels that control over life has been lost. The person is in the process of losing everything he or she has ever known. The potential loss of identity, independence, and control over body functions can lead to a sense of having lost control, dignity, and self-esteem. The person may begin to feel ashamed, humiliated, and like a "burden." There is a need for control—a need to remain in a collaborative role related to the person's own living and dying and as an active participant in his or her own care. The nurse can help the person meet this need by taking every opportunity to return the control to the person and, in doing so, bolster that individual's self-esteem. Whenever possible, the nurse can have the person decide when to groom, eat, wake, sleep, and so forth. The nurse never has the right to determine the activities of the individual, especially in relation to visitors and how time is spent.

Composure

In many cultures, dying is an emotional activity, both for the person dying and for those around him or her. The need for composure is what enables the person to modulate emotional extremes appropriately within cultural norms, not to avoid the sadness but to have moments of relief. The nurse may use many of the countercoping techniques discussed earlier to help meet this need.

Communication

The need for communication is broad, ranging from the need for information for making decisions to the need to share information. Although the type and content of communication that is acceptable to the person vary by culture, the nurse has a responsibility to make sure that the dying person has an opportunity for the communication he or she desires (see Chapter 3).

In a study of communication among the patient, family, and hospital staff about terminal illness, Glaser and Strauss (1963) identified four types of communication: closed awareness, suspected awareness, mutual pretense, and open awareness. Each influenced the work on the unit and on the care of the dying person.

Closed awareness is described as "keeping the secret." Health care providers, the family, and friends know that the person is dying, but the person does not know this or does know but keeps the secret as well. Generally, caregivers invent a fictitious future for the patient to believe in, hoping that this will boost the patient's morale. Although this happens less today because of legislation related to patients' rights, it still occurs. In some cultures, it is expected.

In *suspected awareness*, the person suspects he or she is dying, but because the dying is not discussed, it cannot be confirmed. Inquiries on the part of the person are indirect or are avoided by others. Hints are bandied back and forth, and a contest for control of the information ensues.

Mutual pretense is a situation of "let's pretend." Everyone knows the patient has a terminal illness, but no one talks about it; feelings are kept hidden.

Open awareness occurs when the patient, family, friends, and all health care providers openly acknowledge the eventual death of the person. The person may ask, "Will I die?" and "How and when will I die?" The person becomes resigned to dying, and the family grieves with the person rather than for the person. The nurse can encourage open awareness whenever possible, respecting the person's culture at the same time. In some cultures, talking about an anticipated death is deemed helpful. In others, one can be aware of the dying, but talking about it openly may be taboo.

Continuity

Satisfying the need for continuity equates to maintaining for the dying person as normal a life as possible and helping the person transcend the present by leaving a legacy for the future. Too often, a dying person can feel shut off from the rest of the world at a time when he or she is still capable of being involved and active in some way. Loneliness is the result of a loss of continuity with one's life. The nurse may ask about the person's life and about those things most valued, and can work with the family and the dying person on a plan to remain engaged in as many activities and past roles as possible. A father who watches a certain ballgame with his son every Sunday can continue to do this, regardless of the need to be in hospital, in an LTC home, or in an inpatient hospice unit. If the person is at home and is bedridden, it may make more sense to have the bed in a central area rather than in a distant room. Treating the person who is dying as an intelligent adult, holding a hand, or (if culturally acceptable) putting an arm around a shoulder says "I care" and "You're not alone" and "You are important."

One approach people have taken to ensure the continuity of their lives after death is to establish legacies. Legacies can take many different forms and may range from memories that will live on in the minds of others to fortunes bequeathed to family or loved ones (see Chapter 3). A grandmother who is likely to die before a favourite grandchild's wedding can, by participating in planning the wedding (regardless of the age of the grandchild), leave an enduring and special legacy.

Closure

The need for closure creates an opportunity for reconciliation and transcendence. Closure is not about the end of grief. People often continue to feel grief at least intermittently throughout their lives; there is no absolute closure (Doka, 2016). Reminiscence is one way to move through grief and the reconciliation of loss and to evaluate the pluses and minuses of life. It is a means of resolving conflicts, giving up possessions, and saying final goodbyes. Pain and other symptoms that are not well controlled may interfere with this reconciliation, making appropriate interventions by the nurse especially important.

For some, closure means coming to terms with their spiritual selves. If the expressions of the dying person have spiritual overtones, pastoral or spiritual care may be offered but should never be carried out without the person's permission. The nurse can foster transcendence by providing dying people with the time and privacy for self-reflection as well as an opportunity to talk about whatever they need to talk about, especially the meanings of their lives and deaths.

Care, control, composure, communication, continuity, and closure are necessary to meet the needs of the dying person. Their influence is omnipresent in these needs. Without the six C's, attempts to meet the person's needs will be limited.

FAMILY

Nurses are often present and support the family at the time of death and in the moments preceding it. Regardless of their ages, the surviving family members, spouse or life partner, and friends have needs, and nurses have a responsibility to care for them. In one study, newly bereaved persons were asked what they had found most helpful (Richter, 1987). Their answers showed that they most appreciated nurses who did the following:

- Kept them informed
- Asked how they were doing, and offered support
- Put an arm around them when they cried
- Brought them food
- Knew their name
- Cried with them
- Brought a bed and encouraged them to stay in the room with their dying spouses
- Told them to hold their dying spouses' hands
- Held their hands
- Got the chaplain for them
- Let them take care of their spouses
- Stayed with them after the nurse's shift was over

More recently, Lee et al. (2012) received similar answers. Although these actions will not provide comfort to all or always be possible, they can be used as starting points.

A helpful guide for families and friends is *When Someone Close to You Is Dying: What You Can Expect and How You Can Help,* available in English, French, and Spanish on the National Initiative for the Care of the Elderly website (http://www.nicenet.ca). The guide was developed to provide information that families said they needed. It includes information about what the dying person may need, what happens during the last moments of life, pain control, advance care planning and substitute health care decision making, and strategies to support the dying person. The guide is also helpful for nursing students and novice nurses who may have limited exposure to the dying process.

END-OF-LIFE CARE MODELS IN CANADA

In 2002, the federal government identified seven priorities for improving **end-of-life care** and established five working groups to establish a strategy for palliative and end-of-life care (Health Canada, 2002; 2007). The working groups addressed best practices, accessibility, and quality of care; education of health care providers; public information and awareness; research; and surveillance. Work on a national strategy stopped in 2007.

Canada aspires to adopt the following key components of end-of-life care: (1) universal access to psychosocial, spiritual, and physical care for all dying persons; (2) care coordination by a care coordinator or case manager; (3) access to a broad range of basic and advanced care services, such as palliative and hospice care; and (4) end-of-life care in all settings, wherever a dying person resides (Wilson et al., 2008, pp. 323–324).

Many have argued that in Canada, access to hospice palliative care should be a human right (Freeman et al., 2013). Availability of end-of-life care across settings is important because although most deaths occur in hospital, the proportion of deaths that occur in hospital is decreasing (Northcott & Wilson, 2017). This decrease is due to more deaths occurring at home, in a hospice, or in an LTC home.

Access to palliative care and end-of-life care is an issue for Canadians. Surveys of Canadians indicate that between 55% and 71% prefer to die at home, the next preferred option being a hospice or palliative care facility (Northcott & Wilson, 2017). However, meeting these wishes may not be feasible, depending on availability of family members who are able to provide care. Family members often find that there are inadequate resources to support them. Lack of services and funding for palliative care is particularly problematic in rural communities (Kaasalainen et al., 2012).

While most Canadians prefer to die at home, the preferred place of death differs among various cultures, and depending on the illness condition that a person has, some people may prefer to die in hospital. For example, a study in Quebec found that persons with chronic obstructive pulmonary disease preferred to die in hospital, believing that the care there would better meet their needs (Northcott & Wilson, 2017). Nurses working in all health care settings should be knowledgeable about end-of-life care. Box 25.3 describes a study about palliative and end-of-life care in LTC homes.

BOX 25.3 Research for Evidence-Informed Practice: Death and Dying in Long-Term Care Homes

Problem: The need for palliative care tends to be recognized late for a person living and dying in a long-term care (LTC) home, potentially limiting the preparedness of the family and the comfort of the dying resident. This study investigated how culture in LTC homes is related to the awareness of impending death and the use of palliative care.

Methods: The study was an ethnographic study of end-of-life practices in three Ontario LTC homes. Residents, family members, and staff were interviewed; documents were reviewed; and a focus group was conducted. The data were analyzed with a constant comparative technique.

Findings: The following four elements of the culture of LTC homes influenced end-of-life care: (1) high care demands and limited resources to meet usual care needs; (2) the belief that LTC homes are for living; (3) the belief that no one should die in pain; and (4) the belief that no one should die alone. Even though 30% of residents died each year, staff members felt it important to counteract fears and negative ideas about LTC homes ("It's an old stigma that this is a place to come to die" [p. 6]) by focusing on the LTC home as a place to live. This focus on LTC homes as a place to live distracted from the acknowledgment of death, dying, and the palliative status of many residents. The findings were seen as being influenced in Canada by a broader cultural force of death denying.

Application to Nursing Practice: The researchers called for higher staff-to-resident ratios to meet the needs of residents and allow for timely palliative care. The term "palliative care" was narrowly understood to refer to end-of-life care (i.e., care when death is imminent), a view that limited access to palliative care. A palliative approach is consistent with person-centred care to enhance quality of life. However, a reluctance to acknowledge the palliative status of residents may limit the preservation of their quality of life.

Source: Cable-Williams, B., & Wilson, D. M. (2017). Dying and death within the culture of long-term care facilities. *International Journal of Older People Nursing, 12*(1), e1215. doi:10.1111/opn.12125.

HOSPICE PALLIATIVE CARE

Nurses routinely care for older individuals who have irreversible and progressive conditions such as dementia or Parkinson's disease. Other older persons have exhausted all treatment options or have decided that they want no further treatment for conditions such as cancer or end-stage heart or renal disease. An LTC home resident may elect to remain at the LTC home rather than go to an acute care hospital even if faced with an acute event such as a myocardial infarction or a stroke. These people receive what is called palliative care, care that focuses on comfort rather than cure, on the treatment of symptoms rather than disease, and on the quality of life rather than the quantity of life. Palliative care is "an approach that improves the quality of life of patients and their families facing the problems associated with life-threatening illness, through the prevention and relief of suffering by means of early identification and impeccable assessment and treatment of pain and other problems, physical, psychosocial and spiritual" (World Health Organization, 2017). Box 25.4 lists the aims and goals of hospice palliative care.

BOX 25.4   Hospice Palliative Care

- Aims to relieve suffering and improve the quality of living and dying
- Strives to help patients and families do the following:
  - Address physical, psychological, social, spiritual, and practical issues and their associated needs, hopes, and fears
  - Prepare for and manage self-determined life closure and the dying process
  - Cope with loss and grief during the illness and bereavement
- Aims to do the following:
  - Treat all active issues
  - Prevent new issues from occurring
  - Promote opportunities for meaningful and valuable experiences, personal and spiritual growth, and self-actualization
- Is appropriate for any patient and family living with or at risk of developing a life-threatening illness due to any diagnosis and with any prognosis, regardless of age.
- Is appropriate at any time the patient and family have unmet expectations, needs, or both, and are prepared to accept care
- May complement and enhance disease-modifying therapy or may become the total focus of care

Source: Canadian Hospice Palliative Care Association. (2013). *A model to guide hospice palliative care: Based on national principles and norms of practice* (p. 6). Ottawa, ON: Author. Retrieved from http://www.chpca.net/media/319547/norms-of-practice-eng-web.pdf.

Hospice palliative care comprises much of what is done in gerontological nursing and may indeed be the heart of caring. The term "hospice" gets its meaning from the medieval concept of hospitality, in which a community assisted a traveller at dangerous points along his or her journey. The hospice movement has been a vehicle to help return nursing to its roots—humane, compassionate care, an ideal that has been the basis of nursing for centuries. Dying persons are indeed travellers—travellers along the continuum of life—and the community consists of friends, family, and specially prepared people to care (namely, the hospice team).

The scope and specialty of hospice palliative care has grown considerably over the years; research has been conducted, professional organizations have been formed, and standardized curricula have been developed. Whereas palliative care was initially the specialty of community-based hospices, hospice palliative care is now provided by specialized units in hospitals, in LTC homes, as well as in private dwellings. While access to palliative care in Canada is improving, between 70% and 85% of Canadians are unable to access palliative care services, and older Canadians are less likely to have access to these services (Canadian Hospice Palliative Care Association [CHPCA], 2014; Freeman et al., 2013). Access to and funding for palliative care varies among provinces and territories and between urban and rural areas (Canadian Cancer Society, 2016). Palliative care in Canada is "at the margins of the health care system" (Williams, et al., 2010, ¶11).

Given the complexity of hospice palliative care, it is not surprising that it depends on interprofessional care teams made up of both formal and informal caregivers, the dying person, the person's family, and the person's loved ones. Most hospice palliative care is provided at home. The home becomes the primary centre of care, provided by family members or friends who are taught basic nursing care and how to administer the medication needed to provide comfort for the dying person. (A Canadian study of home-based palliative care is described in Box 25.5.) Hospice palliative care supports and guides the dying person and the family. It ensures that the person will not die alone and that the family will not be abandoned. Bereavement services for the family extend for

---

BOX 25.5 Research for Evidence-Informed Practice: Palliative Medication Kits Can Extend Care in the Home for Patients Nearing Death

Problem: While the majority of palliative patients prefer to die at home, poor symptom control in the last days of life can result in unplanned hospital admission.

Methods: Medication kits were placed in the homes of clients in the Winnipeg Regional Palliative Care Program who were expected to die within 2 weeks. Medications were selected for versatility to address more than one symptom and for the ability to be administered bucally, sublingually, or transdermally. The kits contained enough medication to meet short-term needs or to use until a pharmacy could be accessed. The kit was kept in a locked box accessible only to palliative care staff. Up to 15 kits were available to be placed in homes at any given time.

Findings: Of the 457 kits placed in homes between 2004 and 2007, 44% were used. Among the clients for whom the kits were used, there were 175 (87%) home deaths. The rate of home death in the entire program was 29%.

Application to Nursing Practice: The medication kit was a feasible intervention. The availability and use of these kits may overcome problems of not being able to access medication in a timely manner, thus increasing the likelihood that home care clients will have the opportunity to die at home.

Source: Wowchuk, S. M., Wilson, A., Embleton, L., ... Chochinov, H. (2009). The palliative medication kit: An effective way of extending care in the home for patients nearing death. *Journal of Palliative Medicine, 12*(9), 797–803. doi:10.1089=jpm.2009.0048.

---

a period of time on an emergency and regular basis after the death of the person.

Pain control and the opportunity to die at home are the key ideas and activities that people associate with hospice palliative care services. A growing number of inpatient hospice facilities exist as well. These facilities have developed from home-based programs that have added free-standing, small inpatient facilities for people who have symptoms that cannot be managed at home or who have no caregivers. Hospice nurses and others may also care for dying people who are residents in LTC homes, working with staff members to supplement care and provide expertise in symptom management. Palliative care services guided by formal hospice principles may be provided in LTC homes.

The Nurse's Role in Hospice Palliative Care

Nurses provide much of the direct care for a dying person and their family. Additional nursing roles are coordinating the implementation of the interdisciplinary care plan, managing palliative care services, and advocating for the humane care for persons who are dying and their families.

Canadian standards for hospice palliative care nursing were established in 2009 and revised in 2014 (CHPCA, 2014). The Canadian Nurses Association (CNA) offers certification in hospice palliative care nursing. The Canadian Association of Schools of Nursing entry-to-practice competencies describe the special skills, knowledge, and abilities for palliative and end-of-life care that are expected of graduating nurses. The overarching competencies are presented in Box 25.6. Detailed indicators for each competency are available at www.casn.ca.

DYING AND THE NURSE

Nurses are professional grievers; they invest time and caring. If they are working with older persons, they invest especially in those who are frail and reside in acute and LTC settings. Nurses experience the death of patients and residents over and over again. Some consider the death of a patient a failure—that they have "lost" the person they cared for. But good deaths can be viewed as professional successes each time nurses share the special, personal experience of providing care for dying older people and providing gentle care for their survivors. Nurses can use the reminders of their own mortality as motivation to live the best they can with what they have. Nurses can seek support and give support to one another. As grieving persons themselves, nurses may need to tell the story of the dying or of the person to the health care providers around them, either in formal or in informal support groups. They also must listen to the stories of their colleagues over and over again until the stories become part of the fabric of their colleagues' lives.

Caring for older persons requires knowledge of the grieving and dying processes as well as skills in providing palliative care or relieving symptoms. However, working with grieving or dying persons day in and day out is an art that calls for inner strength and coping skills. The most important coping skills for nurses

BOX 25.6	Entry-to-Practice Competencies for Hospice Palliative Care Nursing in Canada

1. Uses requisite relational skills to support decision making and negotiate modes of palliative and end-of-life care on an ongoing basis.
2. Demonstrates knowledge of grief and bereavement to support others from a cross-cultural perspective.
3. Demonstrates knowledge and skills in holistic, family-centred nursing care of persons at end-of-life who are experiencing pain and other symptoms.
4. Recognizes and responds to the unique end-of-life needs of various populations, such as elders, children, multicultural populations, those with cognitive impairment, language barriers, those in rural and remote areas, those with chronic diseases, mental illness and addictions, and marginalized populations.
5. Applies ethical knowledge skillfully when caring for persons at end-of-life and their families while attending to one's own responses such as moral distress and dilemmas, and success with end-of-life decision making.
6. Demonstrates the ability to attend to psychosocial and practical issues such as planning for death at home and after death care relevant to the person and the family members.
7. Identifies the full range and continuum of palliative and end-of-life care services, resources and settings in which they are available, such as home care.
8. Educates and mentors patients and family members on care needs, identifying the need for respite for family members, and safely and appropriately delegating care to other caregivers and care providers.
9. Demonstrates the ability to collaborate effectively to address the patient and family members' priorities within an integrated inter-professional team, including non-professional health care providers, and the patient himself or herself.

Source: Extracted from Canadian Association of Schools of Nursing (CASN). (2011). *Palliative and end-of-life care: Entry-to-practice competencies and indicators for registered nurses.* Ottawa, ON: Author. Retrieved from http://casn.ca/wp-content/uploads/2014/12/PEOLCCompetenciesandIndicatorsEn1.pdf.

may be the ability to find meaning and the ability to disengage (Desbiens & Fillion, 2007). The effective gerontological nurse has developed a personal philosophy of life and of death; although this outlook can and does change over time, it will help when times are difficult. Emotional maturity enables the nurse to deal with disappointment and the postponement of immediate wants or desires. Maturity also means that the nurse can reach out for help when needed. Finally, in order to provide comfort to grieving persons, nurses must be comfortable with their own lives or at least be able to set aside their own sadness and grief while working with the sadness and grief of others.

DECISION MAKING AT THE END OF LIFE

Decision making at the end of life has become a legal, ethical, medical, and personal concern. The lines between living and dying are blurred as a direct result of technological advances; hence, there is ambivalence concerning whether death is to be delayed, fought, or accepted.

The issue of who has the authority to make end-of-life decisions has been the subject of research, debate, and legislation. Legal requirements may vary across provinces and territories. Nurses have an obligation to know the legal requirements in their jurisdictions and to work with the older person and the family to determine how these requirements will fit the family members' cultural patterns and their end-of-life decision making.

The ethical issues of end-of-life care are complex. Nurses observe the CNA *Code of Ethics for Registered Nurses* (2017). The CNA and the Canadian Hospice Palliative Care Association have provided additional resources related to ethics and end-of-life care. (For additional resources, see http://evolve.elsevier.com/Canada/Ebersole/gerontological/.)

ADVANCE CARE PLANNING

Advance care planning is the process of planning for a time when a person may not have the mental capacity to make decisions about health care (Advocacy Centre for the Elderly, 2010) (see Chapter 22). It involves the person's (1) choosing a substitute decision maker and (2) communicating to the substitute decision maker their wishes for future health care, personal care, and living arrangements. Substitute decision makers are required to make decisions based on the incapable person's wishes or (if the person's wishes were not communicated) in the person's best interests. Advance care planning is sometimes referred to as creating a living will or an advance directive; the term "living will" is not a legal term in Canada. The terms used for advance directives and the legal requirements vary across provinces and territories. In some provinces, verbal communication of wishes for future care is sufficient, whereas other provinces require written directives. In all provinces, designating a substitute decision maker requires a written, dated, and signed document. If the person who becomes incapable has not designated a substitute decision maker, a hierarchy of substitute decision makers is mandated by provincial health care consent acts.

Creating an advance directive is voluntary. Nurses and health care facilities may provide patients with information about advance care planning, but they cannot require patients or residents to complete an advance directive (Wahl, 2009a). Institutional policies and practices must be consistent with provincial laws. In Ontario, the Advocacy Centre for the Elderly has identified a number of problems with the implementation of advance directive forms and policies within health care facilities and LTC homes (Wahl, 2009b). For information about advance care planning laws in the provinces and territories, see http://www.virtualhospice.ca/en_US/Main+Site+Navigation/Home/Topics/Topics/Decisions/Advance+Care+Planning+Across+Canada.aspx.

The nurse cannot provide legal information but often serves as a resource person ready to answer many of the questions that people have about end-of-life decision making. The nurse may be called not only to inquire about the presence of an existing advance directive but also to ensure that the directive still reflects the person's wishes and to advocate for those wishes to be followed. The nurse also has the responsibility to make sure that existing or newly created advance directives are appropriately located in the health record.

MEDICAL ASSISTANCE IN DYING

The recognition of a person's right to refuse life-sustaining medical measures has brought up age-old questions concerning a person's right to make decisions about the continuation of life. Some people, especially those who are suffering unremitting pain from a terminal illness, end their lives. Others ask for assistance in ending life in the most painless way possible.

Medical assistance in dying is legal in Canada, in several other countries, and in several US states. In June 2016, the Government of Canada passed *Bill C-14*, legalizing medically assisted dying. In Canada, medical assistance in dying occurs when either "a nurse practitioner (NP) or physician provides assistance by administering a medication to a client, at their request, that causes their death (i.e., clinician-assisted medical assistance in dying); or, an NP or physician prescribes or provides a medication to a client, at their request, so that they may self-administer the medication and in doing so cause their own death (i.e., client self-administered medical assistance in dying)" (College of Nurses of Ontario, 2016, p. 2). The law sets out eligibility criteria and safeguards that must be adhered to. To be eligible, the person must be at least 18 years old; have a grievous and irremediable medical condition; be capable of making their own health-related decisions; request assistance voluntarily; and provide informed consent, having been informed of other options. Medical assistance in dying cannot be requested by a substitute decision maker. The law defines what "grievous and irremediable medical condition" means. Safeguards include requirements for the following: a written request (with limitations on who can witness the request), a second opinion, a waiting period before the request is fulfilled, communication that prescribing physicians and nurse practitioners must have with pharmacists, and format for the completion of a death certificate.

The nurse's role in medical assistance in dying is to provide nursing care. Nurses are not legally permitted to administer medication in medical assistance in dying; only the patient, a nurse practitioner, or a physician may do this. Nurses should refer to their provincial or territorial regulatory body for guidance regarding nurses' roles in medically assisted dying.

Provincial and territorial governments provide information to the public about medical assistance in dying. Information for professional health care providers is available from the provincial and territorial regulatory bodies for nurses, physicians, and pharmacists. (See http://eol.law.dal.ca/?page_id=236 for links to these resources and the law.)

Strong opinions exist about medically assisted dying and about implementing advance directives. Misunderstanding may exist among nurses regarding terminology and the interpretation of the effects the nurse's role may have. Some nurses believe that turning off the ventilator, turning off tube feedings, stopping intravenous fluids, or giving as much pain medication as is needed—even if directed by the patient—where death is the outcome constitutes assisted suicide. Another perspective is that withdrawing such devices allows a natural death to occur, which is very different from actively doing something to cause death. Nurses, individually and collectively, must consider the implication of this issue for themselves and for the profession.

KEY CONCEPTS

- Grief is an emotional and behavioural response to loss. Grief responses are individual; what is appropriate for a person from one ethnocultural group may be considered inappropriate by another person from the same group or from another ethnocultural group.
- Grief is never completely resolved. Instead, the grieving person incorporates the loss into his or her life.
- Dying is a multifaceted, active process. It affects all involved—the person who is dying, the dying person's family, and the professional caregivers.
- The stages or phases of dying and the types of coping are not universal and do not prescribe the way in which a person should die. Such expectations place an added burden on the dying person.
- The dying older person is a living person who has the same needs for good and natural relationships with people as all persons have.
- Hospice palliative care is both a concept and a health care program that focuses on care rather than cure and on the provision of comfort for the dying person and his or her significant others.
- Advance directives allow a person control over life-and-death decisions through written communication and the appointment of someone (i.e., a proxy) to be the person's advocate when the person is unable to personally communicate his or her desires.

- The nurse's role in medically assisted dying is to provide care and support for the dying person and his or her family.

ACTIVITIES AND DISCUSSION QUESTIONS

1. Explore your response to being given a terminal diagnosis. What coping mechanisms work for you? With which awareness approach would you be comfortable?
2. Describe how you would work with a dying person and his or her family when they are very protective of one another.
3. Describe how you would bring up the topic of advance directives.
4. Identify the advance directives that are legally recognized by your province or territory.
5. Describe how you would introduce the topic of dying with a person who is terminally ill.

RESOURCES

Association for Death Education and Counselling
https://www.adec.org

Canadian Hospice Palliative Care Association (CHPCA)
http://www.chpca.net

Canadian Hospice Palliative Care Nurses Group
http://www.chpca.net/join-us/nurses.aspx

Canadian Nurses Association (CNA). *Code of ethics for registered nurses* (2017)
https://www.cna-aiic.ca/en/on-the-issues/best-nursing/nursing-ethics

Canadian Nurses Association (CNA). *Palliative and end-of-life care*
https://www.cna-aiic.ca/en/on-the-issues/better-health/palliative-and-end-of-life-care

Health Canada. *Palliative and end-of-life care resources*
https://www.canada.ca/en/health-canada/services/health-care-system/palliative-end-life-care/resources.html

Health Law Institute, Dalhousie University. *End-of-life law & policy in Canada*
http://eol.law.dal.ca/

End of Life Nursing Education Consortium
http://www.aacn.nche.edu/ELNEC/about.htm

Hospice & Palliative Nurses Association
http://hpna.advancingexpertcare.org/

National Initiative for Care of the Elderly (NICE). *When someone close to you is dying: What you can expect and how you can help*
http://www.nicenet.ca/files/EOL-_Booklet_(v.11).pdf

For additional resources, please visit *http:// evolve.elsevier.com/Canada/Ebersole/gerontological/*

REFERENCES

Advocacy Centre for the Elderly (ACE). (2010). *Advance care planning—Frequently asked questions.* Retrieved from http://www.advocacycentreelderly.org/advance_care_planning_-_frequently_asked_questions.php.

Canadian Cancer Society (2016). *Right to care: Palliative care for all Canadians.* Toronto, ON: Author. Retrieved from https://www.cancer.ca/~/media/cancer.ca/CW/get%20involved/take%20action/Palliative-care-report-2016-EN.pdf?la=en.

Canadian Hospice Palliative Care Association (CHPCA). (2014). *Canadian Hospice Palliative Care Nursing Standards of Practice.* Retrieved from http://acsp.net/media/367211/chpc_ng.standards.2014.14_july_2014.final.pdf.

Canadian Nurses Association (2017). *Code of Ethics for Registered Nurses.* Ottawa, ON: Author. Retrieved from https://www.cna-aiic.ca/html/en/Code-of-Ethics-2017-Edition/index.html#.

College of Nurses of Ontario (2016). *Guidance on nurses' roles in medical assistance in dying.* Toronto, ON: Author. Retrieved from http://www.cno.org/en/trending-topics/medical-assistance-in-dying/.

Coryell, D. (2007). *Good grief: Healing through the shadow of grief.* Rochester, VT: Healing Arts Press.

Desbiens, J., & Fillion, L. (2007). Coping strategies, emotional outcomes and spiritual quality of life in palliative care nurses. *International Journal of Palliative Nursing, 13*(6), 291–300.

Doka, K. J. (2002). *Disenfranchised grief: New direction, challenges, and strategies for practice.* Champaign, IL: Research Press.

Doka, K. J. (2016). *Grief is a journey. Finding your path through loss.* New York, NY: Simon & Shuster.

Freeman, S., Heckman, G., Naus, P. J., et al. (2013). Breaking down barriers: Hospice palliative care as a human right in Canada. *Educational Gerontology, 39*(4), 241–249. doi:10.1080/03601277.2013.750930.

Giacquinta, B. (1977). Helping families face the crisis of cancer. *American Journal of Nursing, 77*(10), 1585–1588.

Glaser, B. G., & Strauss, A. L. (1963). *Awareness of dying.* Chicago, IL: Aldine.

Glaser, B. G., & Strauss, A. L. (1968). *Time for dying.* Chicago, IL: Aldine.

Health Canada (2002). *National action planning workshop on end-of-life care.* Ottawa, ON: Author. Retrieved from https://www.canada.ca/en/health-canada/services/health-care-system/reports-publications/palliative-care/national-action-planning-workshop-end-life-care.html.

Health Canada (2007). *Canadian strategy on palliative and end-of-life care. Final report of the coordinating committee.* Ottawa, ON: Author. Retrieved from http://www.hc-sc.gc.ca/hcs-sss/alt_formats/hpb-dgps/pdf/pubs/2007-soin_fin-end_life/2007-soin-fin-end_life-eng.pdf.

Jett, K. F. (2004). *The Loss Response Model.* Unpublished manuscript.

Kaasalainen, S., Brazil, K., Williams, A., et al. (2012). Barriers and enablers to providing palliative care in rural communities: A nursing perspective. *Journal of Rural and Community Development, 7*(4), 4–19. Retrieved from http://journals.brandonu.ca/jrcd/article/view/868.

Kübler-Ross, E. (1969). *On death and dying.* New York, NY: Macmillan.

Lee, G. L., Woo, I. M., & Goh, C. (2012). Understanding the concept of a "good death" among bereaved family caregivers of cancer patients in Singapore. *Palliative & Supportive Care, 11*(1), 37–46. doi:10.1017/S1478951511000691.

Lewis, I. D., & McBride, M. (2004). Anticipatory grief and chronicity: Elders and families in racial/ethnic minority groups. *Geriatric Nursing, 25*(1), 44–47. doi:10.1016/j.gerinurse.2003.11.014.

Metzger, P. L., & Gray, M. J. (2008). End-of-life communication and adjustment: Pre-loss communication as a predictor of bereavement-related outcomes. *Death Studies, 32*(4), 301–325. doi:10.1080/07481180801928923.

Murray, S. A., Kendall, M., Boyd, K., et al. (2005). Illness trajectories and palliative care. *British Medical Journal (BMJ), 330,* 1007–1011. doi:10.1136/bmj.330.7498.1007.

Neimeyer, R. A., & Holland, J. M. (2015). Bereavement in later life: Theory, assessment, and intervention. In P. A. Lichtenberg, B. T. Mast, B. D. Carpenter, et al. (Eds.), *APA handbook of clinical geropsychology* (Vol. 2, pp. 645–666). Assessment, treatment, and issues in later life. Washington, DC: American Psychological Association. doi:10.1037/14459-025.

Northcott, H. C., & Wilson, D. M. (2017). *Dying and death in Canada.* Toronto, ON: University of Toronto Press.

Pattison, E. M. (1977). The experience of dying. In E. M. Pattison (Ed.), *The experience of dying.* Englewood Cliffs, NJ: Prentice-Hall.

Richter, J. M. (1987). Support: A resource during crisis of mate loss. *Journal of Gerontological Nursing, 13*(11), 18–22. doi:10.3928/0098-9134-19871101-06.

Tal, I., Mauro, C., Reynolds, C. F., et al. (2016). Complicated grief after suicide bereavement and other causes of death. *Death Studies,* e-pub ahead of print. doi:10.1080/07481187.2016.1265028.

Thompson, N., Allan, J., Carverhill, P. A., et al. (2016). The case for a sociology of dying, death, and bereavement. *Death Studies, 40*(3), 172–181. doi:10.1080/07481187.2015.1109377.

Wahl, J. (2009a). *Advance care planning and end of life decision-making: More than just documents.* Toronto, ON: Advocacy

Centre for the Elderly. Retrieved from http://www.advocacy centreelderly.org/appimages/file/Advance%20Care%20Planning %20&%20End%20of%20Life%20Decision%20Making.pdf.

Wahl, J. (2009b). *Advance care planning in Ontario*. Toronto, ON: Advocacy Centre for the Elderly. Retrieved from http://www.advocacycentreelderly.org/appimages/file/Advance%20 Care%20Planning%20in%20Ontario.pdf.

Ward, L., Mathias, J. L., & Hitchings, S. E. (2007). Relationships between bereavement and cognitive functioning in older adults. *Gerontology*, 53(6), 362–372. doi:10.1159/000104787.

Weisman, A. (1979). *Coping with cancer*. New York, NY: McGraw-Hill.

Weisman, A. (1984). *The coping capacity: On the nature of being mortal*. New York, NY: Human Sciences Press.

Williams, A. M., Donovan, R., Stajduhar, K., et al. (2015). Cultural influences on palliative family caregiving: Service recommendations specific to the Vietnamese in Canada. *BMC Research Notes*, 25(8), 280. doi:10.1186/s13104-015-1252-3.

Williams, A. M., Crooks, V. A., Whitfield, K., et al. (2010). Tracking the evolution of hospice palliative care in Canada: A comparative case study analysis of seven provinces. *BMC Health Services Research*, 10, 147. doi:10.1186/1472-6963-10-147.

Wilson, D. M., Birch, S., Sheps, S., et al. (2008). Researching a best-practice end-of-life care model for Canada. *Canadian Journal on Aging*, 27(4), 319–330. doi:10.3138/cja.27.4.319.

Worden, J. W. (2008). *Grief counseling and grief therapy: A handbook for mental health practitioners* (4th ed.). New York, NY: Springer.

World Health Organization (2017). *WHO definition of palliative care*. Geneva, Switzerland: Author. Retrieved from http://www.who.int/cancer/palliative/definition/en/.

Zisook, S., Iglewicz, A., Avanzino, J., et al. (2014). Bereavement: Course, consequences, and care. *Current Psychiatry Reports*, 16(10), 482. doi:10.1007/s11920-014-0482-8.

Upon completion of this chapter, the reader will be able to:

- Compare the major features, advantages, and disadvantages of several residential options available to the older person.
- Assist an older person in making an informed choice when planning a move.
- Describe factors influencing the provision of long-term care (LTC).
- Discuss the characteristics of LTC homes and the impact of the culture-change movement.
- Name several strategies to ease the transition between settings for the older person.

GLOSSARY

Aging in place Continuing to live in one's home; not having to move to receive services as needs change.

Capitation system "A way of paying for health care for a group of people. Under this scheme, [a health care organization or provider] receives a lump sum payment per person from a provincial or regional government [and] uses the funds to provide services to meet the health needs of all people on its roster in its geographic area" (Canadian Health Services Research Foundation, 1999, p. 2).

Co-payment The amount paid by residents for accommodation in an LTC home or by recipients of home care services.

Ward room A basic or standard room in an LTC home. A ward room is usually a room with three or four beds or a two-bed room that shares an adjoining bathroom with another two-bed room, depending on when the home was built.

THE LIVED EXPERIENCE

My parents are older, I just lost my mom 2 years ago. And she lived in her home till the day she died. Two months before she died, I left [work] to take care of her. And I see a lot of these people and I know how I want my parents taken care of. So I see a lot of them [my parents] in the residents 'cause they were old and so I care for them in that way.

A nurse in an LTC home (McGilton et al., 2014, p. 920)

This is my home. We are all like a family, and I will die here. The girls that help me during the day, we treat one another like family members. We have some days when we are grumpy, some days we are happy, and we don't hold our feelings back, like you would do with your own family at home.

An 85-year-old resident of an LTC home

A mobile youth-oriented society may find it difficult to fully comprehend the insecurity older people feel when moving from one location to another. In addition to the stress of relocation and the initial anxiety of adapting to a new setting, older people often move to a more restrictive environment at a time of crisis. This chapter discusses residential care options across the continuum and related implications for nursing practice. The major issues are the choice and control an older person has over relocation, assistance to the person with making personally appropriate choices, strategies to ease the transition to different settings, and the creation of environments that enhance care outcomes in whatever situation the older person encounters.

AGE-FRIENDLY COMMUNITIES

"Home" is basic shelter, a place to establish security, and the place where a person "belongs." A home should provide the highest possible level of independence, function, and comfort for the older person. Most older people prefer to remain in their own homes, **"aging in place"** rather than relocating, particularly to a residential care setting. Being able to age in place depends on appropriate support for changing needs, so that the older person can stay wherever he or she wants. Developing age-friendly communities and creating more opportunities to age in place can enhance the health and well-being of older people.

In a project organized through the World Health Organization (WHO), 33 cities, including 4 Canadian cities, implemented and evaluated age-friendly principles. The response to this project was overwhelming, so the WHO created a global network of age-friendly communities (WHO, 2007). In Canada, the Age-Friendly Communities Initiative, based on WHO program principles, is led by the Public Health Agency of Canada in collaboration with other federal, provincial, territorial, and nongovernmental partners. Several provinces have age-friendly programs (Public Health Agency of Canada [PHAC], 2016). Many municipalities both formally and informally adopted age-friendly initiatives by assessing their communities and designing community-level interventions to enhance the potential for older people to remain in their homes and familiar environments. The WHO

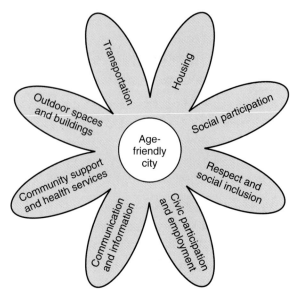

FIGURE 26.1 Elements of age-friendly cities and communities. *Source:* World Health Organization (WHO). (2008). *Global age-friendly cities: A guide* (p. 9). Geneva, Switzerland: Author. Retrieved from http://www.who.int/ageing/publications/Global_age_friendly_cities_Guide_English.pdf.

model of the elements of age-friendly cities and communities is shown in Fig. 26.1. Age friendliness is determined not only by the physical environment but also by the social environment and by health and social services. A checklist of essential features for each element is provided by the WHO (see Resources section at the end of the chapter). Box 26.1 describes a study that was conducted as part of the Age-Friendly Cities project in Quebec.

RESIDENTIAL OPTIONS IN LATER LIFE

Some older people, by choice or by need, move from one type of residence to another. A number of options exist, especially for people with sufficient financial resources. Residential options range from remaining in one's own home; to senior retirement communities; to shared housing with family members, friends, or others; to residential care communities such as assisted-living settings; and (for those with the most needs) to long-term care (LTC) homes (Fig. 26.2). Ten percent of older Canadians would like to move but cannot. These people have higher levels

BOX 26.1 Research for Evidence-Informed Practice: Older Persons' Housing Needs and the Meaning of Home in Older Life

Problem: Most older Canadians live in houses and want to age in their own homes. Alternative housing options are available, including seniors' communities. Some research indicates that available alternatives do not meet older persons' needs. There is little research about older persons' perspectives on aging in place and the meaning of home. The aim of this study was to examine the meaning of home and older persons' housing needs from their perspective.

Methods: A multimethod study was conducted in Quebec. One part of the study was composed of 49 focus groups made up of older persons, caregivers, and service providers. The second part was a case study about not-for-profit community-based housing for older persons, using 11 in-depth interviews. Thematic analysis was conducted.

Findings: One of the study themes was the social aspect of the meaning of home. Participants wanted to have access to services and amenities—access to public transportation

and being able to walk to services such as grocery stores, banks, and clinics. However, zoning regulations and the manner in which communities are now built mean that this access is unlikely. Concentrating housing and services for older persons in one area was seen as problematic. Participants were reluctant to live in seniors' neighborhoods, describing these areas as "ghettoized." They wanted to live in neighborhoods with people of all ages. Pedestrian safety and being able to walk to green spaces were important.

Application to Nursing Practice: Collaboration between health care providers, provincial and municipal governments, and nongovernmental organizations is necessary for achieving age-friendly communities that meet older persons' needs. Concentrating services and housing for older persons may seem efficient, but doing so would isolate those older persons.

Source: Bigonnesse, C., Beaulieu, M., & Garon, S. (2014). Meaning of home in later life as a concept to understand older persons' housing needs: Results from the 7 Age-Friendly Cities pilot project in Québec. *Journal of Housing for the Elderly, 28,* 357–382. doi:10.1080/02763893.2014.930367.

Independence

- Home ownership
- Single-room occupation (SRO)
- Condominium ownership
- Apartment dwelling
- Shared housing/co-housing
- Adult lifestyle communities
- Life lease

Independence to partial dependence

- Public/subsidized housing
- Residence with family
- Supportive housing/living
- Assisted living
- Residential facility
- Retirement homes/ residences/communities

Partial dependence to complete dependence

- Extended care
- Hospice care
- Complex continuing care
- Residential respite care
- Long-term care homes (special care homes, personal care homes, nursing homes)
- Acute care facilities
- Rehabilitation facilities

Independence ←————————————————————————————→ Dependence

FIGURE 26.2 Continuum of residential options based on the level of assistance needed. *Source:* Adapted from Ebersole, P., Touhy, T., Hess, P. et al. (2008). *Toward healthy aging: Human needs and nursing response* (7th ed., p. 438, Fig. 17-1). St. Louis, MO: Mosby.

of psychological distress, greater need of assistance, and lower levels of health and social involvement. They also are less likely to own their own home (Strohschein, 2012). There are many different models of housing, and older people may seek assistance from gerontological nurses when choosing what kind of living situation will be best for them. The terms used to describe the different models vary from province to province; the legislation and regulations vary as well. (In some cases, there are none). Information about care facilities in Canada is available on the Seniors Canada website (http://www.seniors.gc.ca), via the *Care Guide* online directory of older-person care (https://www.caregide.com), and through the provincial websites.

INDEPENDENT LIVING OPTIONS

With the aging of the "baby boomers," architects and engineers are focusing on home designs that adjust to the changes that accompany aging, thereby enabling older people to stay in their homes safely even if they experience illness and functional decline. These new designs are marketed as "transgenerational" or "universal" designs and can benefit everyone, not just older people. Designs and modifications may include safety fittings in the bathroom, walk-in showers, wider doorways, remote-controlled devices for lights and window coverings, raised countertops, polyurethane or cork flooring, and adjustable-height sinks. Available online, *Safe Living Guide—A Guide to Home Safety for Seniors* (Public Health Agency of Canada [PHAC], 2015) includes strategies for home adaptations that improve safety and accessibility. Additional information, including information about financial assistance programs, is available from the Canada Mortgage and Housing Corporation (CMHC) website at https://www.cmhc-schl.gc.ca/en/co/acho/index.cfm.

SOCIAL HOUSING

Social housing, also referred to as subsidized housing or public housing, includes municipally owned and operated housing; nonprofit housing; cooperative housing; and privately owned housing, all for which the government provides a rent supplement for low-income tenants. The subsidies ensure that the tenant does not spend more than 30% of income on rent (Government of Alberta, 2014). Social housing options include for-profit and not-for-profit properties as well as provincial cooperative housing. Social housing is an important option for older people, because poverty is an issue for 12.5% of older Canadians. The rates of poverty are higher among women, people who live alone, immigrants, and Indigenous persons (see Chapter 22).

Since 1996, social housing programs and their administration have been the sole responsibility of the provinces and territories. Some programs reserve social housing units for older persons. Unfortunately, the waiting lists for social housing are long. For example, the Ontario Non-Profit Housing Association (2016) reported that there were 171,360 households on waiting lists at the beginning of 2015; 32% of those households were those of older persons. The average wait time for new applicants is 5.2 years and is much higher than this in urban areas.

LIFE LEASE

Life lease is an arrangement in which a resident neither owns nor rents a home but has a lifelong lease for one. The lease requires a single upfront payment and monthly fees for the management and upkeep of the property. The lease contract gives residents the right to occupy their units and use common areas and facilities until they die or move. Some life lease projects are co-located with assisted-living facilities or LTC homes, and leaseholders can access care services through these facilities for a fee. People aged 55 years and older are the major market for life lease projects, under which older people can move into smaller and usually more affordable housing (Canada Mortgage and Housing Corporation [CMHC], 2007).

Life lease projects are run by for-profit or not-for-profit organizations. The exact number of life lease projects in Canada is not known, because there is no requirement for registration. Manitoba is the only province with legislation specific to life lease housing. Advocates for older persons are lobbying for legislation to ensure that residents' rights are protected. Issues for legislation include protecting civil and human rights; regulating the provided care services; prohibiting illegal promises of automatic admission to LTC homes; and addressing a number of consumer protection issues (Rosenbaum, 2007). The Advocacy

Centre for the Elderly suggests that restricting life lease projects to not-for-profit organizations would ensure a focus on the well-being of lease holders (Rosenbaum, 2007).

ADULT LIFESTYLE COMMUNITIES

Adult lifestyle communities or neighbourhoods are also known as retirement communities, resort communities, and 55-plus communities. Housing is typically in the form of condominiums—as high rises, townhouses, or detached homes. The communities are designed for newly retired persons and often include recreation facilities (e.g., golf courses, trails, swimming pools, fitness centres, and clubs). Most of these communities are "gated," may have security, and have age restrictions that limit ownership and residency to persons of a certain age (such as 50, 55, or 60 years of age).

SHARED HOUSING

Shared housing among adult children and their older relatives is a preferred choice for many because of cultural preferences or need. The sharing may relieve the economic burdens of maintaining a home after widowhood or retirement on a fixed income. Cultural influences predict the frequency of multigenerational residences. Among Asians and South Asians, shared housing is often an expectation. Relocating from one's own home to the home of an adult child can have many benefits; without adequate preparation, however, it can also be stressful for both the family and the older person. Interventions to support healthy relocation and transition are discussed later in the chapter. Box 26.2 presents some factors to consider when adding an older person to the household is planned.

A variation of multigenerational housing is the "granny flat." Granny flats can be apartments added to existing homes, or small housing units on family property that provide privacy and the sharing of time and resources. Such arrangements allow an older person to live separately from the family but close enough to the family to obtain assistance if needed.

COHABITATION OR COHOUSING

Another model of shared housing is that of opening homes to others, or *cohabitation*. Older people often live in houses that they purchased in their younger years and that have ample space geared to family life, but about one-half of the space is underused. The cohousing model is more formalized in the United States and Europe, where there are services to match older people who are looking for houses to share. People who share homes report feeling safer and less lonely. Studies on home sharing focus on its effects on well-being, finances, health, social life, and daily satisfaction. Most successful is the intergenerational model, in which an older person shares his or her home with a younger person.

Cohousing is a model in which older persons own or rent individual homes that are clustered around a "common house" where residents share kitchen, dining room, playroom, and workshop areas; guest rooms; home office support; craft areas; and a laundry area. Each home is self-sufficient, but residents often share meals in the common area. Cohousing in Canada includes multigenerational communities as well as older persons' communities. This model is a growing option in North America (Canadian Cohousing Network, 2016).

COMMUNITY SERVICES FOR AGING IN PLACE

ADULT DAY SERVICES

Adult day services are community-based group programs designed to provide social and health services to older persons who need supervised care in a safe setting during the day. These programs also offer caregivers respite from the responsibilities of caregiving. Most adult day centres operate during normal business hours 5 days a week, but some offer services in the evening, overnight, and on weekends. The three types of adult day centres are social (meals, recreation, some health-related services), medical-health (social activities and more-intensive health and therapeutic services), and specialized (assistance for older persons with dementia or developmental disabilities). Adult day services are provided by publicly funded and volunteer organizations, and some communities offer ethnocultural-specific programs. Fees vary, and subsidies are available in many programs. Adult day services can make it possible for older persons to remain in the community and postpone moving

BOX 26.2   Planning to Add an Older Person to the Household

Questions to Ask
- What are the needs of the new household member and of the family?
- Where will space be allotted for the new member?
- How will the new member be included in existing family patterns?
- How will responsibilities be shared?
- What resources in the community will assist the older person in the adjustment phase?
- Is the environment safe for this new member?
- How will family life change with the older relative in the household, and how do family members feel about it?
- What are the differences in socialization and sleeping patterns between the older person and other family members?
- What are the older person's strong needs and expectations?
- What are the older person's skills and talents?

Necessary Modifications
- Semiprivate living quarters for the older relative if possible.
- Regularly scheduled visits to other relatives to give each family member time for respite and privacy.
- Adult day health programs and activities arranged for the older person to help him or her keep contact with members of his or her own generation. Consider how the older person will feel about giving up familiar surroundings and friends.

Potential Areas of Conflict
- Space (especially if someone has given up his or her space to the older relative).
- Possessions. Some older people may want to move their possessions into the house; others may not find them

attractive or may insist on replacing them with new things.
- Entertainment and times when older persons and young persons feel the need or desire to exclude the others from social events.
- Responsibilities and chores. Older persons may feel useless if they do nothing, and they may feel that they are in the way if they do anything. Younger family members may feel that their position is being usurped or may be angry if they are expected to wait on the older person.
- Expenses. The increased costs of home maintenance, food, clothing, and recreation may not be shared appropriately.
- Vacations (whether to go together or alone). Younger family members may feel uneasy about not taking the older person out and may be resentful if they must.
- Child rearing (disagreement over child rearing policies).
- Child care. Grandparental babysitting may be welcomed by the family but resented by the older person. If it is not allowed, however, the older person may feel a lack of trust in his or her capability.

Decrease Areas of Conflict by the Following:
- Respecting the older person's privacy.
- Discussing space allocations.
- Discussing the older person's furnishings before the move.
- Making it clear in advance when social events include everyone or exclude someone.
- Clearing decisions about household tasks (with everyone's responsibility geared to his or her ability).
- Having the older person pay a share of expenses and maintain a separate phone (reduces strain and increases the person's feelings of independence).

to LTC homes (Kelly et al., 2016). Use of adult day services is associated with less use of hospital services (Kelly, 2017). Access may be limited in rural and remote areas (Morgan et al., 2015).

HOME AND COMMUNITY CARE

Home care helps older persons live in the community by providing health services at home rather than in hospital or an LTC home. Approximately one million Canadians receive publicly funded home care services at any given time (Canadian Home Care Association [CHCA], 2016). Most home care recipients are over

65 years of age (Turcotte, 2014). Home care is delivered by nurses and other regulated health care providers, nonregulated workers, volunteers, friends, and family members. The goals of home care are listed in Box 26.3.

Home care provides nursing, personal care, physiotherapy, occupational therapy, speech therapy, social work, dietitian services, homemaking, respite, Meals on Wheels, friendly visiting, medical supplies and equipment, and case management. Services can be delivered via information and communication technologies (e.g., Telehomecare).

BOX 26.3 Goals of Home Care

- Help people maintain or improve their health status and quality of life
- Assist people in remaining as independent as possible
- Support families in coping with a family member's need for care
- Help people stay at or return home and receive needed treatment, rehabilitation, or palliative care
- Provide informal and family caregivers with the support they need

Source: Health Canada. (2016). *Home and community health care.* (Goals, ¶ 3). Retrieved from https://www.canada.ca/en/health-canada/services/home-continuing-care/home-community-care.html.

Home care is seen as a desirable way for an older person to receive health care while aging at home and as a way to decrease government costs of institution-based health care services (Box 26.4). Home care meets the following three needs: short-term acute care, long-term supportive care, and specialized services such as rehabilitation and palliative care. Some people receive short-term acute home care services as a substitute for (or a complement to) acute hospital-based care. These people receive a higher proportion of professional services. Other home care recipients, most of whom are older, receive long-term home care that helps them to maintain their functioning and to avoid admission to acute or LTC care. They are more likely to receive supportive services from nonprofessional staff.

Providing adequate access to home care services is a challenge across the country because of rising costs and limited funding; a shortage of health care and social care providers; and a lack of high-quality information for evaluation and quality improvement (CHCA, 2016). These issues are compounded in rural, remote, and northern settings (Kitchen et al., 2011).

Under the *Canada Health Act*, home care is an extended service, not an insured service. Home care programs vary from province to province. It is estimated that about 500,000 Canadians purchase home care services that are not funded by the government (CHCA, 2016). The financial cost of home care, paid for by service recipients and families, is about 25% of that paid for by governments (Hermus et al., 2012).

BOX 26.4 Research for Evidence-Informed Practice: Health Promotion for Frail Older Home Care Clients Enhances Quality of Life at No Extra Cost

Problem: Some studies indicate that there may be cost savings associated with home care, but these studies do not consider costs beyond reduced admissions to hospital and long-term care homes. There is a lack of evidence about the effect of home-based health promotion for frail older people.

Methods: This randomized controlled trial compared the usual home care services to the addition of proactive nursing health promotion for frail older home care clients. Health promotion included initial and ongoing assessment, identification and management of risk factors for functional decline, healthy-lifestyle education, an empowerment approach to the management of persistent illnesses, referral and coordination of community services, and caregiver support. Ongoing support was provided through home visits and telephone contact and in the context of a therapeutic relationship. Of the 288 participants, 242 completed a 6-month follow-up.

Findings: The health promotion group experienced a statistically significant improvement in mental and emotional health and decreased symptoms of depression. Social support was significantly increased, but there was no difference between the health promotion group and the control group with respect to coping styles. There was no difference between the two groups in regard to the costs of health and social services.

Application to Nursing Practice: Proactive health promotion by nurses results in improvements in the quality of life and mental well-being of frail older persons who receive home care, at no additional cost to the health care system. This research reinforces the importance of the nurse–client relationship and a client-centred, empowering practice.

Source: Markle-Reid, M., Weir, R., Browne, G., et al. (2006). Health promotion for frail older home care clients. *Journal of Advanced Nursing,* *54*(3), 381–395. doi:10.1111/j.1365-2648.2006.03817.x.

However, the **co-payment** and public–private mix of home care costs vary among provinces.

SUPPORTED LIVING OPTIONS

SUPPORTIVE HOUSING

Supportive housing consists of apartment buildings designated for older persons; they provide on-site personal support services such as homemaking services and on-call staff. Social and recreation programs and dining services may be provided. These programs are often operated by charitable or nonprofit organizations. Supportive housing may be provided in conjunction with social housing for older persons. Depending on the provincial model, government funding for care services for frail older residents is available. Residents are tenants whose rights are determined by provincial tenancies acts.

ASSISTED-LIVING FACILITIES AND RETIREMENT HOMES

Assisted-living facilities (ALFs) are nonmedical community-based residential settings that house adults and provide services such as meals, medication supervision or reminders, activities, transportation, and assistance with activities of daily living (ADLs). About 2.6% of Canadians aged 65 years and older live in ALFs (Statistics Canada, 2015a). These residences provide a rented single room or a bedsitting room and access to shared facilities. They are designed for older people who do not need care in an LTC home but who need more support than is available in shared housing. This kind of facility is known by different names across the country, including the following: assisted living, retirement homes, seniors' residences, personal care homes, residential homes, and retirement residences.

Most ALFs are operated by for-profit corporations, and some are operated by nonprofit or charitable organizations. They are not part of the health care system, and costs are not covered through provincial health insurance. Residents are tenants who pay separate fees for accommodation and care. Most ALFs offer two or three meals per day, light weekly housekeeping, and laundry services, as well as optional social activities. Many facilities have transportation services and Internet access. Some also have exercise facilities, movie theatres, pharmacies, and swimming pools. The ALF rent varies, depending on the market. In 2015, the average rent in Ontario was $2,210 per month; the highest average rent was in Ontario ($2,978), and the lowest was in Quebec ($1,527) (CMHC, 2016). In addition, health care services can be purchased, which can significantly increase costs but also allows individuals with financial resources to remain

in the setting longer as their functional abilities decline.

The governance, regulation, and funding of assisted living vary across provinces and territories. British Columbia and Ontario have provincial regulations that apply specifically to retirement homes. The Canadian Accreditation Council (2011) publishes standards for the accreditation of ALFs.

Many older persons and their families prefer ALFs to LTC homes because ALFs are more homelike and offer more opportunities for control, independence, and privacy. However, many tenants of ALFs have long-term health care needs that are associated with chronic, persistent, or degenerative illnesses; with time, these residents may require more care than the ALF is able to provide. Services (e.g., home health, hospice, homemakers) can be brought into the ALF, but there is some question as to whether such services are an adequate substitute for 24-hour supervision by registered nurses.

Depending on the physical layout of an ALF and how that ALF advertises its services, older persons and their families may not be able to differentiate between an ALF and an LTC home. As stated by Romano et al. (2008), "Although 'nursing' care may be offered by the retirement home, it is up to the individual retirement home operator to decide whether this care will be provided by or under the supervision of a regulated health professional: it is perfectly legal to provide what is advertised as 'nursing' care by unregulated, unsupervised workers" (Romano et al., 2008, p. 29).

With the growing numbers of older persons with dementia residing in ALFs, "many retirement homes have locked units and are operating as *de facto* long-term care homes" (Meadus & Romano, 2009). The legality of locked units in ALFs is questionable (Romano et al., 2008).

Nurses should be familiar with assisted-living options in their communities and be knowledgeable about the rights of ALF tenants. Nurses should help the person with dementia and their family to investigate the available services as well as staff training when making decisions as to the most appropriate housing and support for older persons with dementia. An evidence-informed guideline, *Dementia Care Practice Recommendations for Assisted Living Residences and*

Nursing Homes (Tilly & Reed, 2008), is available at the U.S. Alzheimer's Association website. The recommendations in the guideline are consistent with those in the guideline for dementia care in LTC homes. (See Chapter 21 for further information about dementia.)

Further research is needed on care outcomes of tenants in ALFs and the role of both unregulated and regulated health care providers in these facilities. However, the nonmedical nature of ALFs is the primary factor in keeping costs down. Consumers are advised to inquire as to exactly what services will be provided and by whom if an ALF resident becomes more frail and needs more-intensive care. The Advocacy Centre for the Elderly provides a consumer guide to choosing an ALF at http://www.advocacycentreelderly.org/ace_library.php.

HEALTH CARE FACILITY–BASED LIVING OPTIONS

LONG-TERM CARE HOMES

Long-term care homes (also called nursing homes, special care homes, and personal care homes) are the settings for the delivery of around-the-clock care for people who need specialized care that cannot be provided elsewhere. When run appropriately, LTC homes meet this important need for older people and their families. According to 2013/2014 data, there are 1,519 LTC homes in Canada and 149,488 residents (Statistics Canada, 2015b). About 4.5% of older Canadians live in an LTC home or a chronic care hospital (BC Medical Journal [BCMJ], 2012). Most LTC homes operate on a for-profit basis; about 20% are operated by municipal, provincial, or territorial governments, and about 20% are operated by religious or charitable organizations (Statistics Canada, 2010a).

There are more than twice as many women as men residing in LTC homes. Just over half of LTC residents are aged 85 years or older (Statistics Canada, 2010a). Inability to perform ADLs is one of the main reasons for moving to an LTC home, and most residents require significant assistance with ADLs and with instrumental activities of daily living. More than two-thirds of the residents are cognitively impaired. The prevalence of dementia is high. In Ontario, 90% of residents have some form of cognitive impairment, 40% have a mental health problem or disorder, and 46% have responsive behaviours related to cognitive impairment or mental disorder (Ontario Long Term Care Association [OLTCA], 2016).

Long-term care homes provide care for persons with various circumstances and health conditions—persons recently discharged from hospitals, frail persons, persons with dementia, and dying older persons who lack a caregiver or whose caregivers cannot meet their needs for education in end-of-life care. The development of new models of care provision are priorities in this setting (see Chapter 25).

Costs of Care

Like home care, LTC is an extended service, not an insured service. The cost of care is about $50,000 per year. While there are some entirely private-pay LTC homes, this is the exception. Provincial and territorial governments provide partial funding for LTC home services. In all provinces and all territories except Nunavut, residents pay facilities fees to cover the costs of accommodations and lodging. On average, about 70% of costs are publicly funded, but this varies significantly across the country (McDonald, 2015). The three payment models for facilities fees are (1) a per diem based on public pension incomes available to residents, (2) a per diem that is subsidized depending on the resident's income, or (3) a per diem that is subsidized depending on the resident's assets and income. The maximum fee for a **ward room** varies from $1,112 per month in Quebec to $3,254 per month in New Brunswick (The Care Guide, 2017). In some jurisdictions, spouses (especially low-income couples) who still live in the community may face financial hardship (McDonald, 2015). In addition to the facilities fee, the resident pays medical and personal expenses (e.g., dentures, hearing aids, specialized wheelchairs, foot care, personal hygiene products, and over-the-counter medications); the amount of this out-of-pocket expense varies (McDonald, 2015). Insurance for LTC is available for purchase in Canada.

Regulations and Quality of Care

Long-term care homes are highly regulated, but the related laws, regulations, and standards vary across provinces. Differences in regulatory approaches affect the design and atmosphere of LTC homes in a given province. For example, a comparison of LTC homes in Ontario with those of Nova Scotia found that units within the LTC homes in Nova Scotia were smaller and had a more homelike atmosphere than those in Ontario. Similarly, care in the Nova Scotia homes was less routinized, with more resident choice. The researchers attributed these differences to the differences in regulations (Braedley & Martel, 2015).

Although LTC homes recognize the need to ensure quality, the lack of additional funding to meet new regulations and standards and the increasingly complex needs of LTC home residents can make achieving quality a struggle. Criteria and standards often create a bureaucratic structure and a punitive environment for caregivers for LTC home residents. Facilities are inspected regularly on an unannounced basis to determine compliance with regulations and to investigate quality-of-care indicators. In most jurisdictions, data on quality indicators and complaints are publicly available on provincial government websites.

Regulations have also been created to protect the rights of the residents of nursing homes. Residents in LTC homes have rights under both federal and provincial laws. The staff of the home must inform residents of these rights and must protect and promote those rights. The rights to which the residents are entitled should be conspicuously posted in the LTC home. Box 26.5 lists LTC residents' rights as set out in Ontario's *Long-Term Care Homes Act.*

The Culture Change Movement in Long-Term Care Homes

Across North America, the movement to transform LTC homes from the typical medical model into homes that nurture quality of life for older people and support and empower caregivers is changing the face of LTC. Encouraged by the Pioneer Network, a United States–based national not-for-profit organization that serves the culture change movement, many facilities are changing from a rigid institutional approach to a person-centred approach (http://www.pioneernetwork.net). "Culture change is the process of moving from a traditional nursing home model—characterized as a system unintentionally designed to foster dependence by keeping residents, as one observer put it, 'well cared for, safe, and powerless'—to a regenerative model that increases residents' autonomy and sense of control" (Brawley, 2007, p. 9).

Older people in need of long term care want to live in a homelike setting that does not look and function like a hospital. They want a setting that allows them to make the decisions that they are used to making for themselves, such as when to get up, take a bath, eat, or go to bed. They want caregivers who know them and understand their individuality and their preferences. Box 26.6 presents some of the differences between an institution-centred culture and a person-centred culture.

Examples of philosophies and programs of culture change are the Eden Alternative, founded by Dr. Bill Thomas (http://www.edenalt.org); the Green House Project (www.thegreenhouseproject.org); and the Wellspring Model, developed by Wellspring Innovative Solutions, in Seymour, Wisconsin (http://www.wellspringis.org).

The Eden Alternative is best known for the addition of animals, plants, and children to LTC homes. However, truly transforming an LTC home requires the involvement of all levels of staff and also changes in values, attitudes, structures, and management practices.

The Alzheimer Society of Canada (2011) developed *Guidelines for Care: Person-Centred Care of People with Dementia Living in Care Homes.* Some of the principles of culture-change activities are as follows:

- Staff empowerment
- Resident involvement in decision making
- Individualized rather than routine task-oriented care
- Relationship building
- Sense of community and belonging
- Meaningful activities
- Homelike environment
- Attention to the respect of staff and the value of caring

Making LTC Home Decisions

Gerontological nurses are frequently asked to help older persons and their families make decisions about choosing an LTC home. Gerontological nurse Marilyn Rantz and her colleagues have extensively researched and written about the quality of care in LTC homes. Box 26.7 presents their guide to selecting an LTC home. A systematic review and meta-analysis of quality in LTC homes indicated that on average,

BOX 26.5 Bill of Rights for Long-Term Care Residents in Ontario

1. Every resident has the right to be treated with courtesy and respect and in a way that fully recognizes the resident's individuality and respects the resident's dignity.
2. Every resident has the right to be protected from abuse.
3. Every resident has the right not to be neglected by the licensee or staff.
4. Every resident has the right to be properly sheltered, fed, clothed, groomed, and cared for in a manner consistent with his or her needs.
5. Every resident has the right to live in a safe and clean environment.
6. Every resident has the right to exercise the rights of a citizen.
7. Every resident has the right to be told who is responsible for and who is providing the resident's direct care.
8. Every resident has the right to be afforded privacy in treatment and in caring for his or her personal needs.
9. Every resident has the right to have his or her participation in decision making respected.
10. Every resident has the right to keep and display personal possessions, pictures, and furnishings in his or her room, subject to safety requirements and the rights of other residents.
11. Every resident has the right to do the following:
    i. Participate fully in the development, implementation, review, and revision of his or her plan of care
    ii. Give or refuse consent to any treatment, care, or services for which his or her consent is required by law and be informed of the consequences of giving or refusing consent
    iii. Participate fully in making any decision concerning any aspect of his or her care, including any decision concerning his or her admission, discharge, or transfer to or from a long-term care home or a secure unit, and obtain an independent opinion with regard to any of those matters
    iv. Have personal health information kept confidential and have access to his or her records of personal health information, including his or her plan of care
12. Every resident has the right to receive care and assistance toward independence based on a restorative care philosophy to maximize independence to the greatest extent possible.
13. Every resident has the right not to be restrained, except in the limited circumstances provided for under this *Act* and subject to the requirements provided for under this *Act.*
14. Every resident has the right to communicate in confidence, receive visitors of his or her choice, and consult in private with any person without interference.
15. Every resident who is dying or who is very ill has the right to have family and friends present 24 hours per day.
16. Every resident has the right to designate a person to receive information concerning any transfer or any hospitalization of the resident and to have that person receive that information immediately.
17. Every resident has the right to raise concerns or recommend changes in policies and services on behalf of himself or herself or others without interference and without fear of coercion, discrimination, or reprisal, whether directed at the resident or anyone else.
18. Every resident has the right to form friendships and relationships and to participate in the life of the long-term care home.
19. Every resident has the right to have his or her lifestyle and choices respected.
20. Every resident has the right to participate in the Residents' Council.
21. Every resident has the right to meet privately with his or her spouse or another person in a room that assures privacy.
22. Every resident has the right to share a room with another resident according to their mutual wishes, if appropriate accommodation is available.
23. Every resident has the right to pursue social, cultural, religious, spiritual, and other interests, to develop his or her potential and to be given reasonable assistance by the licensee to pursue these interests and to develop his or her potential.
24. Every resident has the right to be informed in writing of any law, rule, or policy affecting services provided to the resident and of the procedures for initiating complaints.
25. Every resident has the right to manage his or her own financial affairs unless the resident lacks the legal capacity to do so.
26. Every resident has the right to be given access to protected outdoor areas in order to enjoy outdoor activity unless the physical setting makes this impossible.
27. Every resident has the right to have any friend, family member, or other person of importance to the resident attend any meeting with the licensee or the staff of the home.

Note: This list is an example from Ontario-legislated rights of residents of long-term homes. Nurses should check the laws in their province or territory for specific rights.

Source: Long-Term Care Homes Act, 2007, S.O. 2007, c. 8. Retrieved from http://www.e-laws.gov.on.ca/html/statutes/english/elaws_statutes_07l08_e.htm#BK5.

BOX 26.6 Institution-Centred Versus Person-Centred Culture

Institution-Centred Culture
- Schedules and routines are designed by the institution and staff, and residents must comply.
- Focus is on tasks to be accomplished.
- Staff is rotated from unit to unit.
- Decision making is centralized, with little involvement of staff or residents and families.
- Environment is hospital-like.
- Structured activities are provided to all residents.
- Opportunity for socializing is limited.
- Organization exists for employees rather than residents.
- Privacy and individual routines are given little respect.

Person-Centred Culture
- Emphasis is on relationships between staff and residents.
- Individualized plans of care are based on residents' needs, usual patterns, and desires.
- Staff members have consistent assignments, know the residents' preferences, and recognize each resident's uniqueness.
- Decisions are made as close to the resident as possible.
- Staff members are involved in decisions and plans of care.
- Environment is homelike.
- Meaningful activities and opportunities for socialization are available around the clock.
- A sense of community and belonging ("like family") exists.
- The community is involved (e.g., through children, pets, plants, and outings).

Source: Adapted from The Pioneer Network. Retrieved from http://www.pioneernetwork.net.

BOX 26.7 Selecting a Long-Term Care Home

Central Focus
- Residents and families are the central focus.

Interaction
- Staff members are attentive and caring.
- Staff members listen to what residents say.
- Staff members and residents smile at one another.
- There is a prompt response to resident and family needs.
- Meaningful activities are provided at various times of the day and evening to meet individual preferences.
- Residents engage in activities with enjoyment.
- Staff members talk to cognitively impaired residents; these residents are involved in activities designed to meet their needs.
- Staff members do not talk down to residents, talk as if they are not present, or ignore yelling or calling out.
- Families are involved in care decisions and daily life in the home.

Milieu
- Calm, active, friendly
- Presence of community—volunteers, children, plants, animals

Environment
- No odour; clean and well maintained
- Rooms personalized
- Private areas
- Protected outside areas
- Equipment in good repair

Individualized Care
- Restorative programs for ambulation, activities of daily living
- Well-dressed and groomed residents
- Resident and family councils
- Pleasant mealtimes, good food, choices for residents
- Adequate staff to serve meals and assist residents
- Flexible meal schedules, food available 24 hours per day
- Ethnic food preferences

Staff
- Well trained; high level of professional skill
- Professional in appearance and demeanour
- Registered nurses involved in care decisions and care delivery
- Active staff development programs
- Physicians and advanced-practice nurses involved in care planning and staff training
- Adequate staff (i.e., more than the minimum required) on each shift
- Low staff turnover

Safety
- Safe walking areas indoors and outdoors
- Monitoring of residents at risk for injury
- Adequate safety equipment and training in its use

Source: Adapted from Rantz, M. J., Mehr, D. R., Popejoy, L., et al. (1998). Nursing home care quality: A multidimensional theoretical model. *Journal of Nursing Care & Quality, 12*(3), 30–46.

not-for-profit LTC homes scored higher on quality indicators (including staffing ratio, prevalence of pressure injury, and use of physical restraint) and had fewer deficiencies upon regulatory assessments (Comondore et al., 2009). However, as the authors noted, quality in the not-for-profit and for-profit sectors is variable. The most appropriate method of choosing an LTC home is to personally visit the facility, meet with the director of nursing or resident care, observe care practices, discuss the potential resident's needs, and use a format such as the one presented in Box 26.7 to ask questions.

IMPROVING TRANSITIONS ACROSS THE CONTINUUM OF CARE

Older people have complex health care needs and often require care in multiple settings across the continuum of care. "Care transition" refers to the movement of patients from one health care practitioner or setting to another as their condition and care needs change. Transitional care requires a set of clinical and communication activities that should occur when older persons move from one care setting to another. An older person may be treated by a family practitioner; hospitalized and treated by an intensivist or nurse practitioner; discharged to an LTC home and followed by another practitioner; and then discharged home or to an ALF, where the family practitioner may or may not continue to follow him or her. Many health care providers practise in only one setting and are not familiar with the specific requirements of other settings. "Many factors contribute to gaps in care during critical transitions, including poor communication, incomplete transfer of information, inadequate education of older persons and their family members, medication errors, limited access to essential services, and the absence of a single point person to ensure continuity of care" (Naylor & Keating, 2008, p. 65). Language and health literacy issues and cultural differences exacerbate the problem.

Transitions between settings happen often. There is increasing evidence that older persons experience serious care deficiencies when undergoing transitions. Older people who are at high risk for transitional care problems include persons with multiple medical conditions or mental disorders, isolated persons (without family or friends), non-English speakers, immigrants, and persons with low incomes (Graham et al., 2009).

A significant number of older people who are admitted to an acute care hospital end up in another setting, typically an LTC home. Many people wait for a long time in an acute care hospital until there is space available for them in an LTC home or until home care becomes available so that they can go home or move to an ALF. This situation of staying in an acute care hospital when acute care is no longer needed, while waiting for an appropriate place to live or to receive less-intensive care, is called an alternate level of care (ALC). About 13% of Canadian hospital beds are occupied by a person awaiting discharge (Sutherland & Crump, 2013). Thirty-five percent of patients who are designated as ALC patients are aged 85 years or older, and 25% have dementia. The most common destination after discharge is an LTC home (Sutherland & Crump, 2013). Unnecessary functional decline is a common outcome for patients who are designated ALC patients (McCloskey et al., 2014).

Integrated care was developed as an alternative to LTC homes for frail older people who want to live in their communities independently and with a high quality of life. Integrated care programs are seen as a possible way to reduce unnecessary waiting. Examples of integrated care in Canada include two programs in Quebec (Integrated Services for Frail Elders, and the Program of Research to Integrate the Services for the Maintenance of Autonomy) and one program in Alberta (Comprehensive Home Option of Integrated Care for the Elderly) (MacLean et al., 2007). These programs provide a comprehensive continuum of primary care, community and home-based care, social care, and specialty care, provided by a case manager and an interprofessional team. Funding is done through a **capitation system** in which the team is provided with a monthly sum to provide all services. Integrated Services for Frail Elders (SIPA) was evaluated in an experimental study that included frail and nonfrail older persons. The researchers found that SIPA enrollees used fewer institution-based services (e.g., less time in acute care, less time waiting for an LTC bed, and fewer emergency visits). Costs were similar for the overall sample. However, for participants who were frail, there was a cost saving associated with the SIPA program (Béland et al., 2006).

BOX 26.8 Suggested Elements of Transitional Care Models

- Interdisciplinary teams guided by evidence-based protocols
- Comprehensive geriatric assessments
- Performance measured and evaluated
- Information systems such as electronic medical records that span traditional settings
- Targeting of high-risk patients
- Improved communication between patients, family caregivers, and health care providers
- Improved communication between sending clinicians and receiving clinicians
- Well-designed and structured patient transfer records
- Simplified posthospital medication regimens; identification of high-risk medications
- Reconciled pre- and posthospitalization medication lists

- Improved patient and family knowledge of medications prior to discharge
- Educational materials adapted for language and health literacy
- Scheduled follow-up care appointments prior to discharge
- Discussion of warning signs that require reporting and medical evaluation
- Discharge followed up with home visits, telephone calls, or both
- Care coordination by advanced nurse practitioners
- Assessment of informal support
- Involvement, education, and support of family caregivers
- Knowledge of community resources and appropriate referrals to resources and financial assistance
- Discussion of palliative and end-of-life care; communication of advance directives

---

Transitions during the course of hospitalization can also be problematic for older patients. Minimizing the number of transfers from unit to unit during a single hospitalization is associated with more consistent nursing care, fewer adverse incidents (e.g., health care–associated infections, falls, or medication errors), shorter hospital stays, and lower overall costs (Kanak et al., 2008). In addition to taking on the roles of case managers and transition coaches, nurses play a role in many elements of successful transitional care models, such as medication management, family caregiver education, comprehensive discharge planning, and adequate and timely communication amongst providers and sites of services (Box 26.8).

RELOCATION

Relocation is a stressor and sometimes a crisis, both for the older person and for his or her family. Relocation to an LTC home is one of the more stressful kinds of relocations and one that many older people fear. With each move, for the adaptation to be satisfying, the person must begin to claim personal space by somehow placing his or her stamp of individuality on the new surroundings. Because the older person is particularly likely to move or be moved, the subject of relocation is significant. Nurses in hospitals, the community, and LTC homes frequently care for older people who have experienced relocation. The first

issue to address in any move is whether it is necessary and whether it will provide the least restrictive lifestyle appropriate for the individual. Assessing the impact of relocation and determining methods to mitigate any negative reactions are additional nursing actions.

Research indicates that relocation is associated with increased morbidity and mortality but that it does not necessarily result in serious effects on mental or physical health (Holder & Jolley, 2012). The research calls into question the validity of a commonly accepted nursing diagnosis of *relocation stress syndrome,* a catastrophic reaction to relocation. Research indicates that individuals are better able to meet the challenges of relocation if they have a sense of control over the circumstances and have the confidence to carry out the needed activities associated with a move. Advance notice, preparation, choice, and self-efficacy (i.e., "the beliefs in one's capability to organize and execute the courses of action required to manage prospective situations" [Bandura, 1997, p. 2]) may be an important variable in a positive adjustment to a relocation. The Self-Efficacy Relocation Scale, developed by Rossen and Gruber (2007), can be used to assess the self-efficacy of individuals who are relocating, identify potential pre-relocation adjustment issues, and guide interventions to promote positive relocation outcomes.

To assist older persons with relocation decisions and adjustments, nurses should become aware of resources available to the older person; assess the older person's relocation needs; individualize a realistic relocation plan; promote coping while making a relocation decision; help the person prepare for the move; and facilitate continuity of care (Hertz et al., 2016). After relocation, nurses should tailor interventions to the older person's values and preferences; promote the person's sense of control, autonomy, and mastery; provide social support and activities; promote the person's coping with relocation; orient the person to their new surroundings; maintain continuity of care; and ensure that the person's physical and psychosocial needs are met (Hertz et al., 2016). Family members will need considerable support when an older person moves into an LTC home. No matter the circumstances, family members often feel that they have in some way failed the older person. (See Chapter 23 for a more in-depth discussion of these issues.)

 IMPLICATIONS FOR GERONTOLOGICAL NURSING AND HEALTHY AGING

This chapter and this book in general discusses the care of the older person in a variety of settings. Many theories, frameworks, implications, research, evidence-informed practice recommendations, and resources for gerontological nursing and healthy aging have been presented. Nurses with competence in the care of older people will be in great demand as the population ages. Gerontological nurses have always assumed a leadership role in improving care for older persons and in promoting healthy aging. Through their expertise, commitment, dedication, advocacy, and compassion, gerontological nurses who work with older persons in all settings will continue to be leaders in creating models that truly change the culture of existing systems. Our hope is that nurses find joy and fulfillment in nursing older persons. Irene Burnside (1980, p. 32), quoting Martin Buber, wrote, "No one can say thank you the way an old person can." May you hear many "thank yous" in your practice.

KEY CONCEPTS

- A familiar and comfortable environment allows an older person to function at his or her highest capacity.
- Eight elements of age-friendly communities enhance the ability of older people to remain in their homes and familiar environments.
- Nurses must be knowledgeable about the range of housing and residential options for older people so that they can assist older people and their families in making appropriate decisions.
- Access to supports needed by the older person to remain in the community, including home care and adult day programs, is inconsistent from region to region. Accessibility issues are compounded in rural and remote regions and for Indigenous people.
- Long-term care (LTC) homes and home care are integral parts of the LTC system, providing sub-acute, chronic, long-term, and palliative care.
- Culture change in LTC homes is a growing movement to develop models of person-centred care and improve care outcomes and quality of life for residents.
- Nurses play a key role in ensuring optimal outcomes during transitions of care.
- Relocation has variable effects, depending on the individual's personality, health, cognitive capacities, sense of control, opportunities for choice, self-esteem, and preferred lifestyle.

ACTIVITIES AND DISCUSSION QUESTIONS

1. Pick three objects in your living space that are important to you, and explain why they are significant. What would be the effect on you if you were unable to move them to a new home?
2. Using the World Health Organization *Checklist of Essential Features of Age-Friendly Cities* (see Resources), look in your neighbourhood or community for one or more of the eight elements of age-friendly communities. Compare your findings with those of a classmate.
3. Ask an older relative about the items or conditions in his or her home that make him or her feel secure and comfortable.

4. How might your life be affected, positively or negatively, by having an older family member join your household? What might change for you and for the older relative? How would this experience compare with that of moving the older relative to an assisted-living facility or a long-term care (LTC) home?

5. Discuss with an older person the various moves that person has made and how he or she felt about them and adjusted to them.

6. Discuss how the care needs of an older person in assisted living might differ from those of an older person living in an LTC home. What is the role of a registered nurse in each of these settings?

7. Contact three retirement homes in your community, and make inquiries to each regarding a possible move to the home by an older person. What questions did you ask? What is the cost? What are the provisions for health care? What activities and assistance are available? Which home would you recommend for your grandmother, and why?

8. From your experience in the acute care setting, what would you suggest to improve transitions to other care settings? Discuss any experience you or your friends or family may have had with transitions after hospital discharge.

9. If you were the director of nursing, what would your LTC home be like (for instance, in its design, staffing, quality of care, and training)?

RESOURCES

Alzheimer Society of Canada (2011). *Guidelines for care: Person-centred care of people with dementia living in care homes*
http://www.alzheimer.ca/sites/default/files/files/national/culture-change/culture_change_framework_e.pdf

CBC News. Canada's nursing homes (interactive map of LTC home statistics and funding)
http://www.cbc.ca/news2/interactives/map-nursing-homes/

Eden Alternative
http://www.edenalt.org

Public Health Agency of Canada (PHAC). *Age-friendly rural and remote communities: A guide*
https://www.canada.ca/en/public-health/services/health-promotion/aging-seniors/publications/publications
-general-public/friendly-rural-remote-communities-a-guide.html

World Health Organization (WHO)
Age-friendly environments program
http://www.who.int/ageing/age-friendly-environments/en

Checklist of essential features of age-friendly cities
http://www.who.int/ageing/publications/Age_friendly_cities_checklist.pdf

Global age-friendly cities guide
http://www.who.int/ageing/publications/Global_age_friendly_cities_Guide_English.pdf

For additional resources, please visit *http://evolve.elsevier.com/Canada/Ebersole/gerontological/*

REFERENCES

Alzheimer Society of Canada. (2011). *Guidelines for care: Person-centred care of people with dementia living in care homes.* Toronto, ON: Author. Retrieved from http://www.alzheimer.ca/sites/default/files/files/national/culture-change/culture_change_framework_e.pdf.

Bandura, A. (1997). *Self-efficacy: The exercise of control.* New York, NY: W.H. Freeman.

BC Medical Journal (BCMJ). (2012). Statistics Canada: Almost 5% of seniors in long term care. *BC Medical Journal, 54*(9), 450. Retrieved from http://www.bcmj.org/pulsimeter/statistics-canada-almost-5-seniors-long-term-care.

Béland, F., Bergman, H., Lebel, P., et al. (2006). Integrated services for frail elders (SIPA): A trial of a model for Canada. *Canadian Journal on Aging, 25*(1), 25–42. doi:10.1353/cja.2006.0019.

Braedley, S., & Martel, G. (2015). Dreaming of home: Long-term residential care and (in)equities by design. *Studies in Political Economy, 95*(1), 59–81. doi:10.1080/19187033.2015.11674946.

Brawley, E. (2007). What culture change is and why an aging nation cares. *Aging Today, 28*, 9–10.

Burnside, I. (1980). Why work with the aged? *Geriatric Nursing, 2*(3), 29–33.

Canada Mortgage and Housing Corporation (CMHC). (2007). *An examination of life lease housing issues.* Ottawa, ON: Author. Retrieved from http://www.cmhc-schl.gc.ca/odpub/pdf/65427.pdf?fr=1288922994809.

Canada Mortgage and Housing Corporation (CMHC). (2016). *Seniors' housing report. Canada highlights.* Ottawa, ON: Author. Retrieved from https://www03.cmhc-schl.gc.ca/catalog/productDetail.cfm?cat=160&itm=31&lang=en&sid=0gGmUtvFRnR8OcOHDne3zKKSiU7sYJ3Bh3rKA5SqYair2uLMTeNptcY1XQoDegq7&fr=1492222255054.

Canadian Accreditation Council. (2011). *Adult standards.* Retrieved from http://www.cacohs.com/adult-standards.htm.

Canadian Cohousing Network. (2016). *About cohousing*. Retrieved from http://cohousing.ca/about-cohousing/.

Canadian Health Services Research Foundation. (1999). *Integrated health systems in Canada: Three policy syntheses: Questions and answers*. Ottawa, ON: Author. Retrieved from http://www.chsrf.ca/Migrated/PDF/ResearchReports/Commissioned Research/ps-ihsqanda_e.pdf.

Canadian Home Care Association (CHCA). (2016). *CHCA on the issues—overview*. Retrieved from http://www.cdnhomecare.ca/content.php?doc=94.

Comondore, V. R., Devereaux, P. J., Zhou, Q., et al. (2009). Quality of care in for-profit and not-for-profit nursing homes: Systematic review and meta-analysis. *British Medical Journal, 339*, b2732. doi:10.1136/bmj.b2732.

Government of Alberta. (2014). *Seniors' self-contained housing program*. Retrieved from http://www.seniors-housing.alberta.ca/housing/seniors_self_contained_housing.html.

Graham, C., Ivey, S., & Neuhauser, L. (2009). From hospital to home: Assessing the transitional care needs of vulnerable seniors. *The Gerontologist, 49*(1), 23–33. doi:10.1093/geront/gnp005.

Hermus, G., Stonebridge, C., Thériault, L., et al. (2012). *Home and community care in Canada: An economic footprint*. Ottawa, ON: The Conference Board of Canada. Retrieved from http://www.conferenceboard.ca/cashc/research/2012/homecommunitycare.aspx.

Hertz, J., Koren, M. E., Rossetti, J., et al. (2016). Management of relocation in cognitively intact older persons. *Journal of Gerontological Nursing, 42*(11), 14–23. doi:10.3928/00989134-20160901-05.

Holder, J. M., & Jolley, D. (2012). Forced relocation between nursing homes: Residents' health outcomes and potential moderators. *Reviews in Clinical Gerontology, 22*(4), 301–319. doi:10.1017/S0959259812000147.

Kanak, M. F., Titler, M., Shever, L., et al. (2008). The effect of hospitalization on multiple units. *Applied Nursing Research, 21*(1), 15–22. doi:10.1016/j.apnr.2006.07.001.

Kelly, R. (2017). The effect of adult day program attendance on emergency room registrations, hospital admissions, and days in hospital: A propensity-matching study. *The Gerontologist, 57*(3), 552–562. doi:10.1093/geront/gnv145.

Kelly, R., Puurveen, G., & Gill, R. (2016). The effect of adult day services on delay to institutional placement. *Journal of Applied Gerontology, 35*(8), 814–835. doi:10.1177/0733464814521319.

Kitchen, P., Williams, A., Pong, R. W., et al. (2011). Socio-spatial patterns of home care use in Ontario, Canada: A case study. *Health and Place, 17*(1), 195–206. doi:10.1016/j.healthplace.2010.09.014.

MacLean, L. B., Vendenbeld, L., & Miller, J. (2007). *Managing the frail elderly in the community and preventing admission to hospital: An overview of the peer-reviewed evidence*. Kelowna, BC: Interior Health Authority. Retrieved from http://www.interiorhealth.ca/uploadedFiles/Information/Research/Managing_Frail_Elderly_Community.pdf.

McCloskey, R., Jarrett, P., Stewart, C., et al. (2014). Alternate level of care patients in hospitals: What does dementia have to do with this? *Canadian Geriatrics Journal, 17*(3), 88–94. doi:10.5770/cgj.17.106.

McDonald, M. (2015). Regulating individual charges for long-term residential care in Canada. *Studies in Political Economy, 95*(1), 83–114. doi:10.1080/19187033.2015.11674947.

McGilton, K. S., Boscart, V., Brown, M., et al. (2014). Making tradeoffs between the reasons to leave and reasons to stay employed in long-term care homes: Perspectives of licensed nursing staff. *International Journal of Nursing Studies, 51*(6), 917–926. doi:10.1016/j.ijnurstu.2013.10.015.

Meadus, J. E., & Romano, L. (2009). *Written submission to the Standing Committee on Justice Policy: Bill 115, An Act to Amend the Coroners Act*. Toronto, ON: Advocacy Centre for the Elderly. Retrieved from http://www.acelaw.ca/appimages/file/Bill_115_-_Coroners_Amendment_Act_-_March_2009.pdf.

Morgan, D. G., Kosteniuk, J. G., Stewart, N. J., et al. (2015). Availability and primary health care orientation of dementia-related services in rural Saskatchewan, Canada. *Home Health Care Services Quarterly, 34*(3–4), 137–158. doi:10.1080/01621424.2015.1092907.

Naylor, M., & Keating, S. (2008). Transitional care: Moving patients from one care setting to another. *The American Journal of Nursing, 108*(9), 58–63. doi:10.1097/01.NAJ.0000336420.34946.3a.

Ontario Long Term Care Association. (2016). *About long-term care in Ontario: Facts and figures*. Retrieved from http://www.oltca.com/oltca/OLTCA/LongTermCare/OLTCA/Public/LongTermCare/FactsFigures.aspx#/Ontario%27s%20long-term%20care%20residents%20(2015).

Ontario Non-Profit Housing Association. (2016). *2016 waiting list survey report*. Toronto, ON: Author. Retrieved from https://www.onpha.on.ca/web/Policyandresearch/2016_Waiting_List_Survey/Content/PolicyAndResearch/Waiting_Lists_2016/2016_Waiting_Lists_Survey.aspx?hkey=08cff4ce-7f97-4af4-910c-c64954d28a4a.

Public Health Agency of Canada (PHAC). (2015). *The safe living guide—A guide to home safety for seniors*. Retrieved from https://www.canada.ca/en/public-health/services/health-promotion/aging-seniors/publications/publications-general-public/safe-living-guide-a-guide-home-safety-seniors.html.

Public Health Agency of Canada (PHAC). (2016). *Age-friendly communities*. Retrieved from https://www.canada.ca/en/public-health/services/health-promotion/aging-seniors/friendly-communities.html.

Romano, L., Wahl, J. A., & Meadus, J. (2008). *The law as it affects older persons*. Toronto, ON: Advocacy Centre for the Elderly. Retrieved from http://www.acelaw.ca/appimages/file/Law_as_it_Affects_Older_Adults_July_2008.pdf.

Rosenbaum, P. (2007). *Life leasing in Ontario. Submission to the Ministry of Municipal Affairs and Housing*. Toronto, ON: Advocacy Centre for the Elderly. Retrieved from http://www.advocacycentreelderly.org/appimages/file/Life%20Leases%20-%20June%202007.pdf.

Rossen, E., & Gruber, K. (2007). Development and psychometric testing of the relocation self-efficacy scale. *Nursing Research, 56*(4), 244–251. doi:10.1097/01.NNR.0000280609.16244.de.

Statistics Canada. (2010). *Residential care facilities—2007/2008.* Ottawa, ON: Author. Retrieved from http://dsp-psd.pwgsc.gc.ca/collections/collection_2010/statcan/83-237-X/83-237-x2010001-eng.pdf.

Statistics Canada. (2015a). *Living arrangements of seniors.* Retrieved from http://www12.statcan.gc.ca/census-recensement/2011/as-sa/98-312-x/98-312-x2011003_4-eng.cfm#bx2.

Statistics Canada. (2015b). *Long-term care facilities survey, 2013.* Retrieved from http://www.statcan.gc.ca/daily-quotidien/150504/dq150504b-eng.htm.

Strohschein, L. (2012). I want to move, but cannot: Characteristics of involuntary stayers and associations with health among Canadian seniors. *Journal of Aging & Health, 24*(5), 735–751. doi:10.1177/0898264311432312.

Sutherland, J. M., & Crump, R. T. (2013). Alternative level of care: Canada's hospitals, the evident and options. *Healthcare Policy, 9*(1), 26–34. doi:10.12927/hcpol.2013.23480.

The Care Guide. (2017). *Costs of Long Term Care.* Retrieved from http://www.thecareguide.com/residence-options/long-term-care/costs/cost-of-long-term-care.

Tilly, J., & Reed, P. (Eds.). (2008). *Dementia care practice recommendations for assisted living residences and nursing homes.* Washington, DC: Alzheimer's Association. Retrieved from http://www.guideline.gov.

Turcotte, M. (2014). *Canadians with unmet home care needs.* Ottawa, ON: Statistics Canada. Retrieved from http://www.statcan.gc.ca/pub/75-006-x/2014001/article/14042-eng.htm.

World Health Organization (WHO). (2007). *Global age-friendly cities: A guide.* Geneva, Switzerland: Author. Retrieved from http://www.who.int/ageing/publications/Global_age_friendly_cities_Guide_English.pdf.

Index